Breast Cancer

Darius S. Francescatti • Melvin J. Silverstein
Editors

Breast Cancer

A New Era in Management

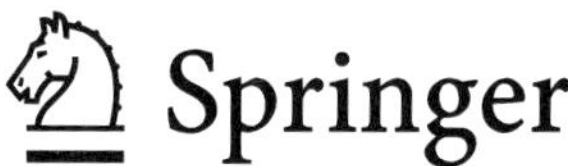

Editors
Darius S. Francescatti
Department of Surgery
Rush University Medical Center
Chicago, IL, USA

Melvin J. Silverstein
Hoag Breast Program
Hoag Memorial Hospital Presbyterian
Newport Beach, CA, USA

Keck School of Medicine
University of Southern California
Los Angeles, CA, USA

ISBN 978-1-4614-8062-4 ISBN 978-1-4614-8063-1 (eBook)
DOI 10.1007/978-1-4614-8063-1
Springer New York Heidelberg Dordrecht London

Library of Congress Control Number: 2013947468

Printed on acid-free paper

Springer is part of Springer Science+Business Media (www.springer.com)

Preface

I am neither statistician nor economist. I am a simple surgeon. Yet as a breast surgeon trained as a general surgeon and recertified an embarrassing number of times, it seems an appropriate time to share a few personal reflections on the state of our profession as we embark on a new century of progress in the care of the breast patient. Within this modest book the reader will discover familiar names as well as topics both familiar and perhaps not so familiar. This book was fashioned to reflect, in a word, change; change in treatment, change in thought, and change in the direction of our investigation into breast disease from one that, in a sense, has become for many of us a purely statistical analysis. The compilation of data and statistical analysis is a subject both beneficial and necessary and yet one that would not exist save for the initial spark of investigative curiosity of individual thought. Surgical investigators rely upon anatomy, physiology, biology, pathology, and applied sciences to pursue their insights into understanding the pathophysiology of breast cancer. Hopefully this will lead to the discovery of a truly limited minimally interventional approach to both the diagnosis and treatment of breast cancer. The foundation to accomplish this goal has been laid by many individual investigators around the world and, within the pages of this book, the reader can read and reflect on the works of many recognized investigators as well as those newly emerging. New approaches to diagnosis and treatment are presented alongside thoughtful discussion of standard surgical treatment. This book will hopefully promote the thought that things are not always, and seldom are, as they seem. To all the authors, on behalf of Dr. Silverstein and myself, I thank you for your contribution. To our readers, it is our hope that in reading this book the information and data will not simply be assimilated, stored unused, and forgotten but will perhaps act as a catalyst for new thought and discovery in the field of breast surgery.

Chicago, IL Darius S. Francescatti
Newport Beach, CA Melvin J. Silverstein

Contents

Contributors

Rosalinda Alvarado Johns Hopkins Medicine, Suburban Hospital, Bethesda, MD, USA

Dominique Amy, M.D. Department of Radiology, Centre Du Sein, B du Rhone, France

Preya Ananthakrishnan, M.D. Division of Breast Surgery, Columbia University College of Physicians and Surgeons, New York, NY, USA

Deanna J. Attai, M.D. Center for Breast Cancer, Inc, Burbank, CA, USA

Susan K. Boolbol, M.D., F.A.C.S. Division of Breast Surgery, Appel-Venet Comprehensive Breast Service, Beth Israel Medical Center, New York, NY, USA

David Brenin, M.D. Department of Surgical Oncology, University of Virginia, Charlottesville, VA, USA

Tony Hsiu-Hsi Chen Graduate Institute of Epidemiology and Preventive Medicine, National Taiwan University, Taipei, Taiwan

Sherry Yueh-Hsia Chiu Department and Graduate Institute of Health Care Management, Chang Gung University, Taoyuan, Taiwan

Catherine Dang, M.D. Department of Surgery, Cedars-Sinai Medical Center, Los Angeles, CA, USA

Peter B. Dean, M.D. Department of Diagnostic Radiology, University of Turku, Turku, Finland

IARC, World Health Organization, Lyon, France

Jill R. Dietz, M.D., F.A.C.S. Cleveland Clinic Foundation, Cleveland, OH, USA

Frederick M. Dirbas, M.D. Division of Surgical Oncology, Department of Surgery, Stanford University School of Medicine, Stanford, CA, USA

Breast Clinical Cancer Program and Breast Cancer Clinical Research GroupStanford Cancer Institute, Stanford, CA, USA

Giancarlo Dolfin, M.D. Department of Ginecologia, Oncologia Clincia, Torino, Italy

Edward J. Donahue, M.D., M.S. Department of General Surgery, St. Joseph's Hospital and Medical Center, Phoenix, AZ, USA

Kambiz Dowlatshahi, M.D. Department of Surgery, Rush University Medical Center, Chicago, IL, USA

Stephen W. Duffy, M.Sc. Queen Mary University, London, London, UK

Sheldon Marc Feldman, M.D., F.AC.S. Division of Breast Surgery, Columbia University College of Physicians and Surgeons, NewYork, NY, USA

Amanda B. Francescatti, M.S. Department of Surgery, Rush University Medical Center, Chicago, IL, USA

Darius S. Francescatti, M.D. Department of Surgery, Rush University Medical Center, Chicago, IL, USA

Beth C. Freedman, M.D. Department of Breast Surgery, St. Luke's Roosevelt Hospital Center, New York, NY, USA

Alyssa Gillego, M.D. Department of Surgery, Beth Israel Medical Center, New York, NY, USA

Armando E. Giuliano, M.D., F.A.C.S., F.R.C.S.E.D. Department of Surgery, Cedars-Sinai Medical Center, Los Angeles, CA, USA

Steven E. Harms, M.D., F.A.C.R. Department of Radiology, The Breast Center of Northwest Arkansas, University of Arkansas School for Medical Sciences, Fayetville, AR, USA

The Breast Center of Northwest Arkansas, Fayetville, AR, USA

Alan B. Hollingsworth, M.D., F.A.C.S. Department of Surgery, Mercy Women's Center, Mercy Hospital, Oklahoma City, OK, USA

Anna Katz, M.D. Advocate Condell Medical Center, Libertyville, IL, USA

Michael D. Lagios, M.D. Breast Cancer Consultation Service, Tiburon, CA, USA

Stanford University School of Medicine, Stanford, CA, USA

Gary Levine, M.D. Hoag Breast Care Center, Newport Beach, CA, USA

Jennifer H. Lin, M.D. Department of Surgical Oncology, John Wayne Cancer Institute, Santa Monica, CA, USA

January Lopez, M.D. Department of Radiology, Hoag Breast Care Center, Newport Beach, CA, USA

Ruta Rao, M.D. Department of Medicine, Rush University Medical Center, Chicago, IL, USA

Melvin J. Silverstein, M.D. Hoag Breast Program, Hoag Memorial Hospital Presbyterian, Newport Beach, CA, USA

Keck School of Medicine, University of Southern California, Los Angeles, CA, USA

Robert A. Smith, M.D. American Cancer Society, Atlanta, GA, USA

László Tabár, M.D., F.A.C.R. Department of Mammography, Falun Central Hospital, Falun, Sweden

Tibor Tot, M.D., Ph.D. Department of Pathology and Clinical Cytology, Central Hospital Falun, Falun, Sweden

Amy Ming-Fang Yen School of Oral Hygiene, Taipei Medical University, Taipei, Taiwan

Part I
Early Diagnosis

Chapter 1
Risk Assessment

Alan B. Hollingsworth

History and Rationale

The history of breast cancer risk assessment can be traced to the early 1700s when the observation was made in Italy that nuns were more likely to die of breast cancer than the general population. Although nulliparity has since been confirmed as a breast cancer risk factor, quantification of this risk is not as straightforward as it might seem, especially when other risks or protective factors are present.

In general, risk factors can be divided into reproductive/endocrine risks, environmental risks, tissue abnormalities (including prior biopsies, cellular changes, or mammographic density), and family history/genetic risk. And, some of these risks may be overlapping, e.g., tissue risks may simply be phenotypic expressions of other risks, presenting a challenge when merging isolated risks into mathematical models. Gender is a given risk, as is advancing age. Countering the power of risk factors are "protective factors," which lower the probability of developing breast cancer.

Risk assessment is the art of combining the relative power of known risks (and protective factors) in order to arrive at a numerical calculation that describes the absolute probability of developing breast cancer over a defined period of time. The rationale behind such an exercise is to select patients for proven interventions that can lower disease incidence and/or mortality.

While clinicians usually think of this process as designed for the individual patient, calculations are more accurate in predicting the number of cancers developing over time in large patient cohorts. When it comes to an individual, risk assessment must address a difficult challenge: if cancer occurs, it is an all-or-nothing event—100 % versus 0—a reality with a capital "R." This Reality cannot be established

A.B. Hollingsworth, M.D., F.A.C.S. (✉)
Department of Surgery, Mercy Women's Center,
4300 McAuley Blvd, Oklahoma City, OK 73120, USA
e-mail: alan.hollingsworth@mercy.net

D.S. Francescatti and M.J. Silverstein (eds.), *Breast Cancer: A New Era in Management*,
DOI 10.1007/978-1-4614-8063-1_1,

through today's technology or mathematics. At best, we can only estimate probabilities for the individual.

It must be considered, too, that risk assessment as a formal exercise is in its infancy. After all, the majority of eventual breast cancer patients will have had none of the standard major risk factors at the time of their diagnosis. For instance, only 20 % will have had a positive family history. Risks are present, of course, but unidentified. Additionally, the widespread attention given to risk factors for breast cancer has had the unintended effect of transmitting a false sense of security to eventual breast cancer patients who do not have the publicized risks.

Relative Risks and Related Concepts

A *relative risk* is a fraction, often expressed as a single number generated *by dividing the numerator*—the probability of an "event" in an "exposed" population—*by the denominator*—the probability of that same event in an "unexposed" population. For purposes here, the "event" is a diagnosis of breast cancer. If the two groups have the same number of participants, then relative risk can be calculated by dividing the raw numbers, i.e., the number of cancers in the "exposed" group by the number in the "unexposed":

$$\text{RR} = \frac{p\ (\text{disease}/\text{exposed})}{p\ (\text{disease}/\text{unexposed})}$$

where p = probability.

While the concept is intuitive, it is easy to forget that the denominator can be just as important as the numerator in determining the final relative risk (RR).

A related concept is *Odds Ratio (OR)*, and here things are not so intuitive. Even the stated definition is confusing, perhaps because "odds" is not used in the colloquial sense of "likelihood," nor the more intuitive "probability." In statistics (and horse-racing), "odds" is the probability of an "event" occurring divided by the probability of this event *not occurring*, expressed as a fraction:

$$\text{Odds} = \frac{p}{1-p}$$

If probability of an event is 50 % (1/2), then "odds" are 1:1, *not* 1:2. As another example, if probability is 66.6 % (2/3), then statisticians and racing handicappers will say that "odds" are 2:1.

Therefore, an OR is the odds of an event in one group divided by the odds of an event in a second group. Stated alternatively, OR is the odds of disease among exposed individuals divided by the odds of disease among the unexposed:

$$\text{Odds Ratio (OR)} = \frac{p\ (\text{disease}/\text{exposed})\ /\ 1\text{-}p\ (\text{disease}/\text{exposed})}{p\ (\text{disease}/\text{unexposed})\ /\ 1\text{-}p\ (\text{disease}/\text{unexposed})}$$

These definitions may now be clear, yet still leave one dangling as to how the two concepts of RR and OR relate to in clinical medicine. To offer an example, if the probability of an event in Group A (exposed population) is 20 % and in Group B (unexposed) is 1 %, then *RR = 20*:

$$\text{RR} = pA/pB, \text{ in this case } 20/1 = 20$$

However, the Odds Ratio is 0.2/(1 − 0.2) divided by 0.01/(1 − 0.01), which is an *OR of 24.75*:

$$\text{OR} = pA/(1\text{-}pA)/pB/(1\text{-}pB), \quad \text{in this case } 0.2/0.8 \text{ divided by } 0.01/.99 = 24.75$$

In this example, the choice of RR = 20 is a risk level in clinical medicine seen only with very strong associations (usually considered causations), such as the risk seen with cigarette smoking and lung cancer, or the risk seen with BRCA gene-positivity and breast cancer. Yet, there is only a modest difference between RR and OR.

When "events" are quite likely to happen, such as probabilities of 99.9 % in one group versus 99 % in another, the OR can be very high while the same data yields an RR barely over 1.0. In clinical medicine, however, where researchers are usually studying events that are infrequent among a large group of participants, well below the RR of 20 in the example above, the difference between OR and RR is usually negligible.

In case–control studies where odds are the usual currency, OR is used primarily, and logistic regression works with the log of the OR, not relative risks. RRs are then used more commonly in cohort studies and randomized controlled trials.

The *Hazard Ratio (HR)* considers "events" over the course of the study, a slightly different concept than RRs which are calculated at a study's conclusion. Thus, it is most helpful to think of HRs as "RRs averaged over time." Hazard Ratios are commonly used in survival analyses and time-to-event treatment studies, where two groups are followed over time, and the two curves plotted. Then, statistical software is used to calculate the HR.

Underlying all of the above is whether or not differences in study groups are statistically significant. Traditionally, *p*-values are used for hypothesis testing, but *p*-values provide little information about the precision of results, that is, the degree to which results would vary if measured multiple times. More recently, emphasis has been placed on reporting a range of plausible results, known as the *95 % Confidence Interval (CI)* that accompanies the "official" RR, OR, or HR. Although any confidence level can be chosen, 95 % is common in the medical literature, implying that if the study were to be repeated 100 times, then "truth" would occur within the range of the reported Confidence Interval 95 times out of 100.

Considering that RR of 1.0 means "no effect," the CI should not cross the 1.0 line, or it is considered a failure to reach statistical significance. Furthermore, the tighter the range in CI the better, and this is usually achieved by having a larger number (*n*) of participants in a study. Simply stated, *p*-values make a statement about power, while CIs provide a statement about range.

Three examples with HR unchanged include the following: (1) a Hazard Ratio of 2.1 with a CI of 2.09–2.2 would be both statistically significant coupled with a tight range; (2) an HR of 2.1 but with a CI of 0.8–2.5 would fail to reach significance because the 1.0 line of "no effect" has been crossed; (3) an HR of 2.1 but with a CI of 1.01–9.9 might be statistically significant, but the wide CI should give pause in the critical analysis of the data, suggesting the need for a larger study (greater "*n*").

Although the definitions are distinct for RR, OR, and HR, for the purposes of this chapter, these comparative concepts are discussed as a single entity—relative risks.

With RR being a fraction that has already undergone mathematical division, we no longer see the numerator (# of cancer cases in an *exposed* population) or the denominator (# of cancer cases in the *unexposed* population) outside the context of a study's publication. Yet, understanding the origin of RRs can be very revealing.

Using nulliparity as an example, if not having children has a relative risk of 1.5 (RR = 1.5) in a given study, then that study might have had 150 breast cancer cases in the nulliparous group and 100 in the control group. Or, there might have been three cases in the nulliparous group and two in the control group. Relative risks alone tell us nothing about the total number of study participants.

Relative risks can be hard to interpret, too, when continuums are involved. For example, nulliparity (the numerator) is a straightforward dichotomy (nulliparous vs. parous), but what about the denominator? If one includes all parous women, there will be a wide range of risk levels in the denominator. Some women will have had a first full-term pregnancy at age 15 with many children to follow (below average risk) while others will have had a first full-term pregnancy over the age of 35 wherein the risk may actually be higher than nulliparity. It is not uncommon for epidemiologists to use two different reference populations for the denominator in order to calculate relative risks as part of the process of validating risk factors.

In this example of nulliparity, we see a continuum at work only on the denominator side of the equation. But what if both numerator and denominator are a continuum?

Mammographic density as a risk factor involves a continuum from 0 to 100 % dense tissue, with risk rising in proportion to density (ignoring some limitations here regarding ethnicity, age, etc.). This continuum affects both the numerator and the denominator. So, is there a relative risk for a 50 % density pattern (numerator)? Yes, if compared to a zero density pattern (denominator), the patient with 50 % density has an approximate twofold risk (RR = 2.0) over a patient with very low density. However, compared to the patient with 100 % density (different denominator), the patient with 50 % density pattern is *half* as likely to develop breast cancer (RR = 0.5). Relative risks are—well—*relative*.

To continue with the density example, it is commonly stated that women with extreme mammographic density (>75 % dense) have a fourfold risk for developing breast cancer (RR = 4.0), but compared to what? In fact, this RR = 4.0 is generated only by comparing women at the highest density (numerator) to women with the lowest density pattern or fatty replacement (denominator), i.e., women *well below average* density, an attribute that applies to only 10–15 % of the population. Epidemiologists call this low-density group the "referent," where RR = 1.0, as they convert this continuum into their modeling strategies. Compared to the average patient with 50 % density, however, extreme density could also be expressed as a twofold risk (RR = 2.0).

These examples demonstrate the inadvisability of focusing on relative risks in patient counseling. And, in the mathematical models to be discussed below, the user will not even see the relative risks at work behind the scenes.

It should be obvious that there is no such thing as RR = 0. If a proposed risk factor is found to impart no risk (numerator and denominator are the same), then RR = 1.0. If the factor is protective, RR will be less than 1.0; and, if the factor proves to be a risk, RR will be greater than 1.0.

Examples of Relative Risks (Approximated from Multiple Studies)

Reproductive/endocrine/hormonal risks:	
Age at menarche 10–11, compared to 12–13	RR = 1.5
Age at menarche 9, compared to 12–13	RR = 2.0
First full-term pregnancy at age 25–29, compared to 20	RR = 1.5
First full-term pregnancy at age 30–35, compared to 20	RR = 2.0
First full-term pregnancy, age greater than 35, compared to 20	RR = 2.5
Nulliparity	RR = 1.5–2.0
Age at menopause after 55, compared to 50	RR = 1.5
Postmenopausal estrogen HRT	RR = 0.8 (protective) to 1.5
Postmenopausal estrogen + progesterone HRT	RR = 1.3–2.0 (risk declines after cessation of Rx)
Oophorectomy at age 35–40	RR = 0.5–0.7

Environmental risks:	
Mantle radiation for Hodgkin's disease at ages 10–19	RR = 40.0
Mantle radiation for Hodgkin's disease at ages 20–29	RR = 15.0
Mantle radiation for Hodgkin's disease, age 30 and over	RR = 1.0
Alcoholic beverages (2–3 drinks/day)	RR = 1.5
Cigarette smoking	RR = 1.0–2.0

Tissue risks (cellular, histologic, mammographic):	
Multiple, chronic cysts (gross cystic change)	RR = 1.5–2.0
Proliferative changes on benign breast biopsy	RR = 1.5–2.0
Proliferative/atypical cellular changes on cytology	RR = 2.0–4.0
Atypical hyperplasia on breast biopsy	RR = 4.0
Atypical lobular hyperplasia with ductal extension	RR = 7.0
Lobular carcinoma in situ (diagnosed at age 35)	RR = 9.0
Lobular carcinoma in situ (diagnosed at age 60)	RR = 3.0
Mammographic density (extreme compared to low)	RR = 4.0
Mammographic density (extreme compared to average)	RR = 2.0

Family history/genetics:	
First-degree relative with breast cancer	RR = 2.0
One second-degree relative with breast cancer	RR = 1.0–1.5
First-degree relative with breast cancer diagnosed at 65	RR = 1.5
First-degree relative with breast cancer diagnosed at 35	RR = 3.0
First-degree relative with bilateral breast cancer at 35	RR = 5.0
Two first-degree relatives with breast cancer	RR = 4.0
BRCA gene-positivity, when diagnosed at 20	RR = 25–40 (for the next 10 years)
BRCA gene-positivity, when diagnosed at 60	RR = 8 (for the next 10 years)

Caveats to Relative Risks

There are many qualifiers and caveats to relative risks, some of which are suspect from the table above. Calculated risk can be impacted greatly by age at exposure to the risk, duration of exposure, duration of follow-up, control group used for the ratio's denominator, or even legitimate variations in risk power from one study to the next. However, a few points are worth making since today's clinician is drawn into risk discussions routinely, often by provocative data as espoused by the media (where risks are usually described in relative terms, given the vastly larger percentages compared to increases in absolute risk).

In addition to the aforementioned problem of continuums in relative risks, there is a normal, expected diminution of relative risks over time. This is sometimes misrepresented as "a risk that loses power over time." This may be true in relative terms, but it does not necessarily mean that the actual (absolute) risk is declining. Baseline risk (the denominator) is, in fact, increasing over time, closing the gap, while the numerator might continue in a linear fashion (Fig. 1.1).

Additional variables can play into declining RRs as well. Note the sharp decline in RRs in the list above associated with mantle radiation in Hodgkin's disease, starting out at a level comparable to BRCA gene-positivity (RR = 40), declining to no risk at all (RR = 1.0), depending on the "age at exposure" to the radiation. In fact, "age at exposure" has been the major contributor to risk in all radiation-related risk studies with negligible power over the age of 30–40, which should help minimize fears about miniscule radiation exposure with mammography for women over 40.

If one makes the cardinal error of multiplying a relative risk X baseline lifetime risk to arrive at an individual's lifetime risk, one will quickly see that something is wrong. Using the RR = 40 above, one might be tempted to multiple 40 × "12 %" baseline to arrive at an individualized risk, but this would yield a 480 % probability for breast cancer. The first problem with this approach is what we have already seen with regard to declining RRs over time. Secondly, the "12 %" overstates baseline risk since the "one-in-eight" figure is drawn from general population risk that includes all women with known risk factors in addition to those with no known risks. For women with no known risk factors, lifetime baseline risk is approximately 7 %.

Even if relative risks are accurate and handled with care, problems arise for those patients with more than one risk factor. For instance, in a patient with extreme

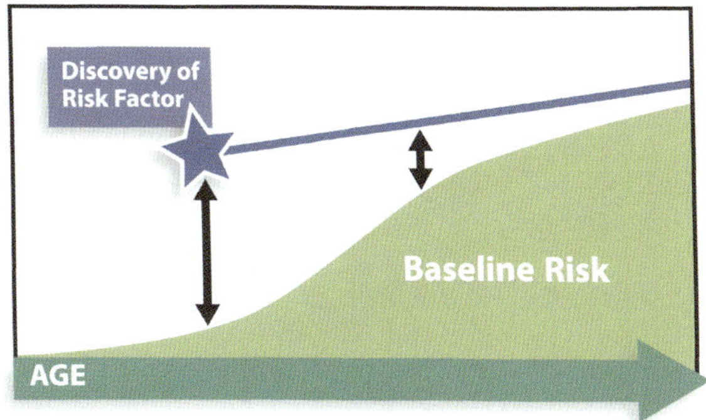

Fig. 1.1 Conceptual representation of diminishing relative risk (RR, ⇞) after discovery of a linear absolute risk, as a result of nonlinear changes in baseline risk

mammographic density plus a first-degree relative with breast cancer, are these risks additive, synergistic, or overlapping? It may be that the risk imparted by the family history is reflected in the mammographic density, and it would be an error to count the same risk twice. The best way to address this would be through the direct study of risks in pairs. In fact, this has been done, albeit infrequently.

Relative risks when factors are paired:	
First-degree relative with breast cancer and nulliparity	RR = 2.7
First-degree relative with breast cancer and first full-term pregnancy after 30	RR = 4.0
First-degree relative with breast cancer and gross cystic change	RR = 3.0
Nulliparity and atypical hyperplasia	RR = 5.0

The most familiar pairing of risk factors came from Drs. Page and DuPont in their landmark work with tissue risks, with the finding of synergism between a positive family history and atypical hyperplasia. To confirm this synergism, these investigators included the use of two different denominator populations to validate the relative risk of:

First-degree relative with breast cancer and atypical hyperplasia on biopsy RR = 9.0.

Subsequent studies have not been able to replicate this synergism, however, leaving atypical hyperplasia with a relative risk of 4.0, with or without a positive family history. This translates to substantial differences in absolute risk when these RRs are converted for patient counseling. Thus, one sees support for the argument that risk assessment should deal in generalities and "ranges of risk," rather than the current trend of mathematical models that carry absolute risk determinations to the right of the decimal point, offering illusory exactitude.

Converting Relative Risks to Absolute Risks

When it became clear that relative risks were a poor way to communicate with patients, several groups began constructing models in the 1980s that would allow clinicians to discuss risk in absolute terms. As it would be impractical to render a final risk assessment based on the direct study of countless combinations of risks as "pairs," "triplets," "quadruplets," etc., the creators of these models had to combine RRs mathematically instead. Although multiplication of RRs is the core principle, the mathematical merger is far more complex. Relative risks based on age (e.g., age at menarche) had to be managed on a "sliding scale" with a reference age serving as "normal." The contributing RRs are not seen by the user. Only absolute risks are generated. Once the models are created from a data set, then they are confirmed with a different cohort, and ideally, prospectively validated as well.

With absolute risk levels that these models generate, a problem arose immediately with regard to patient counseling—how does the newly calculated risk compare to baseline when there are two distinct baseline references? We have, first of all, a "general population" baseline risk *that includes women with risk factors* (the well-known "one in eight" or 12 %) and, secondly, the "no risk" baseline of 7 % that is composed of women without any known risk factors.

If one had to pick a single baseline, it would seem that a comparison should be made to the "no-risk" population as this is the approach when RRs are being calculated in the first place. This was tried with one of the more popular models and the feedback was overwhelmingly negative in that outcomes seemed to exaggerate risk. Many women undergoing routine evaluation with minimal apparent risk were deemed "at increased risk." So, a switch was made to "general population risk," called "average risk," which includes the women with known risks. Now, many users of the model are surprised when a patient thought to be "at modest risk" proves to be the same, or below, general population risk.

This confusion over two acceptable definitions of baseline risk has no easy answers. One approach is to use both reference points, comparing the calculated absolute risk in the patient to both a "no risk" baseline and a "general population" baseline, all to provide better perspective.

Absolute Lifetime Risks

Patients and clinicians are most interested in lifetime risks. The first problem here is that we rarely have solid data for lifetime risks. Even the remarkable 55-year follow-up in a cohort of women who received thymic radiation as infants (RR = 3.0) leaves us wondering about the remaining risk for the last 20–40 years of life for these women. With few exceptions, risk calculations are derived from relative risk studies where follow-up is less than "lifetime." Therefore, lifetime risks tend to be projections.

Then, there are several ways in which lifetime risk can be misstated, either exaggerating or minimizing true risk. As a ground rule, "lifetime" risk for the individual patient implies *remaining* lifetime risk. Key point: We "pass through" risks as we age, so *lifetime cumulative risk* might be "one in eight" for an entire life measured

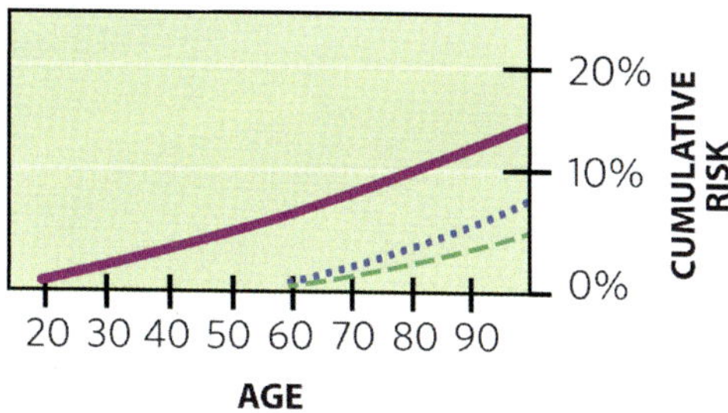

Fig. 1.2 Cumulative lifetime risk for breast cancer is often stated as "1 in 8" or 12 %, but this is total lifetime risk (*solid line*). Since we pass through risk as we age, *remaining* lifetime risk diminishes over time. A 60-year-old faces a 7 % baseline remaining lifetime risk (through age 80) for breast cancer when considering "general population" risk (*dotted line*), and even less (4 %) when considering the "no known risk" population (*dashed line*)

from age 0 to 100, but it does not apply to the 60-year-old who has passed through nearly half of that risk already (Fig. 1.2):

This concept carries through all strata of risk. For example, it is commonly stated that if a patient tests positive for a BRCA gene mutation, she will be at a 55–85 % risk for the development of breast cancer (as well as high risk for ovarian cancer). This might be true for an "entire lifetime," but it must be age adjusted for the individual. If the patient is asymptomatic at age 60 when found to harbor a BRCA mutation, her remaining risk for breast cancer is more in the range of 20–30 % over the next 30 years, not 85 %.

It is also possible to *underestimate* the risk by using short-term studies and not adjusting for patient age. The 30 y/o who is newly diagnosed with lobular carcinoma in situ (LCIS) will learn—either on her own or from other sources—that her risk for invasive breast cancer is "20 %," a one-size-fits-all number found on multiple Web sites without any reference to risk as a function of time. This "20 %" is a risk elevation that may not seem that much different than the 12 % that all women face, giving the patient a false sense of security. But this 20 % is derived from studies with 20-year follow-up, and all indicators so far point to a 1 %/year risk that extends at least 30 years. More recently, the problem of LCIS risk counseling has worsened, often through third-party payors who, perhaps unwittingly, base their "*less* than 20 % lifetime risk for LCIS" on studies that had *less* than 20-year follow-up (at 1 %/year, a 15-year study = 15 % risk). At the other end of the spectrum, a 70-year-old is likely facing only a 10 % remaining lifetime risk for breast cancer after a diagnosis of LCIS, assuming normal life expectancy, compared to a 3–4 % baseline risk. *A floating percentage for absolute risk is meaningless outside the framework of time.*

(Note for the mathematical purist: If a study reveals 15 % risk over 15 years, admittedly, the yearly risk is not exactly 1 %/year. Each incident case of cancer leaves a smaller pool of unaffected individuals and a slightly different percentage each year, albeit only a very small difference when the total "*n*" is large. When "%/year" data is offered in this chapter, it is meant only as a close estimate used to counsel patients.)

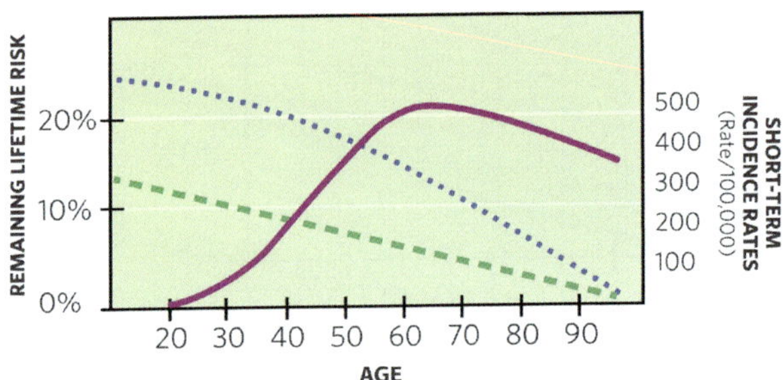

Fig. 1.3 Instead of the rising curve of cumulative lifetime risk, "remaining" lifetime risk in the general population declines as noted by the *dashed line*, while a "high risk" curve declines as noted by the *dotted line*. For illustrative purposes, 5-year incidence rates, smoothed to a *solid-line curve*, are overlaid to approximate short-term probabilities for breast cancer that are rising through age 60

Regarding these long-term calculations for risk, the mathematical models below will automatically calculate *remaining* lifetime cumulative risk over a defined period of time, thus preventing the error of quoting a "total" lifetime risk. However, nothing can overcome this paradox: *As a patient ages, her remaining lifetime risk is declining, while her short-term incidence for breast cancer is rising and peaking* (Fig. 1.3).

This paradox will lead to some improbable management guidelines when it comes to interventions, some based on short-term calculations, while others based on "lifetime" risks. But first, a look at the more commonly used mathematical models.

The Mathematical Models

In the 1980s, with the prospect of tamoxifen as a risk-reducing agent, the need arose for a mathematical model that would standardize risk assessment, allowing an objective entry threshold to a large-scale clinical trial, as well as serving to calculate the size of the trial necessary for statistical significance.

The Gail Model (later modified to the National Cancer Institute Breast Cancer Risk Assessment Tool, or Gail 2) was adopted for the NSABP P-01 trial that randomized patients to receive either tamoxifen or placebo. The threshold for entry was a Gail-calculated 5-year absolute risk of 1.67 % or greater, a risk level achieved simply by being age 60. While this confused many (How can a "normal risk" 60 y/o be labeled "high risk?"), the NSABP was dealing with the aforementioned paradox of peak short-term incidence vs. declining lifetime risk. In supporting this approach, it should be noted that clinical trial design mandates the greatest amount of information in the shortest time possible, so the initial focus needed to be on short-term risk and short-term outcomes.

Importantly, the trial not only proved the efficacy of reducing breast cancer risk with tamoxifen but also prospectively validated the Gail model as a tool to assess breast cancer risk. This validation came through comparing the number of predicted (expected) cancers for the control group versus those actually observed. The Gail model, derived from data generated by the Breast Cancer Detection and Demonstration Project (BCDDP), was also validated when applied to well-known studies such as the Cancer and Steroid Hormone Study (CASH), and the Nurses' Health Study (NHS). In 1999, the Gail model was modified to Gail 2 or NCI-Gail using age-specific incidence rates obtained from the Surveillance, Epidemiology, and End Results (SEER) database.

A proliferation of proposed models followed with varying degrees of validation. Clinicians do not necessarily need to know the details of each model, with regard to the internal relative risks at work; however, some degree of familiarity with the models, including strengths and weaknesses, is important given our dependence on these models for current interventional guidelines.

Risk assessment programs at breast screening centers and cancer centers have proliferated along with the models, and the skill in risk analysis comes not through simple data entry into the models, but through understanding which models are most appropriate for a given patient. It is equally important for the practitioner of risk assessment to develop the skill of estimating risks *without models* such that errors in data entry can be recognized, rather than blindly transmitting misleading risk information to patients who are making serious decisions about interventions.

Brief summaries of the breast cancer risk assessment models are listed below:

Gail-NCI model (download at http://www.cancer.gov/bcrisktool/): This model is the easiest to use and the most thoroughly validated for predicting the risk of *invasive* cancer. Note a distinction here that other models, including the first version of the Gail model, calculate the risk for both invasive disease and DCIS. Gail-NCI incorporates reproductive/endocrine risks, family history, and tissue risks. However, it has a number of caveats: family history is limited to first-degree relatives with breast cancer; there is no provision for the ages of these relatives when diagnosed, nor is there a provision for family members with ovarian cancer. Thus, the model carries the disclaimer that it is inappropriate to use the Gail model if one suspects a BRCA gene mutation. Also, there is no provision for assessing the risk of LCIS. The model conveniently calculates 5-year absolute risks or lifetime risks or anything in between. There have been efforts all along to improve the model, and more emphasis is now being paid to ethnicity. The model can overestimate the risk if a patient has had a large number of benign breast biopsies in the past. And, some experts believe it can underestimate the risk for women with atypical hyperplasia where histology has been confirmed by expert pathology review. Finally, a rarely discussed weakness is the fact that the Gail model does not include the number of women in the family *without* breast cancer, information that can reveal truncated family histories wherein breast cancer risk and BRCA mutation probabilities might be understated.

Claus model (or Claus tables or Jonker-extended Claus): This model estimates the risk for both invasive cancer and DCIS. It is derived from the aforementioned CASH study and is based solely on family history, so it is not the best model if the patient has reproductive/endocrine risks and/or tissue risks. The Claus model incorporates much more family history detail than the Gail-NCI by including both maternal and paternal lines, both first- and second-degree relatives, and importantly, age of onset in those affected relatives. Although limited in that it only accommodates two relatives with breast cancer, the Claus model is most useful when the risk is solely due to family history, maternal or paternal, and when affected relatives are at the extremes of age. The extended Claus now considers bilateral breast cancer, ovarian cancer, and three or more relatives with breast cancer.

Tyrer-Cuzick, a.k.a. IBIS Breast Cancer Risk Evaluation Tool (download at http://www.ems-trials.org/riskevaluator/): This model estimates the risk for both invasive cancer and DCIS. Originating from the United Kingdom and used in the UK prevention trials, it has been criticized as applicable only to that population with no provision for ethnicity. Although it takes more time for data entry than Gail or Claus, an issue minimized by frequent use, this is largely because the model is so much more inclusive of various risks. Conceptually, it is an extension of the Gail approach as it includes family history, prior biopsy information, and reproductive/endocrine risks. That said, reproductive/endocrine risks include the use of hormone replacement therapy and birth control pills where the literature supporting underlying relative risks is controversial. Importantly, the Tyrer-Cuzick model includes age at menopause, which can be a powerful protective factor, ignored by most models, wherein early-age surgical menopause greatly impacts risk calculations. Late menopause is a risk factor as well. With regard to family history, there is enough requested detail, including bilateral breast cancers and ovarian cancer history, that a pedigree is drawn and BRCA gene mutation probabilities determined. However, most US genetic counselors use other BRCA mutation probability models, given that the Tyrer-Cuzick underestimates BRCA probabilities in some studies. The model also incorporates more specific information about tissue risks than the Gail model, properly excluding biopsies that showed no proliferative changes, then separating proliferative disease from atypical hyperplasia, and accommodating a history of LCIS. Although this more specific histology is considered a strength, the model has been criticized for overestimating the risk associated with atypical hyperplasia. Some experts believe the model overestimates risk in general, especially if applied to populations in the United States.

BRCAPRO (http://www4.utsouthwestern.edu/breasthealth/cagene/default.asp): A favorite among many genetic counselors, it is also one of the models (along with Claus and Tyrer-Cuzick) preferred by the American Cancer Society for selecting patients who qualify for high-risk screening with breast MRI. Perhaps even more time-consuming for data entry than the Tyrer-Cuzick model, BRCAPRO focuses on familial/hereditary risk, rather than reproductive/endocrine risks or tissue risks, thus limiting its use when nonhereditary risks predominate. However, it overcomes this limitation by including an "umbrella" function, calculating risks for other models as well. It is thus a tool to predict breast cancer risk (invasive cancer risk in non-BRCA carriers) as well as a method to calculate probabilities for BRCA mutations.

BOADICEA—Breast and Ovarian Analysis of Disease Incidence and Carrier Estimation Algorithm—(download at http://www.srl.cam.ac.uk/genepi/boadicea/boadicea_bwa.html): This model is similar in design and intent to BRCAPRO, originating from the University of Cambridge (UK). It accommodates data such as bilateral breast cancer, as well as family histories that include prostate and pancreatic (needed for BRCA probabilities). The model was introduced too late to be utilized in the clinical trials leading to acceptance of high-risk screening with MRI. However, since that time, it has achieved an approval rating from the United Kingdom's National Institute for Health and Clinical Excellence (NICE) for use in selecting patients for MRI. Like BRCAPRO, the BOADICEA model is best used in patients where the risks are familial/hereditary. Results are given in an easy-to-read format of "risk over specified units of time" for both breast (invasive) and ovarian cancer, as well as BRCA mutation probabilities.

Extemporaneous or Informal Models: With no perfect risk model available (and for that matter, impossible), there is a temptation to improve available models on an informal basis. Online models have been developed by organizations, institutions, and individuals, usually starting with one of the standard models, and then refining according to personal preferences. These models all suffer from the lack of prospective validation, though some have been calibrated to historical cohorts. That said, one of the most intriguing models is the *Harvard Center for Cancer Prevention Risk Assessment Tool*, which includes modifiable lifestyle factors, an attractive feature for those interested in lowering their calculated risk. The introduction of these informal models has clouded an already confusing arena where even the so-called standard models have undergone modifications over time.

As a result of multiple models having multiple variations, a single individual can generate such a wide range of calculated risk that it becomes difficult to maintain interventional recommendations based on exact percentages. And, it promotes "model shopping" as well, i.e., the search for a higher number to justify certain interventions. This raises the question—again—as to whether or not these percentages are nothing more than false clarity, given that Reality for the individual is "all or nothing."

Risk Assessment Software for Breast Screening Centers: Several software options are available that perform risk assessment "automatically" at breast screening centers based on information provided as part of patient registration. These programs have much to offer as long as a risk assessment counselor can double-check accuracy of information provided by the patient. These software applications are not models in and of themselves, but include several of the standard models for both risk assessment and calculation of BRCA probabilities. Information is presented in patient-friendly formats, and corresponding letters are generated for primary care physicians. Some systems address genetic predispositions for other types of cancer, beyond breast and ovarian, and thus may be useful for genetic counselors.

Limitations of All Mathematical Models

Returning to the theme of individual Reality as opposed to populations, it should be kept in mind that when a model has been "validated," we are usually talking about its accuracy in predicting the number of cancers in a large cohort where a more specific term is "calibration," i.e., comparing the number of cancers observed to the number expected. However, for the individual patient, these models have a discriminatory power euphemistically described as "modest." Discriminatory power for the individual is reported in c-statistics (c = concordance), a.k.a. "accuracy," a combination of sensitivity and specificity, expressed as area under the curve (AUC). The Gail model, for instance, has been variably measured to have a c-stat ranging from 0.58 to 0.67. Flipping a coin to determine if an individual is going to get breast cancer would have a c-stat of 0.5. Ideally, we would like to see c-stats above a yet-to-be-achieved 0.80, if not higher (levels that have been achieved with the BRCA probability models), thus the ongoing search for new and improved risk assessment models as well as ongoing modifications of the old models.

Given the "modest" predictive capability of the mathematical models for an individual, some have considered that interventional guidelines should be based on general classes of risk, rather than calculated percentages, e.g., "near-baseline risk," "high risk," and "very high risk." Alternatively stated, perhaps mathematical models should be reserved for planning clinical trials rather than individual counseling. Taking this hesitancy one step further to overt objections, at a 2005 NCI workshop on cancer risk prediction models, the viewpoint was expressed by some that these models may be "misleading, frightening, or even unethical."

That said, if there were no interventions available, then breast cancer risk modeling would be an academic exercise without utility. However, not only are interventions available with proven outcomes, but also these interventions are often recommended through formal guidelines that utilize percentages derived from the mathematical models.

Interventions Based on Risk Assessment

Preventive Surgery

In the 1980s, when epidemiologists began to develop mathematical models to calculate the risk for breast cancer, preventive mastectomy was the only intervention available. No defined risk threshold has ever been proposed for this procedure, given the highly personal nature of a woman's request for surgical prevention.

However, risk analysis today plays an important role for high-risk patients who are considering surgery so that they can understand their personal risk in comparison to general population risk, as well as learning about alternatives.

In spite of the widespread use of the subcutaneous approach with implant reconstructions introduced in the 1960s and 1970s, the degree of risk reduction was not quantified well until recently. A "90 %" relative risk reduction is now commonly quoted, largely based on Mayo Clinic studies, most applicable to those undergoing the subcutaneous approach. Thus, if a patient calculates to be at 40 % absolute (remaining) lifetime risk, surgical prevention will reduce the risk of future cancer to 4 % lifetime (90 % of the 40 %, or an absolute reduction of 36 %). Although this subcutaneous approach is often called "inadequate if one is going to seek surgical prevention," 90 % risk reduction still exceeds any nonsurgical risk-reducing intervention.

With improvements in reconstruction techniques, total bilateral mastectomy (inclusion of nipple-areolar complexes) for prevention has been favored by many patients and surgeons, especially for those who harbor a BRCA gene mutation. In fact, some BRCA-positive cohorts undergoing this more complete approach for prevention have no breast cancers yet reported in their series. With longer follow-up, one can anticipate a 95–99 % relative risk reduction, slightly more complete than the subcutaneous approach, although the differences are a matter of small degree once these relative risk reductions are converted to absolute risk reductions.

Variations have been proposed for surgical prevention, all with the intent of improving cosmesis while maintaining efficacy. These include areola-sparing and nipple-sparing approaches—the latter essentially a subcutaneous approach, but avoiding the maligned historical label by emphasizing a more complete removal of breast parenchyma. One would anticipate risk reduction with these approaches to come close to that afforded through total mastectomies.

In addition to a reduction in the incidence of breast cancer through surgery, a reduction in disease-specific mortality has been demonstrated when preventive mastectomy is utilized in the BRCA-positive population. And, there is little reason to believe otherwise for patients who opt for preventive mastectomy based on significant risk elevations due to other factors. Nevertheless, it is difficult to state that preventive mastectomy is ever "recommended" by the surgeon; rather, it should be considered a patient-driven procedure after the patient has been fully informed of her comparative risk and her alternatives.

Pharmacologic Risk Reduction

At the time of this writing, two drugs are FDA approved for breast cancer risk reduction—(1) *tamoxifen* for both premenopausal and postmenopausal women, and (2) *raloxifene* for postmenopausal women only. It is anticipated that aromatase inhibitors (AIs) will soon join the armamentarium for breast cancer risk reduction.

Although worldwide clinical trials, some ongoing, have demonstrated the ability of selective estrogen receptor modulators (SERMs) and AIs to lower the risk of breast cancer, FDA approval for the two SERMs came primarily through two NSABP trials (P-01 and P-02), both of which used the Gail model for entry. Patients were invited to participate if there was a prior diagnosis of LCIS or a calculated *absolute* 5-year Gail risk of 1.66 % or greater (a number that looks deceivingly like a relative risk, but this is not the case). To summarize conclusions:

- *Tamoxifen* taken for 5 years has a durable benefit that appears to last at least 15 years after cessation of therapy. It is the only drug known to lower the risk in premenopausal women (by 44 % in the P-01 trial), while relative risk reduction in postmenopausal women was 50 %. Subgroups based on tissue risk (atypical hyperplasia or LCIS) benefitted to a greater extent than patients with other risk factors.
- *Raloxifene* is for postmenopausal use only, with risk reduction slightly less than tamoxifen, deduced by combining data from both P-01 and P-02 (38 % relative risk reduction for invasive cancer; 39 % for DCIS), but with a more favorable side effect profile—no increase in uterine cancer, no increase in cataract formation, and less thrombogenic potential than tamoxifen such that thrombotic risks with raloxifene approximate other hormonal therapies such as HRT and BC pills. Optimal duration for raloxifene therapy is yet to be determined, though it is recommended indefinitely when used for its other FDA indication—treatment and prevention of osteoporosis in postmenopausal women.

At this point in time, pharmacologic risk reduction is reflected only through fewer ER-positive tumors. A variety of agents and natural products have been suggested to reduce the risk of both ER+ and ER− tumors, and some, such as vitamin D, are already being used in clinical studies evaluating surrogate endpoints, in the hope of generating large-scale clinical trials.

High-Risk Surveillance with Breast MRI

In a meta-analysis of five international screening trials, sensitivity for mammography in head-to-head comparison with breast MRI was a surprisingly low 40 %. Given the ability of breast MRI to detect at least twice as many breast cancers through asymptomatic screening, guidelines have been adopted by the American Cancer Society (ACS), the National Comprehensive Cancer Network (NCCN), the American College of Radiology (ACR), and the Society of Breast Imaging (SBI).

While several of the MRI indications are based on descriptors of risk without "percentages"—BRCA positivity or probability, other genetic predispositions, and chest wall radiation at a young age—the category that prompted widespread interest in formal risk assessment was the recommendation for annual mammography *and* annual MRI, beginning at age 30, for women with a lifetime risk of "*20–25 % or greater*," as defined by BRCAPRO or other models that are largely based on family history (Claus and Tyrer-Cuzick, specifically). The Gail model was relegated to a lower status, not for its lack of validation, but due to the fact that none of the international screening studies used the Gail for entry. As for "20–25 % or greater," the semantics allowed "20 % or greater" as synonymous, thus imparting the goal of reaching 20 % lifetime risk as a formal risk assessment exercise.

But the difficulties of "20 % lifetime" involve much more than the variability that occurs from one model to the next. Lifetime risks do not necessarily translate into short-term yields which are the basis of MRI cost-effectiveness; and, as a corollary, lifetime risks are age discriminatory. Younger women have higher lifetime risks because they have not yet passed through a significant amount of that risk. Older women often do not qualify for MRI, even though cancer yields would be higher than younger high-risk women. Here is an example how age discrimination works, and how yields will vary, when lifetime risks are used:

30 y/o with two first-degree relatives with breast CA, ages 45 and 48 at diagnosis (BRCA-neg).

Lifetime risk = 34 %; 10-year risk = 3.5 % (Claus model utilized).

60 y/o with the same family history.

Lifetime risk = 18 %; 10-year risk = 10 %.

60 y/o with no risk factors.

Lifetime risk = 7 %; 10-year risk = 3.7 %.

The 30 y/o easily qualifies for annual breast MRI based on her lifetime risk. But the 60 y/o who is *three times as likely to develop breast cancer during the next 10 years and thus benefit more clearly from breast MRI* does not qualify. Worse perhaps, the 60 y/o with no risk factors has the same probability for breast cancer as the easily qualifying 30 y/o for the next 10 years. Yet, the 60-year-old is actively discouraged by the guidelines, which expressly advise *against* MRI in women with less than 15 % lifetime risk.

Furthermore, these lifetime risks put our MRI recommendations at odds with our SERM risk reduction recommendations. Currently, patients can easily qualify for long-term drug therapy to reduce breast cancer risk yet be denied screening with breast MRI where the sensitivity benefits extend across all age groups.

There are other corollaries to the scenario above. For example, patients who barely qualify for MRI initially will lose their candidacy as they age if one uses the same mathematical model. A lifetime risk of 22 % slowly and inexorably drops over time, and then a decade later, when the probability of cancer is actually higher in the short term, the patient will no longer qualify for screening MRI as she dips to 18 % remaining risk. This problem has been compounded by third-party payors who have adopted the "20 % lifetime risk" with more fervor than clinicians, and often want only Gail model predictions, even if the Gail is not the most appropriate model to use. In the United Kingdom, guidelines for screening MRI include an option for 10-year risk calculations, thus lessening the power of the paradox wherein rising short-term risks occur in the face of declining lifetime risks. A thorough understanding of this paradox is necessary not only for patient counseling but also for the design of clinical trials as well as the establishment of guidelines based on risk levels.

BRCA Genetic Testing

Although details concerning BRCA genetic counseling and testing are beyond the scope of this book, the student or the clinician should be familiar with the basic principles of hereditary breast-ovarian cancer syndrome. If an individual is found to harbor a deleterious mutation in either the *BRCA-1* or the *BRCA-2* gene, the lifetime risk for breast cancer, depending on the accompanying family history, might be as high as 85 % (total lifetime, to be adjusted downward based on *remaining* risk as well as phenotypic expression seen in the family). BRCA-positivity trumps all prior risk calculations made using the standard models above.

The surgeon will encounter BRCA-positive, asymptomatic patients who opt for preventive surgery, an approach that can be justified after a comprehensive informed consent, given proven mortality reductions. However, the surgeon should also be facile in discussing alternatives of risk reduction and aggressive surveillance with MRI. Also, the surgeon will encounter patients newly diagnosed with breast cancer who are found to be BRCA positive after the diagnosis, wherein genetic test results may impact the choice of locoregional therapy.

While some models like BRCAPRO include both a standard risk calculation and BRCA probabilities, there are additional models and tables used solely to identify patients for BRCA testing. It is best to identify patients or their family members who qualify for BRCA testing up front to settle this issue early in the risk assessment process. If counseling is performed in a single session, the patient should be advised that her risk could go up dramatically if she is found to harbor a BRCA mutation. Or, her risk might be as low as general population risk, nullifying her positive family history, if an affected family member tests BRCA positive then the patient tests negative. And, a final scenario is as follows: If BRCA testing reveals that a family harbors no detectable mutation, risk calculations made with the standard models listed above remain unchanged for all family members, though there is usually an emotional benefit here in maintaining this status quo as opposed to the higher risks.

The other major risk for carriers of a BRCA mutation is ovarian cancer, with BRCA-1 risk being in the range of 45 % lifetime, and BRCA-2 carriers having a 15–20 % lifetime risk. Although ovarian cancer screening with CA-125 and transvaginal ultrasound are available as options, there is no evidence yet of mortality reduction with such a strategy, so preventive salpingo-oophorectomy remains the mainstay (with some evidence that the cancers are actually arising in the fimbriated end of the fallopian tube). As with preventive mastectomy, preventive salpingo-oophorectomy does not reduce the risk to zero as one can still develop primary peritoneal carcinoma after oophorectomy, more likely in those with a BRCA-1 mutation (5–7 % probability).

A secondary benefit of preventive oophorectomy is *breast cancer* risk reduction when early menopause is induced, even with estrogen add-back to assist with menopausal quality-of-life issues and bone density. There is a common misconception among premenopausal patients, stated as "hormones after removing my ovaries will

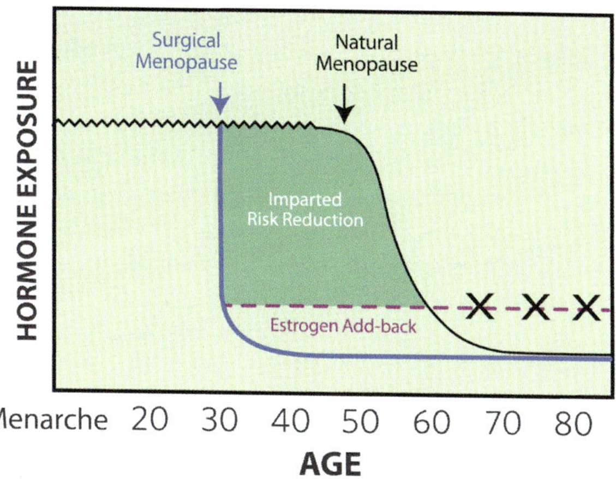

Fig. 1.4 Surgically induced menopause significantly reduces "total lifetime hormone exposure" to breast tissue as well as reducing possible additional risk imparted by cyclic variations each month (*waved line*). Some researchers believe that the early stages of carcinogenesis for both ER-positive and ER-negative tumors are taking place during this phase of life, manifest clinically decades later. While surgically induced menopause has to be weighed in light of its negative features as well, its impact on breast cancer risk reduction is represented by the *shaded area*. The degree of risk reduction is related to the age at which surgery is performed, and its power to reduce the risk easily supersedes any potential risk imparted by estrogen-alone add-back that is noncyclic, at lower levels than the natural premenopausal state, and can often be discontinued by age 50

increase breast cancer risk," when, in fact, the net risk reduction with early-age oophorectomy supersedes any theoretical risk imparted by hormone replacement therapy (HRT) (Fig. 1.4).

In fact, in one of the largest observational studies to date, researchers from Prevention and Observation of Surgical Endpoints (PROSE) reported *no increased risk at all* at 5 years with HRT following oophorectomy in premenopausal women, regardless if HRT was estrogen alone (when hysterectomy was included with salpingo-oophorectomy) or estrogen plus progesterone (in patients who only had salpingo-oophorectomy). While longer term studies are needed, especially in the form of prospective randomized trials, it is reasonable to assume that, even at maximal theoretical risk of HRT through age 50, it would not be enough to neutralize the dramatic reduction in risk achieved through early-age oophorectomy.

Breast cancer relative risk reduction after surgically induced menopause may be as high as 50–70 % when oophorectomy is performed at age 35, with a concomitant decrease in mortality due to breast cancer. The closer one gets to age 50, the less impact oophorectomy has on breast cancer risk, remembering that, by then, prevention of ovarian cancer is the primary goal.

This oophorectomy-based breast cancer risk reduction is seen with both BRCA-1 and BRCA-2 mutation carriers, even though tumors associated with the former are usually ER negative. When it comes to SERM risk reduction, tamoxifen lowers the risk in BRCA-2 patients to the usual degree, but less so in BRCA-1 patients such that some do not recommend tamoxifen for risk reduction in BRCA-1 positive patients. This impact of oophorectomy on what would be ER-negative tumors implies an endogenous hormonal contribution buried early in the carcinogenesis pathway, incompletely addressed by tamoxifen. As of this writing, there is no published data yet on the impact of raloxifene in BRCA mutation carriers.

Two common misconceptions have prevented many candidates from undergoing BRCA testing: (1) fear of discrimination, which is, in fact, prohibited by Genetic Information Non-discrimination Act (GINA) legislation, at least when it comes to health insurance and employer discrimination, and (2) the belief that "nothing can be done," since the mutation itself cannot be corrected. While it is true that the mutation is in every cell in the body and this cannot be corrected, evidence-based outcomes easily justify a variety of interventions for BRCA-positive patients.

Although multiple models are available to determine BRCA probabilities, testing is expensive, so the key to insurance coverage is often based on knowing the guidelines used by the third-party payor in question. Many third-party payors and counselors now follow NCCN guidelines for BRCA testing (accessible at http://www.nccn.org/professionals/physician_gls/f_guidelines.asp#site).

Even if not directly involved in BRCA counseling, the clinician should be aware of red flags that prompt consideration for a referral to the appropriate provider: early-onset breast cancer (even without supporting family history), multiple relatives with breast cancer (some of which are usually early onset), triple-negative breast cancers, family or personal history of ovarian cancer, male breast cancer, Ashkenazi Jewish ethnicity, bilateral breast cancers, or independent primaries in the same breast. Other cancers besides breast and ovarian are associated with BRCA mutations, most notably pancreatic cancer that is now included in NCCN guidelines, while prostate cancer, other GI cancers, and melanoma are sometimes contributory as well.

In surveys designed to determine the understanding of BRCA testing by clinicians, the area still with the most confusion is the result from complete BRCA gene sequencing that states "mutation of uncertain significance." This particular outcome from Myriad Genetics (www.myriad.com) is accompanied by information about the mutation in question, specifically how often Myriad has seen the result in the past and how it has played out in those families who have agreed to research testing. Until further notice, this *"uncertain"* result is treated as a *"negative,"* even if the patient in question has already developed cancer. One does *not* proceed to test other relatives for this "uncertain" mutation. Sometimes, the result will be downgraded in the future to "benign polymorphism," though usually, the result stands. It is very rare for such a result to be converted later to a deleterious mutation.

For the surgeon, it is important to know that BRCA reporting in newly diagnosed breast cancer patients can be obtained within a week. Results may help with planning surgical approaches. While lumpectomy can be performed in BRCA-positive patients with reasonable short-term outcomes, the risk of a second event, often due to a new primary, has been documented at 40 % within 10 years after lumpectomy and radiation. Thus, some BRCA-positive patients who are newly diagnosed with breast cancer will opt for bilateral preventive surgery with reconstruction. Another approach, while awaiting BRCA counseling and testing, is to perform lumpectomy with sentinel node biopsy, allowing the patient to proceed with systemic therapy as soon as possible. Then, if BRCA results later indicate positivity, the patient has time to consider whether or not she would like to continue with planned radiation as part of her conservation package, or proceed with bilateral preventive surgery.

BRCA testing is the closest thing in risk assessment to the aforementioned all-or-nothing Reality. For patients who test positive early in life, the resultant breast cancer risk plus the ovarian cancer risk, without intervention, approaches "all" (though some patients never develop any type of cancer). For patients who come from a BRCA-positive family and then test negative, the risk is lowered dramatically—not to the ideal of "zero"—but at least to a risk more in line with the general population (controversy still surrounds whether or not a modest risk elevation persists due to epigenetic factors).

Other Predisposition Genes

BRCA-1 and BRCA-2 counseling is going to become more complex, given that different levels of risk are being identified within the "gene-positive" population, sometimes based on the nature of the mutation itself, but other genes may harbor mutations or single-nucleotide polymorphisms (SNPs) that impact the power of BRCA-related risk.

While BRCA-1 and BRCA-2 are the most commonly discussed, and most highly penetrant, predisposition genes, other genetic syndromes carry strong predispositions for breast cancer such that affected patients and first-degree relatives fall into the guidelines established for high-risk screening with breast MRI. These include Li-Fraumeni, Cowden, and Bannayan–Riley–Ruvalcaba syndromes. Hereditary Diffuse Gastric Cancer Syndrome (CDH1) and Peutz-Jeghers Syndrome (STK11) likely impart similar breast cancer risk.

In addition, other less penetrant genes, such as CHEK2 where risk levels seem to be dependent on accompanying family history, are being evaluated for routine clinical use. PALB2, BRIP1, ATM, and the newly discovered Abraxas gene may prove to be in this category as well, while a growing number of genes have been identified with lesser degrees of risk elevation. An elevated risk for breast cancer has recently been described in patients with Lynch syndrome (hereditary non-polyposis colorectal cancer).

Miscellaneous Issues in Risk Assessment

Protective Factors

The mathematical models do not always include protective factors. However, if oophorectomy is performed prior to age 45, for whatever reason, even with estrogen add-back, there is significant risk reduction. This protective benefit has been most thoroughly documented in the BRCA literature as noted above; however, it is a recognized phenomenon for premenopausal patients undergoing surgical menopause and has even led to research efforts to prevent breast cancer through the use of GnRH agonists with estrogen add-back. It is important for the physician or other health care provider to recognize this particular protective factor, as many women thought to be at high risk are surprised to learn during formal risk assessment that they are actually at "normal or below normal" risk.

Raloxifene, while FDA approved for both osteoporosis and breast cancer risk reduction, is utilized more commonly for osteoporosis. Many women are, in fact, unaware that they are experiencing risk reduction for breast cancer in addition to the primary indication for osteoporosis, even without traditional risk factors. Unless the risk assessment counselor checks the medication list, this pharmacologic protective factor may go unnoticed.

Other protective factors exist, but are not recognized by the available models, often because they are continuums that are difficult to quantify, such as extended durations of breast-feeding. Modifiable risk factors are especially intriguing, as the risk may be reduced without pharmacologic intervention. Postmenopausal obesity is such a risk, as is daily alcohol intake of two or more drinks. Risk reduction potential is not as powerful as taking a SERM, but these modifiable risks have other health benefits as well. Risk assessment models are therefore being proposed, such as the Harvard Center for Cancer Prevention Risk Assessment Tool, which focus on these modifiable risks.

Population Attributable Risk

Attributable risk is that proportion of a population who will develop the disease in question due to the risk factor under study. An example is the following: Although it was originally hoped that the BRCA genes would be accountable for a large proportion of breast cancers, independent of family history, the attributable risk turns out to be in the range of 5–7 %.

This high-risk status for the BRCA genes, but low attributable risk, brings up another paradox. A major risk can have minor attributable risk, while a minor risk may have major implications at the population level. For instance, the absolute risk imparted to an individual who opts for HRT using both estrogen and progesterone (E+P) is rather small, especially if therapy is limited in duration. In fact, the risk seems to disappear after cessation of therapy, pointing to E+P as a promoter, rather than a causative agent. Nevertheless, if one uses an RR=1.5 as the risk for 5 years of E+P in a 50 y/o with no other known risk factors, the absolute risk for those 5 years increases from 1.25 % baseline to a 1.875 %, an increase in absolute risk of breast cancer of only 0.625 % over a 5-year period. So why did a media storm follow the publication of the Women's Health Initiative wherein the Hazard Ratio in the initial report was only 1.26 for the E+P group (closer to 1.5 when actual compliance was considered)? It is because of population attributable risk. If many millions of women are taking E+P, then a large number of breast cancers can be attributed to this risk factor. (Note: The HR of 1.26 in this report was accompanied by a 95 % CI of 1.00–1.59, with that 1.00 limit being the prompting significance that halted the trial.) This is another example of the population and the individual in an odd relationship, a never-ending issue that is gaining more importance in this era of guideline-based medicine. But as a general rule, relative risks less than 2.0 are going to have little impact on an individual's absolute risk calculated for a 20-year period or less.

Risk Assessment Subsequent to a Diagnosis of Breast Cancer

There are "local-regional" risks to consider after a diagnosis of breast cancer, independent of systemic risks. First, there are the risks associated with the primary tumor, which include recurrence at the lumpectomy site or a locoregional event. Then, there is the risk of a new primary, either on the ipsilateral side or the contralateral side. Combining all these possibilities into a single probability of a "second event" is made complex by the fact that the risk of local recurrence of the primary diminishes over time, while the risk for a new primary is roughly linear.

Although the standard mathematical models are sometimes used to compute risks of second primaries in patients already diagnosed with breast cancer, this is not appropriate. All the standard models were designed for first primaries only, and have no validity beyond that event. Therapy chosen for the first primary can have a major impact on the risk for a second primary.

That said, a substantial body of literature exists for guidance concerning the risk of a second primary, usually in terms of a contralateral primary. Flat statements like "the risk of a second primary is 10 %" are meaningless without framing the risk within a defined period of time. Given identical tumors, a 70-year-old does not have the same risk for a second primary as does a 35-year-old.

As with general risk assessment in predicting primary events, it is probably best to offer 10- or 20-year time frames for calculating and communicating the risk of second events. However, if one is pressed to offer lifetime calculations, a starting point for risk of contralateral cancer in the general population is 0.5–0.7 %/year applied to years of remaining life expectancy. Although disease-specific mortality from the first primary must also be considered, this is a difficult subject in counseling, and many choose to frame the risk of a second primary as, "Assuming the first cancer does not recur (systemically), your risk for a second event is *X* %." As such, risk calculations for second events are going to be more realistic in those patients who had early-stage disease with their primary tumor.

Then, if the patient complies with 5 years of tamoxifen, one can cut the calculated risk by 30–50 % in relative terms; and, if an aromatase inhibitor is utilized, one can cut the calculated risk by 50–70 % in relative terms. This is preliminary counseling information for AIs that is subject to final results in pending clinical trials. Note the use of "ranges" of risk and risk reduction in the suggestions above, intended to acknowledge the countless variables that preclude precise calculations in individual risk assessment.

It is likely that women at higher risk prior to the first cancer will be at higher risk for a second primary (thus, the attempts to use standard models). This principle has been demonstrated most convincingly in the BRCA-positive population where risks for a second primary are far greater than other breast cancer patients. Even in this instance, however, blanket statements like "60 % risk for contralateral cancer" are meaningless without a time frame. Additionally, "age of onset at diagnosis of the primary" contributes to the probability of developing contralateral breast cancer, somewhat independent from the mere difference in life expectancy.

For example, when diagnosed first below age 40, a second primary on the opposite side in a BRCA-positive patient occurs at a rate of approximately 2.5 %/year; if diagnosed first between 40 and 50, contralateral risk is 1.5 %/year, and, after 50, approximately 1 %/year. Yes, for women diagnosed below age 40 with BRCA-related breast cancer, with 25 years of follow-up, the risk of a second primary is 60 %. But without these qualifiers, the "60 %" is misleading. Compare this "60 %" to the BRCA-positive patient diagnosed with her first primary after age 50 where 25-year follow-up reveals a 20 % probability of developing a second primary, slightly above the usual breast cancer patient, but well below the oft-quoted "60 %."

Overall, there is a wide range for second primaries, not only given vastly different life spans depending on the age at diagnosis but also differences in the %/year probability based on the age of onset as well, plus risks present prior to the first diagnosis—all of which must be combined with specific treatments and prognosis of the primary. It has been a welcome event to see attempts at models recently proposed for the specific purpose of calculating second events.

Summarizing Future Directions in Risk Assessment

Given the uncertainties of breast cancer risk assessment and the proliferation of risk-based literature in response, we can anticipate that the "state of the art" will become more complex over time. Risk factors have been linked to certain biologic types of breast cancer (luminal A, luminal B, basal-like, HER2+, etc.), and a substantial body of literature already exists with regard to predicting ER-positive tumors, which might have application in more accurate patient selection for SERM risk reduction. Then, it has been proposed that we might need different models for the premenopausal years versus the postmenopausal years, given the selective impact of such risks as high BMI, clearly a risk in postmenopausal women, but possibly protective with regard to premenopausal cancer development. Patient age at the time of exposure to a risk has already been demonstrated with regard to radiation exposure, and it is likely that other environmental risks are more potent when exposure occurs during the window after menarche and prior to first full-term pregnancy.

It should be remembered, though, that we are capable of generating models so complex as to be of little value for the mainstream clinician, if not for the breast cancer specialist as well. And, we have to confront the fact that these mathematical models are only modest predictors of breast cancer at the individual level. Does complexity ever erase the fact that we are up against the "all-or-nothing" Reality for the individual patient?

Still, in attempting to improve models at the individual level, as measured by c-statistics, a wide variety of approaches have been published, usually selecting the Gail model as the prototype upon which to improve, a limitation if other models are more appropriate for a particular individual. These studies often provide (1) c-stats for the Gail model alone in the study population, (2) c-stats for the additional tool by itself, and then (3) c-stats for the Gail supplemented by the additional tool. In some instances, the proposed tool has performed equal to the Gail model, only to find that, when combined with the Gail, overall c-stats barely improve. The following measures to improve risk assessment are currently generating interest:

Endogenous hormone and metabolite levels in serum and/or urine
Bone density
Asymptomatic Cytology Retrieval (nipple aspirate fluid, lavage, or random FNAs) and/or ductal fluid proteins
SNPs
Mammographic Density

Many efforts are under way as well to identify specific carcinogens responsible for breast cancer, though these potential risks are not yet well delineated and may need to be matched to various SNPs or mutations in genes with only modest penetrance. In the interim, these environmental risks might be reflected through anatomic-based tools, such as abnormal findings in ductal cytology and/or fluid proteomics, serving as common denominators for all risks.

As these efforts continue to improve upon breast cancer risk assessment, it is helpful to keep in mind an important difference between using risk calculations to select patients for pharmacologic risk reduction versus selecting patients for screening recommendations. In the former case, where the SERM is being used to impact a *future* event, it is critical to know the *future* risk of said event occurring over a designated time frame.

However, in the case of high-risk screening using adjunct imaging, the risk of a *future* event is not really the issue. Future risk is merely a surrogate for the probability of immediate yields, with the limitations already noted earlier in this chapter. Rather than future risk, the critical issue in screening ought to be the risk of a cancer being present, but mammographically occult, at a single moment in time. Ideally, if a blood or a urine test were devised with enough accuracy for all women to alert the radiologist that an occult cancer was present on a negative mammogram at *that moment in time*, then risk assessment as performed today would play little or no role in selecting patients for aggressive screening strategies.

In stark contrast to these mathematical models selecting patients for high-risk screening, breast cancer risk assessment has been proposed as a tool to "do less," introducing the potential of discouraging patients from screening opportunities. Such proposals, most notably for the controversial group aged 40–49, made in the name of cost-effectiveness, are tenuous when one considers that the majority of breast cancer cases develop in women with no known risk factors. Furthermore, the difference in 10-year *absolute risk* for the majority of individuals "at risk" versus those "without known risk" is usually negligible when *calculated for the decade of the 40s*. To be specific, from age 40 to 49, absolute breast cancer risk is 1.6 %, so a woman at twofold relative risk would have a 3.2 % likelihood of breast cancer during this decade. Do we tell the patient with "1.6 %" that her risk is too low for screening mammography, while "3.2 %" is high risk? Again, we are fighting a paradox: what might be optimal for the population as a whole, especially with limited financial resources, is not necessarily what is best for the individual.

Breast cancer, unlike several other types of cancer, has a biology that appears vulnerable to early detection as evidenced by mortality reductions seen in prospective, randomized mammography screening trials. Yet, this vulnerability to early detection may be far greater than we currently imagine, given that the oft-quoted 25–30 % mortality reductions have been accomplished using a tool (mammography) that has only modest sensitivity, a parameter more accurately defined today through multi-modality imaging as opposed to the traditional 12-month follow-up. Only two factors influence screening efficacy as it relates to mortality reduction, once all epidemiologic biases have been accounted for—*biology* of the tumor and *sensitivity* of the screening tool. (Many other factors have to be considered, of course, but these relate to cost and feasibility, not mortality reduction.)

Since most now believe that the *biology* of breast cancer is vulnerable to early detection, we are left with a single issue to impact mortality—*sensitivity of the screening tool*. To date, there is no evidence that the biology of breast cancers discovered by ultrasound, molecular imaging, or MRI is any different than mammographically detected cancers, and these newer modalities all contribute significantly to finding the cancers missed by mammography. "Earlier" diagnosis than mammography is not the goal. The goal is finding those tumors large enough to be detected by mammography, but missed due to the subtle growth pattern of the tumor or the mammographic density or both. Thus, it is compelling to do more, rather than less, in our screening strategies.

In summary, multiple mathematical models are available to assess both cancer risk and BRCA gene mutation risk, serving as guides to therapeutic interventions with proven benefits. And while there is considerable momentum to provide breast cancer risk assessment to our patients, we are still left with several paradoxes that limit usefulness, most notably, the "all-or-nothing" phenomenon of dealing with the individual patient as opposed to predicting the number of breast cancer cases in a large cohort.

As we propose advances toward "personalized medicine," we face greater challenges in our ability to prospectively validate individualized approaches. For instance, for a single patient, if we were to identify three historical factors, three SNPs imparting risk, and three risks in ductal fluid proteomics, we would be limited in our ability to find a large cohort of women with these same nine risks and a control group without these nine risks. Thus, progress in risk assessment becomes its own paradox, and it speaks to the need to consider general categories of risk, without so much emphasis on fixed percentages that can vary widely from one mathematical model to another.

The transition to descriptors and categories of risk, rather than fixed percentages, has already been the case in selecting patients for BRCA testing. Originally, a "10 % risk for mutation" (20 % in the United Kingdom) was the defining threshold for testing consideration, but this has become more of an informal guide, as we increasingly rely on described patterns for the family history, be it NCCN guidelines or third-party payor guidelines, to identify candidates for testing.

Finally, given the paradoxes and complexities covered in this chapter, we should heighten our focus on the need to improve screening and diagnosis such that all women benefit equally, remembering that baseline risk is considerable.

References

1. Ottman R, Pike MC, King MC, Henerson BE. Practical guide for estimating risk for familial breast cancer. Lancet. 1983;2:556–8.
2. Anderson DE, Badzioch MD. Risk of familial breast cancer. Cancer. 1985;56:383–7.
3. Dupont WD. Converting relative risks to absolute risks: a graphical approach. Stat Med. 1989;8:641–51.
4. Dupont WD, Page DL. Risk factors for breast cancer in women with proliferative breast disease. N Engl J Med. 1985;312:146–51.
5. Gail MH, Brinton LA, Byar DP, et al. Projecting individualized probabilities of developing breast cancer for white females who are being examined annually. J Natl Cancer Inst. 1989;81:1879–86.
6. Claus EB, Risch N, Thompson WD. Autosomal dominant inheritance of early-onset breast cancer. Implications for risk prediction. Cancer. 1994;73:643–51.
7. Bodian CA, Perzin KH, Lattes R. Lobular neoplasia. Long term risk of breast cancer and relation to other factors. Cancer. 1996;78:1024–34.
8. Tyrer J, Duffy SW, Cuzick J. A breast cancer prediction model incorporating familial and personal risk factors. Stat Med. 2004;23:1111–30. Erratum in: Stat Med. 2005;24(1):156.
9. Chen J, Pee D, Ayyagari R, et al. Projecting absolute invasive breast cancer risk in white women with a model that includes mammographic density. J Natl Cancer Inst. 2006;98:1215–26.
10. Tice JA, Cummings SR, Siv E, Kerlikowske K. Mammographic breast density and the Gail model for breast cancer risk prediction in a screened population. Breast Cancer Res Treat. 2005;94:115–22.
11. Bondy ML, Newman LA. Assessing breast cancer risk: evolution of the Gail model (editorial). J Natl Cancer Inst. 2006;98:1172–3.
12. Amir E, Freedman OC, Seruga B, Evans DG. Assessing women at high risk of breast cancer: a review of risk assessment models. J Natl Cancer Inst. 2010;102:680–91.
13. Gail MH, Mai PL. Comparing breast cancer risk assessment models. J Natl Cancer Inst. 2010;102:665–8.
14. Tice JA, Cummings SR, Smith-Bindman R, et al. Using clinical factors and mammographic breast density to estimate breast cancer risk: development and validation of a new predictive model. Ann Intern Med. 2008;148:337–47.
15. Berry DA, Iversen ES, Gudbjartsson DF, et al. BRCAPRO validation, sensitivity of genetic testing of BRCA1/BRCA2, and prevalence of other breast cancer susceptibility genes. J Clin Oncol. 2002;20:2701–12.
16. Freedman AN, Seminara D, Gail MH, et al. Cancer risk prediction models: a workshop on development, evaluation, and application. J Natl Cancer Inst. 2005;97:715–23.
17. Fisher B, Costantino JP, Wickerham DL, et al. Tamoxifen for prevention of breast cancer: report of the National Surgical Adjuvant Breast and Bowel Project P-1 study. J Natl Cancer Inst. 1998;90:1371–88.

18. Vogel VG, Costantino JP, Wickerham DL, et al. Effects of tamoxifen vs. raloxifene on the risk of developing invasive breast cancer and other disease outcomes. The NSABP study of tamoxifen and raloxifene (STAR) P-2 trial. JAMA. 2006;295:2727–41.
19. Vogel VG, Costantino JP, Wickerham DL, et al. Carcinoma in situ outcomes in National Surgical Adjuvant Breast and Bowel Project breast cancer chemoprevention trials. J Natl Cancer Inst Monogr. 2010;41:181–6.
20. Hartmann LC, Schaid DJ, Woods JE, et al. Efficacy of bilateral prophylactic mastectomy in women with a family history of breast cancer. N Eng J Med. 1999;340:77–84.
21. Hartmann LC, Sellers TA, Schaid DJ, et al. Efficacy of bilateral prophylactic mastectomy in BRCA1 and BRCA2 gene mutation carriers. J Natl Cancer Inst. 2001;93:1633–7.
22. Grann VR, Jacobson JS, Thomason D, et al. Effect of prevention strategies on survival and quality-adjusted survival of women with BRCA 1/2 mutations; an updated decision analysis. J Clin Oncol. 2002;20:2520–9.
23. Parmigiani G, Chen S, Iversen ES, et al. Validity of models for predicting BRCA2 and BRCA2 mutations. Ann Intern Med. 2007;147:441–50.
24. Hollingsworth AB, Singletary SE, Morrow M, et al. Current comprehensive assessment and management of women at increased risk for breast cancer. Am J Surg. 2004;187:349–62.
25. Saslow D, Boetes C, Burke W, et al. American Cancer Society guidelines for breast screening with MRI as an adjunct to mammography. CA Cancer J Clin. 2007;57:75–9.
26. Zhang Y, Kiel DP, Kreger BE, et al. Bone mass and the risk of breast cancer among postmenopausal women. N Engl J Med. 1997;336:611–7.
27. Gail MH. Value of adding single-nucleotide polymorphism genotypes to a breast cancer risk model. J Natl Cancer Inst. 2009;101:959–63.
28. Wrensch MR, Petrakis NL, Miike R, et al. Breast cancer risk in women with abnormal cytology in nipple aspirates of breast fluid. J Natl Cancer Inst. 2001;93:1791–8.
29. Vogel VG, editor. Management of patients at high risk for breast cancer. Malden, MA: Blackwell Science; 2001.

Chapter 2
The Impact of Mammography Screening on the Diagnosis and Management of Early-Phase Breast Cancer

László Tabár, Peter B. Dean, Tony Hsiu-Hsi Chen, Amy Ming-Fang Yen, Sherry Yueh-Hsia Chiu, Tibor Tot, Robert A. Smith, and Stephen W. Duffy

Introduction

Throughout history women have detected their own breast cancers and, often after a considerable delay, have brought these palpable tumors to the attention of their physicians. From the days of Hippocrates through to the mid-nineteenth century physicians considered breast cancer to be an incurable and hopeless disease [1]. During the past century there has been a gradual but steady decrease in the average delay from palpation to treatment, which has been reflected in a gradual decrease in tumor

L. Tabár, M.D., F.A.C.R. (✉)
Department of Mammography, Falun Central Hospital, Svärdsjögatan, Falun, Sweden
e-mail: laszlo@mammographyed.com

P.B. Dean, M.D.
Department of Diagnostic Radiology, University of Turku, Turku, Finland

T.H.-H. Chen
Graduate Institute of Epidemiology and Preventive Medicine, National Taiwan University, Taipei, Taiwan

A.M.-F. Yen
School of Oral Hygiene, Taipei Medical University, Taipei, Taiwan

S.Y.-H. Chiu
Department and Graduate Institute of Health Care Management, Chang Gung University, Taoyuan, Taiwan

T. Tot, M.D., Ph.D.
Department of Clinical Pathology, Central Hospital Falun, Falun, Sweden
e-mail: tibor.tot@ltdalarna.se

R.A. Smith
Cancer Control Science Department, American Cancer Society, Atlanta, GA, USA

S.W. Duffy, M.Sc.
Centre for Cancer Prevention, Wolfson Institute of Preventive Medicine, Queen Mary University, London, London, UK

D.S. Francescatti and M.J. Silverstein (eds.), *Breast Cancer: A New Era in Management*, DOI 10.1007/978-1-4614-8063-1_2,

size and a corresponding improvement in survival. Physician- and patient-detected breast cancers still have an average size exceeding 3.0 cm [2]. The development of modern breast imaging methods has resulted in a significant improvement in the spectrum of tumor characteristics, including tumor size, node status, and histologic malignancy grade. When mammography is used as a screening tool, the balance shifts from mainly palpable to mainly impalpable breast cancers, most of which are still localized to the breast [3–5]. Half of the invasive cancers are <15 mm in modern breast centers, with only 20 % poorly differentiated and <15 % node positive [6]. This revolutionary shift in disease presentation provided the opportunity for a considerably improved control of breast cancer, which has been realized through the establishment of comprehensive breast centers specializing in the diagnosis and treatment of breast cancer as early as possible. Their diagnostic and therapeutic team members faced the challenge of maximizing the benefits and minimizing the risks by avoiding the extremes of overtreatment and undertreatment as well as the extremes of overdiagnosis and underdiagnosis. The rationale for using early diagnosis and treatment in the early phase to better control of breast cancer is based upon the continuous improvement in outcome which has followed the steady decrease in average tumor size. The implication is that most breast cancers in their non-palpable, preclinical phase are without viable metastases, and that breast cancer is a progressive disease, which is why early detection and surgical removal in the early phase can decrease the rate of advanced cancers and reduce breast cancer death. The success of the population-based randomized controlled mammography screening trials provides proof that earlier detection and treatment accomplish this goal.

Concurrently with the accumulation of evidence supporting the progressive nature of breast cancer, an opposing theory was proposed by Bernard Fisher, according to which "It is likely that a tumor (breast cancer) is a systemic disease from its inception," [7] a statement which is incompatible with the nature of an adenocarcinoma during its early stages of development. Commenting on this theory, Edwin Fisher stated: "There is no evidence that delay in diagnosis unfavorably influences the survival of patients with breast cancer" [8]. According to Bernard Fisher's theory, "… variations in the treatment of locoregional disease were unlikely to affect survival," and systemic adjuvant therapy should not be delayed [9]. The implication for the surgeon is that local disease control cannot affect survival outcomes, a long-held belief of the National Surgical Adjuvant Breast and Bowel Project (NSABP). Additionally, Fisher predicted, "it is likely that surgery for the disease will continue to diminish in importance as improved methods of detection and tumor cell eradication become more commonly used" [9].

These statements are surprising in the face of scientific data and continually accumulating evidence for the effectiveness of early detection in reducing the rate of advanced cancer and the accompanying disease-specific mortality [10]. Had all breast cancers been truly "systemic" from the time of inception, surgical removal of the primary tumor could not have affected the systematic metastases postulated by Fisher. In particular, the HIP study of Greater New York had demonstrated a significant decrease in breast cancer mortality already in 1971, [11] nearly a decade before Fisher first published his "alternative theory." The largest randomized controlled mammography screening trial used only mammography as a screening method and published in 1985 a 31 % significantly decreased mortality from breast cancer among women invited to screening compared to the control group [12]. Numerous meta-analyses of eight population-based randomized controlled trials and the evaluation of several large-scaled service screening programs have all proved that *breast cancer is a progressive disease, and is not, as advanced by Fisher*, "a systemic disease from its inception." The randomized controlled trials demonstrated a significant decrease in breast cancer death among women invited to screening, [10–17, 21] and the service screening evaluations showed a significant decrease in breast cancer death among women who attended screening regularly [18–20].

The primary results of the randomized trials of screening, with additional research on tumor progression, have demonstrated that the interruption of disease progression results in reduced mortality from breast cancer and that the time at which the progression is arrested is crucial [22]. Despite the magnitude of this evidence, it was ignored by Fisher and Anderson in 2010 when they published that "no scientific evidence has been presented to challenge the alternative hypothesis, any of its tenets, or the paradigm that currently governs the treatment of breast cancer" [23].

Comments

1. If breast cancer were "a systemic disease from its inception," then it would not be possible to cure breast cancer patients by surgery alone, no matter what the tumor size or the node status is at the time of operation, because viable metastases would already be present throughout the body. The long-term follow-up of the NSABP B-04 and B-06 trials themselves provide evidence to the contrary. Both demonstrated a significantly better outcome for women with node-negative cancers compared with node-positive cases, irrespective of the treatment methods chosen (see Figs. 2.1 and 2.2, printed with permission from NEJM) [24, 25]. Although not discussed in these publications, the better survival of the node-negative cases indicates that surgical treatment is more effective earlier in the natural history of the disease before the establishment of metastases. The three therapeutic choices in the B-04 trial were radical mastectomy, total mastectomy combined with irradiation, and total mastectomy [24]. In the B-06 trial the choices were total mastectomy, lumpectomy, or lumpectomy combined with postoperative irradiation [25]. It is noteworthy that *the outcome in each arm was equally poor (not equally good!)*, regardless of the three choices of therapy.

   Conclusion: These observations from the NSABP trials provide good evidence that the long-term outcome of the breast cancer patients will be determined by whether the treatment is given early or late in the natural history of the disease. Had the NSABP trial results been correctly interpreted, both the mammography screening trials and the NSABP trials would have arrived at the same conclusion, as follows: *The current therapeutic regimens are most effective at an earlier stage of breast cancer, when the probability of systemic metastases is lower.*

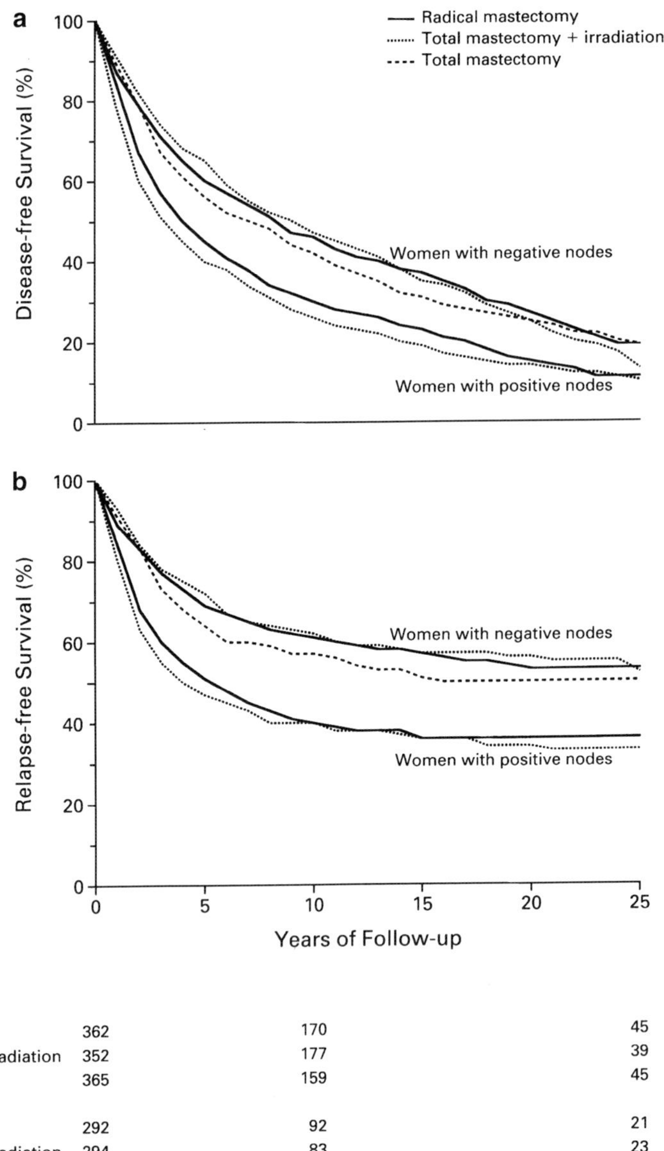

No. at Risk			
Negative nodes			
Radical mastectomy	362	170	45
Total mastectomy + irradiation	352	177	39
Total mastectomy	365	159	45
Positive nodes			
Radical mastectomy	292	92	21
Total mastectomy + irradiation	294	83	23

Fig. 2.1 Disease-free survival (Panel **a**) and relapse-free survival (Panel **b**) during 25 years of follow-up after surgery among women with clinically negative axillary nodes and women with clinically positive axillary nodes. There were no significant differences among the groups of women with negative nodes or between the groups of women with positive nodes in either analysis. Printed with permission from NEJM

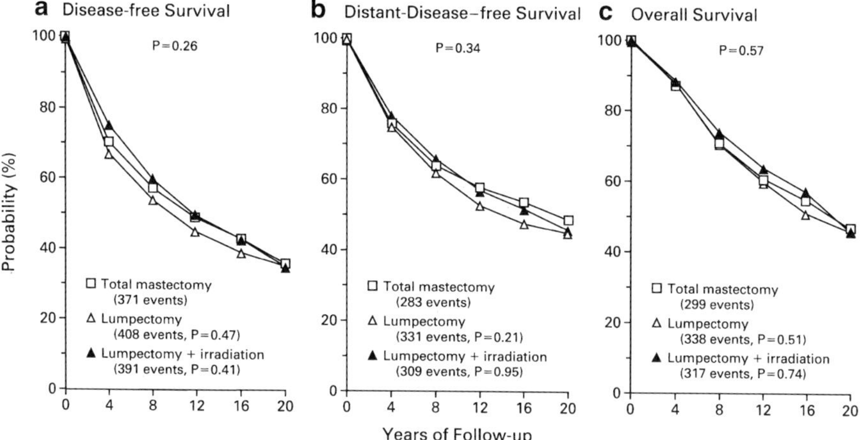

Fig. 2.2 Disease-free survival (Panel **a**), distant-disease-free survival (Panel **b**), and overall survival (Panel **c**) among 589 women treated with total mastectomy, 634 treated with lumpectomy alone, and 628 treated with lumpectomy plus irradiation. In each panel, the *P* value above the curves is for the three-way comparison among the treatment groups; the *P* values below the curves are for the two-way comparisons between lumpectomy alone or with irradiation and total mastectomy. Printed with permission from NEJM

2. Fisher's "alternative theory" also implies that finding non-palpable breast cancers at screening will not lead to a decrease in breast cancer death, but the large volume of evidence, including their own, does not support this theory.

   Results from randomized controlled trials: To date there have been ten randomized controlled mammography screening trials (eight population based) which tested the influence of early detection upon the disease-specific mortality from breast cancer. Meta-analyses of these trials have shown a highly significant, long-term mortality benefit from invitation to screening [10, 13, 14]. Very-long-term follow-up (29 years) of the largest of the mammography screening trials showed a highly significant 31 % decrease in mortality from breast cancer in the women invited to screening compared with the uninvited control group (relative risk [RR]=0.69; 95 % confidence interval [CI]: 0.56–0.84; $P<.0001$). This long-term evaluation also demonstrated a steady increase in the absolute benefit of early detection, in terms of the number of lives saved, which continued well beyond 20 years of follow-up (71 lives saved at 10 years, 141 lives saved at 20 years, 158 lives saved at 29 years) [21]. Thus, the majority of the benefit of mammography screening occurs more than 10 years after screening begins. The more aggressive cancers would have led to breast cancer death in the first 10 years without early detection and surgical removal, while some of the more slowly growing, "indolent" cancers would have led to death after 10–20 years of follow-up in the absence of screening. Claims that mammography screening finds mostly "indolent" cancers [26–28] fail to acknowledge published evidence documenting the propensity for a dedifferentiation of the tumor malignancy grade. The term "ultralow risk tumors" is thus unrealistic and misleading [27].

Results from evaluation of service screening: It should be noted that the randomized controlled trials use the "intention-to-treat" approach, which includes all women with breast cancer, both those who attended and those who declined the invitation to screening. Mortality from breast cancer is decreased to a greater extent in women who attended screening regularly than in the invited group as a whole. Disease-specific mortality among the women who attended screening regularly has been quantified in several ongoing service screening programs. A highly significant reduction of 43 % was observed in Sweden and 49 % in the Netherlands in women who attended mammography screening regularly [15, 19]. This emphasizes the importance of distinguishing between the effect of *invitation to* versus the effect of *regularly attending* mammography screening [20].

The issue of subgroup analysis: The population-based randomized controlled trials were all designed to have sufficient statistical power to evaluate the impact of early detection on mortality from breast cancer within the age group selected. However, when the populations were inappropriately subdivided into age cohorts of unequal size (40–49 vs. 50–69), the younger, smaller cohort with lower breast cancer incidence had insufficient statistical power. The resulting lack of a statistically significant decrease in mortality within individual age subgroups was erroneously interpreted as evidence of no impact at ages below 50 years, despite the existence of clear trends towards fewer advanced tumors and decreased mortality. Meta-analysis of trials shows a significant mortality reduction with the policy of offering screening in women aged 40–49 [10, 29]. Also, when Sweden gradually implemented nationwide screening, the option for the lower age limit was either 40 or 50 years. As it happened, the individual counties independently chose 40 years as the lower age in approximately half of the country. This gave the opportunity to evaluate the impact of screening in a population aged 40–49 which was sufficiently large for statistical significance, comprising more than 16 million women-years with 16 years of follow-up. A highly significant 29 % decrease in breast cancer mortality was documented in the women who attended screening (RR 0.71; 95 % CI, 0.62–0.80). This reduction occurred in a country where treatment guidelines are uniform and closely adhered to, so this mortality reduction was achieved in addition to the benefits of modern therapeutic advances [17].

3. All these results have convincingly demonstrated that the diagnosis and treatment of breast cancer at an earlier phase can prevent death from breast cancer, before viable metastases have been developed, confirming that breast cancer is not a systemic disease from its inception, in contradiction to the "alternative theory," developed by Fisher. The screening trial results unequivocally proved that *breast cancer is a progressive disease*, and that its progression can be arrested by early detection. As a result, the prognosis of the breast cancer patients can be substantially improved by local treatment. *Fisher's proposal that breast cancer is a "systemic disease from its inception" is either mistaken or, as the screening results convincingly show, it is not relevant to the treatment of node-negative,*

- *<15 mm breast cancers.* "Screening has made possible the detection of a large proportion of node negative tumors less than 15 mm size (i.e. before the development of viable metastases) and there is substantial evidence that local–regional therapy is effective in these cases and that adjuvant systemic therapy has negligible scope to improve the survival of patients with these tumors; also, the notion of 'early' breast cancer for tumors up to 50 mm is clearly outmoded" [22].

Key Points

Mammography screening alters the presentation of breast cancers from mainly palpable to mainly non-palpable. Randomized controlled mammography screening trials have convincingly demonstrated the following:

- Early detection through mammography screening and surgical removal at an early phase can prevent death from breast cancer.
- Breast cancer is not a systemic disease from its inception. Therefore, when it is detected as either an in situ or a 1–14 mm invasive tumor, it is primarily a surgical disease.
- Breast cancer is a progressive disease, but this progression can be interrupted by early detection and treatment at a sufficiently early phase.
- The breast cancer patient's long-term outcome will be mostly determined by whether the treatment is given early or late, rather than by the choice of treatment offered to breast cancer patients.
- The revolution in imaging that has enabled the detection of breast cancer at these early stages awaits a similar revolution in histopathology and therapy.
- Therapeutic guidelines for screen-detected breast cancers should not be based on trial results obtained from palpable, clinically detected cancers. There is considerable risk for overtreatment when the adjuvant treatment regimens developed for palpable cancers are also used to treat mammographically detected, non-palpable cancers.
- Long-term follow up of screen-detected cases is necessary for the accurate quantification of absolute benefit of screening, because the true potential of the so-called indolent tumors to dedifferentiate cannot be accurately predicted at the time of treatment.

The Mechanism by Which Screening Affects the Natural History of the Disease

The randomized controlled mammography screening trials have provided the opportunity to study the mechanism by which earlier diagnosis and treatment affect the outcome of breast cancer. In these trials one group was randomized to receive an invitation to screening, but the other, randomly selected group of women (control

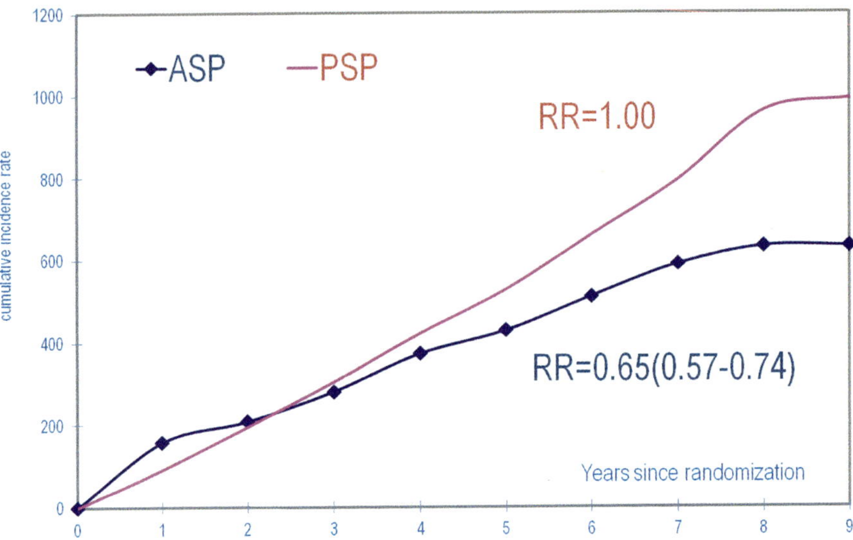

Fig. 2.3 Cumulative incidence rates of advanced breast cancers (Stage II or more advanced) in women invited versus not invited to the Swedish Two-County mammography screening trial. The first screening brought to light both occult and clinically advanced cancers, resulting in the initial slight excess of Stage II+cancers in the invited group. After the first round of screening the advanced cancer rate in women invited to screening fell significantly below that of the control group, because many small invasive cancers were detected at screening and surgically removed before they could grow to a more advanced stage

group) was not invited. The breast cancers in women invited to screening were diagnosed on average at an earlier phase than the self-detected tumors in the control group. Screening has a significant impact on all three first-generation prognostic factors: tumor size, axillary node status, and histologic malignancy grade. In a high-quality service screening program 15–20 % of the cancers will be in situ and more than 50 % of the invasive carcinomas will be <15 mm in diameter. Early detection also results in significantly fewer cases with axillary lymph node metastases and also prevents worsening of the malignancy grade in a certain percentage of the tumors. Since two components of the TNM classification, tumor size and node status, will improve significantly in women invited to screening, the incidence of Stage II and more advanced cancers will decrease in this same group of women (see Fig. 2.3).

There is parallelism between the incidence of advanced cancers and the breast cancer-specific mortality rate in any given population, since most breast cancer deaths occur in women whose tumor was at an advanced stage at the time of detection [10, 12, 30–32]. Thus decreasing the incidence rate of advanced tumors through screening will result in a corresponding decrease in breast cancer mortality in this same group of women. In the Swedish Two-County Trial the advanced cancer rate began to fall starting from year four and onwards in women invited to screening, as did the breast cancer death rate. Both of these declines were a consequence of early detection and treatment in an earlier phase (see Fig. 2.4).

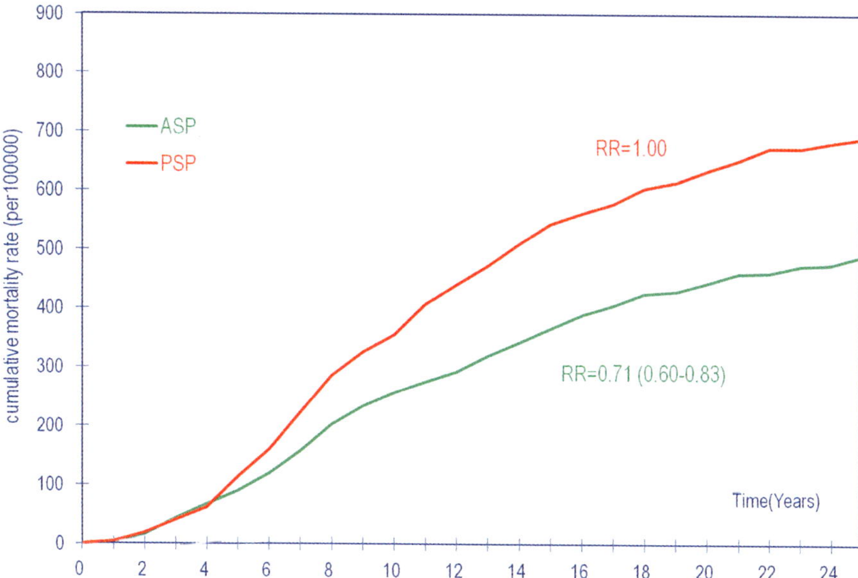

Fig. 2.4 Cumulative breast cancer mortality in women invited to mammography screening (*ASP*) compared to women not invited (control group, *PSP*) at 25-year follow-up after randomization

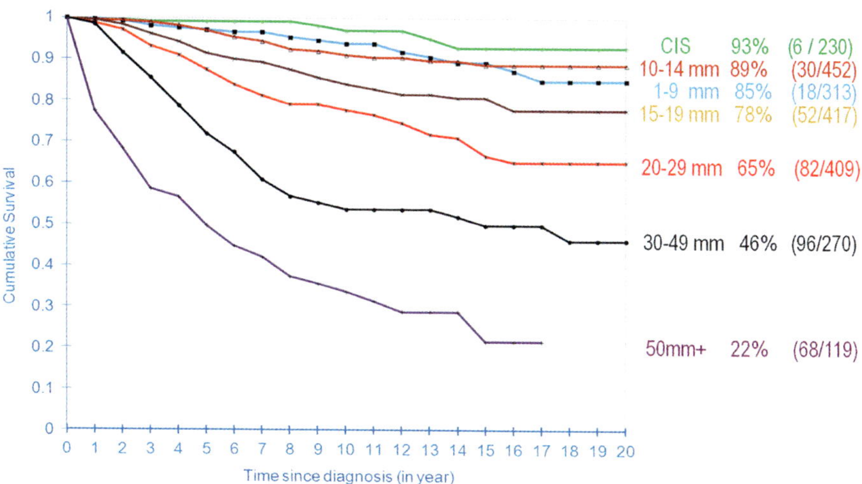

Fig. 2.5 20-year disease-specific survival of women according to tumor size in Dalarna County, Sweden

The effect of tumor size on long-term survival (28 years) in the Swedish Two-County Trial is presented in Fig. 2.5. The beneficial impact of screening is reflected in the excellent long-term survival of women with in situ and 1–14 mm invasive

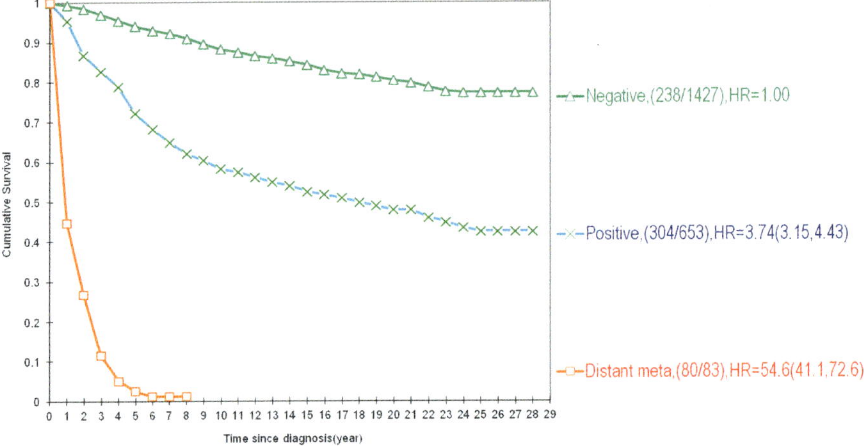

Fig. 2.6 28-year disease-specific survival of women according to axillary node status and the presence of distant metastases in the Swedish Two-County Trial, for all tumor sizes

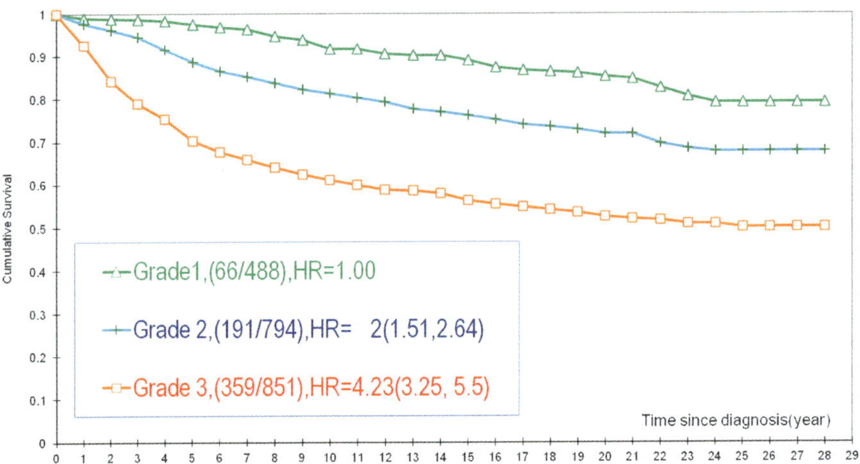

Fig. 2.7 Cumulative survival of women aged 40–69 years according to the histologic grade of invasive breast cancers from the Swedish Two-County Trial, for all tumor sizes

breast cancer. The 28-year survival according to axillary node status and distant metastases for all tumor sizes demonstrates the profound prognostic impact of these parameters (see Fig. 2.6). These survival rates are from the era prior to the widespread use of chemotherapy for primary breast carcinoma; none of the women with <20 mm node-negative tumors received chemotherapy in the Swedish Two-County Trial (1977–1985). Women with lymph node metastases had significantly poorer survival than those without lymph node metastases. The cumulative survival of women aged 40–69 years according to the histologic grade of the invasive cancers is shown in Fig. 2.7.

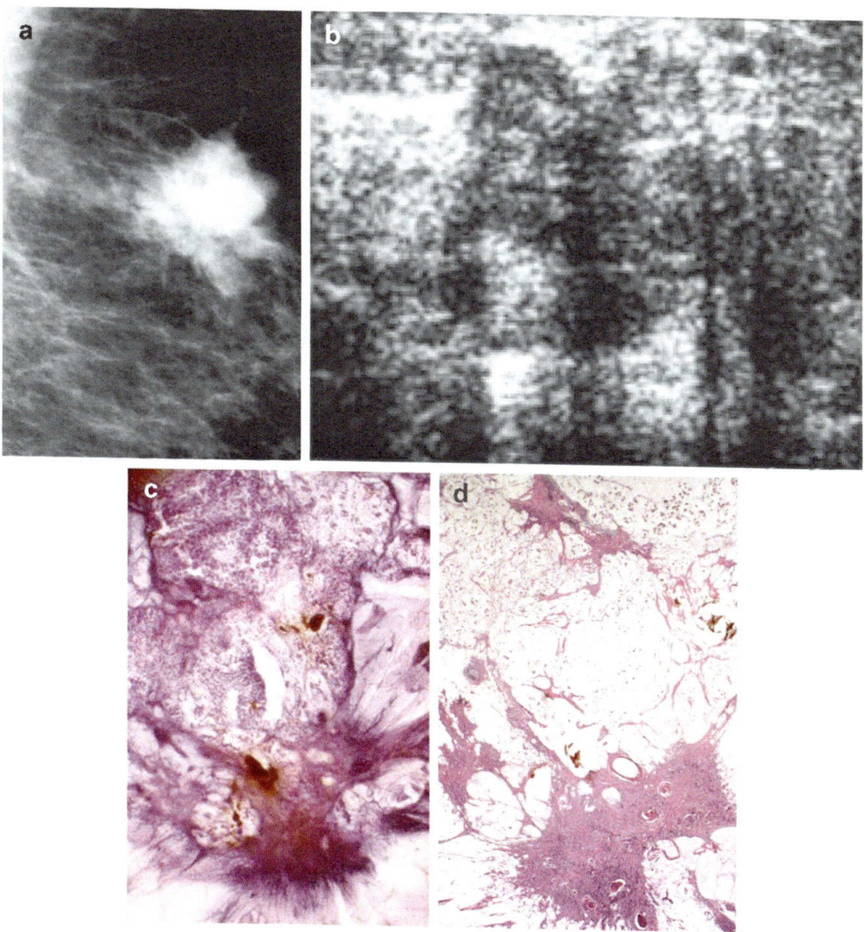

Fig. 2.8 Details of the mammographic (**a**) and ultrasound (**b**) images of a tumor containing both a circular/lobulated and stellate components. Subgross, 3D (**c**) and large thin-section (**d**) histology images show that the stellate component corresponds to a moderately differentiated invasive ductal carcinoma and the lobulated component is a well-differentiated mucinous cancer

Many breast tumors display intratumor heterogeneity, containing two or more histologic types and phenotypes (see Fig. 2.8a–d) [33–35]. Early detection through screening prevents many small, well- or moderately differentiated tumors from developing into more poorly differentiated, larger tumors. The evidence that the histologic malignancy grade worsens as the breast cancer progresses comes from the analysis of both clinical [36] and screening data [37]. The clinical research of Tubiana et al. demonstrated that "during their growth tumors progress towards higher grades" [36]. Duffy et al. used data from a randomized controlled mammography screening trial to perform a more precise measurement of progression by comparing the tumor characteristics in the control group, where the tumors were allowed to grow until clinically detectable, with the tumor characteristics in the group of women invited to mammography screening, where screening aimed at arresting tumor growth [37]. This comparison required the removal of the prevalence screen tumors from both groups in order to eliminate length bias. These two sets of tumors were then equivalent in all aspects except that the tumors in the group invited to screening were diagnosed, on average, earlier. Comparison of tumor size, node status, histologic malignancy grade, and detection mode showed that the proportion of cancers with positive nodes and a higher malignancy grade increased with increasing tumor size [3, 37]. There were also significantly fewer node-positive and poorly differentiated cancers among women invited to screening. There could be two competing explanations for these results: (1) The malignancy grade remains unchanged as the tumor grows, and screening has mostly detected well- and moderately differentiated tumors (length bias sampling). (2) The malignancy grade tends to worsen as the tumor grows, and tumor progression does indeed occur. If this were to happen, one would see a deficit of poorly differentiated tumors in the incident cancers of a group of women invited to screening compared with an uninvited group. When Duffy et al. eliminated the length bias cases from both groups, i.e., the prevalent screen, and could thus compare the incident cancers in those invited and those not invited to screening, they observed that the tumors were significantly smaller and there was a significant deficit of poorly differentiated tumors in the invited group. This demonstrated that screening prevented the deterioration of the malignancy grade of some of the tumors. In summary, tumor progression (worsening of the malignancy potential through the process of dedifferentiation) has been shown to occur in both clinical and screening studies [36, 37].

Detailed analysis of the breast cancer cases from women invited and not invited to a randomized controlled trial demonstrated that the rate of poorly differentiated breast cancer increases in all age subgroups with increasing tumor size, but in premenopausal women this process of dedifferentiation occurs more rapidly, earlier in the preclinical detectable phase, and to a greater extent than in postmenopausal women. All these factors in combination make it necessary that women are invited to screening at a frequency which takes into account the varying tumor growth rates according to different histologic tumor types and women's age [29, 38]. Reversion to less frequent screening, as recommended by the US Public Services Task Force (USPSTF), would tend to increase the number of advanced (more frequently poorly differentiated and node positive) cancers at the time of treatment and increase fatality from breast cancer [39].

The recent publications by Esserman et al. maintain that screening does not decrease the incidence of advanced breast cancers [27, 28]. This is contrary to the published evidence [10, 12, 30–32, 40]. The claim of Esserman et al. that "tumor biology does not change over time" [27] reflects unfamiliarity with appropriate statistical analysis of clinical [36] and screening trial data [37] and fails to account for certain fundamental observations in breast tumor biology, including the consequences of intratumor heterogeneity [35].

Key Points

- Breast cancer screening has a favorable impact on all three first-generation prognostic factors: tumor size, node status, and histologic malignancy grade.
- The favorable prognosis of women with screen-detected breast cancers can be accounted for by smaller tumor size, less node positivity, and lower malignancy grade at the time of treatment.
- The frequency of poorly differentiated breast cancers increases with increasing tumor size.
- The frequency of node positivity increases with increasing tumor size.
- More frequent screening will reduce the number of interval cancers, and also improve the prognostic characteristics of screen-detected cancers.

Multifocal and Diffusely Invasive Breast Cancers: High Fatality Rate and High Recurrence Rate

Our primary goal is to reduce mortality from breast cancer. Mammography screening and the associated improvements in diagnosis and therapy have enabled us to reduce the breast cancer mortality in women attending screening regularly by 40–50 % [19]. Despite this accomplishment, women are still dying from breast cancer. Investigation into the characteristics of the cancers that are still causing breast cancer death requires assessing the *extent* of the disease as a measure of the tumor burden. Two comprehensive whole-breast histologic studies examined the unifocal, multifocal, and diffusely infiltrating nature of breast cancer [41, 42]. The term multifocality includes (a) multiple in situ cancer foci without invasion, (b) a solitary invasive carcinoma associated with multiple in situ foci, and (c) multiple invasive breast cancer foci with or without associated in situ cancer. The invasive cancers with or without an associated in situ component are responsible for breast cancer death; the relative frequency of unifocal/multifocal/diffusely infiltrating invasive breast cancers is approximately 68/27/5 % [109]. In which of these groups is breast cancer most fatal? The fatality ratio of unifocal breast cancers (with or without associated in situ foci) is 9.1 % and most (74 %) of these fatal cancers were >2.0 cm in size. In the era of mammography screening enhanced by the use of multimodality breast imaging, unifocal tumors can be detected and successfully removed before they reach the size of 2.0 cm. The fatality ratio in multifocal and diffusely infiltrating invasive breast cancers is 20 and 26 %, respectively, considering all sizes of tumors [43]. Multifocality is an important, independent negative prognostic factor (see Fig. 2.9) and its harmful effect becomes more significant with increasing tumor size. Weisenbacher and coworkers have arrived at the same conclusion [44].

The highly significant size-related survival difference also applies to multifocal breast cancers, suggesting that a combination of imaging methods that enables detection of multifocal cancers with a lower tumor burden (when the largest tumor

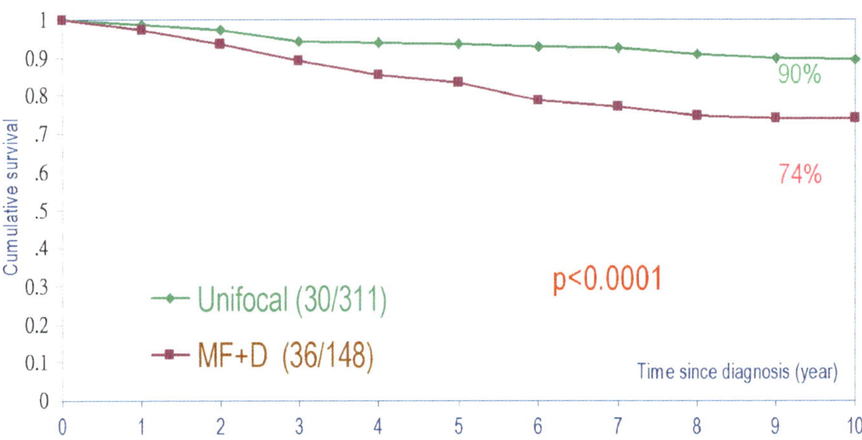

Fig. 2.9 Cumulative survival of women with unifocal invasive versus combined multifocal and diffusely infiltrating breast cancer

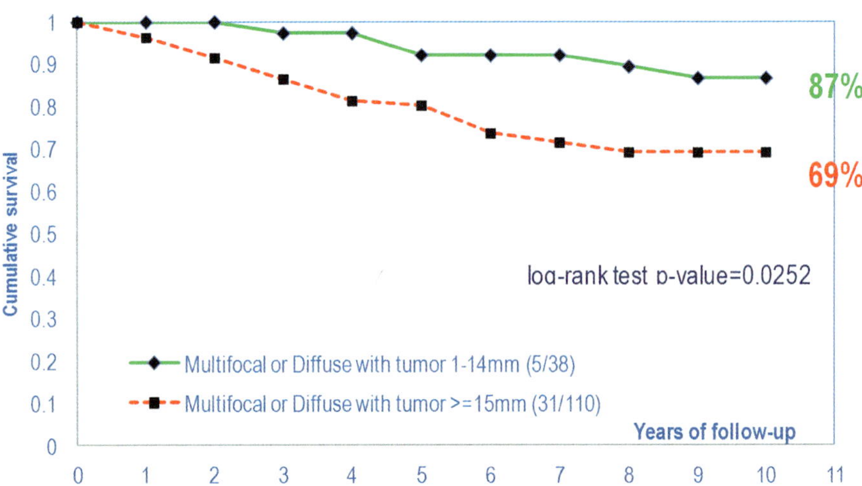

Fig. 2.10 Cumulative survival of women with 1–14 mm multifocal invasive versus >15 mm multifocal invasive breast cancer

focus is <15 mm) will result in a lower fatality rate (see Fig. 2.10). The multimodality approach (mammography, automated breast ultrasound, and especially breast MRI) will detect multifocal cancers having a lower tumor burden, and will correspondingly lower the fatality rate. This emphasizes the importance of using breast MRI to determine the presence and extent of multifocal disease. The use of breast MRI in multifocal and diffusely infiltrating invasive breast cancers is invaluable in describing the true extent of the disease. This is an important part of treatment planning to prevent incomplete resection of breast cancer at primary surgery. Incomplete resection of invasive cancer foci is associated with a poor outcome: "For patients who underwent second surgery, the finding of a residual invasive carcinoma was associated with increased risk for distant recurrence (22.8 vs. 6.6 %; HR 3.5; 95 % confidence interval, 1.8–7.4; $P<.0001$)." These same authors concluded, "there is a need to improve techniques for the presurgical and/or intraoperative determination of margins" [45].

Modern, high-resolution breast MRI has the capability of describing the true extent of the disease in the vast majority of cases, far exceeding that of earlier MRI technology, on which most currently available reviews are based. The COMICE trial, which used 2.4/4.0 mm slice thickness (as opposed to the current practice of 0.7–1.0 mm), was a multicenter trial in which 45 centers supplied an average of only 18 cases each during the 5-year accrual period starting in 2002. This study's failure to detect an impact of preoperative MRI upon reoperation rate may reflect the outdated technology and the extremely low average rate of patient accrual per site, reflecting limited experience in breast MRI interpretation. High-resolution breast MRI was practically nonexistent prior to 2007. For these reasons the COMICE trial results [46], the meta-analysis by Houssami et al. [47], and other earlier studies may have lost their relevance to current breast MRI practice.

The reliance upon local recurrence as a measure of success or failure of breast cancer treatment is subject to serious limitations. Fatality often occurs without local recurrence and the term "local recurrence" as used in the literature does not discriminate among recurrences in unifocal, multifocal, and diffusely infiltrating breast cancers. One classification system uses a cutoff point of 4.0 cm to separate "extensive" from "non-extensive" breast cancer [42]. Using this arbitrary cutoff point, "A disease extent ≥4 cm was shown to be an independent marker for local recurrence; the cumulative 10-year local relapse rate for the group with a disease extent ≥4 cm was 20.5 %, and for the rest 6.7 % (p value = 0.003)" [48].

The seriousness of multifocal and diffusely infiltrating breast cancers has not been generally appreciated for two main reasons. First, the current TNM classification system does not account for multifocality, using only the size of the largest invasive focus as the major descriptive factor. This seriously underestimates the actual tumor burden of multifocal tumors. We have proposed a quantitative evaluation of tumor burden in terms of total tumor volume and surface area [43].

Second, the current practice of histopathology of breast specimens has serious limitations; "conventional techniques may not reflect the extent of neoplasia when the neoplasia is impalpable or grossly indistinct as in the case of dense breast tissue." Additionally, "complete specimen examination is rarely performed in clinical practice." "In a typical 8-cm diameter lumpectomy specimen, assuming four conventional pathology margin sections are removed in a single plane, only 16 % of the circumference is examined microscopically" [49] (see Fig. 2.11). "People blame MRI instead of the limitations of conventional pathology *and* a failure of small section pathology to correlate with MRI and mammography." (Lee Tucker, M.D., F.A.P.C., personal communication 2012).

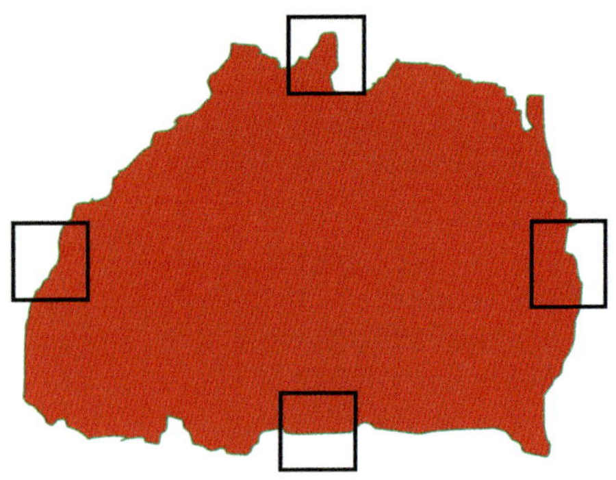

Fig. 2.11 Conventional pathology samples only 16 % of the circumference in a typical 8 cm lumpectomy specimen (courtesy of Lee Tucker M.D., F.C.A.P.)

We recommend that *large-section histopathology should be standard* for all breast cancer surgical specimens, as it also provides better correlation with breast imaging (see Fig. 2.12a–m).

Key Points

Despite the remarkable improvements in the diagnosis and therapy of breast cancer that resulted in a significantly decreased mortality from the disease, it is unfortunate that women are still dying from breast cancer.

- The fatality rate is highest for multifocal and diffusely infiltrating breast cancer cases and lowest for unifocal tumors.
- Multifocality is an important, independent negative prognostic factor whose harmful influence increases with increasing tumor size.
- Even multifocal invasive breast cancers can be detected in a relatively early phase with a lower tumor burden and a correspondingly lower fatality rate, provided that the most sensitive imaging methods are used preoperatively. The combination of currently available imaging methods, especially breast MRI, has this capability.
- The use of preoperative MRI helps to prevent incomplete resection of breast cancer at primary surgery because it provides more accurate determination of tumor size and extent than either mammography or breast ultrasound.
- The failure to remove invasive breast cancer foci is associated with a poorer outcome.
- The current TNM classification system should be upgraded to provide a better quantitative evaluation of the tumor burden by categorizing unifocal, multifocal, and diffusely infiltrating breast cancers separately.
- Large-section histopathology of all breast cancer surgical specimens should be the standard of care.

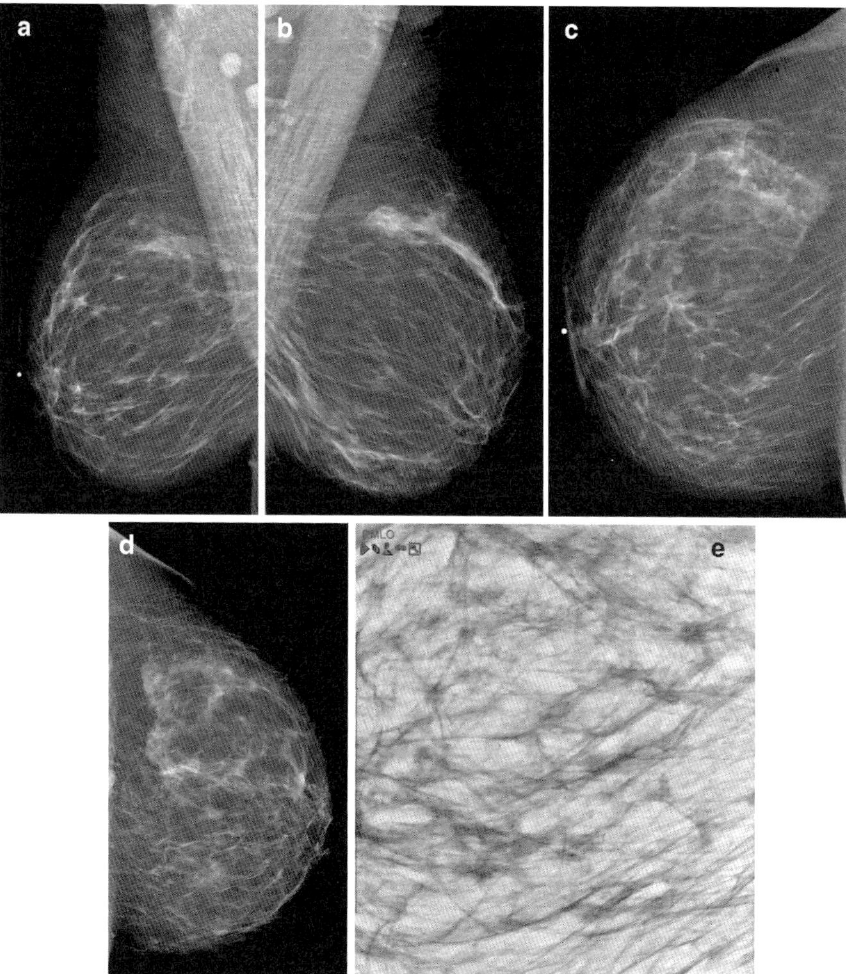

Fig. 2.12 (**a**–**e**) This 49-year-old woman felt a lump under her right areola. A slight degree of skin retraction could be provoked over the tumor. Physical examination confirmed the presence of a hard tumor, but also revealed a "thickening" in the upper and central portions of the right breast. The mammograms show a retroareolar asymmetric density corresponding to the palpatory finding. In addition, there are a large number of small stellate lesions spread throughout the upper-medial portion of the right breast, pathologic lymph nodes in the right axilla, and an oval tumor mass in the upper portion of the left breast. (**f**–**i**) Breast MRI of the right breast shows at least 30 independent tumor foci in the upper-medial portion of the breast with washout pattern (histologically proven invasive breast cancer foci) and a solitary, oval lesion with benign features in the left breast (histologic examination of the core biopsy specimen: fibroadenoma). (**j**–**m**) Correlation of the right mastectomy specimen slices with large-section histology. Multifocal cancer: at least 25 invasive tumor foci (well and moderately differentiated), the largest measuring 33 mm × 15 mm, and the smallest focus being 8 mm. The second and third largest foci measure 20 mm × 12 mm and 10 mm × 8 mm. In addition LCIS and Grade 1 and 2 in situ carcinoma are found over a 45 mm × 11 mm area. Six out of 17 surgically removed axillary lymph nodes showed metastases at histologic examination

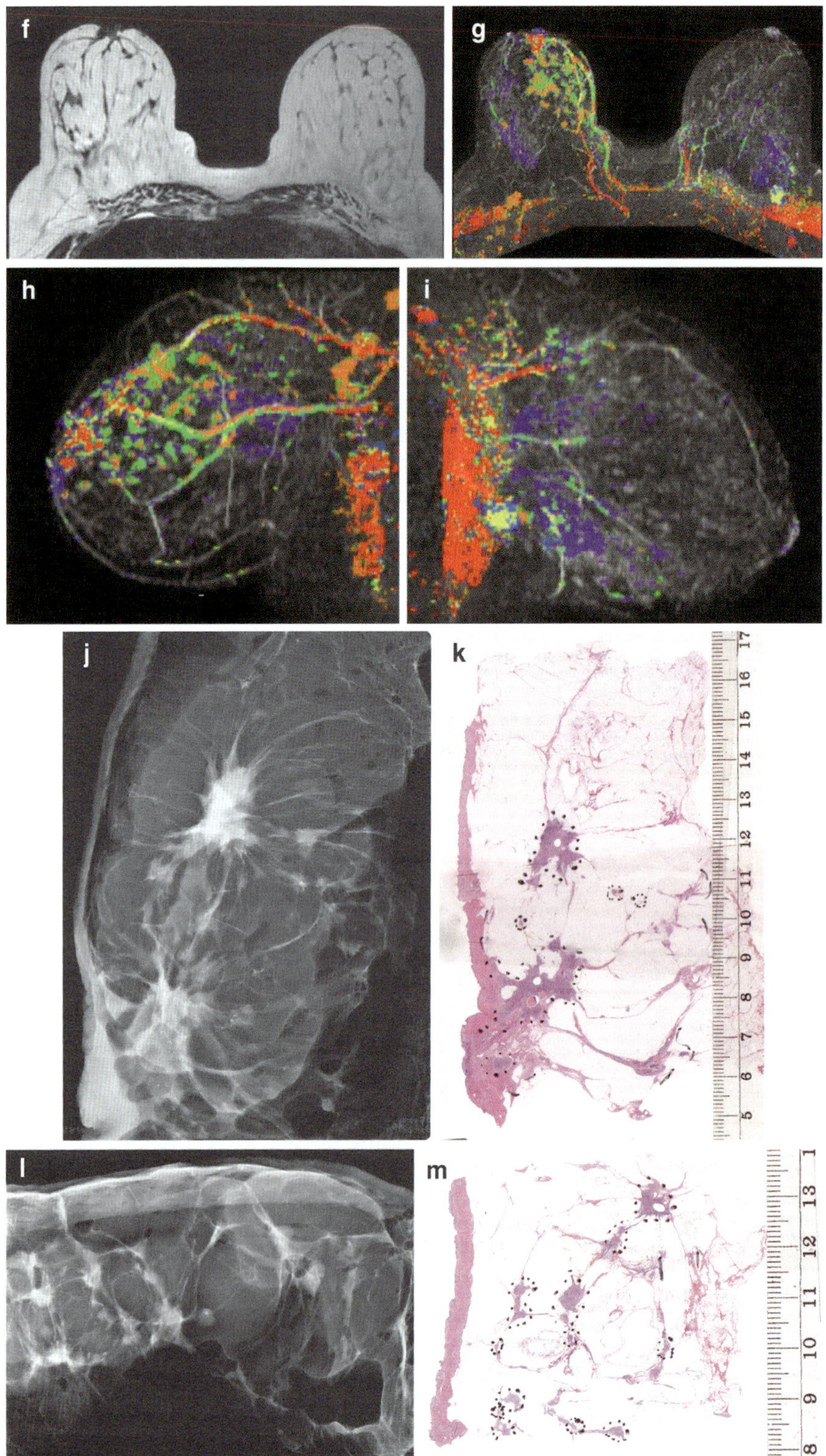

Fig. 2.12 (continued)

The Need for Improved Terminology Reflecting the Site of Origin of Breast Cancer

Breast cancer originates either from the epithelial cells lining the acini within the terminal ductal lobular unit (TDLU) or from the cells lining the milk ducts (see Fig. 2.13). The majority of breast cancers originate from the TDLUs, not from the ducts. Figure 2.14 shows the relative distribution of the crushed stone-like and powdery microcalcifications on the mammogram, both of which are the mammographic presentations of in situ tumor growth which arise from and are localized within the TDLUs. Despite the fact that these in situ tumors arise within the lobules and not from the ducts, they are paradoxically termed "ductal" carcinoma in situ. When this population of cancer cells invades the surrounding breast tissue, forming a stellate or circular/oval-shaped tumor mass, the invasive tumor is also erroneously called "ductal."

In situ breast cancers are usually detected at mammography. There are more than ten distinctly different mammographic presentations of in situ cancer subtypes (see Figs. 2.15a–c and 2.16a–x), but current terminology bundles them all under the same name: DCIS. This simplification unfortunately leads to misunderstanding and confusion. Additionally, the term DCIS is a misnomer, since the vast majority of in situ carcinomas do not arise from the milk ducts and are not situated within these ducts.

Breast cancers actually arising within the major milk ducts have a histopathologic appearance (see Fig. 2.17a, b) very similar to that of metastatic prostate cancer (Fig. 2.17c–e) and metastases of breast cancer to the axillary lymph node(s) (Fig. 2.18a, b). Although the histopathologic appearance shown in Figs. 2.17c–e and 2.18a, b will be termed by pathologists as invasive cancer, i.e., when found in the prostate or in the axillary lymph node(s), the similar histopathologic appearance is termed "DCIS" when found in the breast. The unpredictable clinical course and

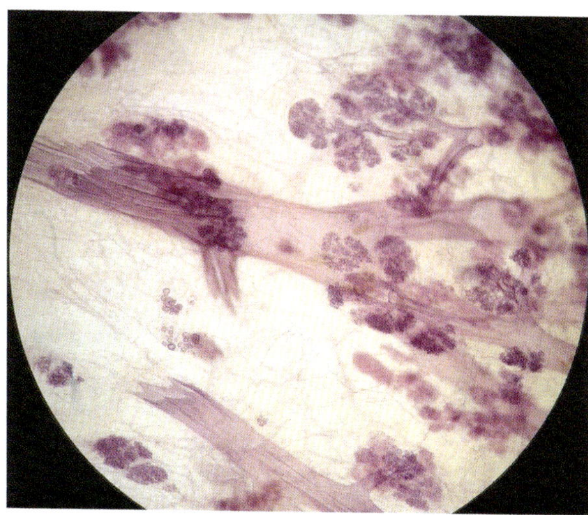

Fig. 2.13 3-Dimensional histology image of major milk ducts and several terminal ductal lobular units (TDLUs). The majority of breast cancers originate from the TDLUs

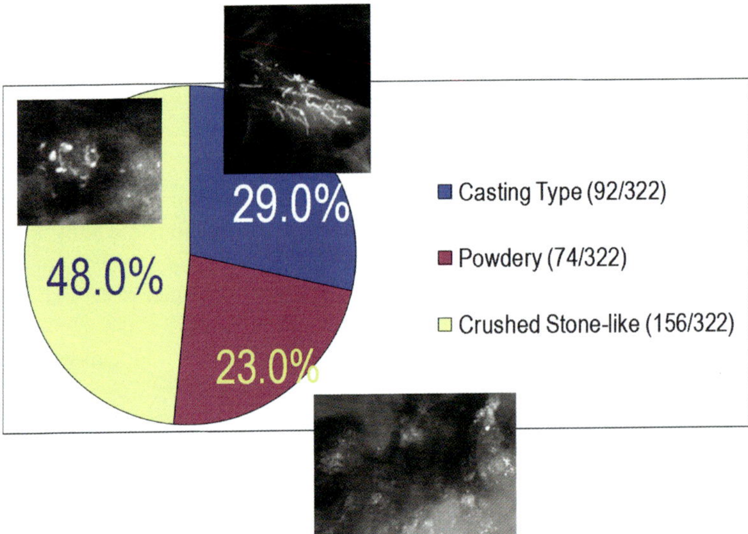

Fig. 2.14 Relative distribution of histologically proven calcified in situ carcinoma cases according to their presentation on the mammogram. The crushed stone-like and powdery microcalcifications constitute the majority of in situ cases. Both of them are the mammographic presentations of in situ tumor growth arising from and localized within the TDLUs

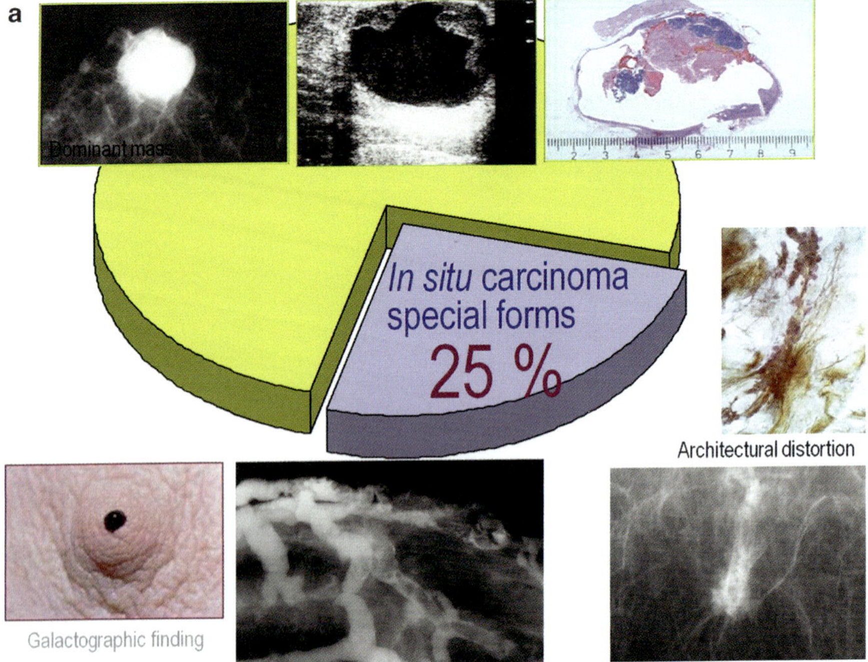

Fig. 2.15 (**a**) About 25 % of the mammographically demonstrable in situ carcinomas lack calcifications on the mammogram. In these cases the mammogram shows either a dominant mass or a architectural distortion; the third option is a galactographic finding. (**b**) In 75 % of the

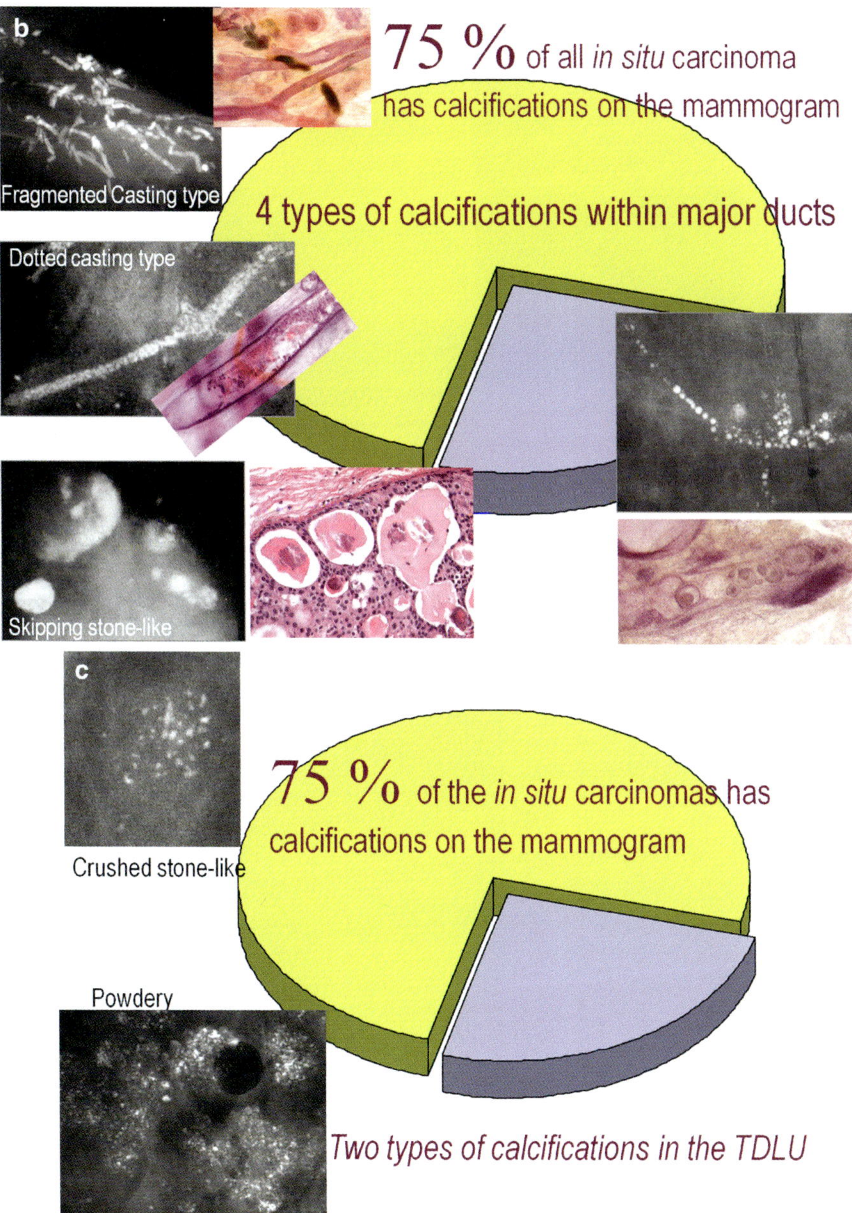

Fig. 2.15 (continued) mammographically demonstrable in situ breast cancer cases calcifications are seen on the mammograms. There are four different mammographic appearances of the calcifications associated with the malignant processes localized within the major ducts. (**c**) In 75 % of the mammographically demonstrable in situ breast cancer cases calcifications are seen on the mammograms. There are two different mammographic appearances of the calcifications associated with the malignant process localized within the terminal ductal lobular units (TDLUs)

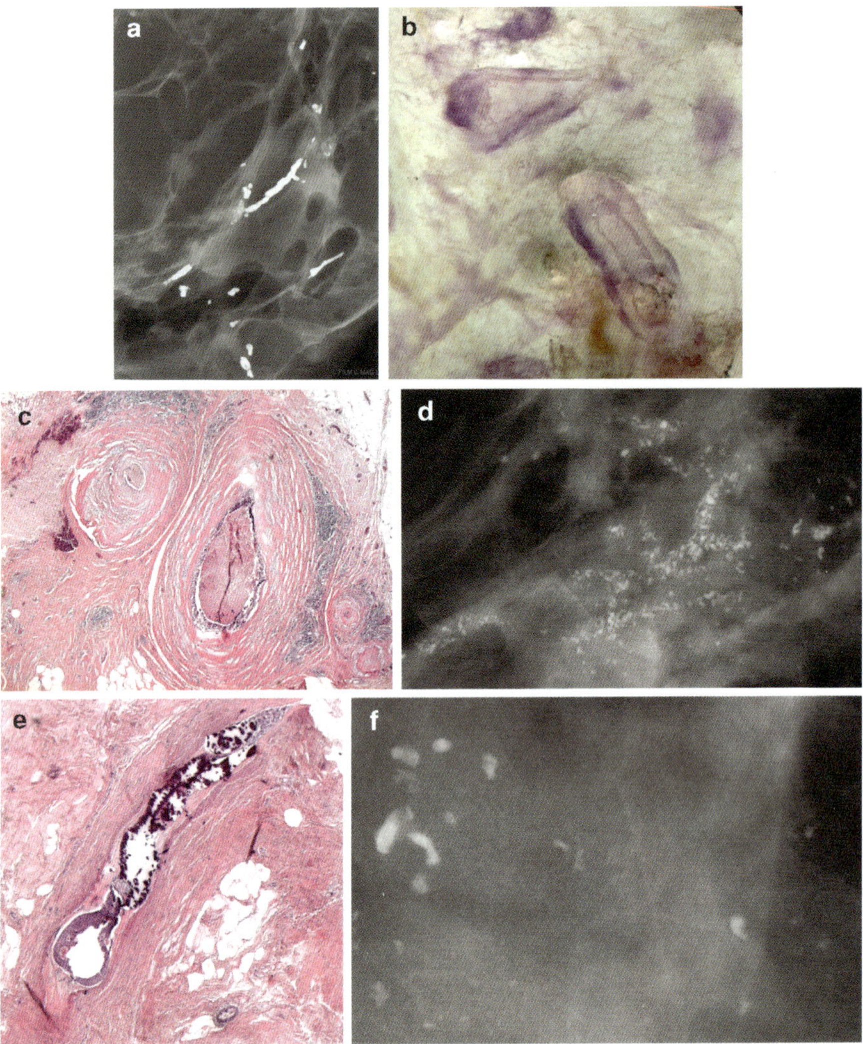

Fig. 2.16 A collage demonstrating the mammographic and histologic heterogeneity of *in situ* carcinoma of the breast. Regrettably, there is still only one term in current use to describe all these different diseases, and that term is "DCIS." (**a**–**c**) Fragmented casting-type calcifications in Grade 3 in situ carcinoma with solid cell proliferation. (**d**, **e**) Dotted casting-type calcifications seen in high-grade carcinoma in situ with micropapillary cell proliferations and necrosis within the major ducts. (**f**, **g**) Skipping stone-like calcifications seen in high-grade carcinoma in situ with micropapillary cell proliferations without necrosis, but with fluid production in the major ducts. (**h**–**j**) A mixture of crushed stone-like and skipping stone-like calcifications spread over two-thirds of the right breast. The Grade 2 and 3 in situ carcinoma contiguously fills the major ducts and branches as well as a large number of TDLUs. (**k**, **l**) Pearl necklace-like calcifications: Grade 1 in situ carcinoma with cribriform cell architecture and large psammoma body-like calcifications in the major ducts. (**m**, **n**) Multiple clusters of crushed stone-like calcifications localized within TDLUs: Grade 2 in situ carcinoma with solid cell proliferation, central necrosis, and amorphous calcifications in

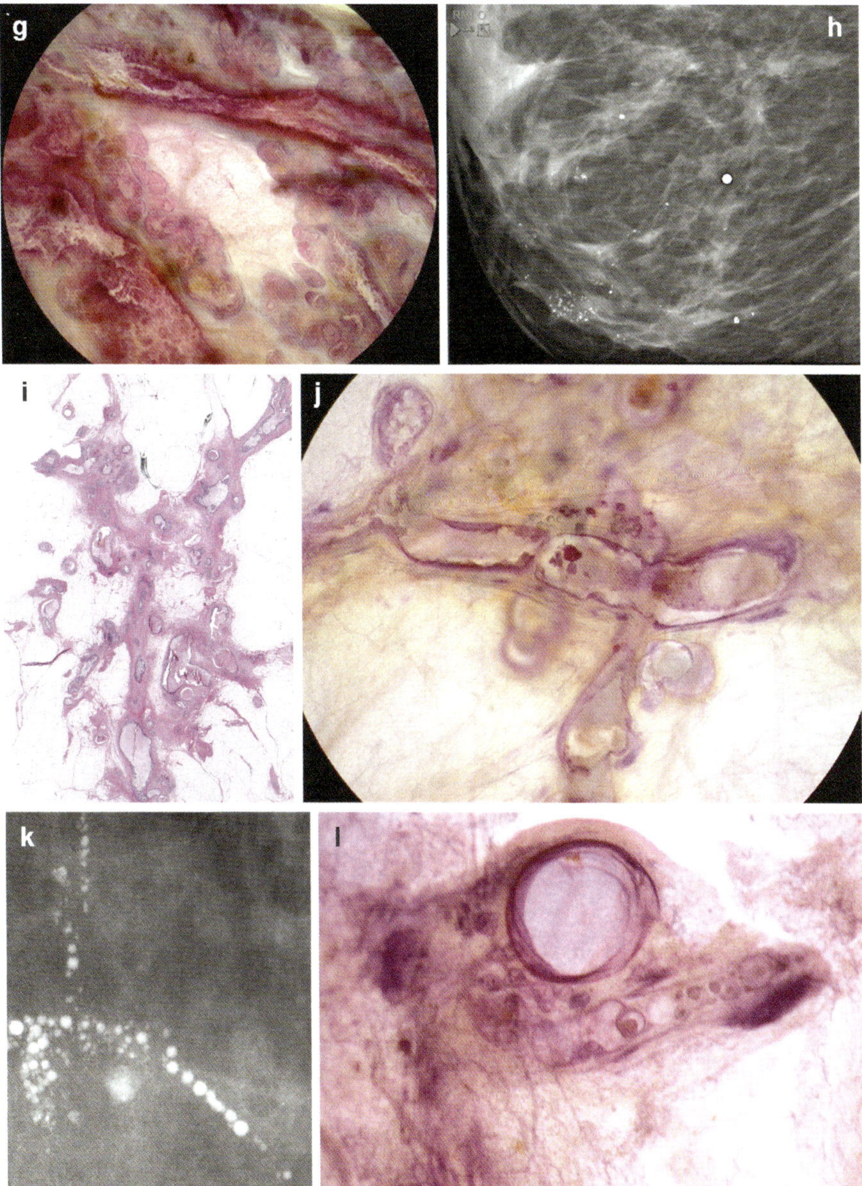

Fig. 2.16 (continued) the extremely distended acini. (**o**, **p**) Multiple clusters of powdery calcifications: Grade 1 in situ carcinoma associated with psammoma body-like calcifications in the TDLUs. (**r**, **s**) Paget's disease. In this case the mammogram is normal, and the high-grade in situ carcinoma was occult for mammography. In most of the Paget's disease cases the mammograms show malignant-type calcifications within the major ducts. (**t–v**) Palpable tumor and architectural distortion with no associated calcifications on the mammogram. The histology shows a large number of cancer-filled, tortuous ducts with high-grade micropapillary cancer in situ, no necrosis, and extreme fluid production. (**w**, **x**, **z**) Architectural distortion associated with calcifications within the cancer-filled, distended, tortuous ducts

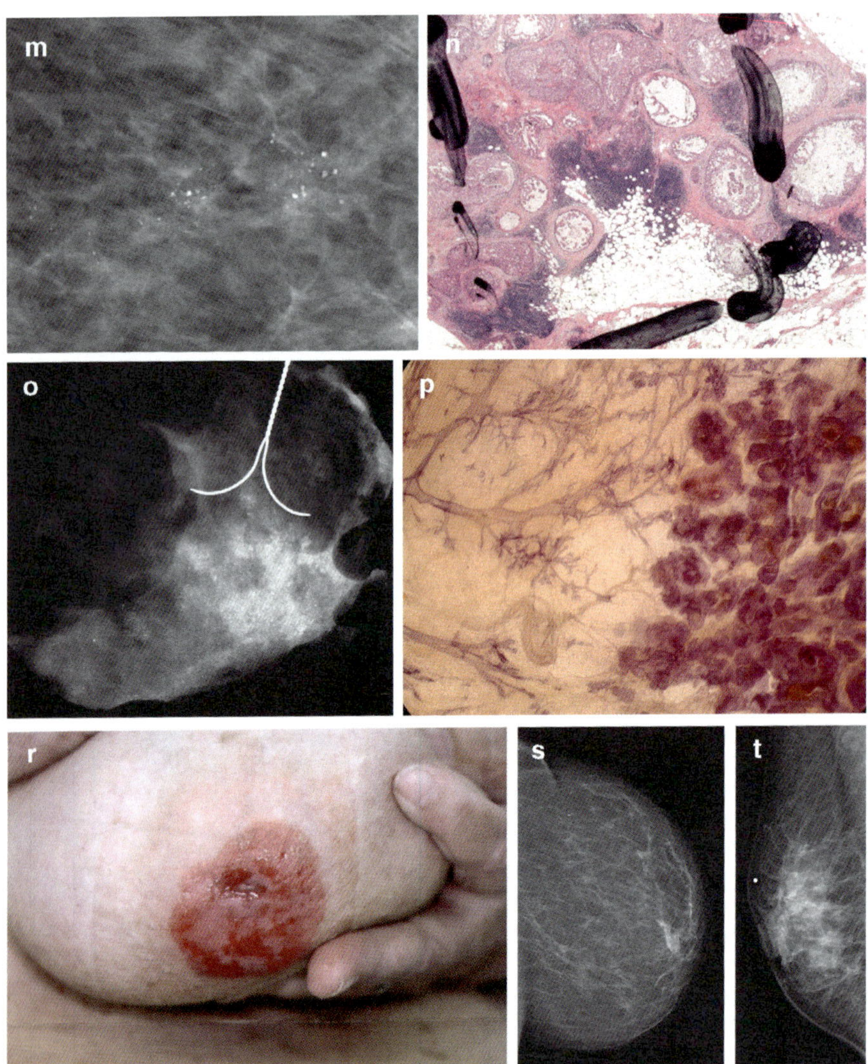

Fig. 2.16 (continued)

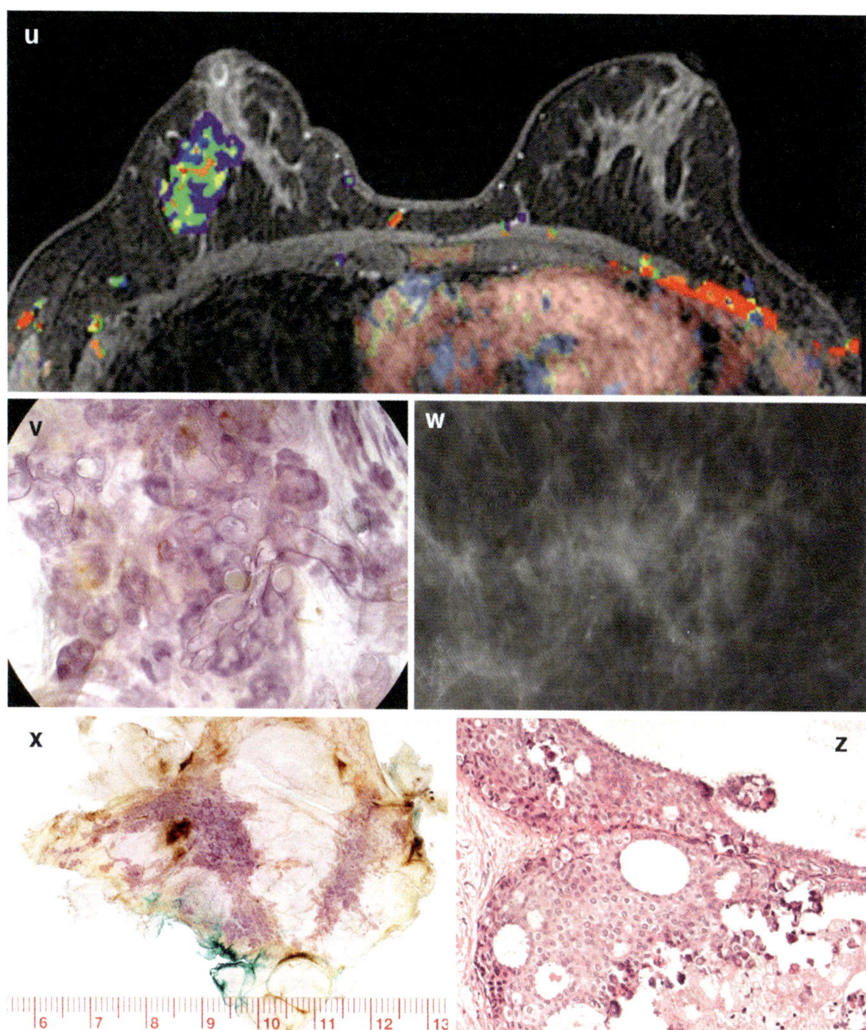

Fig. 2.16 (continued)

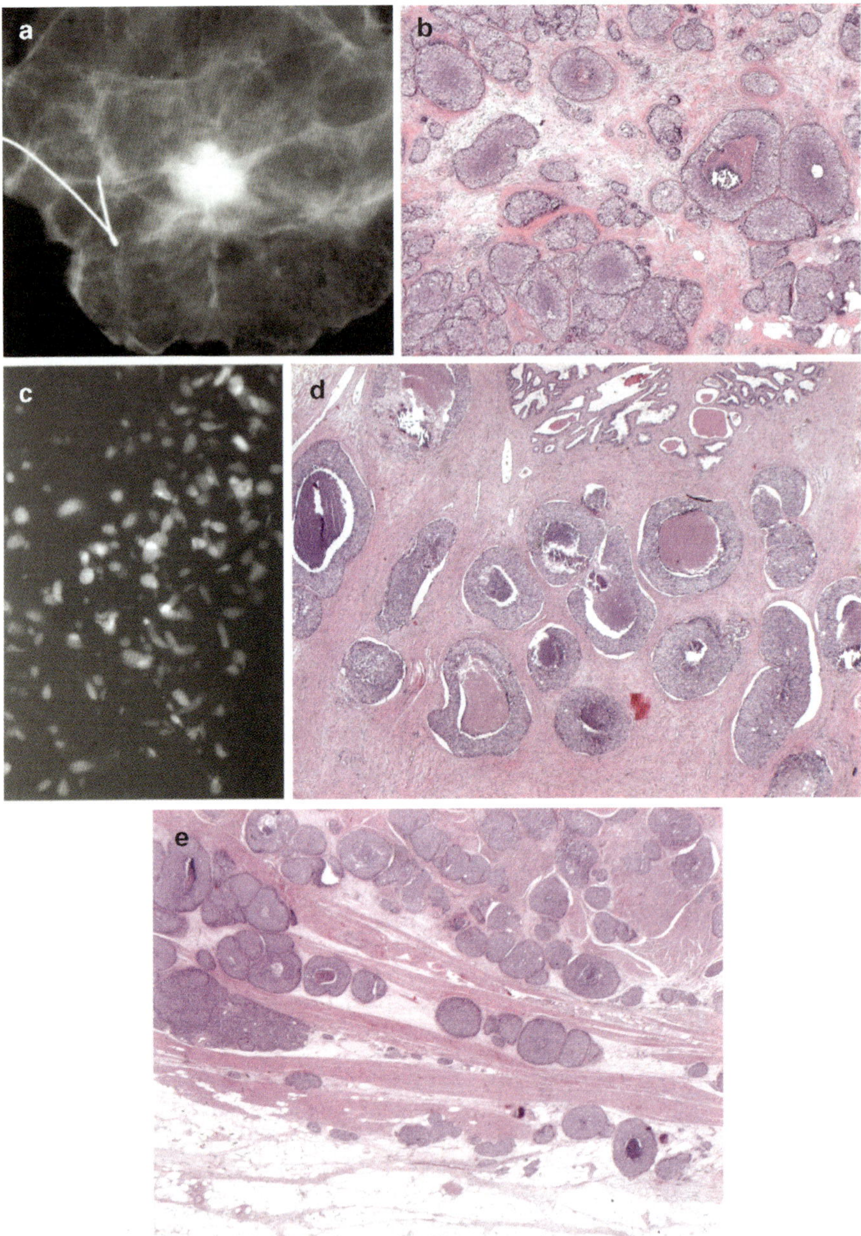

Fig. 2.17 (**a**, **b**) Segmentectomy specimen radiograph containing breast cancer. The histology image (**b**) is very similar to the histology of the prostate cancer shown in (**d**). (**c**) Specimen radiograph of a prostate cancer (ductal adenocarcinoma of the prostate *DAP*). (**d**) Intermediate power histology image of this prostate cancer. (**e**) This DAP infiltrates the surrounding organs in the lesser pelvis; the cancer-filled ducts can be seen among the muscle fibers of the urinary bladder

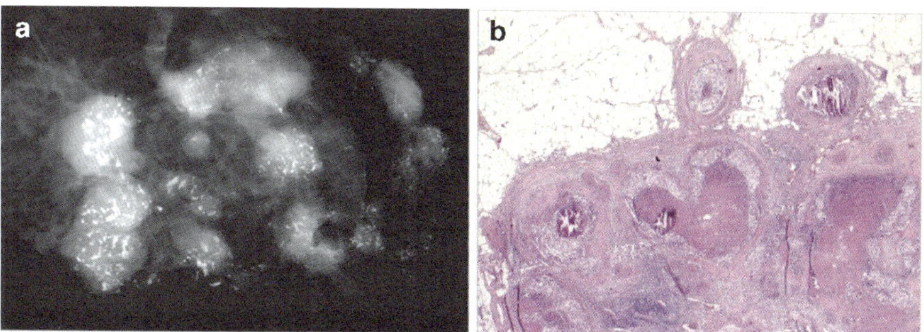

Fig. 2.18 (**a**, **b**) Radiograph of an axillary specimen containing 12 pathologic lymph nodes with malignant-type calcifications. The histology of one of the axillary lymph nodes contains "duct-like structures," mimicking the histologic image of prostate cancer (DAP) shown in Fig. 2.17d and the so-called in situ breast cancer shown in Fig. 2.17b

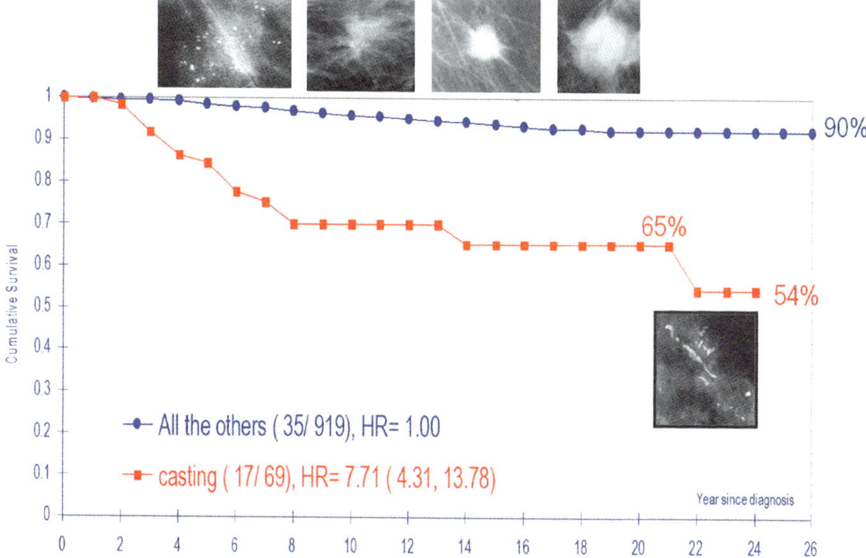

Fig. 2.19 26-year cumulative survival of women aged 40–69 years with 1–14 mm invasive breast cancers by mammographic tumor features. Dalarna County, Sweden. 1–14 mm invasive breast cancers originating from the TDLU (AAB) have excellent (90 %) long-term survival, compared to the subtype of ductal origin (DAB), presented on the mammogram as casting-type calcifications (65 % long-term survival)

also the occasional fatal outcome of these cases indicate that, contrary to its name "ductal carcinoma in situ" of the breast, the special breast cancer subtype originating from the major ducts may behave as an invasive cancer and can prove fatal (see Figs. 2.19, 2.20, and 2.21) [50].

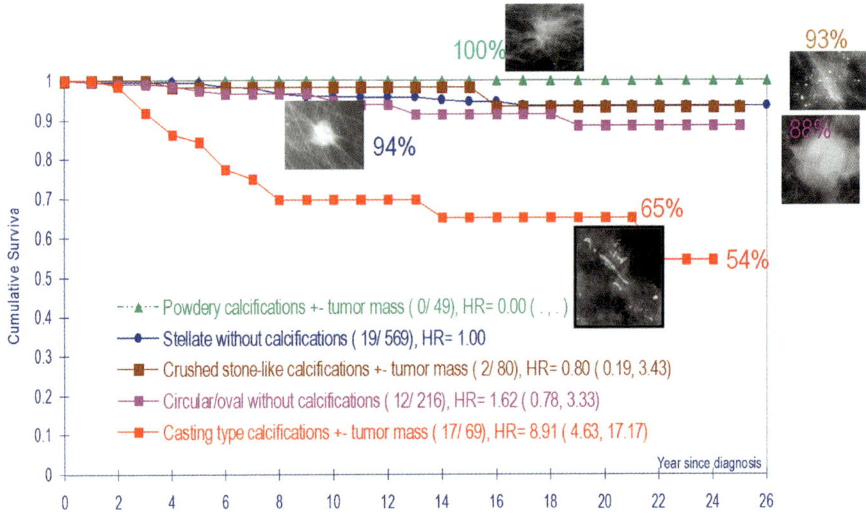

Fig. 2.20 Cumulative survival of women aged 40–69 years with 1–14 mm invasive breast cancers as a function of the five mammographic tumor features

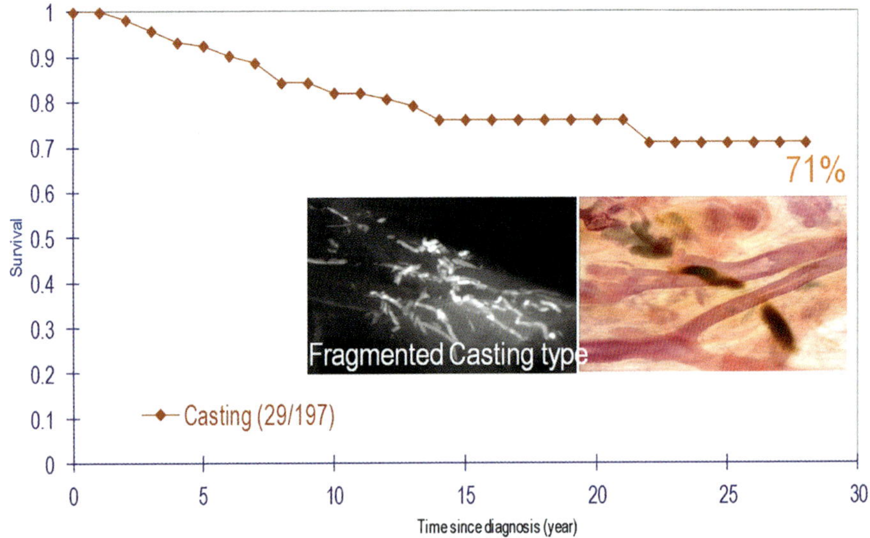

Fig. 2.21 Cumulative survival of breast cancer cases with casting-type calcifications on the mammogram. Women 40–69 years old, diagnosed in Dalarna county, Sweden, between 1977 and 2006

Taking the logical and consistent nomenclature that is used to describe prostate cancer and using it to describe breast cancer as well can resolve these terminological inconsistencies and the resulting confusion. Our proposed terminology emphasizes the site of origin of the cancer: *a*cinar *a*denocarcinoma of the *p*rostate (AAP) would correspond to *a*cinar *a*denocarcinoma of the *b*reast (AAB), in which the cancer originates from the TDLU. Similarly, *d*uctal *a*denocarcinoma of the *p*rostate (DAP) would correspond to *d*uctal *a*denocarcinoma of the *b*reast (DAB), in which the breast cancer originates from the major milk ducts. The striking difference between the long-term outcome of breast cancers of similar size originating from the TDLUs (AAB) and the cancers originating from the major ducts (DAB) justifies the radical change in terminology (Figs.2.19 and 2.20).

The Mammographic Appearance of 1–14 mm Invasive Breast Cancers Has Important Prognostic Significance

The mammogram can be viewed as a low-resolution, grayscale image of the underlying histopathology of the breast. The mammographic presentations of breast cancers originating from the TDLUs (AAB) are as follows: crushed stone-like clustered calcifications (most often Grade 2 in situ carcinoma) [51], clustered powdery microcalcifications (characteristic of Grade 1 in situ carcinoma), and stellate or circular/oval tumor masses representing invasive carcinoma. The in situ and 1–14 mm breast cancers of acinar origin (i.e., from the TDLU) have excellent long-term prognosis. In the minority of cases when the cancer originates from the cells lining the milk ducts (DAB), the mammographic presentation and the patient's long-term prognosis are considerably different [50] (see Figs. 2.19 and 2.21). The myriad of prognostic features (histologic types and first-generation prognostic factors/biomarkers/gene profiling) should be correlated with the "mammographic prognostic features" described above (Figs. 2.22, 2.23, and 2.24).

Patient management planning routinely utilizes specific prognostic factors including tumor size, histologic malignancy grade, lymph node status, and a series of second-generation tumor characteristics (receptor status, HER2/neu status, gene expression profiling, etc.). The predictive value of these prognostic factors is, however, less successful in distinguishing screen-detected 1–14 mm invasive breast cancers, which have an excellent prognosis, from those with a potentially poor long-term outcome, when classified according to the current TNM criteria. This deficiency can be remedied by *adding the mammographic tumor features* to the treatment planning of these small, early-stage tumors, because four out of the five mammographic appearances are characteristic of tumors originating from the TDLU (AAB) and have a good/excellent long-term outcome. Within the AAB subgroup, multifocal cases have a poorer prognosis than the unifocal AAB cancers.

The fifth mammographic feature, the eminently characteristic "casting-type" calcifications on the mammogram (see Fig. 2.16a–d), represents cancer originating from the major ducts (DAB) and indicates a breast cancer subtype having a high fatality rate (71 % long-term survival) (see Fig. 2.21) despite its histologic description as a node-negative 1–14 mm invasive cancer associated with Grade 3 in situ carcinoma [50–55].

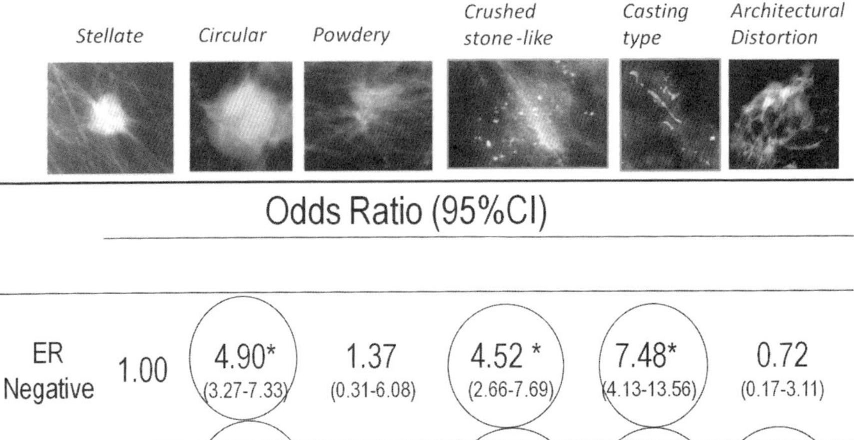

Fig. 2.22 Comparison of the mammographic prognostic features with the tumor biomarkers estrogen and progesterone receptors. There is a significant correlation between receptor negativity and the circular/oval shape of the tumor on the mammogram, and also with the presence of crushed stone-like and casting-type calcifications on the mammogram

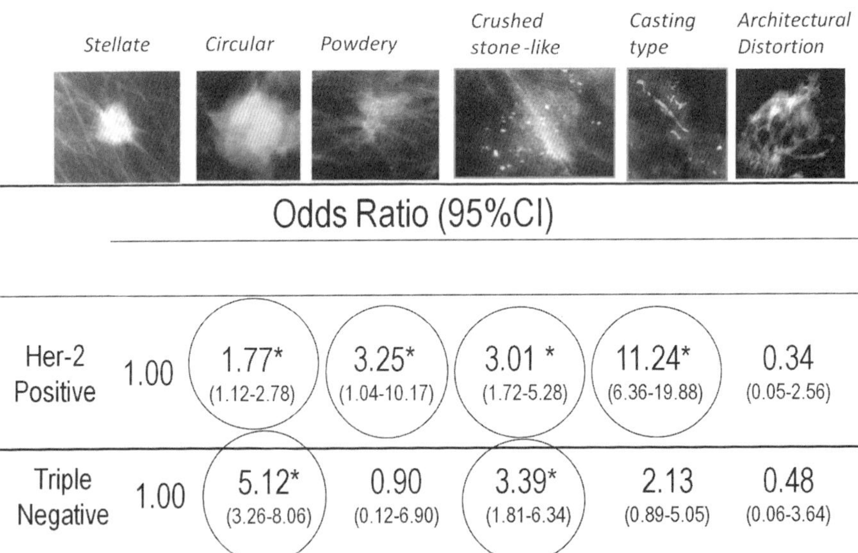

Fig. 2.23 Comparison of the mammographic prognostic features with the tumor biomarkers Her-2 and triple negativity. Her-2-positive and triple-negative tumors correlate significantly with the circular/oval shape of the tumor on the mammogram, and also with the presence of crushed stone-like calcifications on the mammogram

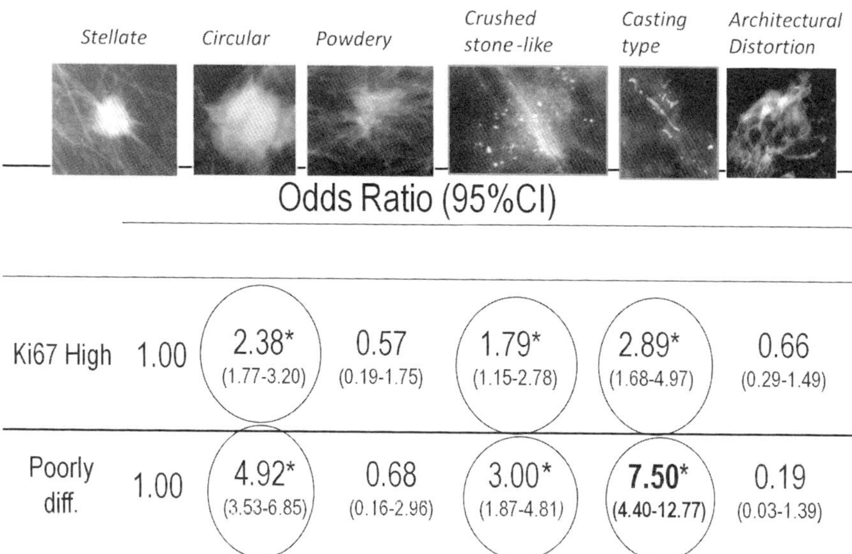

Fig. 2.24 Comparison of the mammographic prognostic features with high Ki67 value (proliferation index) and poorly differentiated malignancy grade. Tumors with high proliferation index and poorly differentiated tumors correlate significantly with the circular/oval shape of the tumor on the mammogram, and with the presence of crushed stone-like and casting-type calcifications on the mammogram

The efficacy and reproducibility of the mammographic tumor features for predicting patient outcome in consecutive, in situ, and 1–14 mm invasive breast cancer cases have been demonstrated in Europe and in the USA. There was poor prognosis for the cases with casting-type calcifications on the mammogram, and excellent prognosis for the remaining mammographic categories, providing further evidence that the current practice of predicting the long-term outcome of breast cancers in their earliest detectable phases can be significantly improved by including the mammographic tumor features in treatment planning [54]. The poor long-term survival of T1a and T1b breast cancers having casting-type calcifications on the mammogram (RR=6.50, 95 % CI: 3.61–11.72) indicates that we are dealing with a much larger tumor burden than would be expected from 1–14 mm tumors. This large tumor burden with its poor prognosis can be explained by the theory of neoductgenesis, according to which the "Grade 3 in situ carcinoma" is a mixture of both in situ and a poorly differentiated duct-forming invasive cancer, which accounts for its high fatality rate [50, 55]. Including the mammographic tumor features to evaluate the small, 1–14 mm invasive breast cancers will enable planning targeted therapy for the 10 % of breast cancers which have the greatest potential fatality, i.e., those associated with casting-type calcifications on the mammogram. In the remaining 90 % of small breast cancers, distinction has to be made between unifocal and multifocal cases. In unifocal cases the necessity for using adjuvant treatment following surgery needs to be seriously reconsidered, since the long-term survival of these patients has been excellent with local therapy alone.

The integration of imaging morphology into the TNM classification in the 1–14 mm tumor size range has great potential for more accurate outcome prediction, facilitation of specifically targeted therapy, and curtailment of needless therapy.

Key Points

Despite the excellent prognosis of most patients with small breast cancers, a small number of women still die from tumors of <15 mm in size a few years after diagnosis.

- The first- and second-generation prognostic tumor features in current use do not discriminate between fatal and nonfatal invasive breast cancers <15 mm.
- The inclusion of mammographic tumor features provides significantly improved outcome prediction for these patients.
- Invasive breast cancers originating from the acini of the TDLU (i.e., cancers with good/excellent outcome) have a characteristically different mammographic appearance from those originating within the major ducts (i.e., cancers with poor outcome).
- The integration of imaging morphology into the TNM classification of the in situ and 1–14 mm invasive tumor size range would facilitate more accurate outcome prediction, specifically targeted treatment and curtailment of unnecessary therapy.

The Mortality Benefit in Relative and Absolute Terms and Related Issues

1. *The relative mortality benefit*. Evaluation of randomized mammography screening trials and service screening has shown a significant 25–30 % relative decrease in breast cancer mortality in women invited to screening and 43–49 % among women who attended screening at regular intervals [10–21, 29, 40, 56, 57]. These results have been available for decades and have not changed with time. The accuracy of these results is based upon *comprehensive individual patient data* detailing both diagnosis and treatment. These data include precise knowledge of each tumor's detection mode (detected at screening, in the interscreening interval, among invited but not attending women or among non-invited women), time of detection (whether the breast cancer case was diagnosed prior to the beginning of screening or during the screening period), and the ability to isolate breast cancer deaths attributable to cancers that were diagnosed before screening was offered to the population. *None of the publications questioning the benefit of early detection on mortality from breast cancer have had access to individualized patient data, making their claims that modern mammography screening plays*

little or no role in reducing breast cancer death simply a biased guess. The harsh critics of screening mammography, Jørgensen, Zahl, and Gøtzsche, "were unable to find an effect of the Danish screening programme on breast cancer mortality," using only registry data and admitted that "we compared open cohorts because our data did not allow identification of individual women" [58]. Their methodological shortcomings caused them to inflate the number of breast cancer deaths in the screening period by including cases diagnosed before screening began. The same severe biases affect other critics who rely upon registry data [59–62].

The lack of precision in Jørgensen, Zahl, and Gøtzsche's analysis is reflected in their use of "hedging" text: [58] i.e., "is unlikely," "It may be reasonable," "suggest," "may have," "would be expected," and "could be." Welch et al. state, "We were forced to make an assumption to capture the downstream benefit of screening" [61] while Haukka et al. admit, "Without individual data it is impossible to completely separate the effects of improved treatment and health service organization from that of screening ... There will also be some contamination of post-screening mortality from breast cancer diagnosed prior to screening" [62]. Indeed, there is more than "some" contamination. We demonstrated in a 10-year period that more than half of all breast cancer deaths are attributable to diagnoses before the beginning of that 10-year period [32]. Yet, despite inadequate data and unjustified assumptions, all these authors still consider their estimates on breast cancer mortality worthy of publication and freely allow themselves to speculate on the impact of treatment versus screening. These comments are made without accurate data and should not have been published in peer-reviewed journals.

Access to individual patient data is crucial for an accurate evaluation of the true impact of screening, because more than 50 % of the breast cancer deaths occurring in a 10-year screening period are from cases diagnosed before the start of that period (see Fig. 2.25a, b) [18, 63]. One cannot expect mammography to have an impact on patients who were treated before mammography was used, yet these patients were included in the biased calculations of Jørgensen, Zahl, and Gøtzsche [58].

2. *The absolute mortality benefit.* Following the evaluation of the randomized controlled trials, case–control studies and large population-based service screening programs have also demonstrated a statistically significant decrease in breast cancer mortality as a result of diagnosis and treatment at an earlier phase of the disease. Attention has subsequently turned to estimating the absolute benefit in terms of deaths prevented. Several estimations have been made of the number of women needed to undergo repeated mammography screening examinations over a 10-year period in order to prevent one breast cancer death. Differences among the results are due to several factors:

   (a) *Calculations based on meta-analysis* of screening results always use the number of women invited, not the number actually screened. This considerably underestimates the benefit [26, 60, 64, 65]. If a woman does not attend mammography screening, she should not be included in a group that ostensibly measures the value of screening, yet this error has been repeated over and over.

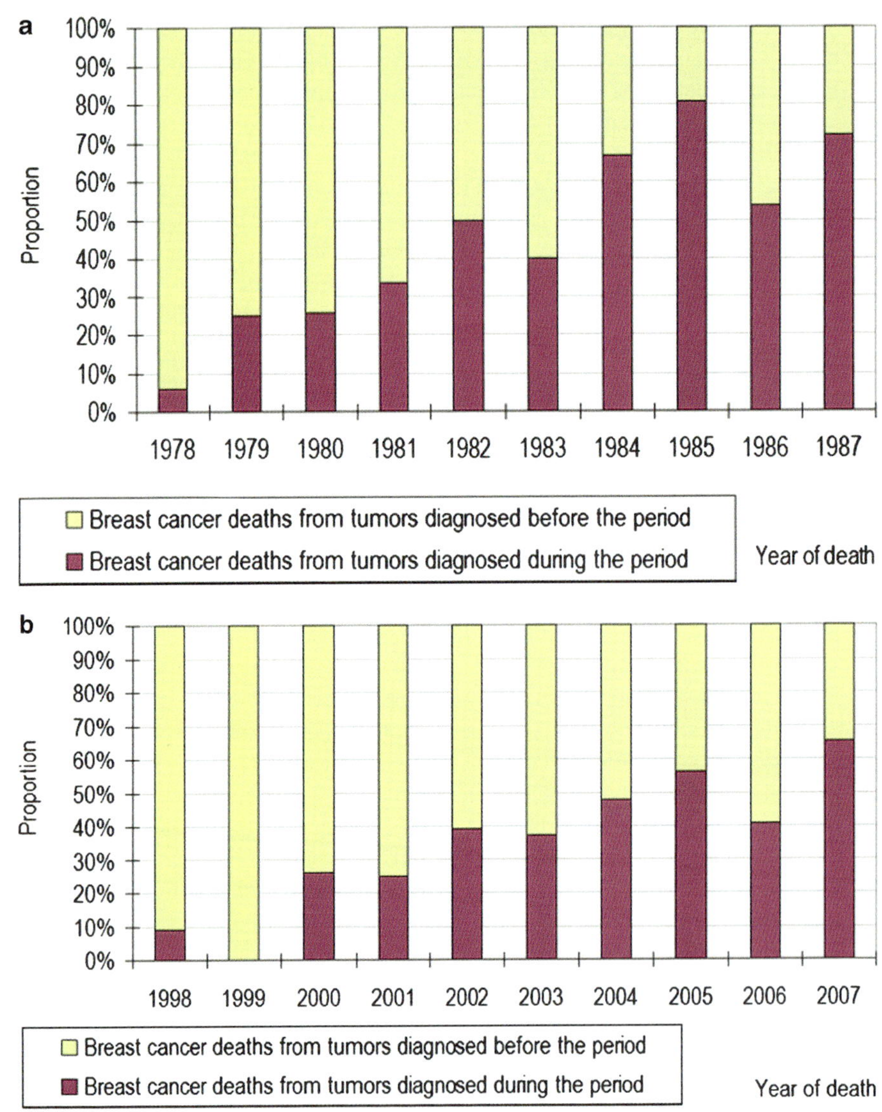

Fig. 2.25 (**a**, **b**) Proportion of breast carcinoma deaths between 1978–1987 and 1998–2007, Dalarna, Sweden, according to the date of diagnosis occurring before (*yellow columns*) or during (*red columns*) these periods. Irrespective of the starting date of mammography screening, a majority of the breast cancer deaths occurring within the decade in question were from breast cancers detected prior to that decade (*yellow columns*)

(b) *Short-term follow-up*. Mammography screening prevents breast cancer death which would otherwise have occurred over the next 2–3 decades if screening had not taken place. Although some benefit may be seen as soon as 4–6 years after screening has started, the majority of the benefit occurs after the first decade of follow-up [21]. Thus, an evaluation with a follow-up limited to only 10 years will seriously underestimate the absolute mortality benefit of screening. Combination of the above two errors magnifies the underestimation of the true benefit, particularly if the relative benefit of screening has already been erroneously underestimated [66]. The resulting miscalculation can produce a tenfold error as pointed out by Wald et al. and Duffy [41, 67, 68].

It is perhaps illuminating to consider one of the most high-profile publications claiming that the absolute benefit of screening is small, the Nordic Cochrane review [26]. The authors claim that 2,000 women need to be screened for 10 years to prevent one breast cancer death. Although screening 2,000 women five times at 2-year intervals is a small price to pay to save one woman's life, this estimate is inaccurate for the following reasons:

- Their estimate is based on invitation to screening rather than on the screening examination itself. Gøtzsche et al. thus biased their calculations by including many women who did not actually receive any screening at all. Their estimate was calculated from an arbitrary assumption of a 15 % reduction in breast cancer mortality which was never observed, not even by the same authors [66]. They simply assume that 15 % is "reasonable" in the absence of supporting data.
- Their estimate is derived from a follow-up time which is far too short to observe the full benefit of screening, as described above.
- The authors then apply their unrealistic 15 % mortality reduction estimate to a population dominated by 40–49-year-old women, mainly from the UK Age Trial. These women will have a much smaller absolute mortality from breast cancer than the 50–70-year age groups usually targeted for screening. These errors and biases, in combination, cause Gøtzsche and Nielsen to seriously underestimate the absolute benefit of mammography screening.

Several recent studies avoided the above errors by calculating the benefit based on women actually undergoing regular screening and having a sufficiently long-term follow-up [17, 21, 69–71]. The benefit of mammography screening can be expressed in terms of one breast cancer death prevented by regular mammography screening examinations of 300 women aged 40–74 years over a period of 10 years, with follow-up for 20 or more years [70, 71]. These results demonstrate how important long-term follow-up is for determining the full absolute mortality benefit from screening. There is a steady increase of the number of lives saved at ever-longer follow-up [21].

3. *The issue of overdiagnosis*. Overdiagnosis of breast cancer can be defined as cases detected at screening which would never have been detected if screening had not taken place. This topic has attracted considerable attention in recent years. The opponents of screening have estimated rates of overdiagnosis of 15–54 % and some have used these estimates as a reason to advocate cessation of mammography screening programs [28, 72–75]. However, studies with adequate statistical evaluation (such as adjusting for lead time and correcting for

changes in background incidence) of individualized patient data have found rates of overdiagnosis less than 10 % [69, 70, 76–85].

None of the publications claiming high rates of overdiagnosis have had access to individualized patient data, seriously limiting the reliability of the results of such analyses. Jørgensen and Gøtzsche [75] did not even base their estimation on registry data, but resorted to estimating trends by "eyeballing" previously published graphs of breast cancer incidence. Such crude methodology introduces a wide margin of error. Furthermore, these authors failed to adjust for lead time, and assumed that the excess number of breast cancers detected in the early years of screening was entirely due to overdiagnosis, and refuse to acknowledge that screening detects cancers in their early phase that would have surfaced clinically in future years. Additionally, the ongoing, gradually increasing breast cancer incidence is one of the essential factors requiring statistical adjustment in overdiagnosis calculations [70]. However, this adjustment was also inadequately performed, as can be seen from the excess incidence observed in unscreened as well as screened age groups [75]. All of these errors in combination can lead to highly unrealistic estimates, as indeed has happened [70, 84, 85]. Welch and Black, when seeking evidence to support their claim that early detection leads to overdiagnosis, stated: "A persistent excess in the screening group years after the trial is completed constitutes the best evidence that overdiagnosis has occurred" [74]. No such evidence for considerable "overdiagnosis" has been found in studies that have avoided the above-mentioned errors [69, 80].

A sufficiently long follow-up time is also necessary to adequately assess the magnitude of potential overdiagnosis. A randomized controlled trial that was followed for 29 years [82] had equal cumulative breast cancer incidence in the invitation and control arms of the study (RR = 1.00, 95 % CI 0.92–1.08). This complete lack of excess breast cancer incidence at 29 years of follow-up in the population invited to mammography applied to every age group, and was unaffected by the inclusion or the exclusion of in situ cases. Although there was an overall excess of in situ carcinomas in the group of women invited to screening, this excess was balanced by the deficit in invasive cancers, because some of the surgically removed in situ cancers would have progressed to the invasive stage. The substantial excess of node-negative cancers <20 mm in the invited population was balanced by a corresponding excess of advanced cancers in the control population. The significant deficit in advanced cancers in the invited group explains the long-term and highly significant decrease in breast cancer mortality in the trial [82].

The issue of overdiagnosis in the age group 40–49 was recently studied from individualized data of the nationwide service screening program in Sweden, and concluded: "We found no significant overdiagnosis for women aged 40–49 in the Swedish service screening programme with mammography" (RR = 1.01, 95 % CI: 0.94–1.08) [83].

4. *All-cause mortality*. There is a broad consensus that mammography screening accomplishes its main objective, a significant reduction in breast cancer-specific mortality [14]. Some opponents of screening have insisted that, rather than breast cancer mortality, all-cause mortality should define the true measure of the success of screening, even though the screening examination is restricted to the

organ in question (in this case the breast) [86–89]. In fact, all-cause mortality is an inappropriate endpoint, since it depends on the unrealistic expectation that "deaths from road-traffic accidents or hip fractures were in some way indicative of the effect of breast-cancer screening" [90]. Since screening for breast cancer is unlikely to affect mortality in women who do not develop the disease, the cause of death investigation should be restricted to those women diagnosed with breast cancer [91].

Rather than all-cause mortality, mortality analysis should therefore be focused upon the following: (1) evaluation of the impact of *invitation to* and *attendance at* screening on breast cancer death, which has been discussed in detail above and (2) investigation of death from other causes in *women with breast cancer*, in order to ascertain (a) whether there was any misclassification of cause of death in breast cancer cases and (b) whether or not treatment of breast cancers detected at screening might increase the risk of death from other causes (e.g., cardiovascular death from radiotherapy, death from chemotoxicity).

We have already established that a considerable body of evidence accumulated over the past three decades demonstrated that invitation to and exposure to screening substantially reduces breast cancer mortality. With respect to misclassification of death, or collateral death associated with therapy, no significant evidence of an increased rate of death from other causes was found in women invited to screening in the Swedish Two-County Trial, and thus there was no evidence of bias in cause of death classification [91]. The first overview of all Swedish randomized mammography trials agreed, concluding: "The cause of death pattern in the invited group was, except for breast cancer, very similar to that in the control group, showing that the groups were comparable" [92].

5. *Investigation of all causes of death in women diagnosed with breast cancer.* There was a significant 19 % reduction in death from all causes *in breast cancer cases* in the invited group (RR 0.81, CI 0.72–0.90, $p<0.001$) [91]. Indeed, a difference in disease-specific mortality and all-cause mortality associated with screening is expected since death from breast cancer is a leading cause of premature death in women among all causes of death.

Key Points

- Invitation to mammography screening substantially reduces mortality from the disease (intention-to-treat approach).
- The number of breast cancer deaths prevented is greater for women who attend screening at regular intervals compared to those who do not attend.
- No significant evidence of an increased rate of death from other causes was found *in women with breast cancer* in the group invited to screening; thus there was no evidence of bias in the cause of death classification.
- There was a significant reduction in death from all causes *in the breast cancer cases* in women invited to screening.

Is There Really a Controversy About Breast Cancer Screening?

Evidence-based medicine requires careful collection of reliable individual patient data and adherence to well-established evaluation methods. The eight population-based randomized mammography screening trials, carried out in several countries with different health care systems, provide an excellent example of careful data collection and competent evaluation. In stark contrast, the criticism emerging from the Nordic Cochrane Center (Director: Peter C. Gøtzsche) lacks access to individual patient data and fails to adhere to well-established evaluation methods. These elementary limitations were immediately apparent to competent investigators, some of whom published rather harsh criticism.

1. Nicholas Day, Professor of Public Health, University of Cambridge, UK, wrote the following: "the Lancet paper by Gøtzsche and Olsen … is not simply controversial, it contains a number of serious statistical mistakes which invalidate its conclusions, and uses a selective approach to the studies and data it assesses. It is a worthless piece of work which if it had been produced by one of our masters students, would have been sent back with demands for a complete rewrite" [93].
2. David Freedman, Professor of Statistics, University of California at Berkeley concluded after an extensive overview of all the trials: "The basis for the Gøtzsche–Olsen critique turns out to be simple. Studies that found a benefit from mammography were discounted as being of poor quality; remaining negative studies were combined by meta-analysis. The critique therefore rests on judgments of study quality, but these judgments are based on misreading of the data and the literature." "There is good evidence from clinical trials that mammographic screening reduces the death rate from breast cancer. The critique by Gøtzsche and Olsen has little merit and has generated much confusion" [94].
3. Nicholas Wald, Professor of Epidemiology and Institute Director, Wolfson Institute of Preventive Medicine, Barts and The London School of Medicine and Dentistry, wrote the following about the first paper on breast cancer screening emerging from the Nordic Cochrane Centre: "Gøtzsche and Olsen's paper lacks scientific merit." "The Lancet should not have published this paper" [95].
4. The trialists of the Two-County Swedish study, having been subjected to a considerable amount of unjustified criticism, were obliged to respond frequently in peer-reviewed journals. The Swedish Cancer Society initiated comprehensive overviews of this influential trial [13, 96], confirming the accuracy and transparency of the published data and disproving the unjustified accusations of the opponents of screening. The following citation summarizes the viewpoint of the trialists concerning the accusations of Olsen and Gøtzsche (OG) and colleagues: "Because of serious flaws such as those noted above, we conclude that OG's review provides no grounds for the medical community to alter the conclusion that has been based on millions of person-years of experimental evidence, i.e., that breast cancer screening leads to a substantial reduction in mortality from the

disease. Health care professionals should have confidence that more meticulous and credible reviews have been carried out by numerous independent expert panels in Europe and the United States and consistently reached the same conclusion: early breast cancer detection and treatment results in decreased breast cancer mortality. Clinicians should have confidence in the current recommendations issued by leading organizations, and they should impart that confidence to their patients. We should remain vigilant to avoid any setbacks to the progress we've made in encouraging women to get regular mammograms. Women who have developed confidence in breast cancer screening should not be intimidated, and overworked staff who go to great lengths to make screening work should not have their morale damaged by poor quality reviews such as that of OG. It would be wrong to use this error-prone analysis to discourage an early detection procedure that has been shown in trial after trial to reduce breast cancer mortality" [97].

5. Daniel Kopans, Professor of Radiology, Harvard Medical School, summarized his view with the following title: "*The most recent breast cancer screening controversy about whether mammographic screening benefits women at any age: nonsense and nonscience*" [98].
6. A group of 41 screening experts, exasperated by the steady flow of nonscientific criticism, published a letter in The Lancet [99]. "Although the wider scientific community has long embraced the benefits of population-based breast screening, there seems to be an active anti-screening campaign orchestrated in part by members of the Nordic Cochrane Centre. These contrary views are based on erroneous interpretation of data from cancer registries and peer reviewed articles. Their specific aim seems to be to support a pre-existing opposition to all forms of screening" [100]. "We consider the interpretation by Jørgensen, Keen, and Gøtzsche [101] of the balance of benefits and harms to be scientifically unsound. Women would be better served by focusing efforts on how best, and not whether, to provide breast screening" [99]. Gøtzsche and Jørgensen responded with the following suggestion: "stopping the mammography screening programme would reduce the breast cancer incidence in the screened age group" [102]. In response three of the Lancet letter's authors stated: "We regard the proposal to reduce the apparent incidence of breast cancer by failure of detection as unethical" [103].
7. Peter Gøtzsche has recently published a book summarizing his personal view of breast cancer screening, entitled "*Mammography Screening. Truth, Lies and Controversy*," in which he declares: "The most effective way to decrease women's risk of becoming a breast cancer patient is to avoid attending screening" [104]. Jack Cuzick, Professor of Epidemiology at the Wolfson Institute of Preventive Medicine, Barts and The London School of Medicine and Dentistry, in a review of this book made the following comment: "Gøtzsche's desire to abandon screening altogether ... has detracted from efforts to improve breast cancer screening, so that it can make its maximal contribution to controlling this devastating disease" [105].

In summary, the term "controversy" hardly seems to apply to mammography screening. The scientific establishment and health care professionals who care for breast cancer patients support the detection and treatment of breast cancer in its early phases. What ought to be regarded as controversial is the regular opportunity provided by scientific journals and mass media for a group of pseudo-skeptics to repeat over and over again the same flawed science and logic to question the value of screening.

The Alleged Harm of Attending Versus the Actual Harm of Not Attending Mammography Screening

The balance between the benefits and risks of mammography screening has been under continuous evaluation for the past four decades, ever since the publication of the first successful randomized controlled trial in 1971 [11]. During these decades the evidence has been steadily accumulating for the multiple benefits of attending mammography screening. These benefits include considerably and significantly decreased breast cancer mortality, less need for radical treatment (mastectomy, axillary dissection, systemic treatment), and assuring most women that, at a given point in time, they have no detectable breast cancer [106]. Additionally, the vast majority of those whose impalpable breast cancer is detected will have a normal life expectancy without the disease having a major impact on their life quality. Despite this accumulating evidence there has been much recent discussion about the alleged harms of mammography screening [73, 107–117]. These include radiation exposure, discomfort from breast compression, anxiety from screening or from assessment procedures and their outcome, overdiagnosis, and the detrimental effects of treatment. The magnitude of these potential harms has been exaggerated in many reports, where the benefits of screening are either discounted or seriously underestimated [72–75, 86, 104, 114, 116].

Feig and Duffy have carefully reviewed these arguments and have concluded: "Adverse consequences of screening such as callbacks for additional imaging, false positive biopsies, potential over-diagnosis, and any hypothetical radiation risk do not outweigh the benefits from early detection" [106]. Although anxiety from screening, callback for further assessment of the finding at screening, and waiting for the results are important issues, they do not appear to have a negative effect upon subsequent attendance of women who are not diagnosed with breast cancer [107]. The subject of "overdiagnosis," which is currently touted as the most important "harm" of screening, has been discussed in detail in the previous section. The influence of the introduction of mammography screening upon breast surgery has been extensively studied, particularly upon mastectomy rates. There is a claim that screening is associated with an increase in mastectomy rates [117]. Objective studies have repeatedly demonstrated a decline in mastectomy rates corresponding to the decline in advanced cancer rate as a direct consequence of screening [118, 119]. "Women with screen-detected breast cancer in the UK have half the mastectomy rate of women with symptomatic cancers i.e., 27 versus 53 %" [99].

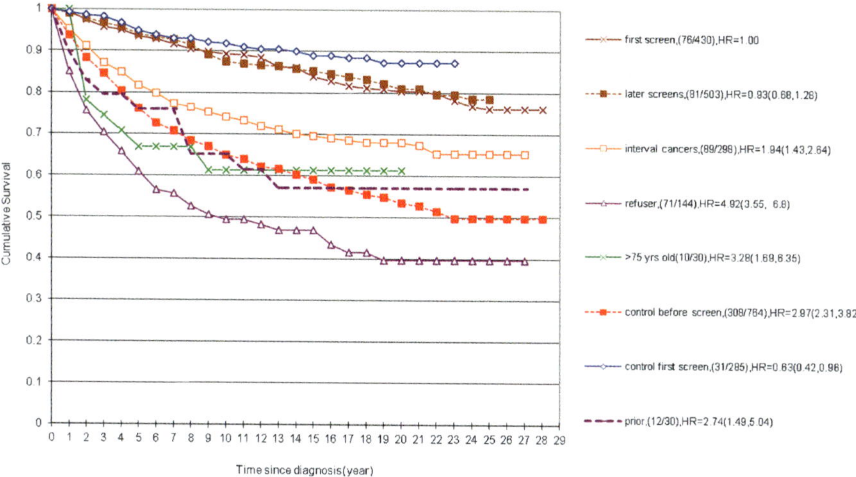

Fig. 2.26 28-year disease-specific survival of women according to the mode of detection in the Swedish Two-County Trial

The harm of *not* attending mammography screening has seldom been discussed in the medical literature. A recent review of prospectively collected data provides insight into the consequences of delaying the diagnosis of breast cancer until it becomes symptomatic. This study on 1977 women aged 40–49 diagnosed with breast cancer compared the tumor characteristics, treatment regimens used, and long-term outcome of women with symptomatic versus women with mammographically detected breast cancer [2]. Women whose cancers were self-detected or physician-detected had significantly more mastectomies (47 vs. 25 %), larger average tumor size (3.02 vs. 1.63 cm), significantly worse disease-specific survival (log-rank test = 22.04 $p<.001$), and overall survival (log-rank test = 20.67 $p<.001$) than did women whose asymptomatic cancers were detected mammographically. In the randomized controlled trials, the women in the control groups did not have access to mammography screening, presented with palpable tumors, and had significantly higher breast cancer mortality. Delay in diagnosis will occur in some women attending mammography whose cancer is not detected at the time of screening, resulting in interval cancers. Women who chose not to attend mammography screening had even worse outcomes (see Fig. 2.26) [19].

In the light of these serious harms associated with detection of breast cancer at a later stage it is astonishing and disconcerting that opponents of mammography now are calling for mammography screening to be abolished [72, 104, 120] and recommend that women not perform breast self-examination. The Director of the Nordic Cochrane Center, Peter Gøtzsche, M.D., stated the following in a BBC Radio 4 interview: "What women should do is, as they have always done, if they find something unusual, go and see a doctor, but don't examine yourself regularly. It has no effect ... there is general agreement now that women should not be advised to examine themselves every month. Our advice is that you should not examine your breasts regularly" [121].

Key Points

Of all the harms associated with breast cancer screening, *the greatest harm comes from nonattendance*. Earlier detection of breast cancer through mammography screening results in:

- Significant decrease in advanced breast cancers.
- Significantly better disease-specific survival, relapse-free survival, and overall survival.
- Fewer breast cancer deaths.
- Fewer mastectomies and more lumpectomies (higher frequency of breast-conserving surgery).
- Fewer patients needing advanced forms or more severe forms of adjuvant therapy.

Our efforts should be directed at further improving the efficacy of screening.

References

1. Druitt R, Sargent F. The Principles and Practice of Modern Surgery. A New American from the last and improved London edition. Philadelphia: Blanchard and Lea. 1852, p 513. http://voyagercatalog.kumc.edu/Record/81542/Cite
2. Malmgren JA, Parikh J, Atwood MK, Kaplan HG. Impact of mammography detection on the course of breast cancer in women aged 40–49 years. Radiology. 2012;262:797–806.
3. Tabár L, Duffy SW, Vitak B, Chen Hsiu-Hsi T, Prevost TC. The natural history of breast carcinoma. What have we learned from screening? Cancer. 1999;86(3):449–62.
4. Duffy SW, Tabár L, Fagerberg G, Gad A, Grontoft O, South MC, et al. Breast screening, prognostic factors and survival results from the Swedish two-county study. Br J Cancer. 1991;64:1133–8.
5. Tabár L, Tucker L, Davenport RR, Mullet JG, Chen Hsiu-Hsi T , Ming-Fang Yen A, Yueh-Hsia Chiu S, Gladwell J, Olinger K, Dean PB. The use of mammographic tumour feature significantly improves outcome prediction of breast cancers smaller than 15 mm: a reproducibility study from two comprehensive breast centres. memo. 2011;4: 1–10. Vienna: Springer; 2011. doi:10.1007/s12254-011-0287-y.
6. Tabár L, Vitak B, Chen HH, Duffy SW, Yen MF, Chiang CF, Krusemo UB, Tot T, Smith RA. The Swedish two-county trial twenty years later. Updated mortality results and new insights from long-term follow-up. Radiol Clin North Am. 2000;38(4):625–51.
7. Fisher B. Laboratory and clinical research in breast cancer: a personal adventure: the David A. Karnofsky memorial lecture. Cancer Res. 1980;40(11):3863–74.
8. Fisher ER. Pathobiologic considerations in the treatment of breast cancer. In: Grundfest-Broniatowski S, Esselstyn CB, editors. Controversies in breast disease. New York: Marcel Dekker; 1988. p. 151–80.
9. Fisher B. From Halsted to prevention and beyond: advances in the management of breast cancer during the twentieth century. Eur J Cancer. 1999;35(14):1963–73.
10. Smith RA, Duffy SW, Gabe R, Tabár L, Yen AM, Chen TH. The randomized trials of breast cancer screening: what have we learned? Radiol Clin North Am. 2004;42(5):793–806.
11. Shapiro S, Strax P, Venet L. Periodic breast cancer screening in reducing mortality from breast cancer. JAMA. 1971;215:1777–85.

12. Tabár L, Fagerberg CJ, Gad A, Baldetorp L, Holmberg LH, Gröntoft O, Ljungquist U, Lundström B, Månson JC, Eklund G, et al. Reduction in mortality from breast cancer after mass screening with mammography. Randomised trial from the Breast Cancer Screening Working Group of the Swedish National Board of Health and Welfare. Lancet. 1985;1(8433):829–32.
13. Nyström L, Rutquist LE, Wall S, et al. Breast cancer screening with mammography: overview of the Swedish randomised trials. Lancet. 1993;341:973–8.
14. International Agency for Research on Cancer. Breast cancer screening, IARC handbooks of cancer prevention, vol. 7. Lyon: IARC; 2002.
15. Otto SJ, Fracheboud J, Verbeek AL, Boer R, Reijerink-Verheij JC, Otten JD, Broeders MJ, De Koning HJ, National Evaluation Team for Breast Cancer Screening. Mammography screening and risk of breast cancer death: a population-based case-control study. Cancer Epidemiol Biomarkers Prev. 2012;21(1):66–73.
16. Bjurstam N, Björneld L, Duffy SW, Smith TC, Cahlin E, Eriksson O, Hafström LO, Lingaas H, Mattsson J, Persson S, Rudenstam CM. Säve-Söderbergh. The Gothenburg breast screening trial: first results on mortality, incidence, and mode of detection for women ages 39-49 years at randomization. Cancer. 1997;80(11):2091–9.
17. Hellquist BN, Duffy SW, Abdsaleh S, Björneld L, Bordás P, Tabár L, Viták B, Zackrisson S, Nyström L, Jonsson H. Effectiveness of population-based service screening with mammography for women ages 40 to 49 years: evaluation of the Swedish Mammography Screening in Young Women (SCRY) cohort. Cancer. 2011;117(4):714–22. doi:10.1002/cncr.25650. Epub 2010 Sep 29.
18. Duffy SW, Tabár L, Chen HH, et al. The impact of organized mammography service screening on breast carcinoma mortality in seven Swedish counties. Cancer. 2002;95(3):458–69.
19. Group SOSSE. Reduction in breast cancer mortality from organized service screening with mammography.I. Further confirmation with extended data. Cancer Epidemiol Biomarkers Prev. 2006;15(1):45–51.
20. Feig SA. Effect of service screening mammography on population mortality from breast carcinoma. Cancer. 2002;95(3):451–7.
21. Tabár L, Vitak B, Chen TH, Yen AM, Cohen A, Tot T, Chiu SY, Chen SL, Fann JC, Rosell J, Fohlin H, Smith RA, Duffy SW. Swedish two-county trial: impact of mammographic screening on breast cancer mortality during 3 decades. Radiology. 2011;260(3):658–63.
22. Tabár L, Fagerberg G, Day NE, Duffy SW, Kitchin RM. Breast cancer treatment and natural history: new insights from results of screening. Lancet. 1992;339(8790):412–4.
23. Fisher B, Anderson SJ. The breast cancer alternative hypothesis: is there evidence to justify replacing It? J Clin Oncol. 2010;28(3):366–74.
24. Fisher B, Jeong JH, Anderson S, Bryant J, Fisher ER, Wolmark N. Twenty-five-year follow-up of a randomized trial comparing radical mastectomy, total mastectomy, and total mastectomy followed by irradiation. N Engl J Med. 2002;347(8):567–75.
25. Fisher B, Anderson S, Bryant J, Margolese RG, Deutsch M, Fisher ER, Jeong JH, Wolmark N. Twenty-year follow-up of a randomized trial comparing total mastectomy, lumpectomy, and lumpectomy plus irradiation for the treatment of invasive breast cancer. N Engl J Med. 2002;347(16):1233–41.
26. Gøtzsche PC, Nielsen M. Screening for breast cancer with mammography. Cochrane Database Syst Rev. 2009;(4):CD001877
27. Esserman LJ, Shieh Y, Rutgers EJ, Knauer M, Retèl VP, Mook S, Glas AM, Moore DH, Linn S, van Leeuwen FE, van t Veer LJ. Impact of mammographic screening on the detection of good and poor prognosis breast cancers. Breast Cancer Res Treat. 2011;130(3):725–34.
28. Esserman L, Shieh Y, Thompson I. Rethinking screening for breast cancer and prostate cancer. JAMA. 2009;302(15):1685–92.
29. Swedish Cancer Society and the Swedish National Board of Health and Welfare. Breast-cancer screening with mammography in women aged 40–49 years. Int J Cancer. 1996;68(6):693–9.

30. Fracheboud J, Otto SJ, van Dijck JA, Broeders MJ, Verbeek AL, de Koning HJ, National Evaluation Team for Breast cancer screening (NETB). Decreased rates of advanced breast cancer due to mammography screening in The Netherlands. Br J Cancer. 2004;91(5):861–7.
31. Day NE, Williams DR, Khaw KT. Breast cancer screening programmes: the development of a monitoring and evaluation system. Br J Cancer. 1989;59(6):954–8.
32. Tabár L, Vitak B, Chen HH, Yen MF, Duffy SW, Smith RA. Beyond randomized controlled trials: organized mammographic screening substantially reduces breast carcinoma mortality. Cancer. 2001;91(9):1724–31.
33. Connor AJM, Pinder SE, Elston CW, Bell JA, Wencyk P, Robertson JFR, et al. Intratumoural heterogeneity of proliferation in invasive breast carcinoma evaluated with MIB1 antibody. Breast. 1997;6:171–6.
34. Teixera MR, Pandis N, Bardi G, Andersen JA, Mitelman F, Heim S. Clonal heterogeneity in breast cancer: karyotypic comparisons of multiple intra and extra-tumorous samples from 3 patients. Int J Cancer. 1995;63:63–8.
35. Gerlinger M, Rowan AJ, Horswell S, Larkin J, Endesfelder D, Gronroos E, Martinez P, Matthews N, Stewart A, Tarpey P, Varela I, Phillimore B, Begum S, McDonald NQ, Butler A, Jones D, Raine K, Latimer C, Santos CR, Nohadani M, Eklund AC, Spencer-Dene B, Clark G, Pickering L, Stamp G, Gore M, Szallasi Z, Downward J, Futreal PA, Swanton C. Intratumor heterogeneity and branched evolution revealed by multiregion sequencing. N Engl J Med. 2012;366(10):883–92.
36. Tubiana M, Koscielny S. Natural history of human breast cancer: recent data and clinical implications. Breast Cancer Res Treat. 1991;18(3):125–40.
37. Duffy SW, Tabár L, Fagerberg G, Gad A, Gröntoft O, South MC, Day NE. Breast screening, prognostic factors and survival–results from the Swedish two county study. Br J Cancer. 1991;64(6):1133–8.
38. Tabár L, Tot T, Dean PB. Early detection of breast cancer: large-section and subgross thick-section histologic correlation with mammographic appearances. RadioGraphics. 2007;27:S5–S35.
39. Hendrick RE, Helvie MA. United States Preventive Services Task Force screening mammography recommendations: science ignored. AJR Am J Roentgenol. 2011;196(2):W112–6.
40. Swedish Organised Service Screening Evaluation Group. Effect of mammographic service screening on stage at presentation of breast cancers in Sweden. Cancer. 2007;109(11):2205–12.
41. Holland R, Veling SHJ, Mravunac M, Hendriks JHCL. Histologic multifocality of Tis, T1-2 breast carcinomas. Implications for clinical trials of breast conserving surgery. Cancer. 1985;56:979–90.
42. Tot T. Clinical relevance of the distribution of the lesions in 500 consecutive breast cancer cases documented in large-format histologic sections. Cancer. 2007;110(11):2551–60.
43. Tabár L, Dean PB, Tot T, Lindhe N, Ingvarsson M, Yen AM-F. The implications of the imaging manifestations of multifocal and diffuse breast cancers. In: Tot T, editor. Breast cancer: a lobar disease. London: Springer; 2011. p. 87–152.
44. Weissenbacher TM, Zschage M, Janni W, Jeschke U, Dimpfl T, Mayr D, Rack B, Schindlbeck C, Friese K, Dian D. Multicentric and multifocal versus unifocal breast cancer: is the tumor-node-metastasis classification justified? Breast Cancer Res Treat. 2010;122(1):27–34.
45. Kouzminova NB, Aggarwal S, Aggarwal A, Allo MD, Lin AY. Impact of initial surgical margins and residual cancer upon re-excision on outcome of patients with localized breast cancer. Am J Surg. 2009;198(6):771–80.
46. Turnbull L, Brown S, Harvey I, Olivier C, Drew P, Napp V, Hanby A, Brown J. Comparative effectiveness of MRI in breast cancer (COMICE) trial: a randomised controlled trial. Lancet. 2010;375(9714):563–71.
47. Houssami N, Ciatto S, Macaskill P, et al. Accuracy and surgical impact of magnetic resonance imaging in breast cancer staging: systematic review and meta-analysis in detection of multifocal and multicentric cancer. J Clin Oncol. 2008;26:3248–58.

48. Lundquist D, Hellberg D, Tot T. Disease extent ≥4 cm is a prognostic marker of local recurrence in T1-2 breast cancer. Patholog Res Int. 2011; 2011:860584.
49. Tucker FL. New era pathologic techniques in the diagnosis and reporting of breast cancers. Semin Breast Dis. 2008;11:140–7.
50. Tabár L, Tot T, Dean PB. Breast cancer. Early detection with mammography. Casting type calcifications: sign of a subtype with deceptive features. Thieme: Stuttgart; 2007.
51. Tabár L, Tot T, Dean PB. Breast cancer. Early detection with mammography. Crushed stone-like calcifications: the most frequent malignant type. Thieme: Stuttgart; 2008.
52. Tabár L, Tot T, Dean PB. Breast cancer: the art and science of early detection with mammography. New York: Stuttgart; 2005.
53. Tabár L, Dean PB, Chen HHT, Duffy SW, Yen AM-F, Chiu SY-H. Early detection of breast cancer challenges current standards of care. In: Silberman H, Silberman AW, editors. Principles and practice of surgical oncology. Philadelphia: Wolters Kluwer; 2010.
54. Tabár L, Tucker L, Davenport RR, Mullet JG, Chen H-HT, Yen AM-F, Chiu SY-H, Gladwell J, Olinger K, Dean PB. The use of mammographic tumour feature significantly improves outcome prediction of breast cancers smaller than 15mm: a reproducibility study from two comprehensive breast centers. memo. 2011;4:1–10.
55. Tabár L, Chen HH, Yen MF, et al. Mammographic tumor features can predict long-term outcomes reliably in women with 1-14-mm invasive breast carcinoma. Cancer. 2004;101: 1745–59.
56. Wald NJ, Law MR, Duffy SW. Breast screening saves lives. BMJ. 2009;339:b2922.
57. Smith RA, Duffy S, Tabár L. Screening and early detection. In: Barbiera GV, Esteva FJ, Skoracki R, editors. Advanced therapy of breast disease. 3rd ed. Shelton, Conn: People's Medical Publishing House; 2011.
58. Jørgensen KJ, Zahl PH, Gøtzsche PC. Breast cancer mortality in organised mammography screening in Denmark: comparative study. BMJ. 2010;340:c1241. doi:10.1136/bmj.c1241.
59. Sjönell G, Ståhle L. Mammographic screening does not reduce breast cancer mortality. Lakartidningen. 1999;96(8):904–5. pp. 908–13 (Swedish).
60. Autier P, Boniol M, Gavin A, Vatten LJ. Breast cancer mortality in neighbouring European countries with different levels of screening but similar access to treatment: trend analysis of WHO mortality database. BMJ. 2011;343:d4411. doi:10.1136/bmj.d4411.
61. Welch HG, Frankel BA. Likelihood that a woman with screen-detectedbreast cancer has had her "life saved" by that screening. Arch Intern Med. 2011;171(22):2043–6.
62. Haukka J, Byrnes G, Boniol M, Autier P. Trends in breast cancer mortality in Sweden before and after implementation of mammography screening. PLoS One. 2011;6(9):e22422.
63. Dean P, Tabár L, Yen M-F. Why does vehement opposition to screening come from Denmark, which has one of Europe's highest breast cancer mortality rates? BMJ. 2010. http://www.bmj.com/cgi/eletters/340/mar23_1/c1241. Assessed 1 Jun 2012.
64. Humphrey LL, Helfand M, Chan BKS, Woolf SH. Breast cancer screening: a summary of the evidence for the US Preventive Services Task Force. Ann Intern Med. 2002;137:347–60.
65. Nelson HD, Tyne K, Naik A, et al. Screening for breast cancer: systematic evidence review update for the US Preventive Services Task Force. Ann Intern Med. 2009;151:727–W242.
66. Gøtzsche P, Hartling OJ, Nielson M, Brodersen J, Jørgensen KJ. Breast screening: the facts-or maybe not. BMJ. 2009;338:446–8.
67. Duffy SW. Estimate of breast screening benefit was 6 times too large. http://www.bmj.com/content/338/bmj.b86?tab=responses. Assessed 2 Jun 2012.
68. Wald NJ, Law MR. Breast screening saves lives. BMJ. 2009;339:b2922.
69. Beral V, Alexander M, Duffy S, Ellis IO, Given-Wilson R, Holmberg L, Moss SM, Ramirez A, Reed MW, Rubin C, Whelehan P, Wilson R, Young KC. The number of women who would need to be screened regularly by mammography to prevent one death from breast cancer. J Med Screen. 2011;18(4):210–2.
70. Duffy SW, Ming-Fang Yen A, Chen H-H, Chen S, Chiu S, Fan J, Smith RA, Vitak B, Tabár L. Long-term benefits of breast screening. Breast Cancer Manage. 2012;1(1):31–8.

71. Tabár L, Vitak B, Yen MF, Chen HH, Smith RA, Duffy SW. Number needed to screen: lives saved over 20 years of follow-up in mammographic screening. J Med Screen. 2004;11(3):126–9.
72. Gøtzsche PC, Jørgensen KJ, Zahl PH, Mæhlen J. Why mammography screening has not lived up to expectations from the randomised trials. Cancer Causes Control. 2012;23(1):15–21.
73. Kalager M, Adami HO, Bretthauer M, Tamimi RM. Overdiagnosis of invasive breast cancer due to mammography screening: results from the Norwegian screening program. Ann Intern Med. 2012;156(7):491–9.
74. Welch HG, Black WC. Overdiagnosis in cancer. J Natl Cancer Inst. 2010;102(9):605–13.
75. Jørgensen KJ, Gøtzsche PC. Overdiagnosis in publicly organised mammography screening programmes: systematic review of incidence trends. BMJ. 2009;339:b2587. doi:10.1136/bmj.b2587.
76. Duffy SW, Agbaje O, Tabár L, Vitak B, Bjurstam N, Björneld L, Myles JP, Warwick J. Overdiagnosis and overtreatment of breast cancer: estimates of overdiagnosis from two trials of mammographic screening for breast cancer. Breast Cancer Res. 2005;7(6):258–65.
77. de Gelder R, Heijnsdijk EA, van Ravesteyn NT, Fracheboud J, Draisma G, de Koning HJ. Interpreting overdiagnosis estimates in population-based mammography screening. Epidemiol Rev. 2011;33(1):111–21.
78. Paci E, Miccinesi G, Puliti D, Baldazzi P, De Lisi V, Falcini F, Cirilli C, Ferretti S, Mangone L, Finarelli AC, Rosso S, Segnan N, Stracci F, Traina A, Tumino R, Zorzi M. Estimate of overdiagnosis of breast cancer due to mammography after adjustment for lead time. A service screening study in Italy. Breast Cancer Res. 2006;8(6):R68.
79. Kopans DB, Smith RA, Duffy SW. Mammographic screening and "overdiagnosis". Radiology. 2011;260(3):616–20.
80. Paci E, Duffy S. Overdiagnosis and overtreatment of breast cancer: overdiagnosis and overtreatment in service screening. Breast Cancer Res. 2005;7(6):266–70.
81. Yen MF, Tabár L, Vitak B, Smith RA, Chen HH, Duffy SW. Quantifying the potential problem of overdiagnosis of ductal carcinoma in situ in breast cancer screening. Eur J Cancer. 2003;39(12):1746–54.
82. Yen AM, Duffy SW, Chen TH, Chen LS, Chiu SY, Fann JC, Wu WY, Su CW, Smith RA, Tabár L. Long-term incidence of breast cancer by trial arm in one county of the Swedish Two-County Trial of mammographic screening. Cancer. 2012. doi: 10.1002/cncr.27580
83. Hellquist BN, Duffy SW, Nyström L, Jonsson H. Overdiagnosis in the population-based service screening programme with mammography for women aged 40 to 49 years in Sweden. J Med Screen. 2012;19(1):14–9.
84. Duffy SW, Tabár L, Olsen AH, et al. Absolute numbers of lives saved and overdiagnosis in breast cancer screening, from a randomized trial and from the breast screening programme in England. J Med Screen. 2010;17:25–30.
85. Puliti D, Zappa M, Miccinesi G, Falini P, Crocetti E, Paci E. An estimate of overdiagnosis 15 years after the start of mammographic screening in Florence. Eur J Cancer. 2009;45: 3166–71.
86. Gøtzsche PC, Olsen O. Is screening for breast cancer with mammography justifiable? Lancet. 2000;355:129–34.
87. Olsen O, Gøtzsche PC. Cochrane review on screening for breast cancer with mammography. Lancet. 2001;358:1340–2.
88. Black WC, Haggstrom DA, Welch HG. All-cause mortality in randomized trials of cancer screening. J Natl Cancer Inst. 2002;94:167–73.
89. Juffs HG, Tannock IF. Screening trials are even more difficult than we thought they were. J Natl Cancer Inst. 2002;94:156–7.
90. Duffy SW, Tabár L, Smith RA. Screening for breast cancer with mammography. Lancet. 2001;358(9299):2166. author reply 2167-8.
91. Tabár L, Duffy SW, Yen MF, Warwick J, Vitak B, Chen HH, Smith RA. All-cause mortality among breast cancer patients in a screening trial: support for breast cancer mortality as an end point. J Med Screen. 2002;9(4):159–62.

92. Nyström L, Larsson LG, Wall S, Rutqvist LE, Andersson I, Bjurstam N, Fagerberg G, Frisell J, Tabár L. An overview of the Swedish randomised mammography trials: total mortality pattern and the representivity of the study cohorts. J Med Screen. 1996;3(2):85–7.
93. Day NE. Breast cancer screening. Ugeskr Laeger. 2002;164(2):207–9. Danish.
94. Freedman DA, Petitti DB, Robins JM. On the efficacy of screening for breast cancer. Int J Epidemiol. 2004;33(1):43–55.
95. Wald N. Populist instead of professional. J Med Screen. 2000;7(1):1.
96. Holmberg L, Duffy SW, Yen AM, Tabár L, Vitak B, Nyström L, Frisell J. Differences in endpoints between the Swedish W-E (two county) trial of mammographic screening and the Swedish overview: methodological consequences. J Med Screen. 2009;16(2):73–80.
97. Duffy SW, Tabár L, Smith RA. The mammographic screening trials: commentary on the recent work by Olsen and Gøtzsche. CA Cancer J Clin. 2002;52(2):68–71.
98. Kopans DB. The most recent breast cancer screening controversy about whether mammographic screening benefits women at any age: nonsense and nonscience. AJR Am J Roentgenol. 2003;180(1):21–6.
99. Bock K, Borisch B, Cawson J, Damtjernhaug B, de Wolf C, Dean P, den Heeten A, Doyle G, Fox R, Frigerio A, Gilbert F, Hecht G, Heindel W, Heywang-Köbrunner SH, Holland R, Jones F, Lernevall A, Madai S, Mairs A, Muller J, Nisbet P, O'Doherty A, Patnick J, Perry N, Regitz-Jedermann L, Rickard M, Rodrigues V, Del Turco MR, Scharpantgen A, Schwartz W, Seradour B, Skaane P, Tabár L, Tornberg S, Ursin G, Van Limbergen E, Vandenbroucke A, Warren LJ, Warwick L, Yaffe M, Zappa M. Effect of population-based screening on breast cancer mortality. Lancet. 2011;378(9805):1775–6.
100. Gøtzsche P. Screening for colorectal cancer. Lancet. 1997;349:356.
101. Jørgensen KJ, Keen JD, Gøtzsche PC. Is mammographic screening justifiable considering its substantial overdiagnosis rate and minor effect on mortality? Radiology. 2011;260:621–7.
102. Gøtzsche PC, Jørgensen KJ. Effect of population-based screening on breast cancer mortality. Lancet. 2012;379(9823):1297.
103. Patnick J, Perry N, de Wolf C. Effect of population-based screening on breast cancer mortality. Lancet. 2012; 379(9823): author reply 1298.
104. Gøtzsche PC. Mammography screening: truth, lies and controversy. Milton Keynes, UK: Radcliffe Publishing Ltd.; 2012.
105. Cuzick J. Breast cancer screening – time to move forward. Lancet. 2012;379(9823):1289–90.
106. Feig SA, Duffy SW. Screening results, controversies and guidelines. In: Bassett LW, Mahony M, Apple S, D'Orsi C, editors. Breast imaging. Philadelphia: Saunders; 2010. p. 56–75.
107. O'Sullivan I, Sutton S, Dixon S, Perry N. False positive results do not have a negative effect on reattendance for subsequent breast screening. J Med Screen. 2001;8(3):145–8.
108. Harris R. Variation of benefits and harms of breast cancer screening with age. J Natl Cancer Inst Monogr. 1997;22:139–43.
109. Barton MB. Breast cancer screening. Benefits, risks, and current controversies. Postgrad Med. 2005;118(2):27–8, 33–6, 46.
110. Østerlie W, Solbjør M, Skolbekken JA, Hofvind S, Saetnan AR, Forsmo S. Challenges of informed choice in organised screening. J Med Ethics. 2008;34(9):e5.
111. Kmietowicz Z. Breast screening benefits twice as many women as it harms, shows new analysis. BMJ. 2010;340:c1824. doi:10.1136/bmj.c1824.
112. Roder DM, Olver IN. Do the benefits of screening mammography outweigh the harms of overdiagnosis and unnecessary treatment?–yes. Med J Aust. 2012;196(1):16.
113. Bell RJ, Burton RC. Do the benefits of screening mammography outweigh the harms of overdiagnosis and unnecessary treatment?–no. Med J Aust. 2012;196(1):17.
114. Gøtzsche PC, Nielsen M. Screening for breast cancer with mammography. Cochrane Database Syst Rev. 2011;(1):CD001877. Review.
115. Thornton H. Communicating to citizens the benefits, harms and risks of preventive interventions. J Epidemiol Community Health. 2010;64(2):101–2.
116. Baum M. Should routine screening by mammography be replaced by a more selective service of risk assessment/risk management? Womens Health (Lond Engl). 2010;6(1):71–6.

117. Suhrke P, Mæhlen J, Schlichting E, Jørgensen KJ, Gøtzsche PC, Zahl PH. Effect of mammography screening on surgical treatment for breast cancer in Norway: comparative analysis of cancer registry data. BMJ. 2011;343:d4692. doi:10.1136/bmj.d4692.
118. Lawrence G, Kearins O, Lagord C, et al. Second all breast cancer report. 2011. http://www.ncin.org.uk/view.aspx?rid=612. Accessed 4 Nov 2011.
119. Paci E, Duffy SW, Giorgi D, et al. Are breast cancer screening programmes increasing rates of mastectomy? Observational study. BMJ. 2002;325(7361):418.
120. Jørgensen KJ, Gøtzsche PC. Dags att slopa mammografi screeningen (Time to abolish mammography screening). Lakartidningen. 2012;109(13):690–2. Swedish.
121. Gøtzsche PC. BBC Radio 4 Interview Jan 23. 2012. http://www.bbc.co.uk/programmes/b019rly3.

Chapter 3
The Sick Lobe Concept

Tibor Tot

Introduction

Breast cancer is the most common malignancy among younger women worldwide [1]. Women are at 100 times higher risk of getting breast cancer during their lifetime than men. The lifetime risk of getting the disease is, at least, fivefold higher in carriers of mutated BRCA1 and BRCA2 genes than in the normal population [2, 3]. Certain geographic areas in the USA, Europe, Australia, and Canada are well known for their exceptionally high breast cancer incidence [4]. Female gender, carrying a mutated gene, living in a high-incidence country, and many other known cancer risk factors are characteristics of the entire organism and influence the genetic construction, as well as the milieu, of all the cells in the body. However, breast cancer develops in one quadrant of one breast in the vast majority of cases. This simple observation indicates presence of at-risk tissue in the breast that is more sensitive to oncogenic stimuli than the other structures of the human body. In our view, this at-risk tissue corresponds to a sick breast lobe [5].

T. Tot, M.D., Ph.D. (✉)
Department of Pathology and Clinical Cytology, Central Hospital Falun, Central Hospital, Falun, Sweden
e-mail: tibor.tot@ltdalarna.se

D.S. Francescatti and M.J. Silverstein (eds.), *Breast Cancer: A New Era in Management*, DOI 10.1007/978-1-4614-8063-1_3,

Biological Considerations

Lobar Morphology of the Breast

The breast is a glandular organ with lobar morphology. The lobe is a complex structure beginning with a lactiferous duct opening within the nipple and branching into segmental and subsegmental ducts. The subsegmental ducts end in hundreds and thousands of terminal ductal-lobular units. All of the ducts and terminal units belonging to a single lactiferous duct, together with the surrounding stromal elements, comprise a breast lobe, a pyramid-like structure with its tip in the nipple and base towards the pectoralis muscle. The lobes are individual units that exhibit considerable variation in size and shape. A lobe can comprise everything between 2 and 23 % of the breast volume; a single lobe can be spread over more than one breast quadrant [6–8]. Though the size of a lobe varies depending on the hormonal status of the woman (largest during pregnancy and lactation, rich in terminal units during the reproductive period of life, not fully developed before puberty, and involuted after menopause), the number of lobes is constant. The largest lobes are located in the upper outer quadrant of the breast; these are the lobes completing their development earliest during the woman's lifetime and the last to involute [9].

Stem Cells, Progenitor Cells, and Differentiated Progeny

Cells with stem cell-like properties have been proposed to exist in normal human breast epithelium and in breast carcinomas. Differentiated cells tend to have a short life, but stem cells persist and reproduce themselves throughout the entire life of the organism [10]. Progenitor cells represent stem cells differentiated to a certain extent. Both progenitor cells and stem cells are capable of further differentiation and are often pluripotent, giving rise to different mature cells representing differentiated progeny and comprising various tissues of an organism. Tissue-specific stem/progenitor cells are defined by their ability to produce the differentiated progeny of the tissue [11]. The actual morphology of the tissue is the result of a balance between the renewal and loss of cellular and non-cellular elements [12].

During embryonic development of the mammary gland, the stem cells undergo stepwise differentiation ("commitment"), with the final step of differentiation leading to the appearance of two cell populations: luminal epithelial and basal myoepithelial cells [13, 14]. Evidence suggests the existence of three distinct epithelial progenitor cells in the breast: one capable of producing all the cells of the parenchyma, and two others capable of producing branching ducts or secretory lobules [15]. Thus, the processes of initialisation and arborisation (which happen at an early phase of embryonic development) and the process of lobularisation (characteristic of the pubertal and mature breast tissue) seem to be, to a certain extent, independent of one another.

In order for a cell to become neoplastic, a series of changes are needed to overcome the stringent controls of cell division. A malignant tumour represents a heterogeneous population of mutant cells that share some mutations but vary in genotype and phenotype. The original cancer cell(s) and its progeny exhibit stem cell properties [16, 17]. The cancer cells share their immortal character with tissue-specific stem cells, as they are also slow-dividing, long-lived cells with a capacity for self-renewal and differentiation [18], but only a small proportion of the malignant cells have unlimited proliferation potential and possess the ability to lead to tumour formation. These cells are called cancer stem cells. The more differentiated cancer cells that account for the majority of the tumour cell population may have high, but not unlimited, proliferation potential.

Theoretical Background

The Sick Lobe Theory

Our hypothesis, the sick lobe theory, postulates that breast cancer is a lobar disease, as the in situ and invasive tumour structures originate within a single sick lobe of the breast in the vast majority of cases [5]. The lobes are formed early during embryonic life, suggesting that the sick lobe is malconstructed during its embryonic development. The sick lobe contains a larger number of progenitor cells than the other ("healthy") lobes of the same breast and/or the progenitor cells become mutated during the early development of the lobes and "committed" to undergo malignant transformation [18]. The genetic abnormalities and longevity of such committed progenitor cells make them more sensitive to the mutagenic effects of exogenic and endogenic stimuli; thus, malignant transformation may happen substantially earlier in the lobes carrying such cells than in the lobes free of such cells [12, 19, 20].

The committed progenitor cells may be evenly distributed throughout the entire sick lobe if the committing mutation(s) happens in the initial phase of lobe morphogenesis. If such a mutation happens at the arborisation phase (branching of the main duct into segmental and subsegmental ducts), the presence of committed progenitor cells may be limited to a segmental duct, its branches, and terminal units. If the committing mutation(s) appears late, in the lobularisation phase, the presence of committed progenitor cells will be limited to one or several terminal units [5, 19].

The Theory of Biological Timing

Though the sick lobe develops early during embryonic life, complete transformation of the committed progenitor cells into a cancer within the breast occurs decades later. This difference in timing may be explained by the large number of replications needed for the accumulation of additional mutations and other genetic alterations necessary for malignant transformation. This requirement acts as a biological clock, determining the timing of malignant transformation [12, 19, 20]. Differences in the sensitivity of the committed and non-committed progenitor cells to oncogenic stimuli may explain why the malignant transformation within the sick lobe appears earlier than in other lobes; the transformation in the healthy lobes may not be completed during the woman's lifetime. Rarely, several lobes may carry a large number of sufficiently sensitive committed progenitor cells and develop malignancy at the same time (*synchronous multicentricity*) or at variable times (*asynchronous multicentricity*). The committed progenitor cells within the same sick lobe may not have identical sensitivity to oncogenic stimuli, so that complete malignant transformation may appear earlier in some parts, preceding such transformation at other locations within the same sick lobe (*asynchronous multifocality*). It is also possible that committed progenitor cells in different parts of the same sick lobe may have identical biological timing (i.e., similar sensitivity to oncogenic stimuli and similar number of replications needed for the accumulation of a sufficient number of genetic alterations), leading to the development of malignancy at multiple distant points of the same sick lobe at approximately the same time (*synchronous multifocality*).

If the committed progenitor cells are evenly distributed through the entire sick lobe (altered already at the early phase of initialisation of the lobe during embryogenesis) and biologically timed to undergo malignant transformation at the same time, the cancer will involve the entire sick lobe or large portions of it (*lobar pattern of malignant transformation* within the sick lobe). If the committing mutation happens at the phase of arborisation and the committed progenitor cells are timed to undergo malignant transformation at the same time, the cancer will involve a segmental duct with its branches and terminal units (*segmental pattern of malignant transformation*). If the committing mutation(s) appears late, in the lobularisation phase, the cancer will involve the most peripheral portion of the sick lobe, the terminal units (*peripheral pattern of malignant transformation*) [5, 12].

Supporting Evidence

A growing body of scientific evidence supports the correctness of these theories. The epidemiological, morphological, genetic, radiological, and clinical evidence was collected and published, filling a separate Springer book [21], and as such is beyond the scope of the present chapter. Briefly, as early as in 1855, Rudolf Virchow proposed an embryonal rest hypothesis, stating that cancer arises from the activation of "dominant" cells that are reminders of embryonic tissue [22]. Early morphological observations that breast carcinoma may grow in a triangular area with its tip in the nipple and base towards the pectoralis muscle suggested the lobar nature of the disease [23, 24]. In cases with involvement of the lactiferous ducts, the malignant cells regularly occupy only one of the many ducts [8], suggesting that only one of the many lobes are involved. Epidemiological studies have shown that pre-natal and peri-natal factors influence an individual's risk of developing breast carcinoma during their adult life [25]. Evidence indicates existing genetic alterations in the seemingly normal breast tissue surrounding the cancer, which may be located as far as 4 cm from the malignant focus [26] and exist long time before any microscopic signs of the disease appear [27]. Microcalcifications detected on mammogram may also be localised to a triangular area of breast tissue, and magnetic resonance imaging may show segmental—lobar disease distribution in a considerable number of cases [28]. The entire concept of ductal echography is based on the hypothesis of lobar localisation of the disease [29].

Thus, the theory of the sick lobe and the theory of biological timing are new concepts but rooted in previous observations and studies. In addition to the results of these studies, the new theories connect the process of carcinogenesis to an existing and well-defined anatomical structure, a breast lobe, and provide a possible explanation for the progressive character and morphological heterogeneity of breast carcinoma. These theories place the process of carcinogenesis into a unifying concept with genetic, developmental, and morphological perspectives, understanding breast carcinoma as a life-long process with determined natural history, which may be modified by endogenous and exogenous influences.

Malignant Transformation Within the Sick Lobe with Various Biological Timing: The Complexity of Breast Cancer Subgross Morphology

Cancer In Situ

Cancer in situ represents the earliest histologically detectable phase in the development of breast cancer. After malignancy-committed progenitor cells undergo complete malignant transformation, they not only replace the progenitor cells of the breast ducts and terminal units in the involved portion of the sick lobe but also take over their functions. These functions include, first of all, maintaining the ductal-lobular architecture of the breast parenchyma, maintaining the myoepithelial cell layer and basement membrane surrounding the parenchyma, and maintaining the relationship of the parenchyma to the stroma [5, 20]. Depending on the severity of the genetic alterations acquired during the malignant transformation, the malignant progenitor cells vary in their ability to retain these functions. At the highest level of retained functions (*low-grade cancer in situ*), the malignant progenitors are able to maintain all of these functions and renew the ductal and lobular structures, though these structures will eventually be distended and distorted as they fill with the differentiated cancer cells. At the lowest level of retained functions, the malignant progenitors may not be able to retain the terminal units, new duct-like structures appear in close proximity to each other, defective myoepithelium is formed and focally disappears, and the periductal stroma undergoes remodelling and becomes infiltrated by lymphocytes (*high-grade in situ carcinoma with ductal neogenesis*) [30].

Both low-grade and high-grade in situ cancers may exhibit lobar, segmental, and peripheral patterns of malignant transformation in the sick lobe, but the high-grade

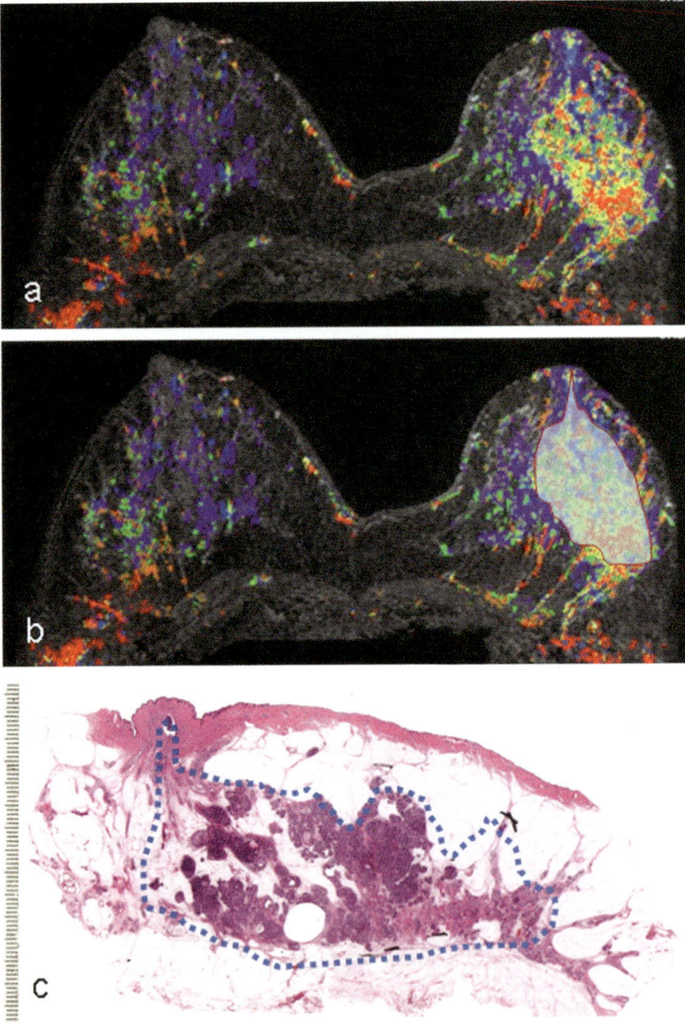

Fig. 3.1 Lobar growth pattern in diffusely growing in situ breast carcinoma. (**a**) Magnetic resonance imaging, (**b**) the same image with diseased area marked, (**c**) corresponding large-format histology section of the lesion with diseased area marked. Note the lobe-like shape of the lesion and involvement of a single lactiferous duct. The radiology images are courtesy of Dr. Mats Ingvarsson. **c** was reproduced from ref. [52]

cancers tend to be associated with a lobar pattern and involve not only terminal units and smaller branches but also the largest ducts within the sick lobe. Involvement of the large ducts gives the appearance of a network of dilated cancer-filled tubes, which is difficult to histologically delineate (*diffuse in situ cancer*) [31–34]. Such a lesion may or may not show signs of ductal neogenesis. One such case is illustrated in Fig. 3.1. Malignant transformation in a segmental pattern will result in a relatively well-delineated cancer area (*unifocal in situ cancer*). The involvement of a single terminal unit will also result in a unifocal process, but the peripheral pattern of malignant transformation in the sick lobe is usually associated with several malignant terminal units, well demarcated and distant from each other (*multifocal in situ cancer*) [31–33]. In approximately one-fourth of cases, in situ carcinoma involves existing benign lesions in the breast or forms similar structures (intracystic papillary carcinoma, tumour forming in situ carcinoma, and others). This subgroup of in situ carcinoma is designated as "special types."

The development of in situ carcinomas may be a synchronous or asynchronous process. If synchronous, the entire sick lobe, a segment of the sick lobe, or many terminal units show histologically detectable in situ carcinomas at an early phase of cancer development. In such cases, the area/tissue volume involved with malignant cells (i.e., the *extent of the disease*) is similar during the early and later phases of the cancer's natural history (though the involved lobe, segment, or terminal units may grow during the process). If the malignant transformation is asynchronous, only a few structures will show histologically detectable signs of malignant transformation at the beginning of the process, but these signs will be more widespread at the end of it. In this case, the extent of the disease also increases with time.

Early Invasive Cancer

Further mutations in the malignant cells and cells of the surrounding tissue may lead to deregulation of the epithelial–stromal balance, resulting in the cancer cells losing their ability to rebuild the ductal-lobular architecture and becoming unable to reproduce the myoepithelial layer and basal membrane. Individual cancer cells and their groups will come into direct contact with the stroma, which has also undergone remodelling during this process. The remodelled stroma limits the lesion to an altered part of the breast tissue called the invasive tumour focus [35]. Such a focus may develop from the in situ cancer at a single place within the breast (*unifocal invasive component*) or on several distant loci (*multifocal invasive component, primary type*). Cancer cells may enter prelymphatic [36] and lymphatic spaces and be transported through these channels to distant parts of the breast tissue, as well as locations outside the breast, such as the lymph nodes. The transported cancer cells may be dormant for years and decades, but they may also leave the channel, interact with the surrounding tissue, and develop secondary invasive foci. If this process is localised to the breast, *multifocal invasive component(s) of secondary (metastatic) type* develops. Of course, in this case, the process no longer respects the boundaries of a sick lobe.

In most cases, invasion appears focally in the sick lobe, and the vast majority of breast carcinomas exhibit both in situ and invasive components. The real extent and distribution of the lesions in the tumours can only be appreciated if the parameters of both in situ and invasive components are combined [33].

Advanced Cancer

Through the proliferation of the cancer cells, the invasive component(s) of the tumour may grow, and the tumour foci may eventually coalesce, resulting in a larger tumour mass and more complex morphology. With further mutations and dedifferentiation, new cell clones may appear within the cancer, leading to *intratumoural and intertumoural heterogeneity* in tumour characteristics. The transported cancer cells may wake from their dormancy and develop additional tumour foci within the breast or metastases in other organs. Through these mechanisms, the cancer gradually enters the advanced phase.

On rare occasions, the remodelling of the stroma is insufficient and the growth-limiting effect of such remodelling is missing. In these cases, invasion may occur simultaneously at many places in proximity to the in situ component. The tumour cells infiltrate the normal stromal structures in an unlimited way, giving rise to a spider web-like invasive component, which is usually extensive (*diffuse invasive component*) [37].

An advanced invasive carcinoma with a diffuse in situ component showing a lobar growth pattern is illustrated in Fig. 3.2.

The Clinical Relevance of Breast Cancer Subgross Morphology

Distribution of the Cases by Size, Extent, and Focality

Purely in situ carcinomas comprise 10–20 % of breast cancer series in countries with ongoing mammography screening. In our material (Central Hospital Falun, Sweden, period 2008–2011), the proportion of in situ cancer was 14 % (107/780) of the consecutive series of newly diagnosed breast cancers. Half of the cases were extensive (52 %, 55/107), in that they occupied a tissue volume measuring at least 4 cm in the largest dimension, and half of them were non-extensive (48 %, 52/107). The lesions were unifocal in 30 % of cases (32/107), multifocal in 30 % (32/107), and diffuse in 40 % (43/107) (Table 3.1).

In addition to purely in situ carcinomas, microinvasive cancers (invasive foci less than 1 mm in size) and invasive carcinomas less than 15 mm size belong to the category of *early breast carcinomas*, as we define [30, 38]. Patients with such tumours have an excellent, over 90 %, 10-year cumulative survival. The proportion of cases in our material that were classified in this category was 48 %: 14 % (107/780) in situ, 33 % (260/780) invasive <15 mm, and two cases of microinvasive cancer. The majority (70 %, 182/260) of the early invasive cancers had a unifocal invasive component, but when the combined morphology of the in situ and invasive components

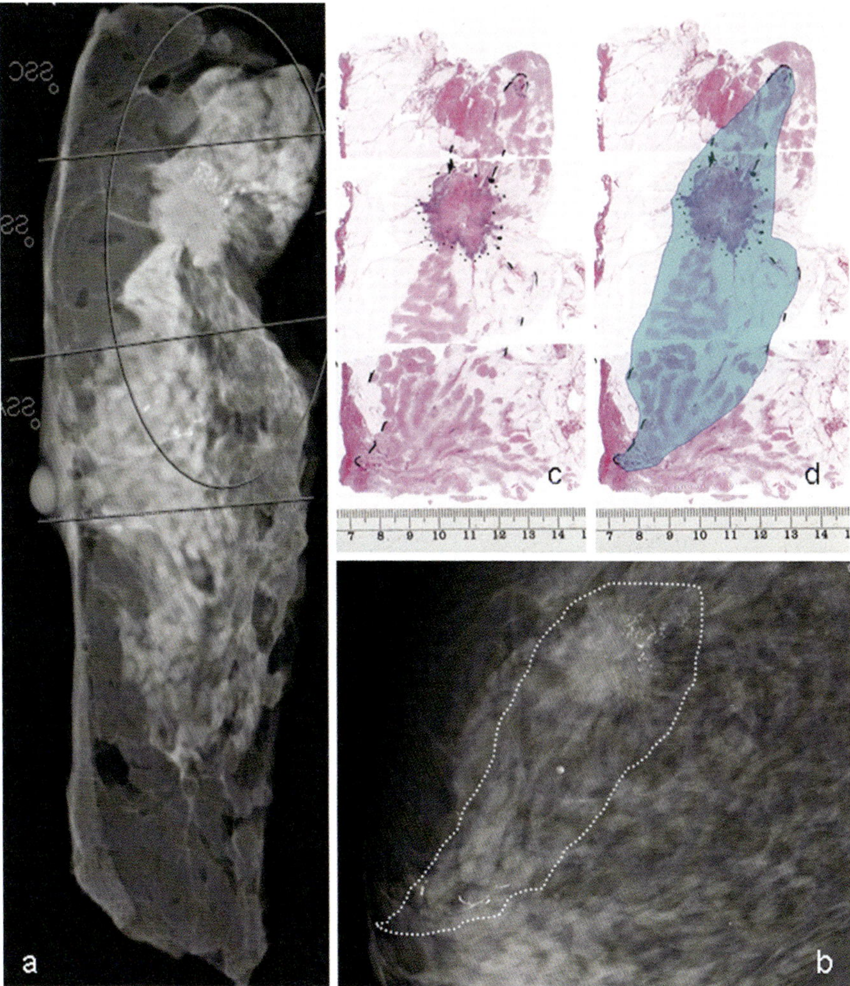

Fig. 3.2 Breast carcinoma with a unifocal invasive component and diffusely growing in situ component occupying a whole breast lobe. (**a**) Radiogram of a slice of the mastectomy specimen, (**b**) mammogram of the lesion with diseased area marked, (**c**) corresponding large-format histology sections (half of the slice reconstructed in three adjacent standard-sized large slides), (**d**) the same histology sections with diseased area marked. Note the lobe-like shape of the lesions and involvement of a single lactiferous duct. The radiology images are courtesy of Dr. Mats Ingvarsson

were taken into account, the majority (59 %) were in fact multifocal or diffuse; 40 % (103/260) of the early cases were extensive and occupied a tissue volume measuring 4 cm or larger (Table 3.1).

More advanced cancers have an invasive component measuring 15 mm or greater. Patients with such tumours have less favourable survival outcomes compared to early breast cancer cases. The proportion of cases in our material that were

Table 3.1 Distribution of cases in a consecutive series of newly diagnosed breast carcinomas in Falun, Sweden, 2008–2011 by tumour size, disease extent, and focality

	Unifocal		Multifocal		Diffuse		
	Extensive	Non-extensive	Extensive	Non-extensive	Extensive	Non-extensive	Total
In situ	0	30 % (32/107)	20 % (21/107)	10 % (11/107)	32 % (34/107)	8 % (9/107)	100 % (107/107)
Early Invasive	0	41 % (107/260)	18 % (48/260)	15 % (38/260)	21 % (55/260)	5 % (12/260)	100 % (260/260)
Advanced	3 % (13/413)	32 % (133/413)	29 % (118/413)	8 % (35/413)	23 % (96/413)	5 % (18/413)	100 % (413/413)
Total	36 % (285/780)		35 % (271/780)		29 % (224/780)		100 % (780/780)

Early invasive = invasive component <15 mm. Advanced = invasive component 15 mm or larger. Extensive = disease extent 40 mm or larger. Non-extensive = disease extent <40 mm

classified in this category was 52 % (413/780). Approximately one-third (35 %, 126/413) had unifocal combined (in situ + invasive) morphology, one-third (37 %, 153/413) had multifocal, and the rest (28 %, 13/413) had diffuse combined lesion distribution; 55 % (227/413) of the cases were extensive and occupied a tissue volume measuring 4 cm or larger (Table 3.1).

In summary, most breast carcinomas exhibit both in situ and invasive components. Although up to 70 % of invasive tumours have only a unifocal invasive component, most breast carcinomas have complex morphology when the distributions of the in situ and invasive components are combined. This complexity is already evident at early stages of the disease. Half of breast cancer cases are extensive and occupy a tissue volume measuring 4 cm or larger in the greatest dimension. This conclusion is in concordance with the results of whole organ studies [24, 39–42], studies using large-format histology in routine diagnostics [23, 32–34, 43–48], and studies relying on modern radiological breast imaging methods [9, 28, 29].

Local Disease Control

Ipsilateral local recurrences following breast-conserving surgery develop most often in the vicinity of the operative area. Postoperative irradiation decreases the incidence of such recurrences; without irradiation this incidence may be as high as 40 %. A recent meta-analysis of more than 10,000 women treated with breast-conserving surgery found that 35 % of patients without and 19.3 % with postoperative irradiation had local recurrences during the 10-year follow-up period [49]. A long-term (25-year) follow-up study in the USA demonstrated a more than six times higher locoregional recurrence rate in patients treated with breast-conserving surgery with postoperative irradiation compared to those treated with mastectomy [50]. In addition to the possibility of incomplete surgical intervention, the recurrence can be explained by the possibility of developing additional malignant foci in the at-risk tissue in which no malignancy was detected at the time of surgery. This possibility clearly indicates the necessity of removing or destroying the entire at-risk tissue within the breast, the entire sick lobe.

According to our previously published series with long-term follow-up, the rates of local recurrence after breast-conserving surgery were almost ten times higher in extensive compared to non-extensive in situ carcinomas of non-special type (19 % versus 2 %). The highest rates were seen in cases of diffuse in situ carcinoma, especially those with signs of ductal neogenesis (27 % recurrence rate) [5]. Similar results were demonstrated by Silverstein and Lagios [51], who showed that mastectomy is needed for the majority of extensive (40 mm or larger) in situ carcinomas to reach a <20 % 12-year local recurrence rate.

According to our previously published series, extensive breast carcinoma (all size categories included) had an almost triple relative risk of ipsilateral local recurrence after breast-conserving surgery and radiotherapy compared to non-extensive cases (RR, 2.7511; CI, 1.3401–5.6478). Likewise, the relative risk of local recurrence was tripled if breast-conserving surgery was performed compared to the risk in mastectomy cases (RR, 2.8182; CI, 1.1955–6.6435) [52]. These results were confirmed by data on disease-free survival in the same series of patients [53]. Thus, our findings indicate the need for mastectomy in extensive breast cancer cases, comprising 40–50 % of the series, which is in concordance with the results of some previous publications on this topic [54, 55]. The introduction of more sensitive preoperative imaging methods, such as magnetic resonance imaging, which allows more precise mapping of the disease, increases mastectomy rates, from 29 to 52.8 % in one study [28]. As magnetic resonance imaging correlates well with histologically detectable malignant structures, this increase in the mastectomy rate is justified.

Using preoperative ductoscopy to find the altered lactiferous duct and mark its branches efficiently assists the surgeon in delineating the area to excise. Such an approach has substantially reduced the incidence of local recurrences [56]. As a special ultrasound approach, ductal echography is also efficient in delineating the sick breast lobe [9]. The concept and the technical details of lobectomy as a successful alternative surgical approach in breast cancer are presented by Giancarlo Dolfin elsewhere in this book.

Survival

Despite the influence of the in situ component, survival is mainly related to the characteristics of the invasive component of the breast cancer. The worst outcome is related to diffuse invasive breast carcinoma [37, 57], but multifocality of the invasive component and the extent of the disease also impact prognosis. Most related publications have reported a greater propensity of metastatic spread to the axillary lymph nodes in multifocal invasive carcinomas compared to unifocal tumours [33, 47, 48, 58, 59]. Our studies have demonstrated that the risk of lymph node metastasis is approximately doubled in multifocal and tripled in diffuse invasive carcinomas compared to unifocal carcinomas [33, 47, 48].

Relatively few studies have been performed to examine the effect of multifocality on breast cancer-related cumulative survival. These studies generated somewhat conflicting results, as the diagnostic criteria and understanding of the multifocality of the process varied among the studies. Some publications have reported a significant influence of multifocality on disease-free survival in breast cancer patients but no significant effect on overall survival [60]. However, four recent independent studies reported a highly significant impact of breast cancer multifocality, which reduced the overall survival of the patients [57, 61–63]. Such an impact of multifocality seems to be independent of other morphological prognostic parameters [57, 62, 63] and the applied therapeutic measures [62]. The impact of tumour multifocality on the cumulative survival of oestrogen-receptor positive and oestrogen-receptor negative patients is illustrated in Fig. 3.3.

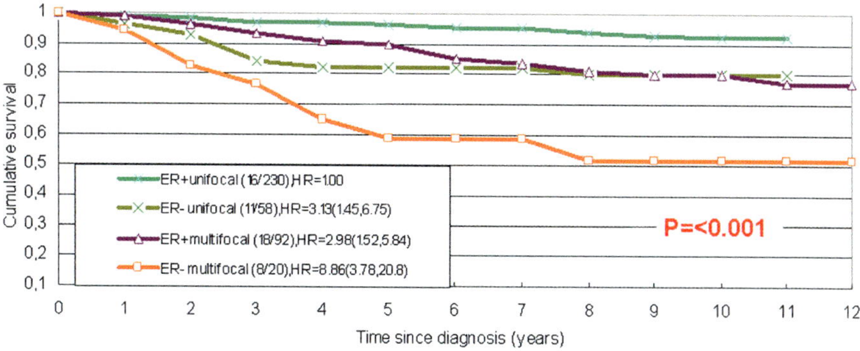

Fig. 3.3 Cumulative survival of patients with oestrogen-receptor positive and oestrogen-receptor negative tumours by focality of the invasive tumour component (Falun, Sweden, 1996–1998)

Conclusions

- Breast cancer is a lobar disease.
- The variations in biological timing of malignant transformation within the sick lobe result in complex breast cancer morphology in most cases.
- Half of breast cancer cases are extensive, occupying an area of malignant transformation measuring 40 mm or more in the largest dimension. Mastectomy seems to be the adequate surgical approach in the majority of such cases.
- For adequate breast-conserving surgery, detailed preoperative mapping of not only the malignant structures within the breast but also the sick lobe is required. Imaging methods, such as magnetic resonance imaging, ductal echography, and ductoscopy, are often helpful in delineating the sick lobe.
- Shifting focus from the palpable lesion and width of the excision margins toward attempting to remove the entire sick lobe is rational.
- Multifocality and diffuse distribution of the invasive component of the tumour is associated with increased metastatic potential and reduced cumulative survival of the patients.
- The subgross morphology of breast cancer has a substantial prognostic impact and has to be taken into consideration when planning individualised therapy.

References

1. Boyle P, Ferlay J. Cancer incidence and mortality in Europe 2004. Ann Oncol. 2005;16(3):481–8.
2. Easton DF, Steele L, Fields P, et al. Cancer risk in two large breast cancer families linked to BRCA2 on chromosome 13q12-13. Am J Hum Genet. 1997;61:120–8.

3. Ford D, Easton DF, Bishop DT, et al. Risk of cancer in BRCA1-mutation carriers. Breast cancer linkage consortium. Lancet. 1994;343:692–5.
4. Clarke CA, Glaser SL, West DW, et al. Breast cancer incidence and mortality trends in an affluent population: Marine county, California, USA, 1990-1996. Breast Cancer Res. 2002;4:R13.
5. Tot T. DCIS, cytokeratins, and the theory of the sick lobe. Virchows Arch. 2005;447:1–8.
6. Going JJ, Moffat DF. Escaping from flatland: clinical and biological aspects of human mammary duct anatomy in three dimensions. J Pathol. 2004;203:538–44.
7. Going JJ, Mohun TJ. Human breast duct anatomy, the 'sick lobe' hypothesis and intraductal approaches to breast cancer. Breast Cancer Res Treat. 2006;97:285–91.
8. Going JJ. Lobar anatomy of the human breast and its importance for breast cancer. In: Tot T, editor. Breast cancer—a lobar disease. New York: Springer; 2011. p. 19–37.
9. Amy D. Lobar ultrasound of the breast. In: Tot T, editor. Breast cancer—a lobar disease. New York: Springer; 2011. p. 153–62.
10. Gudjonsson T, Magnusson MK. Stem cell biology and the pathways of carcinogenesis. APMIS. 2005;113:922–9.
11. Fridriksdottir AJR, Petersen OW, Ronnow-Jessen L. Mammary gland stem cells: current status and future challenges. Int J Dev Biol. 2011;55:719–29.
12. Tot T. The theory of the sick lobe. In: Tot T, editor. Breast cancer—a lobar disease. New York: Springer; 2011. p. 1–17.
13. Villadsen R. In search of stem cell hierarchy in the human breast and its relevance in breast cancer evolution. APMIS. 2005;113:903–21.
14. Villadsen R, Fridriksdottir AJ, Ronnov-Jenssen L, et al. Evidence for stem cell hierarchy in the adult human breast. J Cell Biol. 2007;177:87–101.
15. Smith GH, Boulanger CA. Epithelial stem cells transplantation and self renewal analysis. Cell Prolif. 2003;36 Suppl 1:3–15.
16. Al Hajj M, Wicha MS, Benito-Hernandez A, et al. Prospective identification of tumorigenic breast cancer cells. Proc Natl Acad Sci USA. 2003;100:3983–8.
17. Reja T, Morrison SJ, Clarke MF, Weissmann IL. Stem cells, cancer, and cancer stem cells. Nature. 2001;414:105–11.
18. Agelopoulos K, Buerger H, Brandt B. Allelic imbalance of the egfr gene as key event in breast cancer progression—the concept of committed progenitor cells. Curr Cancer Drug Targets. 2008;8:431–45.
19. Tot T. The theory of the sick breast lobe and the possible consequences. Int J Surg Pathol. 2007;15:369–75.
20. Tot T. The origins of early breast carcinoma. Semin Diagn Pathol. 2010;27:62–8.
21. Tot T, editor. Breast cancer—a lobar disease. New York: Springer; 2011.
22. Virchow R. Cellular-Pathologie. Archiv fur Pathologische Anatomie und Phisiologie fur Klinische Medizin. 1855;8:3–39.
23. Gibbs NM. Large paraffin sections and chemical clearance of axillary tissues as a routine procedure in the pathological examination of the breast. Histopathology. 1982;6(5):647–60.
24. Mai KT, Yazdi HM, Burns BF, Perkins DG. Pattern of distribution of intraductal and infiltrating ductal carcinoma: three-dimensional study using serial coronal giant sections of the breast. Hum Pathol. 2000;31:464–74.
25. Xue F, Michels KB. Intrauterine factors and risk of breast cancer: a systematic review and meta-analysis of current evidence. Lancet Oncol. 2007;8:1088–100.
26. Yan PS, Venkataramu C, Ibrahim A, et al. Mapping geographic zones of cancer risk with epigenetic biomarkers in normal breast tissue. Clin Cancer Res. 2006;12:6626–36.
27. Lakhani SR, Chaggar R, Davies S, et al. Genetic alterations in "normal" luminal and myoepithelial cells of the breast. J Pathol. 1999;189:496–503.
28. Barchie MF, Clive KS, Tyler JA, et al. Standardized pretreatment breast MRI-accuracy and influence on mastectomy decisions. J Surg Oncol. 2011;104(7):741–5.
29. Teboul M, Halliwell M. Atlas of ultrasound and ductal echography of the breast: the introduction of anatomic intelligence into breast imaging. London: Wiley-Blackwell; 1995. p. 380.

30. Tabár L, Chen HT, Yen MFA, et al. Mammographic tumor features can predict long-term outcomes reliably in women with 1-14 mm invasive carcinoma. Cancer. 2004;101:1745–59.
31. Andersen JA, Blichert-Toft M, Dyreborg U. In situ carcinomas of the breast. Types, growth pattern, diagnosis and treatment. Eur J Surg Oncol. 1987;13:105–11.
32. Tot T. The subgross morphology of normal and pathologically altered breast tissue. In: Suri J, Rangayyan RM, editors. Recent advances in breast imaging, mammography and computer—aided diagnosis of breast cancer. Bellingham, WA: SPIE Press; 2006. p. 1–49.
33. Tot T. The clinical relevance of the distribution of the lesions in 500 consecutive breast cancer cases documented in large-format histological sections. Cancer. 2007;110:2551–60.
34. Tot T. General morphology of benign and malignant breast lesions: old parameters in new perspectives. In: Suri J, Rangayyan RM, Laxminarayan S, editors. Emerging technologies in breast imaging and mammography. Valencia, CA: American Scientific Publisher; 2008. p. 1–12.
35. de Neergaard M, Kim J, Villadsen R, et al. Epithelial-stromal interaction 1 (EPSTI1) substitutes for peritumoral fibroblasts in the tumor microenvironment. Am J Pathol. 2010;176(3): 1229–40.
36. Asioli S, Eusebi V, Gaetano L, et al. The pre-lymphatic pathway, the roots of the lymphatic system in the breast tissue: a 3D study. Virchows Arch. 2008;453:401–6.
37. Tot T. The diffuse type of invasive lobular carcinoma of the breast: morphology and prognosis. Virchows Arch. 2003;443:718–24.
38. Tot T, Kahán Z. A new approach to early breast cancer. In: Kahán Z, Tot T, editors. Breast cancer, a heterogeneous disease entity. The very early stages. New York: Springer; 2011. p. 1–22.
39. Clarke GM, Eidt S, Sun L, et al. Whole-specimen histopathology: a method to produce whole mount breast serial sections for 3-D digital histopathology imaging. Histopathology. 2007;50:232–42.
40. Egan RL. Multicentric breast carcinoma: clinical-radiographic-pathologic whole organ studies and 10-year survival. Cancer. 1982;49:1123–30.
41. Gallager HS, Martin JE. The study of mammary carcinoma by mammography and whole organ sectioning. Early observations. Cancer. 1969;23:855–73.
42. Holland R, Veling SH, Mravunac M, et al. Histologic multifocality of Tis, T1-2 breast carcinomas. Implications for clinical trials of breast conserving surgery. Cancer. 1985;56:979–90.
43. Foschini MP, Tot T, Eusebi V. Large section (macrosection) histologic slides. In: Silverstein MJ, editor. Ductal carcinoma in situ of the breast. 2nd ed. Philadelphia, PA: Lippincott, Williams and Wilkins; 2002. p. 249–54.
44. Foschini MP, Flamminio F, Miglio R, et al. The impact of large sections on the study of in situ and invasive duct carcinoma of the breast. Hum Pathol. 2007;38:1736–43.
45. Jackson PA, Merchant W, McCormick CJ, Cook MG. A comparison of large block macrosectioning and conventional techniques in breast pathology. Virchows Arch. 1994;425:243–8.
46. Mechine-Neuville MP, Chenard B, Gairard C, et al. Large sections in routine breast pathology. A technique adapted to conservative surgery. Ann Pathol. 2000;20:275–9.
47. Tot T. The metastastic capacity of multifocal breast carcinomas: extensive tumors versus tumors of limited extent. Hum Pathol. 2009;40:199–205.
48. Tot T, Gy P, Hofmeyer S, et al. The distribution of lesions in 1-14-mm invasive breast carcinomas and its relation to metastatic potential. Virchows Arch. 2009;455:109–15.
49. Early Breast Cancer Trialists' Collaborative Group (EBCTCG), Darby S, McGale P, Correa C, et al. Effect of radiotherapy after breast-conserving surgery on 10-year recurrence and 15-year breast cancer death: meta-analysis of individual patient data for 10,801 women in 17 randomised trials. Lancet. 2011;378(9804):1707–16.
50. Simone NL, Dan T, Shih J, et al. Twenty-five year results of the National Cancer Institute randomized breast conservation trial. Breast Cancer Res Treat. 2012;132(1):197–203.
51. Silverstein MJ, Lagios MD. Choosing treatment for patients with ductal carcinoma in situ: fine tuning the University of Southern California/Van Nuys Prognostic Index. J Natl Cancer Inst Monogr. 2010;41:193–6.
52. Tot T. Subgross morphology, the sick lobe hypothesis, and the success of breast conservation. Int J Breast Cancer. 2011;2011:634021. doi:10.4061/2011/634021. Article ID 634021, 8 p.

53. Lindquist D, Hellberg D, Tot T. Disease extent ≥4cm is a prognostic marker of local recurrence in T1-2 breast cancer. Patholog Res Int. 2011;2011:860584.
54. Faverly DRG, Hendricks JHCL, Holland R. Breast carcinoma of limited extent. Frequency, radiologic—pathologic characteristics, and surgical margin requirements. Cancer. 2001;91: 647–59.
55. Holland R, Hendricks JH, Vebeek AL, et al. Extent, distribution, and mammographic/histological correlation of breast ductal carcinoma in situ. Lancet. 1990;335:519–22.
56. Dooley WC. Routine operative breast endoscopy during lumpectomy. Ann Surg Oncol. 2003;10:38–42.
57. Tot T, Gere M, Gy P, et al. Breast cancer multifocality, disease extent, and survival. Hum Pathol. 2011;42(11):1761–9.
58. Andea AA, Wallis T, Newman LA, et al. Pathologic analysis of tumor size and lymph node status in multifocal/multicentric breast carcinoma. Cancer. 2002;94:1383.1390.
59. Coombs NJ, Boyages J. Multifocal and multicentric breast cancer: does each focus matter? J Clin Oncol. 2005;34:7497–502.
60. Pedersen L, Gunnarsdottir KA, Rasmussen BB, et al. The prognostic influence of multifocality in breast cancer patients. Breast. 2004;13:188–93.
61. Boyages J, Jajashinghe UW, Coombs N. Multifocal breast cancer and survival: each focus does matter particularly for larger tumours. Eur J Cancer. 2010;46:1990–6.
62. Weissenbacher TM, Zschage M, Janni W, et al. Multicentric and multifocal versus unifocal breast cancer: is the tumor-node-metastasis classification justified? Breast Cancer Res Treat. 2010;22:27–34.
63. Chung AP, Huynh K, Kidner T, et al. Comparison of outcomes of breast conserving therapy in multifocal and unifocal invasive breast cancer. Am Coll Surg. 2012;215:137–47.

Part II
Image-Based Intervention

Chapter 4
Lobar Ultrasonic Breast Anatomy

Dominque Amy

Introduction

Surgery is founded on the anatomical study of an organ. The understanding of the functioning and pathology of that organ can only be achieved through a precise investigation of its anatomy. These are fundamental precepts that support scientific investigation.

Since the breast is a superficial organ to which one has direct access, its anatomical approach should be easy. And yet, for decades, there has been a great difference between the description of the mammary gland made by anatomopathologists and those made by the whole body of radiologists, surgeons, and oncologists.

The breast has been extensively studied in laboratory by many authors since the work of Astley Cooper in 1840. The description of its various lobes and ducts has been the subject of numerous publications, but the transposition of these studies into radiological diagnosis and surgery has not been carried out.

J. Going in Professor T. Tot's volume: Breast Cancer 2011, states the obvious fact [1]. The very phrase "normal breast tissue" often used to describe what is inside the mammary gland does not correspond to anatomical fact.

The real question to be answered should be: Is it possible to have direct visualization of a lobe, its ductal axis and lobules and to identify Termino-Ducto-Lobular Units?

The classical techniques used in breast imagery (standard or digital mammography with or without tomosynthesis, galactography, conventional echography, magnetic resonance, etc.) do not allow us to achieve an anatomical investigation but are directed towards the search for a lesion or a tumor.

Mammography, which remains the gold standard in the field of diagnosis is unable to meet this first requirement, the visualization of ducts and lobules which are radio-transparent.

D. Amy, M.D. (✉)
Department of Radiology, Centre Du Sein, B du Rhone, France
e-mail: domamy@unandoo.fr

D.S. Francescatti and M.J. Silverstein (eds.), *Breast Cancer: A New Era in Management*,
DOI 10.1007/978-1-4614-8063-1_4, © Springer Science+Business Media New York 2014

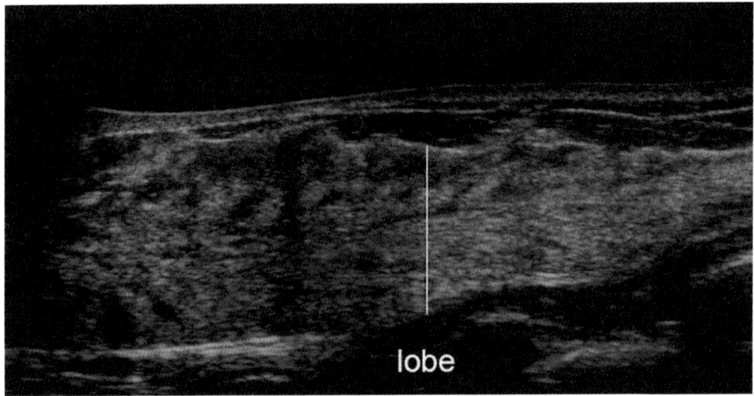

Fig. 4.1 Young woman thick lobe with lobular and ductal hyperplasia and poor fatty tissue

As a direct consequence, the surgeon has no anatomical reference point during the surgical procedure. No imaging technique used today for diagnosis can provide an anatomical waypoint.

And yet, there exists an ultrasound technique described by M. Teboul published in 1995 [2] that describes the technique of ductal echography that makes possible the visualization of lobar, lobular and ductal structures with the ability to localize TDLUs within the lobes in real time. Today this technique is the sole imaging modality capable of providing an accurate anatomical approach to the mammary gland. Punctual echography is performed routinely in the diagnostic imaging evaluation of the breast.

The major advantages offered by ductal ecographic examination of the breast include the following:

- A precise anatomical study of breast structures based on morphological analysis of each of the lobes and the demonstration of the anatomical elements.
- A visual analysis of any modifications in a lobe or duct.
- Early detection of pre-tumorous or suspicious lesions.
- Lobar morphological variations that reflect the menopausal state of the individual patient (Figs. 4.1, 4.2, 4.3, and 4.4).

The Concept of Breast Study

Breast pathology is a pathology of the epithelial cells. Mammary epithelium is located along the acino-ductal axis and is found in every lobe. The lobe of the breast is, in part, composed of fibrous and fatty tissue. The functional breast is limited by the external skin and lies on the internal pectoral muscle.

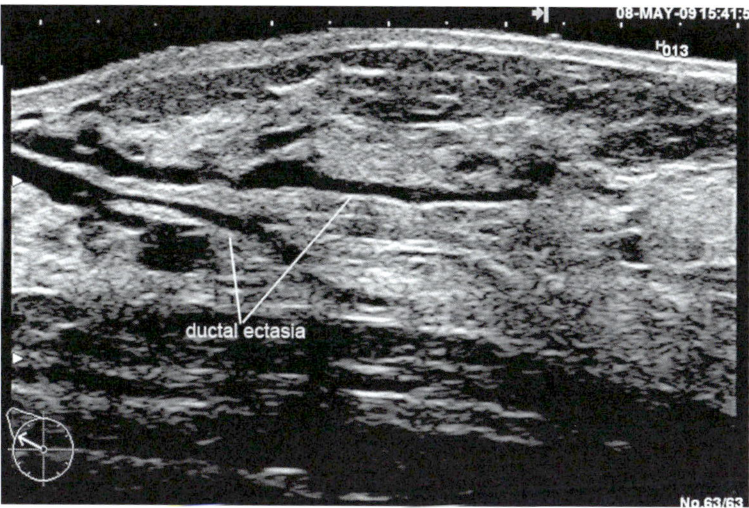

Fig. 4.2 Ultrasonic scan of an adult breast: ductal ectasia in the main ducts

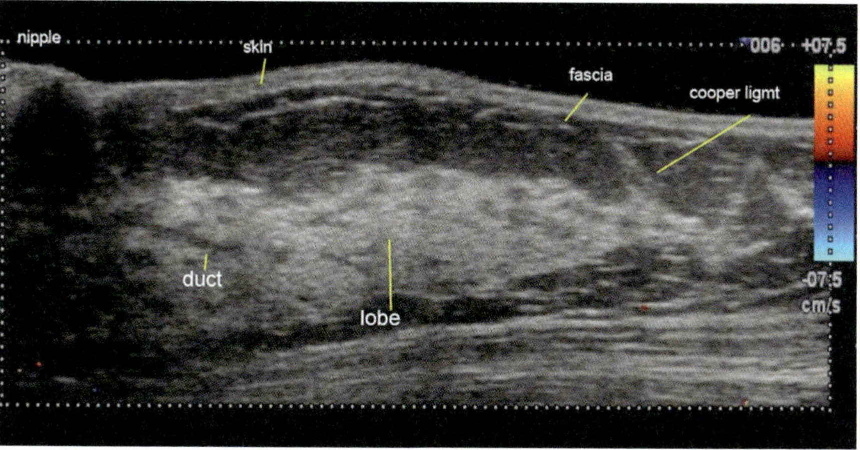

Fig. 4.3 Premenopausal lobar reduction and fatty thickening

The primary goal of DE is the investigation of the ductal axis and its lobules, as well as a study of the entire lobe and ligamentous structures and any pathological modifications (both within and external to the lobe itself).

It is essential to distinguish conventional breast echography from that of ductal echography.

Conventional echography utilizes systematic orthogonal scanning of all breast quadrants with a high frequency probe of limited length. This technique is used by 90 % of the radiologists.

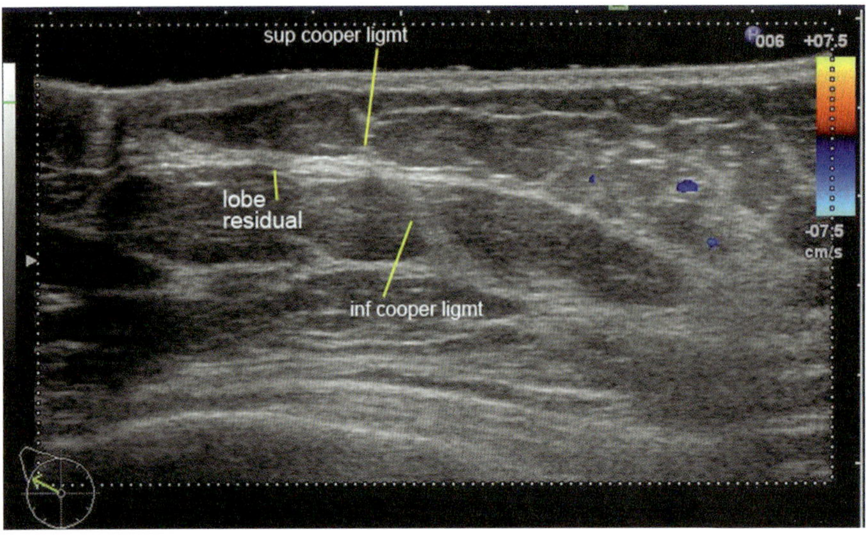

Fig. 4.4 Postmenopausal important lobar involution

Ductal echography in contradistinction employs radial technique with concentric scanning circumferentially performed around the nipple examining each individual lobe by locating first each lobal duct at the N/A junction and following it to its terminos. If done properly, the tail of spence, if present, will be investigated fully. The technique is best performed with a lung transducer and use of a water bag mat will prevent pressure induced obfuscation of potentially diagnostic clues. The examination is carried out on the supine patient and does not take longer than 10 min for the investigation of a lesion-free breast by an experienced sonographer.

This technique allows the anatomical study of the breast and correlates remarkably with the large anatomico-pathological sections achieved by Professor Tibor Tot (Figs. 4.5, 4.6, and 4.7).

Examination of these sections allows the investigation to see with precision:

- The nipple with its internal ductal structures, the areola and the skin.
- Under the skin, a thin layer of fat limited by the fascia superficialis.
- The fascia linked to the skin by fine conjunctival structures: the retinacula cutis.
- Below the fascia the presence of fatty tissue towering above the elongated shape of the mammary lobe.
- The upper surface of the lobe bristling with Cooper's ligaments connecting the lobe to the fascia superficialis.
- The distal part of the lobe ending with ligaments (those connecting the lobes to the sub-clavicular area are called Giraldes ligaments).
- The lower portion of the lobe giving a reversed mirror image of the upper portion with shorter lower ligaments connecting it to the lower fascia.
- The fascia wending its way along the pectoral muscle.

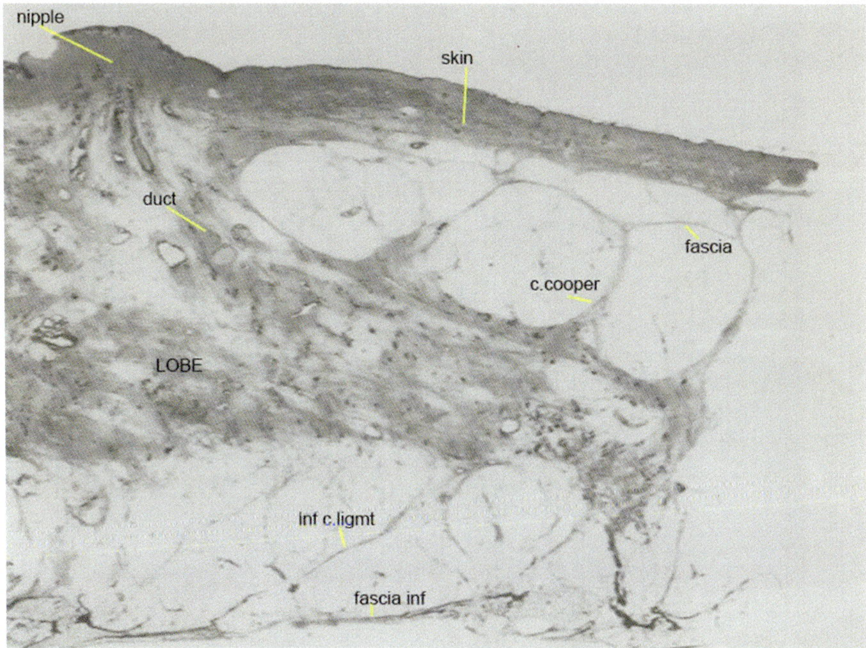

Fig. 4.5 Large anatomopathological breast section: all the anatomic elements are perfectly identified (courtesy of Pr T. Tot Sweden)

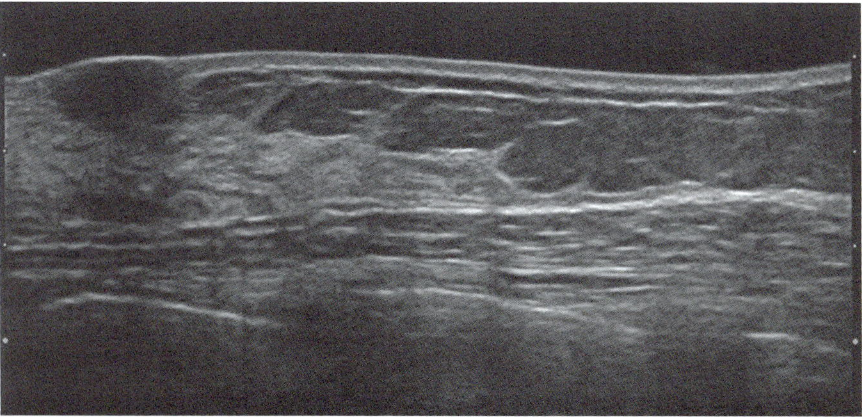

Fig. 4.6 Perfect correlation of the ducto-lobar echography: evidence of the exact similitude with the anatomical description

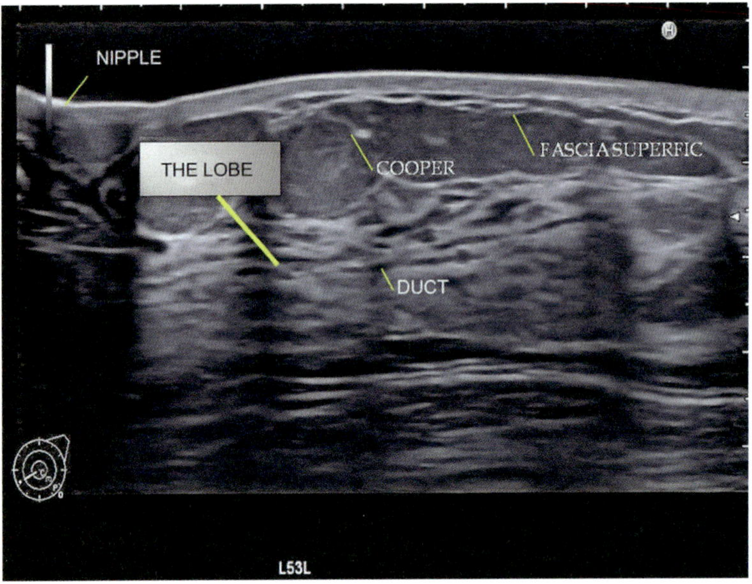

Fig. 4.7 Another ducto-lobar echography

Relationship Between Anatomy and the Development of Breast Cancers

In the early detection of breast cancers, the initial modifications of Cooper's ligaments and the fasciae correspond to the first extra-lobar signs of the development of cancer, as described by Gallager and Martin in their 1969 publications [3] and by Nakama in his 1991 publications [4].

In their first article "early phases in the development of breast cancer," Gallager describes the involvement of the conjunctival tissue in the initial carcinogenic process.

J de Brux in his 1979 book "Histopathology of the Breast" underlines this as well. Lastly, in several publications, Nakama describes the "invasive process of the breast and fixation to the skin." He shows that cancerous cells together with lymphocytes, histiocytes, and fibroblasts migrate along Cooper's ligaments towards the fascia superficialis and the skin.

Therefore it is obvious that it is essential to identify the ligaments and the fasciae to discover early modifications.

On a radial lobar section, T. Tot shows the localization of a small breast cancer at the junction of a Cooper's ligament with the ductal axis (Fig. 4.8).

All the investigations cited confirm localization of lesions (both benign and malignant) in Cooper's ligaments. The Termino-Ducto-Lobular Unit is the nidus where lesions will develop and are to be found at the base of the ligaments.

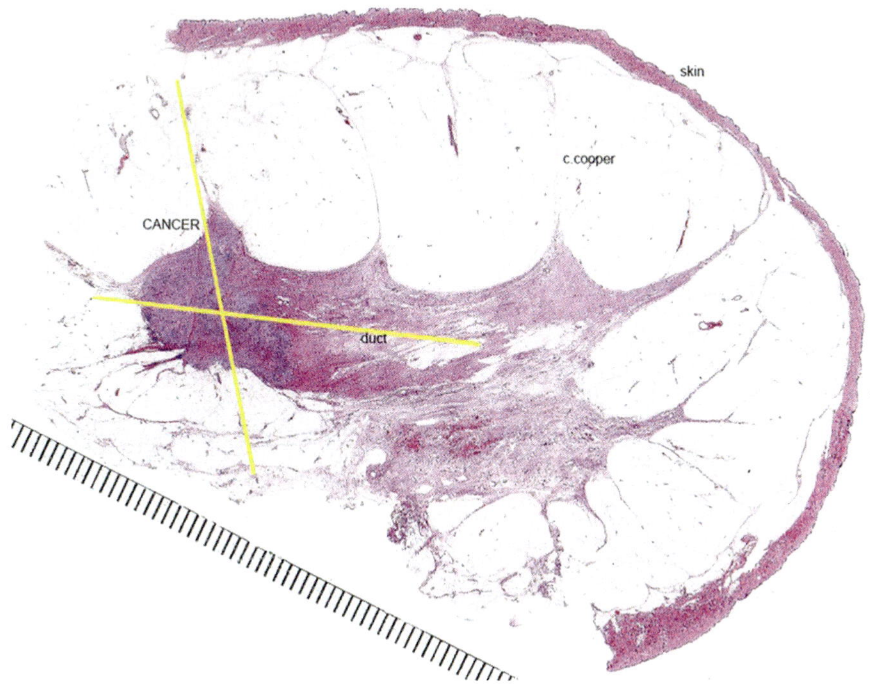

Fig. 4.8 very large lobar anatomopathological section with a small cancer located at the crossing section of a ductal axis and a cooper ligament axis (TDULs) (courtesy of Pr T. Tot)

To be able to identify the millimetric anatomical elements involved in the millimetric pathology of the breast is enormously helpful in the early diagnosis of breast cancer. Therefore one must search for these initial modifications in these very elements.

The remarkable correlation between ultrasound and anatomopathology is visualized in the example displayed below. The discovery of the primary cancer combined with multifocal and multicentric lesions made mastectomy necessary (Figs. 4.9, 4.10, and 4.11): ducto-radial ultrasound, a one centimeter thick image of a large section of the breast and an anatomopathological study on an 8 cm long glass plate.

This investigation was carried out in collaboration with Pr DI Marino and Dr. Rojat-Habib from the Medical University of Marseilles.

Ductal echography allows a precise anatomical study of the ducts (with ectasia here) and of the initial tumor (with two additional younger neoplastic foci on either side of the cancer) along a ductal axis.

No other technique in medical imagery offers this degree of analytical quality and precision particularly in the case of multifocal lesions.

The discovery of multifocal, multicentric, or diffuse lesions opens a new perspective in the understanding of breast cancer. In the light of Prof. Tibor Tot's publications [1, 5–7], cancer must no longer be considered as an isolated event but as a

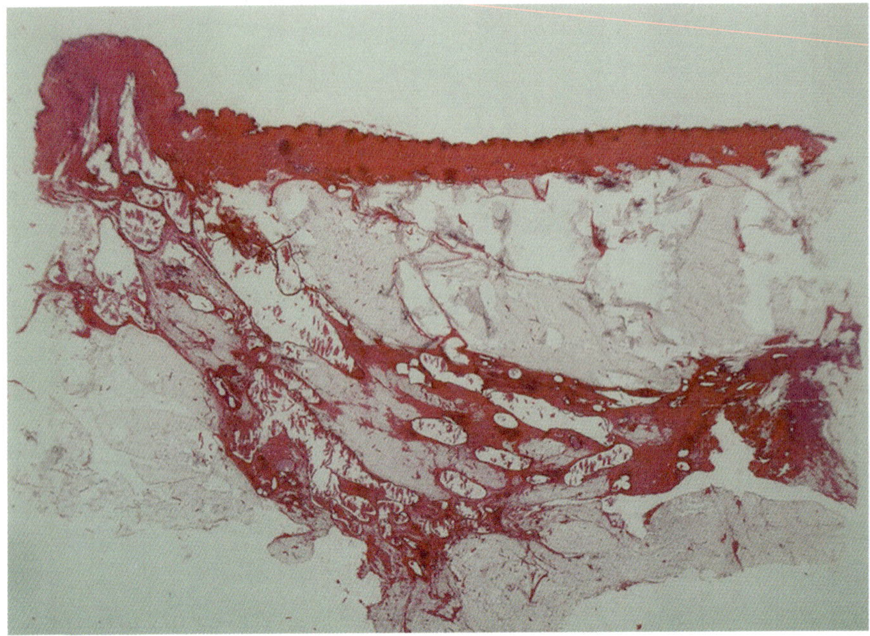

Fig. 4.9 Wide anatomopathologic section of a lobe with ductal ectasia associated with two pathologic fosi (cancer) at the distal lobar extremity. The ductal echographic correlation is remarkable (courtesy Dr. Rojat Habib, France)

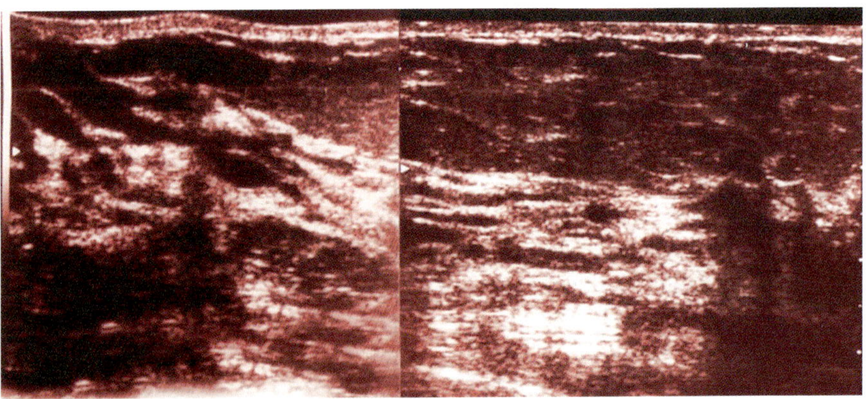

Fig. 4.10 Echographic correlation with Fig. 4.9

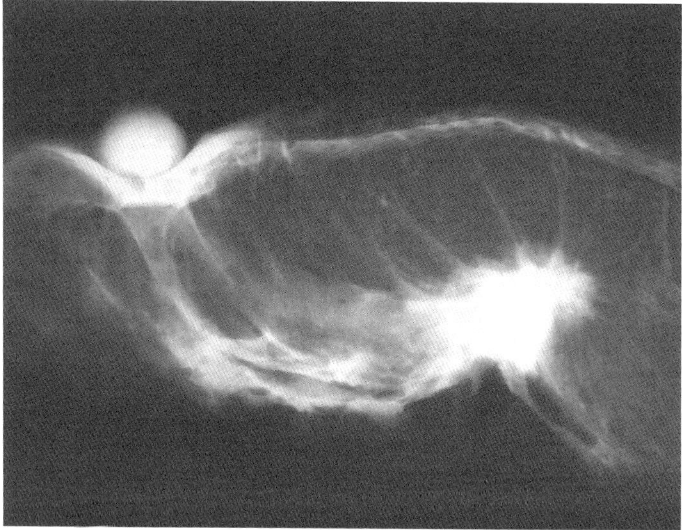

Fig. 4.11 Radiological analysis of a slice (1cm thick)

disease of the breast. Its development can be single, multifocal, multicentric, simultaneous, or delayed, affect a single lobe or several. The standard definition of multifocal or multicentric lesions must be amended: multifocal corresponds to several foci within a same lobe, while multicentric is used when several lobes are affected.

For the radiologist, there remain a small percentage of cancers which are diagnostic nightmares: the rare diffuse lobular cancer which not visible mammography and barely visible on echography. The echographic sections presented opposite illustrate cases of multiple cancers (Figs. 4.12, 4.13, 4.14, 4.15, 4.16, 4.17, 4.18, and 4.19).

Echo-Surgical Implications

The radiologist should incorporate mammography in conjunction with ductal echography to increase diagnostic yield.

Indeed, micro-calcifications which are obvious on a mammogram are rarely visible on echography. It is for accurate mapping of the diseased area, necessary to combine the two techniques. If this is done, at the conclusion of the study, the examiner can produce a more precise map of the lesion(s) in reference to their clockwise location (right breast at 12 o'clock) and the distance (7 cm from the nipple, 2 cm deep). Importantly, these measurements should be taken with the patient in the operating position with the arm at 90°.

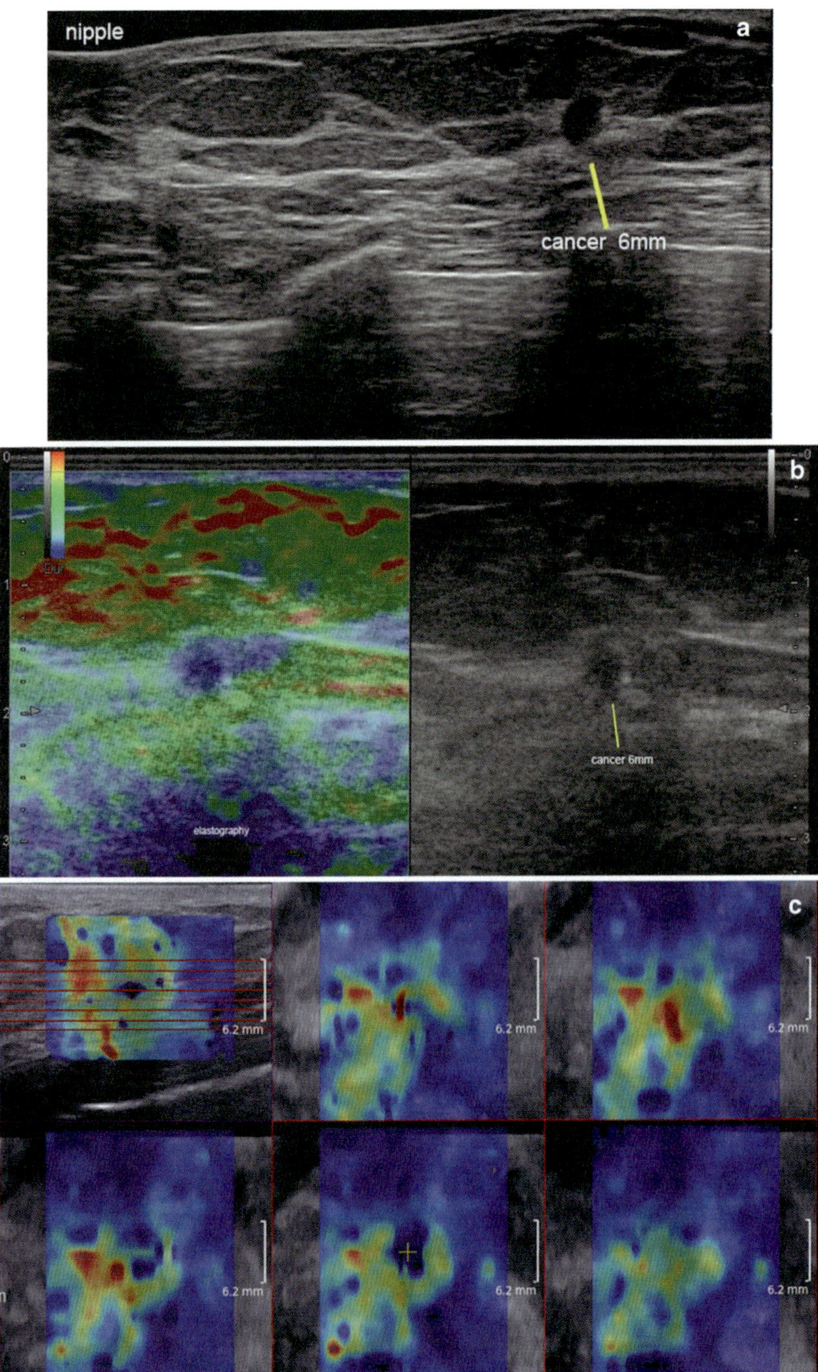

Fig. 4.12 Millimetric breast carcinoma within an involuted lobe. The complementary elastographic analysis (with the two techniques: strain (**a**), (**b**), and shear-wave (**c**)) confirm the malignancy

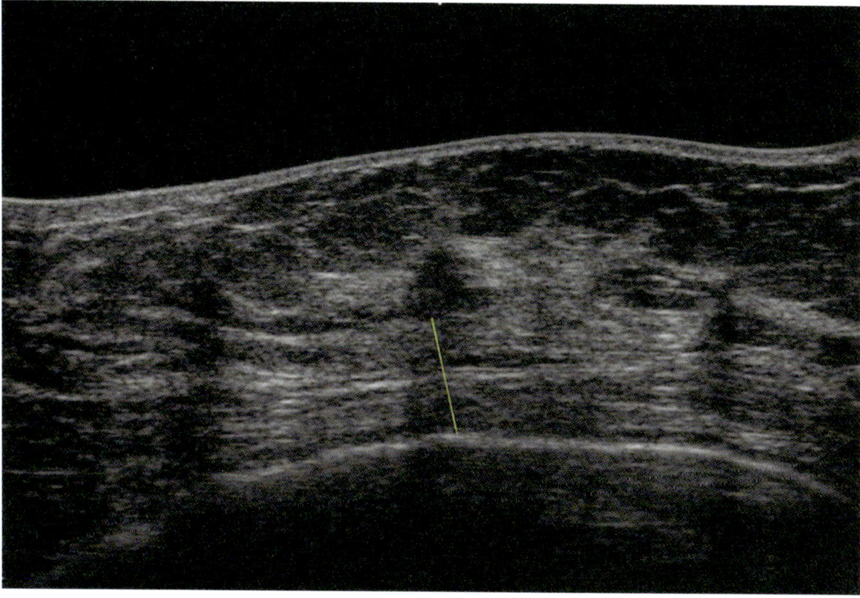

Fig. 4.13 A lobular millimetric carcinoma in a TDLUs located in the middle part of the lobe: hypoechogenic structure along the duct axis

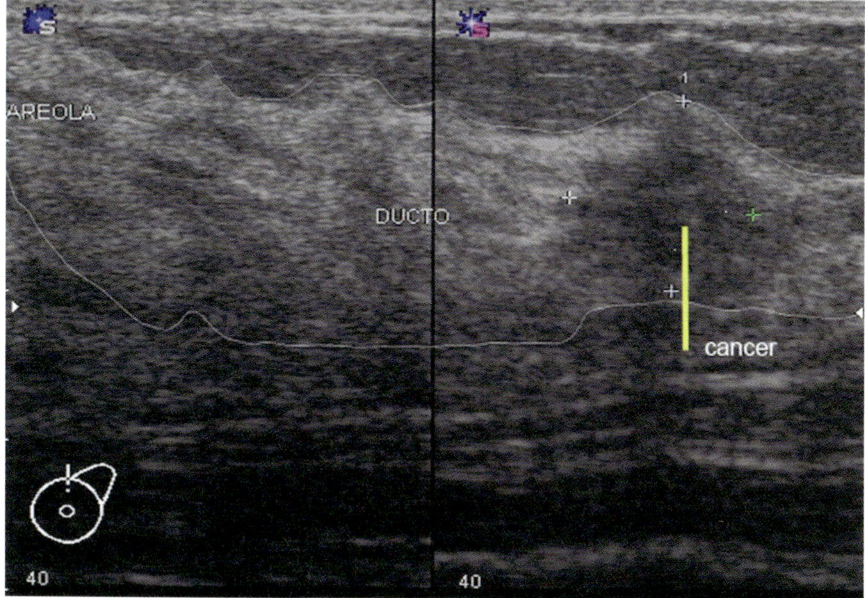

Fig. 4.14 Breast cancer at the lobar extremity: hypoechogenic irregular nodule

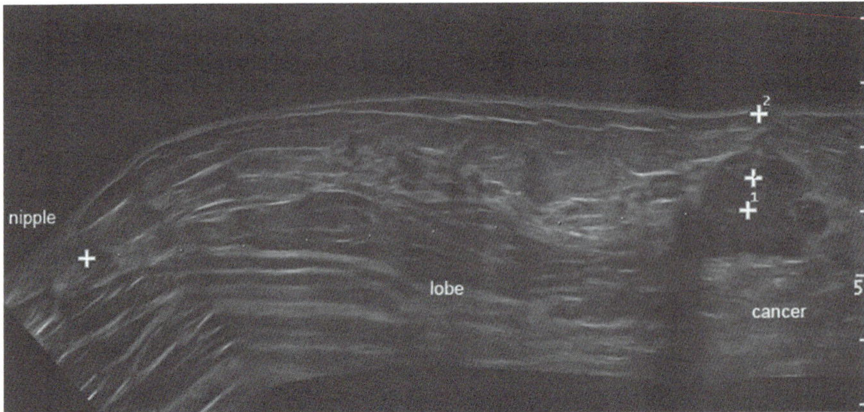

Fig. 4.15 Panoramic seascape ultrasonic scan of a centimetric cancer

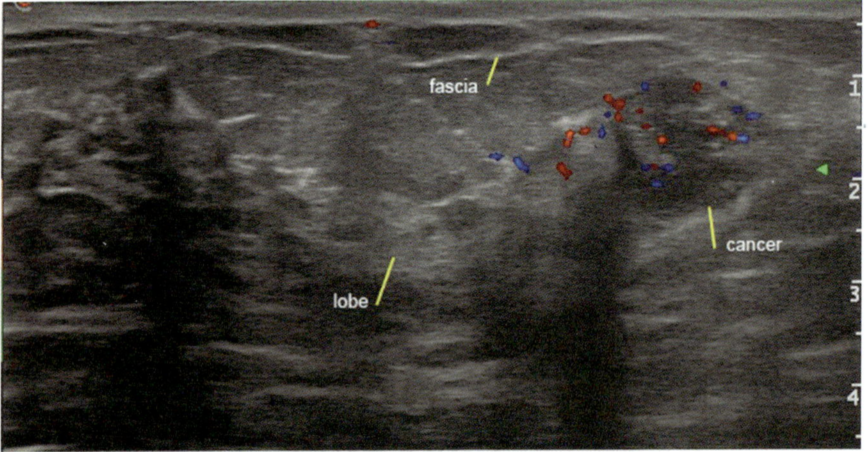

Fig. 4.16 Ducto-radial echography with a centimetric cancer at the lobar distal extremity

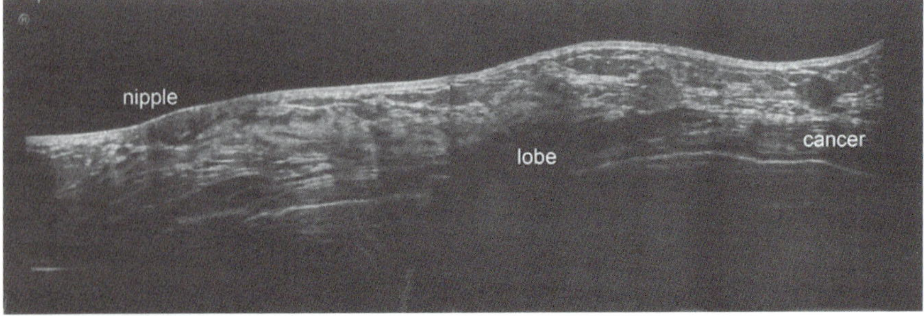

Fig. 4.17 A very long lobe exploration with a sub centimetric carcinoma at the distal extremity

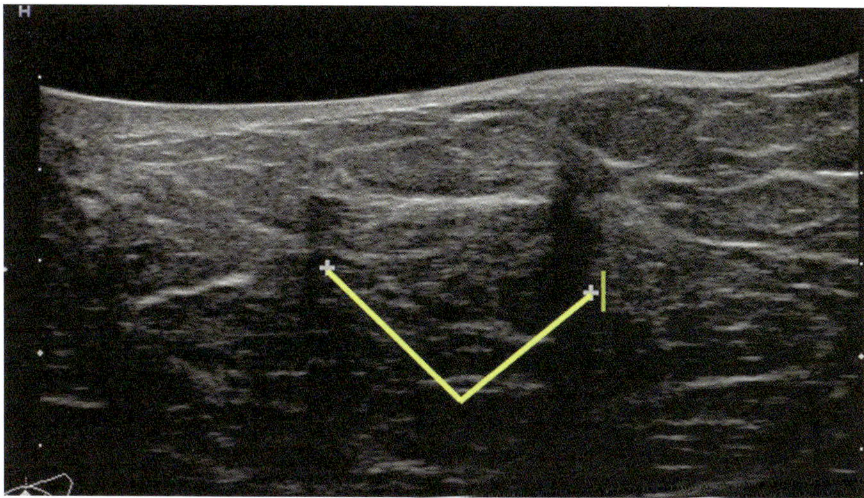

Fig. 4.18 Bifocal millimetric cancer with two hypoechogenic micro nodules in an involuted residual lobe

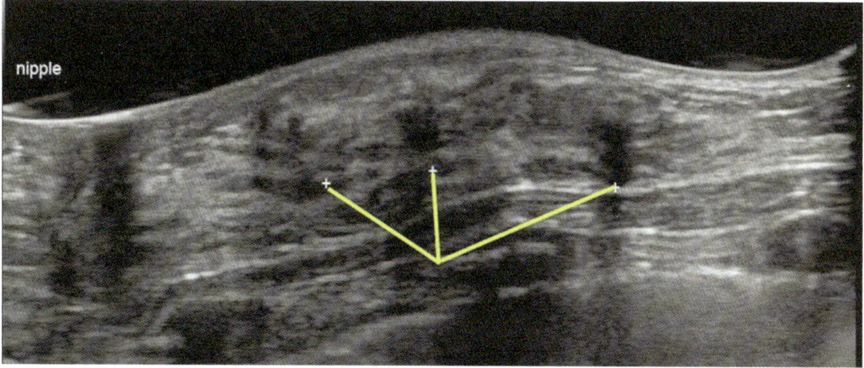

Fig. 4.19 Three millimetric hypoechogenic malignant foci in a young woman right breast, lobe at 10 o'clock

The surgeon will then have a more precise localization of the lesion(s). If he so wishes, real time ultrasound at the time of surgery can confirm the findings. Preoperative knowledge of the condition of the lobe or lobes involved will aid the choice of the most appropriate resection. The analysis of margins around the tumor will be replaced circumference of the resected specimen by the lobal bonder(s).

Because of cancerous cellular migration into Cooper's ligaments, it will be necessary to take into account the relationship of the skin and underlying conjunctival ligamentary tissues viz a viz the cancer.

The information provided by ductal echography will therefore guide and direct the surgical resection as depicted by Prof. Giancarlo Dolfin. This technique will insure a more anatomical resection of the diseased lobe and result in a marked decrease in the reexcision rate.

Conclusion

As a result of the research work carried out by Gallager, Nakama, Going, Teboul, Tot [1, 2, 4, 5, 8] and many others in the decades past, therapeutical progress in the surgical treatment and understanding of breast cancer is ongoing.

The simultaneous development of new echographic techniques (in combination with standard breast imagery) and of the understanding of the disease of breast cancer disease through Pr. T. Tot's research work will enable the surgeon to plan and achiever an optimal cancer resection.

The rediscovery of lobar anatomy of the breast via Ductal Echtography is an enormous stride forward in image analysis of the breast.

The understanding of the stages in the development of the mammary gland, both morphological and physiological, has additional implications in mammary imagery. As an example, galactography should be replaced by ductal echography, a technique that allows to visualization of the entire duct, its contents, the surrounding environment and relationship to the observed lesions.

The ability to visualize cancerous pathology at the millimetric level is a third major advancement.

The ability to detect multifocal and/or multicentric lesions is a reality utilizing the technique of Ductal Echography pioneered by Teboul. In his work "Breast Ultrasound" (2006), STRAVROS recommended searching for other lesions immediately after discovering a first tumor, utilizing the technique of DE.

As importantly, the pathologic confirmations brought by anatomopathologists and most especially by Prof. T. Tot helps researchers in their quest to unravel the secrets of breast cancer.

Through his exceptional work involving several thousand pathologic investigations over 20 years, Prof. T. Tot encourages the widespread use of ductal echography in the image analysis of the breast.

In the conclusion to his latest book, he writes that more than one cancer patient out of two is the carrier of a multifocal and/or multicentric or diffuse cancer. Awareness of those patients will ensure better local therapy. The use of Color Doppler has increased detection and more recently, 3/4 D probes have increased the detection threshold.

Lastly, the use of mammary elastography (strain technique and/or shear-wave technique SWE) in conjunction with 3D acquisition has significantly enhanced the specificity of sonographic investigation. Preliminary results show that modifications in elasticity around the cancer (stroma reaction, desmoplastic reactions, vascular modifications, etc.) can be analyzed and can visually attest to the effectiveness of primary chemotherapy through a reduction in the elastographical alterations around the lesions. Results must be confirmed by additional studies (Fig. 4.12).

The treatment of breast cancer today now more than ever is dependent on a multidisciplinary, highly specialized team approach, in order to achieve a seamless coordination leading to better management of the individual patient.

The combination of early diagnosis based on precise anatomical investigation, adaptive surgical techniques and improved, personalized oncological treatments predicated on genomic analysis will lead to markedly improved outcomes in the treatment of breast cancer.

Acknowledgment Various colleagues throughout the world, who practise Ductal Echography on a daily basis, have welcomed my invitation to have their share in this chapter:
by courtesy of:
Fig. 2: Dr. G. Dolfin, Italy.
Fig. 3/4: Dr. A. Georgescu, Roumania.
Fig. 7: Dr. G. Kern, France.
Fig. 14: Dr. J. Parada, Uruguay.
Fig. 15/16: Dr. J. Amoros, Spain (in memoriam).
Fig. 17: Dr. V. Buljevic, Croatia.

References

1. Tot T, editor. Breast Cancer a lobar disease. London: Springer; 2011.
2. Teboul M, Halliwell M. Atlas ultrasound and ductal echography of the breast. Oxford: Blackwell Science; 1995. p. 115631.
3. Gallager S, Martin J. Early phases in the development of breast cancer. Cancer. 1969;24(6): 1170–8.
4. Nakama S. Comparative Studies on Ultrasonogram with Histological Structure of Breast Cancer: An Examination in the Invasive Process of Breast Cancer and the Fixation to the Skin. In: Kasumi R, Ueno E, editors. Topic in breast ultrasound. Tokyo: Shinohara Publishers Inc.; 1991.
5. Tot T. The diffuse type of invasive lobular carcinoma of the breast: morphology and prognosis. Virchows Arch. 2003;443:718–24.
6. Tot T. Clinical relevance of the distribution of the lesions in 500 consecutive breast cancer cases documented in large—format histologic sections. Cancer. 2007;110:2551–60.
7. Tot T. The theory of the sick breast lobe and the possible consequences. Int J Surg Pathol. 2007;13:68–71.
8. Teboul M. Practical ductal echography. Madrid: Editorial Medgen SA; 2004.

Suggested Reading

Amoros OJ. Cancer du sein: critères échographiques de malignité. J Mensuel Echogr. 2000;10:672–86.

Amy D. Echographie Mammaire: écho-anatomie. J.L mensuel d'échographie LUS 2000. N° 10. 654.62.

Amy D. Millimetric breast carcinoma ultrasonic detection in leading edge conference Pr. Goldbert B; May 2005.

Amy. D. Introduction and principal of elastography. 6th Biennale meeting of the Asian Breast Cancer Society. Hongkong. 2007.

Amy D. Lobar ultrasound of the breast. Chap. 8. In: T. Tot, éditor. Breast cancer a lobar disease. London: Springer-Verlag London Limited; 2011.

Dolfin G, Chebib A, Amy D, Tagliabue P. 30e S2MINAIRE franchosyrien d'Imagerie Médicale. Tartous-Syrie 10–12/06/08 Carcinome mammaire et chirurgie conservatrice.

Durante E. Multimodality imaging and interventional techniques. IBUS Course Abstracts Ferrara Sept 2006.

Going JJ, Al. Human breast ductal anatomy, the sick lobe hypothesis and intraductal approach to breast cancer. 2006.

Stavros T. Breast ultrasound. Philadelphia, PA: Lippincott Williams and Wilkins; 2006.

Chapter 5
The Surgical Approach to the "Sick Lobe"

Giancarlo Dolfin

Introduction

In senology, it is essential to have a good genetic, anatomical, physiological and diagnostic knowledge to choose the best surgical treatment in case of breast carcinoma.

This chapter points out the utility to correlate radial echographic technique diagnosis (introduced by Michel Teboul) and conservative surgical therapy.

To reiterate, breast cancer arises at the epithelium level of one TDLU (Terminal Ductal Lobular Unit) or multiple TDLUs of the same lobe synchronously or asynchronously as well as from the ductal epithelium. From here a single nubis, growth may occur in three main ways:

1. It may invade the surrounding highly vascularized soft tissues, thus appearing as a star-shaped lesion.
2. It may spread via the lymphatic system and cause distant metastasis, and metastasize via blood vessels (particularly in the lobular type).
3. Or it may spread via a ductal dissemination, up to and including the nipple; the involvement of the nipple–areola complex is estimated to be between 11 and 54 %.[1]

As described by Tibor Tot, breast carcinoma is pathology that involves the entire lobe. Tot emphasizes that volume, morphology and orientations of different lobes can be variable and not always regular. This is a practical problem in the accurate

[1] The risk of spreading to the nipple is related to the tumor's size (only 17 % of cases when it is less than 10 mm). When spreads to the nipple, 25 % of cases are invasive cancer, while in 15 % of other cases it is both invasive and in situ. In most cases the tumor is limited to a small area (deeper than 5 mm from surface) and consists of a completely intraductal cellular extension (almost 60 % of the cases).

G. Dolfin, M.D. (✉)
Department of Ginecologia, Oncologia Clinica, Corso Cosenza 35, 10137 Torino, Italy
e-mail: giancarlodolfin@gmail.com

D.S. Francescatti and M.J. Silverstein (eds.), *Breast Cancer: A New Era in Management*, DOI 10.1007/978-1-4614-8063-1_5, © Springer Science+Business Media New York 2014

localization of a cancerous lesion prior to surgery. A more precise method is called for.

To this end, ecography made with scans and introduced by Teboul, enables a more precise localization of the lobar structure, as well as it's major axis detected by the course of the main duct. Lobar structures, usually invisible to the eye and mammographically, become highly visible under ultrasounds.

Utilizing ductal echography, cancerous structural irregularity, including indirect surrounding signs, highlight pathologic area.

The integration of different diagnostic methodologies enables the surgeon to make a more precise resection based on anatomical information provided by ductal echography.

Of equal importance, more than 75 % of detected tumors will be T1 stage, clinically presenting even greater challenges.

In the collective imagination, breast is related to the sexual and relational life and to the wellbeing: always in the foreground of the advertising spots (on papers, on TV, etc.), breast has become an organ with specific esthetic standards of form and volume.

Breast Surgery

The improvement of diagnostic imaging techniques permits earlier diagnosis, therefore the possibility of employing a more limited surgical operation to remove the cancerous area is feasible. High-resolution sonographic equipments and minimally invasive diagnostic techniques such as needle biopsy (cytological or histological samples) have accelerated this process.

In 1988, Enzo Durante reduced its percentage of relapses to 0.6 %, using conservative surgery. His technique incorporated the removal the sick ductal tree up to the nipple. In this operation, the skin incision is made along Langer lines. The breast glandular tissue is then dissected from the skin and muscular fascia. The isolated cancerous segment is then removed, keeping a margin of at least 10 mm from the cancer. By not mobilizing the nipple–areola complex, areola scar tissue occurred.

A variant of this technique has been developed that markedly reduces scar formation. For this reason, it is difficult to comply with the main principle of the surgical radicality. Furthermore, only an anatomically correct resection will transform an inexact surgical resection into a more precise operation based on anatomopathologic waypoints.

In this way, the surgeries led to the concept of a precise lobectomy as a better way to resect a cancerous breast lesion.

Choice of Surgical Treatment

In considering breast lobectomy as a surgical option, for patients two requisites are essential:

1. Unifocal cancer, less than 20 mm
2. The exclusion of multicentricity

   Affected lobules have alterations in structure, morphology, vascularization and these features can be highlighted by ductal echography. Multifocality is defined as neoplastic foci in the same lobe (not in the same quadrant), as defined by Tibor Tot and the "sick lobe theory".

   The technique of operation is based upon an "ultrasound-guided lobectomy" performed "real time" at the time of operation.

   Identified landmarks can demarcate the lesion but not the borders of the affected lobe. Sonographic identification of the lobar main duct will direct the lobar resection.

Two additional factors of importance:

1. The distance from skin, fascia, and nipple with evaluation of their possible involvement.

   Carcinoma must be included in the glandular tissue, without growth into the muscular fascia or skin: if skin is involved it is possible to remove the overlying affected skin as well as the underlying area with its Cooper's ligaments, that run from the cancerous area to the skin.
2. Aquiring nodal analysis should be based on histological analysis of invasion.
   Contraindications to this surgical approach include the following:

   - Multicentric lesions (more than one lobe involved) or previous irradiation of the breast.
   - Collagen disease and associated altered skin vascularization.

Preparation of the Patient in the Operating Room

Evaluation of preoperative ductal echography is essential. The main duct should be identified since it corresponds to the longitudinal axis of the lobe; the duct should be followed from the nipple to the end of the lobe; Fig. 5.1 demonstrates a pathological area at a distance of 50 mm from the nipple and irregularity along the main duct.

The patient is placed on the operating table with the arm at 90°.

At this point a "real-time" ultrasound localization of the cancer and evaluation of the nearby tissues is performed (see Figs. 5.2 and 5.3).

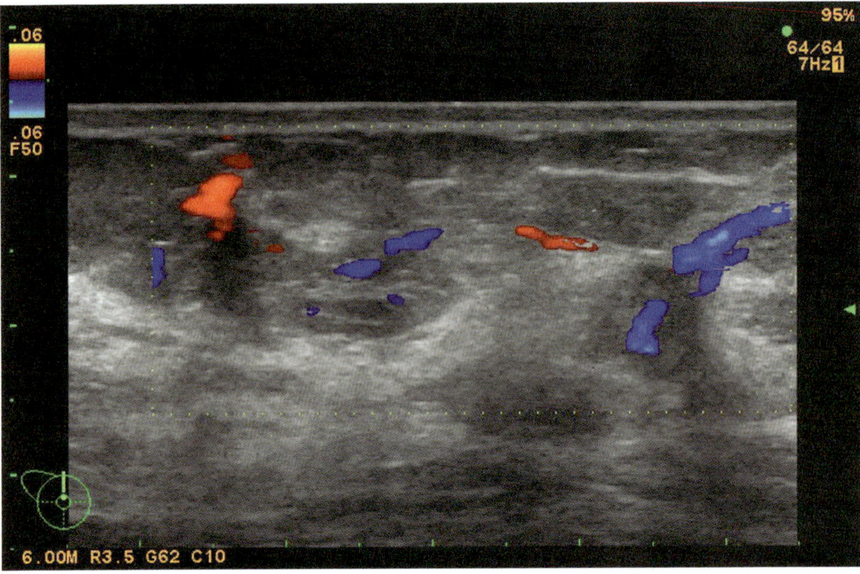

Fig. 5.1 Ducto-radial scan in ultrasound examination of the breast; lobe with a structural anomaly situated at a distance of 50 mm from the nipple; irregular patterns along the main duct and the longitudinal axis of the lobe

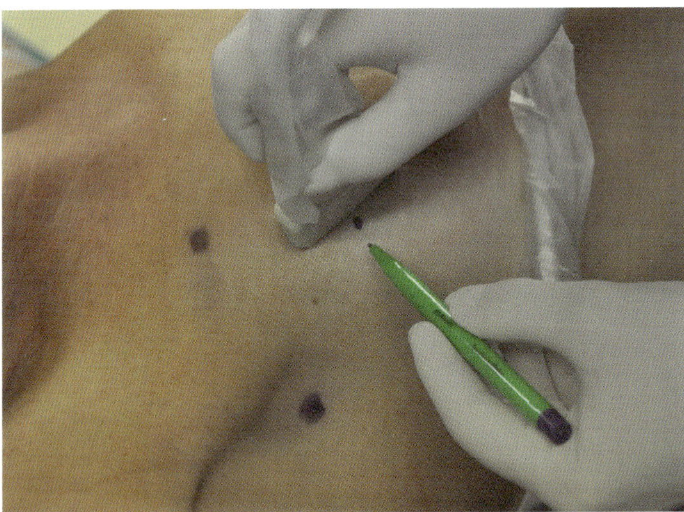

Fig. 5.2 The surgeon controls, with the ducto-radial method scanning, the lesion and the nearby tissues and marks its epidermic correspondence

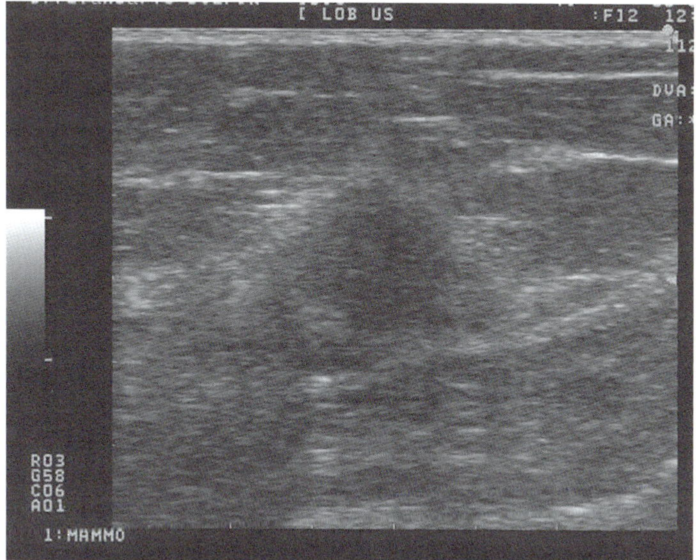

Fig. 5.3 Ultrasonic picture of the lesion

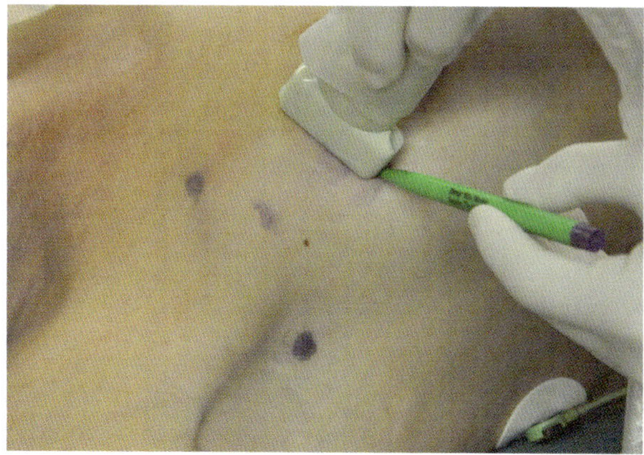

Fig. 5.4 Antiradial scan and draw of the lateral zone, marking the limits of the lesion and nearby modified areas

An outline of the ductal axis and associated abnormalities is then outlined on the overlying skin with a marker. The duct is traced from the nipple areola border to the distal end (see Fig. 5.4).

A transverse evaluation of the lobe is now performed which marks the lateral extent of the resection inclusive of a 10 mm "bulge" around the affected zone (see Fig. 5.5).

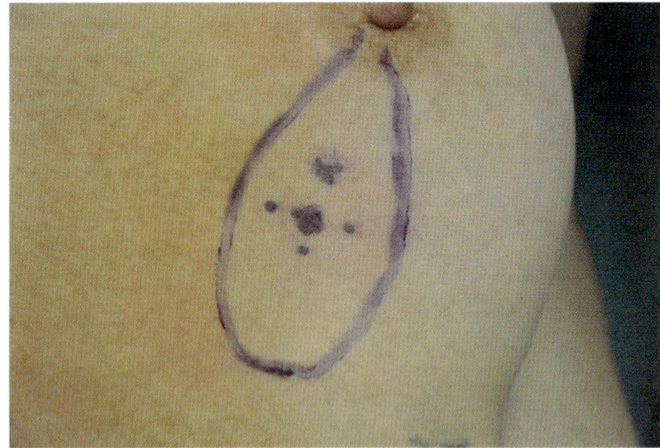

Fig. 5.5 Design of the lateral surgical resection borders, containing the affected lobe, whose borders are distant unless 10 mm from the lesion's localization

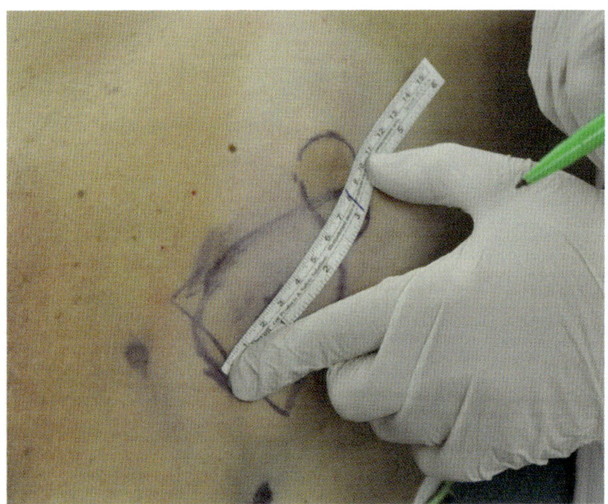

Fig. 5.6 The figure of the glandular area to remove is assimilated to a triangle area

Evaluate the glandular area to be removed (length of duct) and draw a triangular area[2] (apex at N.A.) overlying the duct (base at peripheral limit of duct) (see Fig. 5.6).

It is important to remember one should consider removal of an area of periareolar epidermis (circular sector) corresponding to the surface of the skin area above the lobe to be removed.

Mark the border of the areola. Evaluate the skin area to be removed around the areola. It must be equal to an annulus of epidermis with the inner circumference already marked.

[2] Area of the triangle: half of base times height.

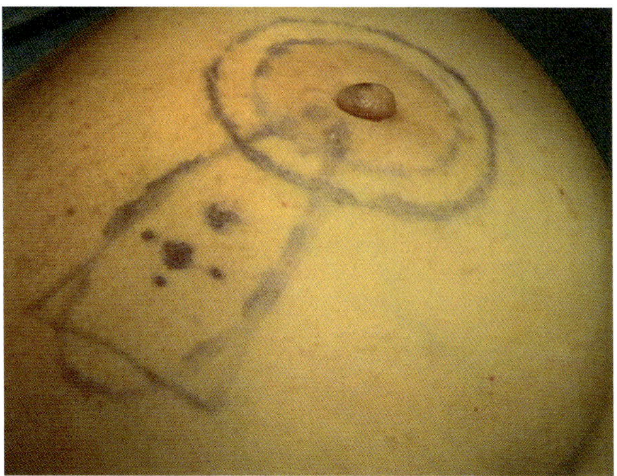

Fig. 5.7 Design of the periareolar circular ring

You can apply the formula of the annulus[3] to obtain the radius (R) of the outer circumference of the annulus: the distance between the nipple and the maior circle.

Then draw points to obtain the second circumference with radius R and one arrives at the expected circular ring. At this point the area to be removed is known. It must be equal to the breast parenchymal area removed (see Fig. 5.7).

Bear in mind that the skin area limited by the picture of the annulus corresponds to the area of the redundant skin that must be removed in order to balance the deficit of glandular tissue removed in the lobar resection.

Procedural Steps

Axillary evaluation if required.

With the breast cone stetched, start with the incision along the areola border and continue the incision along both the superior and inferior line of resection (see Fig. 5.8).

This is followed by the removal of the epithelial strip in the marked zone between the areola line and the outside perimeter, keeping the vascular plexus undamaged (see Fig. 5.9). This is essential for the visibility of the areola–nipple complex (see Fig. 5.10).

The dermis is incised on the outside perimeter along the outlined length to expose the breast parenchyma in order to proceed with the resection of the fixed glandular portion (see Fig. 5.11).

A subcutaneous dissection of the nipple (3–4 mm in depth) is then done. Grasp the zone with a forceps, to mark the central point of resection (see Fig. 5.12a and b).

---

[3] Area of the annulus: area of the large circle minus area of the small circle → $\pi R^2 - \pi r^2$.

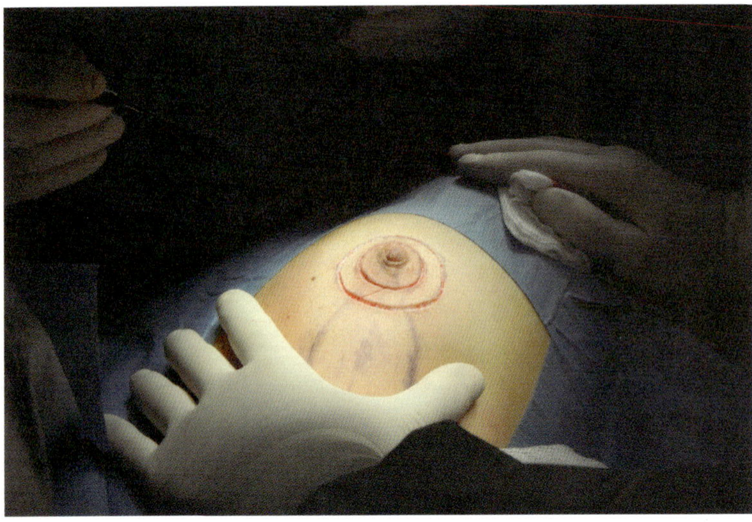

Fig. 5.8 Incision of the two circumferences of the periareolar circular ring

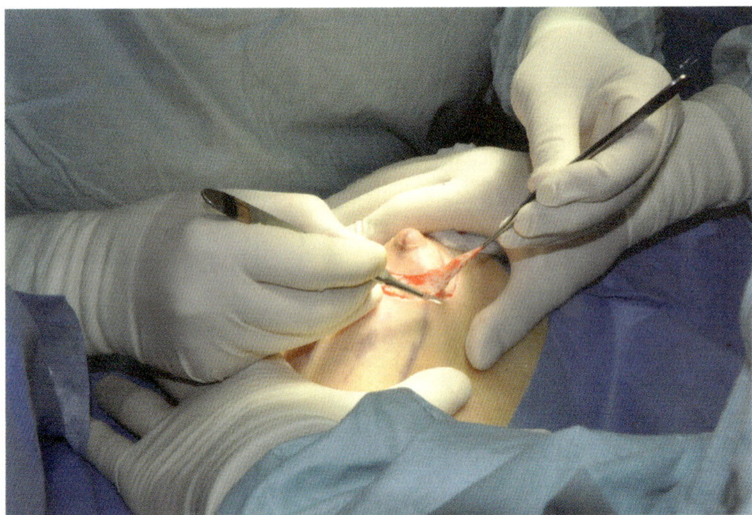

Fig. 5.9 Starting of removal of the epithelium between the two circumferences of the circular ring

Now grasp the point just distal to this and incise between the graspers. Proceed to dissect the segment from its subcutaneous attachments, deep to the fascia or fascial space (Fig. 5.13).

Pulling up on the top of the lobe (see Fig. 5.14) you proceed with the dissective peripheral incision till the end of the lobe and then remove it (see Fig 5.15).

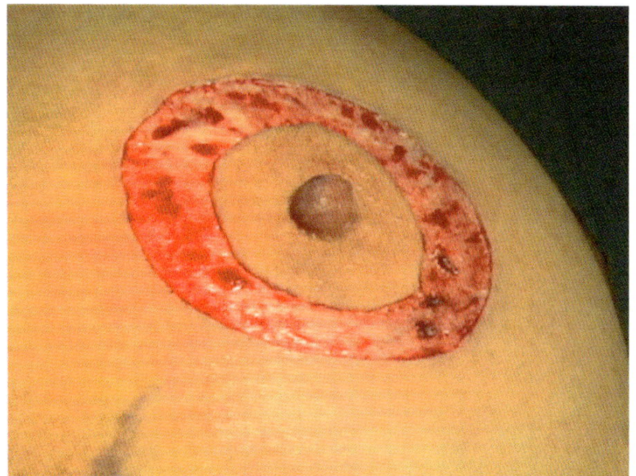

Fig. 5.10 Epithelium removed around the nipple

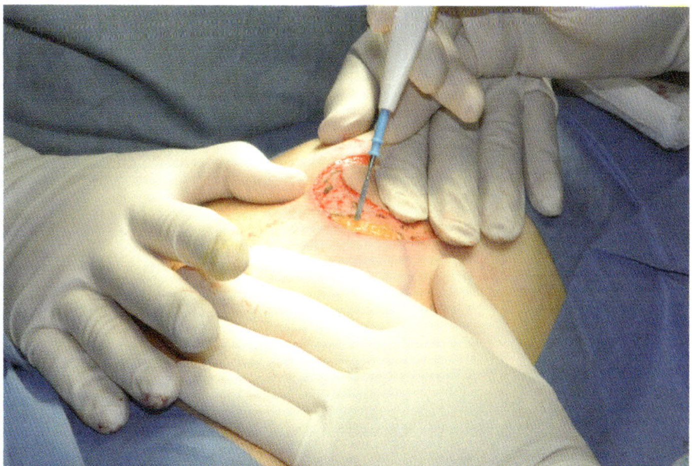

Fig. 5.11 Incision of the outside perimeter

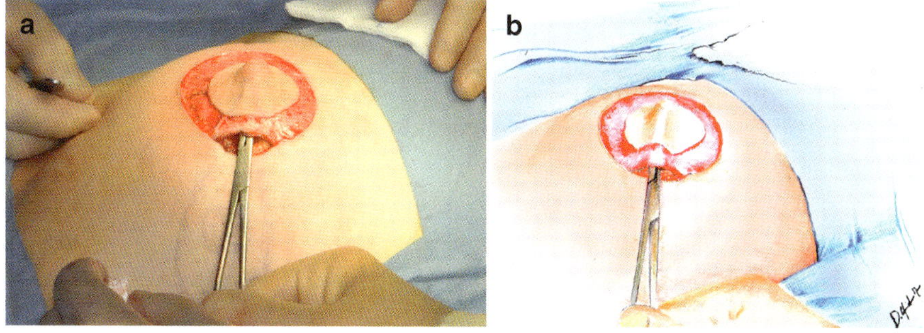

Fig. 5.12 (**a**) Forceps under the nipple. (**b**) Design of the operatory field

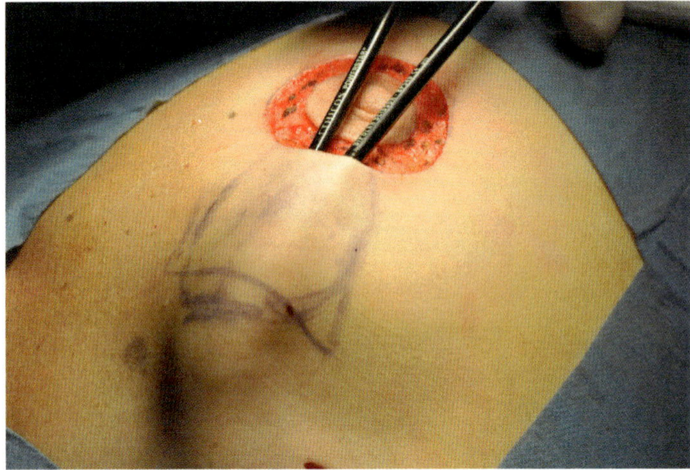

Fig. 5.13 Detachment of the gland from subcutaneous tissue

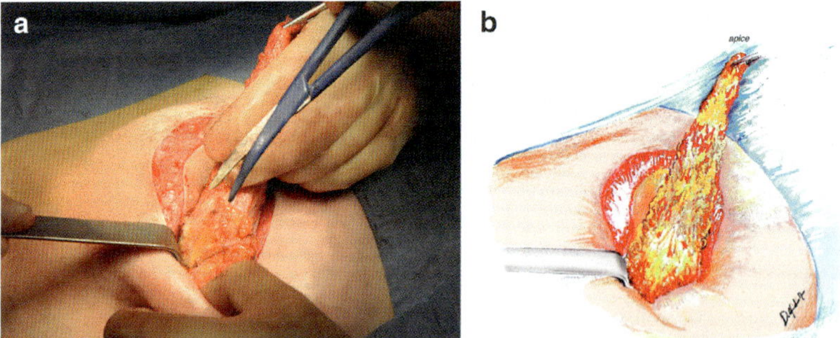

Fig. 5.14 (**a**) Proceeding to remove the lobe cutting with bipolar scissors. (**b**) Design of the lobe during its excision

The muscular fascia can be removed with the specimen if indicated.

Hemostasis is achieved (see Fig. 5.16).

Real-time ultrasound is now used to the dissected specimen at both longitudinal and transverse orientation to evaluate the margin around the cancer (see Fig. 5.17). Compare the resected images with the preprocedure images (see Fig. 5.18).

Macroscopic evaluation of the dissected specimen is provided by the anatomopathologist (see Fig. 5.19). The images show the serial sectioning of the specimen (see Fig. 5.20a and b).

If a close mark is seen under imaging, further tissue can be resected on one or both sides of the specimen. Clips can be placed on the fascial surface at the precise locations of the cancer to facilitate a more targeted radiotherapeutic dose (see Fig. 5.21).

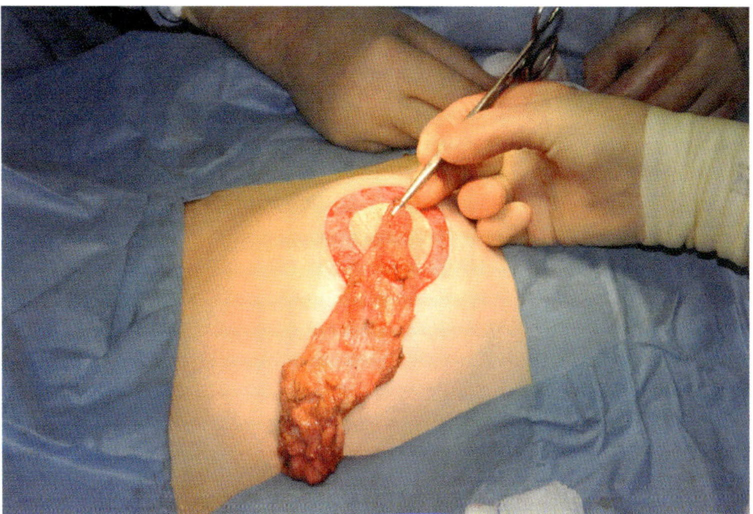

Fig. 5.15 Removed lobe

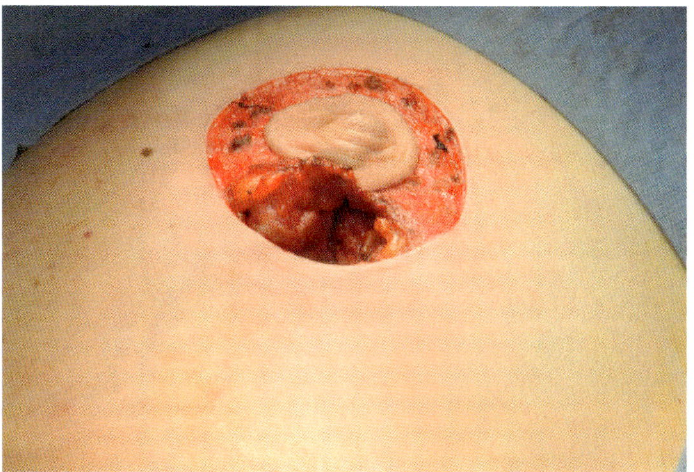

Fig. 5.16 Hemostasis of the operatory field

An anatomic reconstruction of the breast cone can be performed by the mobilization and detachment of the gland borders close to the resected specimen, utilizing oncoplastic technique.

Then proceed with the periareolar "tobacco pouch" suture (see Fig. 5.22) to remodel the skin and suture the areola mucosal border to epidermis (see Fig. 5.23).

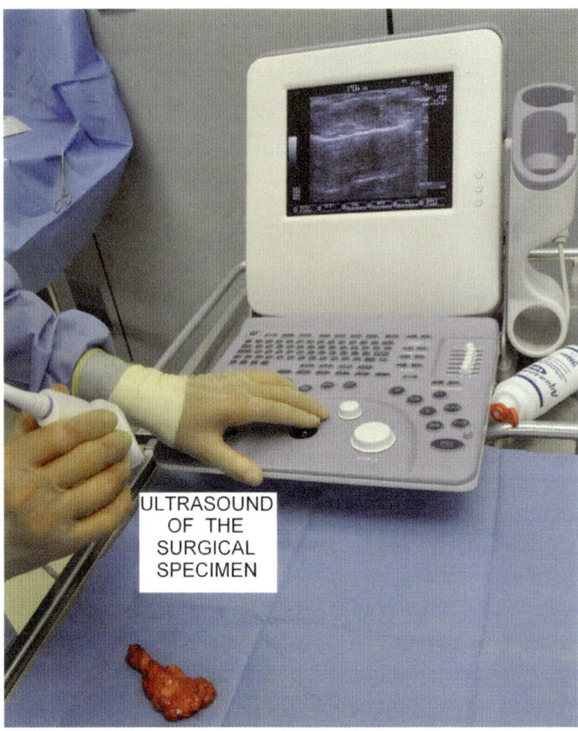

Fig. 5.17 Ultrasonographic control of the specimen

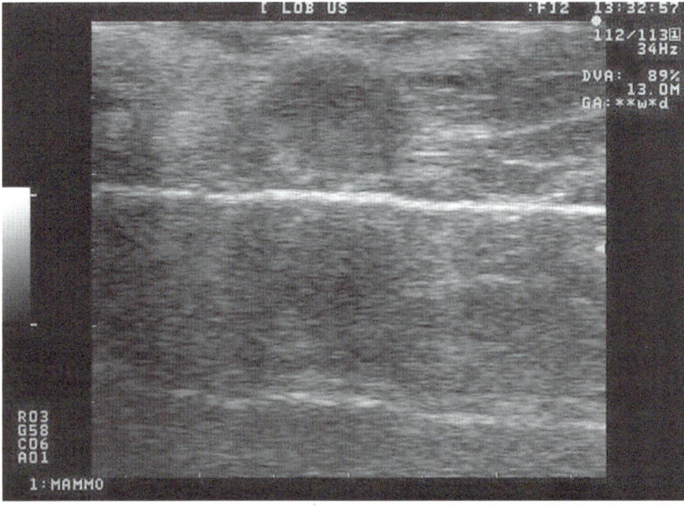

Fig. 5.18 In the echographic image you can immediately see the distance of the suspect area from the borders

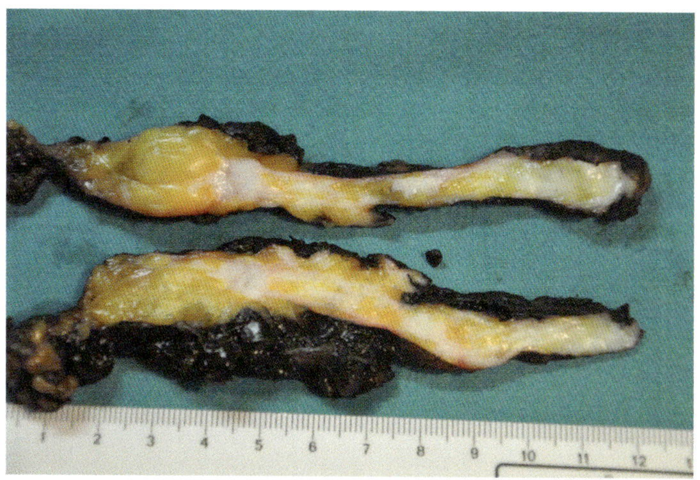

Fig. 5.19 Macroscopic control of the pathologist

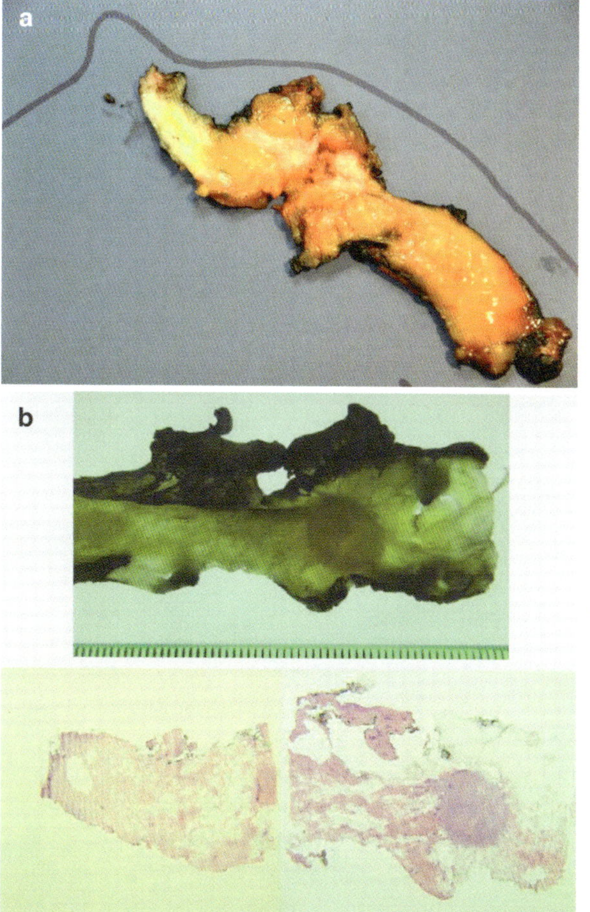

Fig. 5.20 **a** and **b** Successive anatomopathological macrosections findings

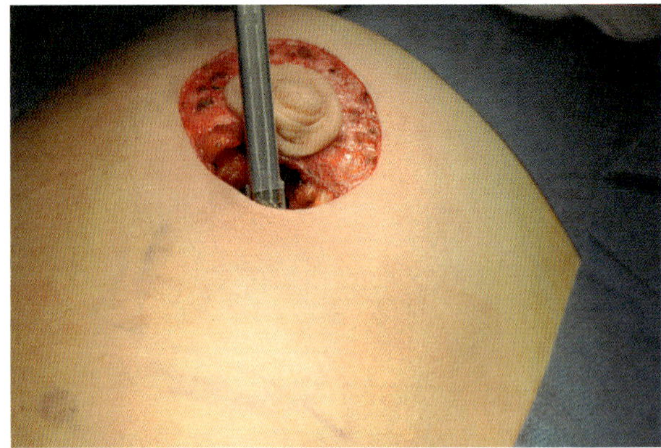

Fig. 5.21 Clips in titanium to let the localization of the removed pathological area

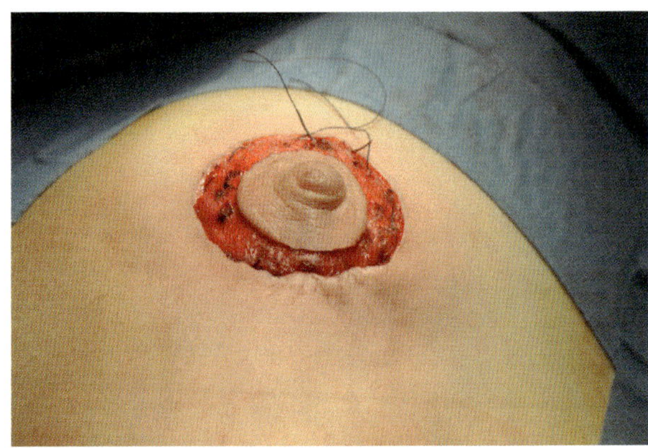

Fig. 5.22 The "tobacco pouch" suture after glandular remodeling

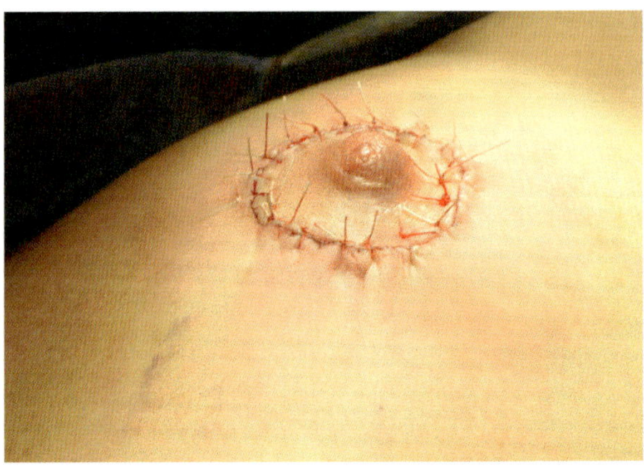

Fig. 5.23 Suture mucosa-epidermis

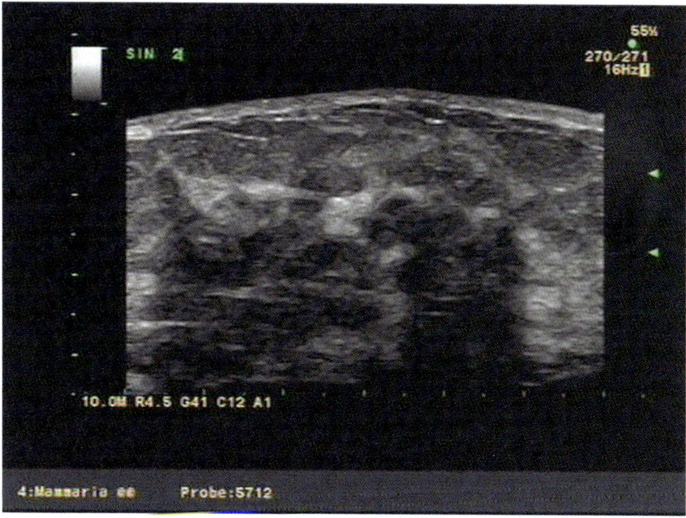

Fig. 5.24 Pathologic lobe at Q1 *left* breast (2 o'clock)

Drains should be avoided if possible to assure a better functional and esthetic result.

*Absorbable materials, attention to skin closure and compression bandages are primary factors for an enhanced cosmetic result.

Case Report

Case # 1

Anamnesis: a 49-year-old patient with family history.

Thickening of the left breast Q1 noted 1 month prior to initial visit.

Ductal echography revealed in left Q1, at 2 o'clock, structural alterations along the entire lobe. The presence of many hypoechogenic areas, particularly 45–55 mm from the nipple, was seen (see Fig. 5.24).

Use of a water bag facilitated visualization of the irregularities, corresponding to neoplastic foci, as well as widespread lobar changes.

These abnormalities are even more apparent if compared to the mirrored image lobe (see Fig. 5.25) of the controlateral side (right Q1 at 10 o'clock).

Mammography (R5) and needle biopsy (positive) were performed prior to operation.

Round block lobectomy operation and dissection of the sentinel lymph node (negative) were performed.

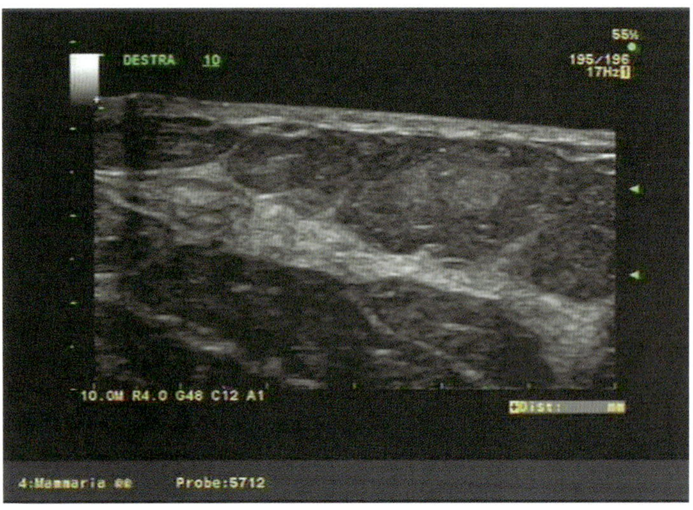

Fig. 5.25 Specular normal lobe at Q1 *right* breast (10 o'clock)

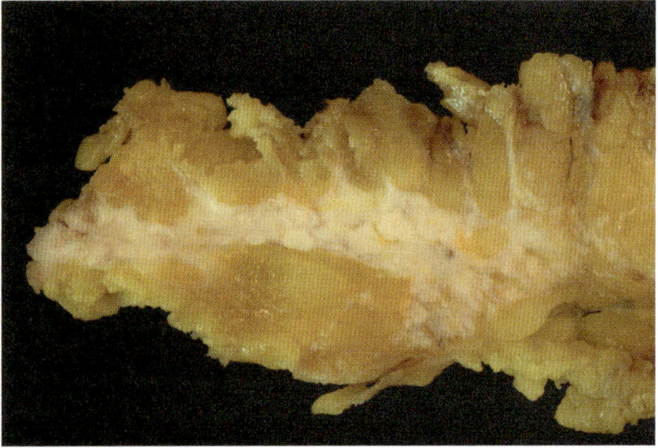

Fig. 5.26 Longitudinal superficial-deep section of the removed lobe at 2 o'clock *left*

Final histological report: infiltrating lobular carcinoma, classic and alveolar variant. GII. Multiple nodes with a max total diameter of 52 mm; pT3 N0; ER 90 % PgR 95 %; Ki67: 25 %; CERB 2: weak focal positivity; P 53: rare positive cells. Presence of infiltrating lobular carcinoma foci in periareolar area (see Figs. 5.26 and 5.27).

Because of neoplastic foci near the under-areolar border of the resected specimen, a skin sparing mastectomy was performed.

The final histological report of the left mastectomy specimen did not reveal residual cancer.

Foci of atypical lobular hyperplasia were noted.

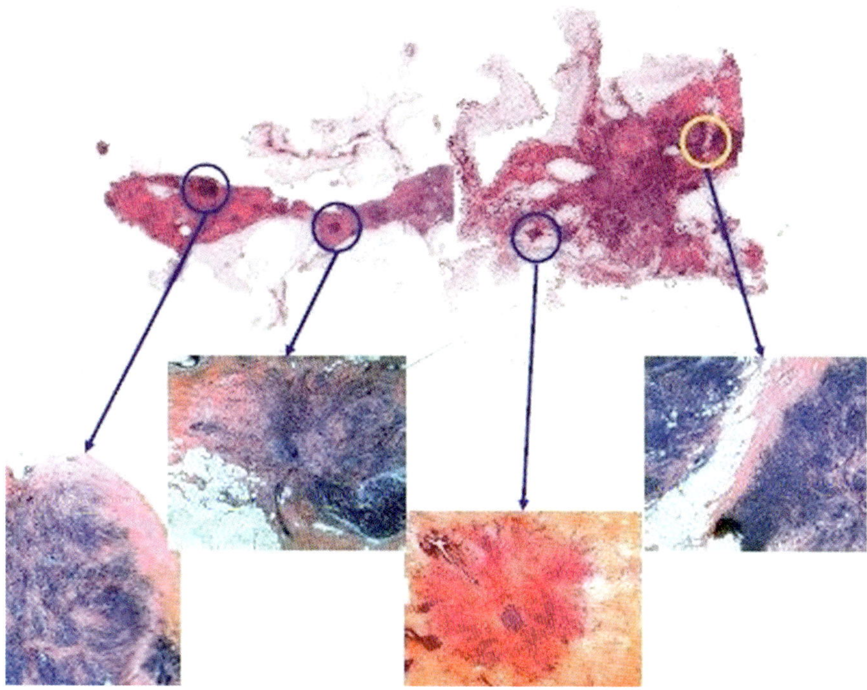

Fig. 5.27 Macrosection of the lobe and hystologic features

Case # 2

Anamnesis: a 45-year-old patient with negative family history.

Ultrasound scanning utilizing the ducto-radial technique revealed two hypoechogenic focal areas at 12 o'clock in the right breast. The first 16 mm in diameter at a distance of 54 mm from the nipple and the second lesion of 8 mm in diameter 82 mm distant (see Fig. 5.28).

Subsequent mammography confirmed these findings (R 5) (see Fig. 5.29).

The needle biopsy was positive in both lesions.

Round block lobectomy and sentinel node biopsy (see Fig. 5.30) were performed and a diagnosis of IDC made, bifocal; GII, pT1c (15 and 10 mm), N0; ER 99 %, PgR 99 % (see Fig. 5.31).

The patient subsequently underwent chemotherapy and radiotherapy with good functional and esthetic results (see Fig. 5.32).

Final Remarks

Oncological evaluation must be based on the anatomical foundation, taking into account the embryological development as well as the natural means of presentation of breast cancer.

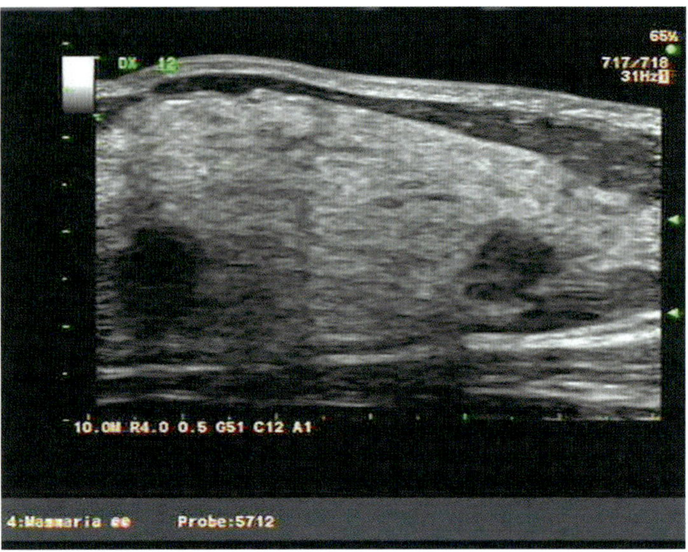

Fig. 5.28 Ultrasound longitudinal scanning of the lobe, with two pathologic areas

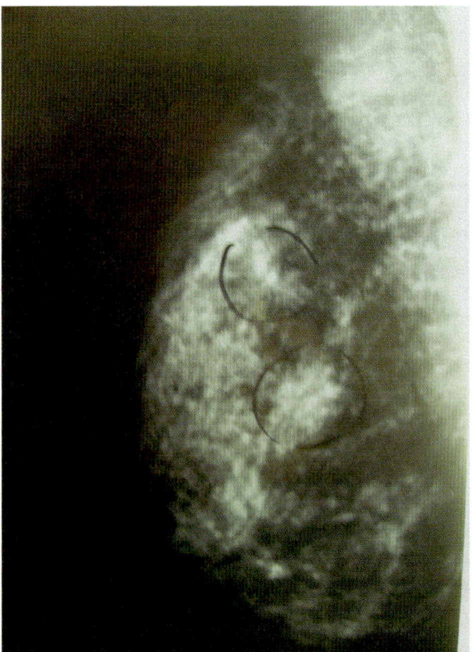

Fig. 5.29 Successive mammography, confirming the same report

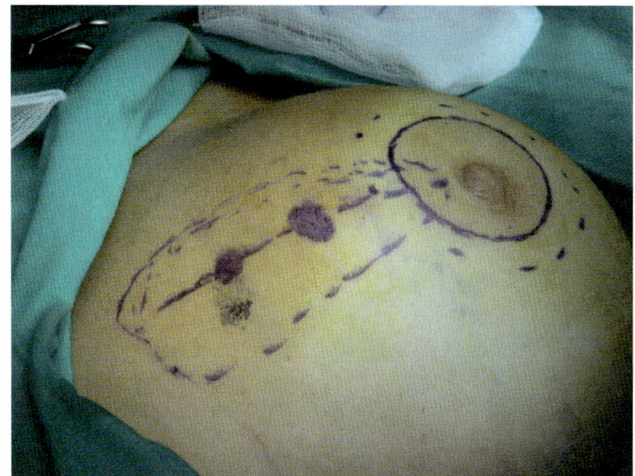

Fig. 5.30 Patient in the operating theater

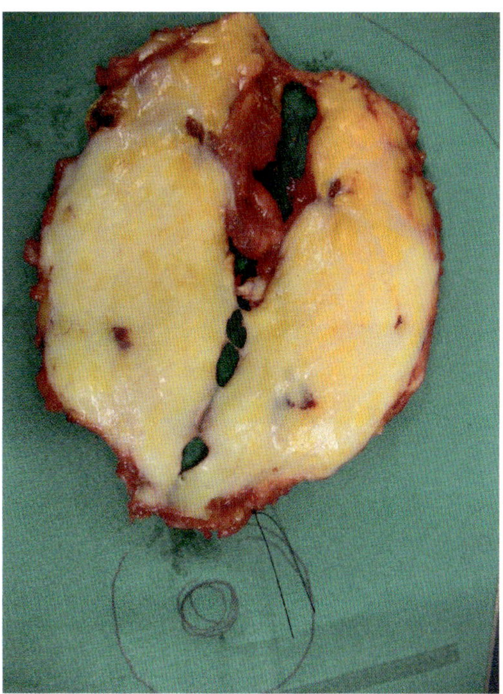

Fig. 5.31 Open lobe with the signs of previous needle biopsy

A full imaging analysis of the breast in question, including ductal echography is requisite prior to any surgical decision.

Because of the use of ductal echography, a better anatomopathological assessment of the extent of disease is now available.

Lobar resection of the breast is a readily mastered surgical technique that can be performed by a surgeon with the appropriate sonographic skills.

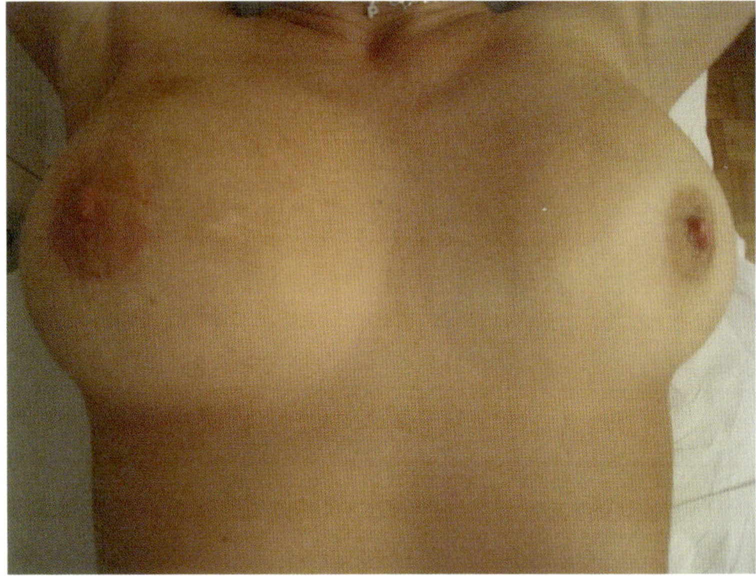

Fig. 5.32 Patient after 5 months from the operation (presence of signs of recent radiotherapy)

Acknowledgment Thanks to Gianni Botta, Anna Maria Dolfin, Elisabetta Dolfin, Grazia Mannini, Chiara Palieri, and Paolo Tagliabue for the help in writing this chapter and for providing the images.

I want to thank also my son Alberto for the translation.

Suggested Reading

1. Amoros J, Dolfin G, Teboul M. Atlas de Ecografia de la Mama. Torino: Ananke; 2009.
2. Amy D. Lobar Ultrasound of the Breast. In: Tot T (ed.) Breast cancer. Springer-Verlag London Limited; 2011. p. 153–162.
3. Dolfin G, Tagliabue P, Dolfin AM, Indelicato S. Chirurgia conservativa: cosa possiamo fare per evitare la mutilazione? Riv It Ost Gin. 2007;14:663–70.
4. Dolfin G, Chebib A, Amy D, Tagliabue P. Carcinoma mammarie et Chirurgie Conservatrice. 30° Seminare Franco-Syrien d'Imagerie Médicale. Tartous, Syrie; 2008.
5. Durante E. Multimodality imaging and interventional techniques. Ferrara, Italy: IBUS Course Abstracts; 2006.
6. Teboul M. Practical ductal echography. Madrid, Spain: Medgen. S.A; 2004.
7. Tot T. DCIS, cytokeratins, and the theory of sick lobe. Virchows Arch. 2005;447:1–8.
8. Tot T. The theory of the sick lobe. In Tot T. Breast cancer. Springer-Verlag London Limited; 2011. p. 1–15.
9. Veronesi U, Cascinelli N, Mariani L, et al. Twenty-year follow-up of a randomised study comparing breast-conserving surgery with radical mastectomy for early breast cancer. N Engl J Med. 2002;347(16):1227–32.

Chapter 6
Ultrasound-Guided Breast Biopsy Tissue Sampling: Technique and Breast Ultrasound Characteristics of Benign and Malignant Lesions

Edward J. Donahue

Ultrasound-Guided Breast Biopsy Tissue Sampling Technique

A 40-year-old woman with a strong family history of breast cancer has been referred for a surgical opinion regarding a nonpalpable left breast density that was visualized on an initial screening mammogram. Compression views have confirmed the presence of a density in the upper inner portion of the left breast. Physical examination in the surgeon's office reveals no palpable abnormalities in the left breast. There is no evidence for nipple inversion, skin dimpling, or nipple discharge.

A focused ultrasound examination of the upper inner left breast reveals a lobulated, soft tissue density that is 9 mm wide and 12 mm tall. The lesion is hypoechoic. Unilateral edge shadowing is present. There is no enhancement. The lesion has the ultrasonic characteristics of a solid lesion, and by accepted criteria is suspicious for malignancy.

Several options are available to the surgeon to diagnosis this suspicious abnormality.

Excisional breast biopsy was the gold standard for diagnosis for nearly 100 years. The emergence of minimally invasive image-guided breast surgery has given surgeons familiar with this new technology an accurate, reproducible, and cost-effective method of diagnosis in the office setting. This chapter reviews the ultrasound-guided biopsy methods and techniques that are now available to the surgeon.

Fine-Needle Aspiration Biopsy

Fine-needle aspiration has been utilized for the evaluation of palpable breast masses for many years. A small gauge hollow needle was inserted into the mass after

E.J. Donahue, M.D., M.S. (✉)
Department of Surgery, St. Joseph's Hospital and Medical Center,
333 West Thomas Road, Phoenix, AZ, USA
e-mail: edonahue@cox.net

D.S. Francescatti and M.J. Silverstein (eds.), *Breast Cancer: A New Era in Management*,
DOI 10.1007/978-1-4614-8063-1_6,

Table 6.1 Supplies for fine-needle aspiration biopsy

Alcohol swabs	
3 cm³ syringe, 10 cm³ syringe	22-gauge spinal needle (for deep lesions)
22 or 23 gauge 2½-inch needle	Glass microscope slides
1 % Xylocaine buffered with bicarbonate spot band-aid	Container filled with 95 % alcohol of formalin

stabilizing the mass with the opposite hand. If fluid was withdrawn from the lump and the mass disappeared, the conclusion was that the lesion would be classified as a simple cyst. If a bloody aspirate was obtained, the aspirated material would be sent to the cytology laboratory for analysis. Conversely, if the needle biopsy was "dry," yielding no fluid, or if the mass was still palpable following aspiration of some fluid, an open excisional biopsy would then be performed to obtain a tissue diagnosis. When surgical biopsy was performed it was not at all unusual for the surgeon to discover that the excised palpable mass was in fact, an uncomplicated cyst that had not been pierced by the needle that had been blindly inserted into the breast. The use of ultrasound guidance for these procedures has transformed a "blind" procedure into an extremely accurate sampling procedure, where the hyperechoic signature of a biopsy needle can be seen within a breast mass during an ultrasound-guided breast biopsy.

The procedures for ultrasound-guided fine-needle cyst aspiration and ultrasound-guided fine-needle aspiration biopsy utilize similar technique and are applicable for both palpable and nonpalpable abnormalities. The same size needle can be used for both procedures and the patient's positioning is the same.

The decision to proceed with cyst aspiration or aspiration biopsy depends upon the clinical history, physical examination, and the findings of the focused ultrasound examination. Ultrasound findings compatible with a simple cyst or a complex cyst would allow the surgeon to discuss plans for a cyst aspiration with the patient prior to the procedure. Recognizing the ultrasonic characteristics of a cyst filled with thick fluid would alert the surgeon to use a larger 16- or 18-gauge needle to perform a successful aspiration. A palpable mass composed of multiple benign cysts (a complex cyst) could be successfully aspirated with multiple ultrasound-guided passes of the needle. In these examples, the use of interventional breast ultrasound would avoid an unnecessary trip to the operating room. Likewise, findings compatible with a solid lesion would allow the surgeon to discuss plans for an office-based image-guided biopsy of the mass with the patient before proceeding with the procedure. The supplies required for a fine-needle aspiration biopsy are listed in Table 6.1. The imaging techniques for ultrasound-guided cyst aspiration and fine-needle aspiration are identical.

Following completion of a focused breast ultrasound examination, the ultrasonic characteristics of the mass are evaluated and the decision is made to proceed with a fine-needle aspiration biopsy (fnab). The patient is positioned supine on the examining table with the ipsilateral arm raised behind head, similar to the position used for breast examination. Lesions located in the lateral portions of the breast can be made more accessible by moving the patient to a decubitus or modified decubitus position. A folded pillow placed under the patient's shoulder may also help to displace the

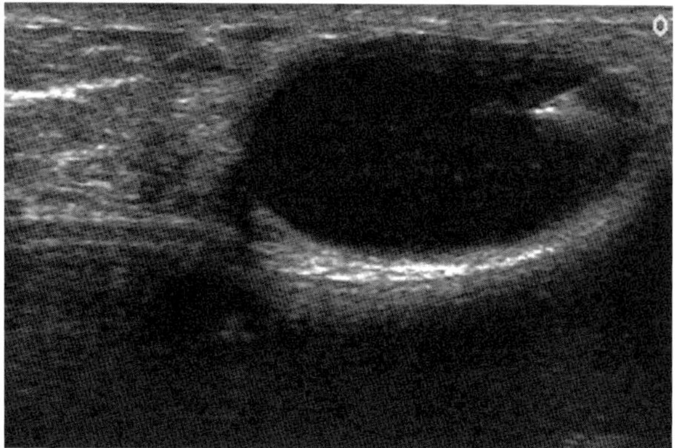

Fig. 6.1

breast medially. Pendulous breasts may have to be manually retracted to facilitate insertion of the needle into the breast.

The skin of the breast is painted with a topical antibacterial solution. Non-sterile gel is applied to the breast. The ultrasound transducer is again placed over the area of concern. The transducer is positioned so that the needle can be introduced into the breast in a manner that maximizes the comfort of the patient and the surgeon. Simple rotation of the transducer while it is centered directly over the mass will allow the surgeon to choose which end of the transducer will serve as the reference point for the safe insertion of the needle into the breast. Insertion of a needle into the nipple–areolar complex should be avoided, as this may cause unacceptable pain to the patient. The lesion should be positioned on the monitor so that the entire path of the needle can be visualized at all times when the needle is within the breast. When this imaging has been accomplished, the hand holding the transducer will keep the transducer immobile directly over the mass. The only moving object during the procedure will be the needle approaching the mass under ultrasound guidance. A skin wheal is created with local anesthetic at a location close to the narrow base of the transducer where the needle will be inserted into the breast. Additional local anesthetic can be injected into the breast along the projected path of the needle. The local anesthetic can be visualized as it enters the breast parenchyma. A 23-gauge 2½-inch needle is attached to the syringe and introduced into the breast in alignment with the long axis of the transducer. If the needle is outside of the plane of the narrow 1.5 mm ultrasound beam, the needle will not be visualized. The needle must be kept in view at all times to avoid inadvertent puncture of surrounding vital structures, such as pleura, pectoralis muscle, or breast implants as seen in Fig. 6.1. This type of needle has sufficient length so that it can reach a targeted cyst/mass that is located within 3 cm of the skin surface. Lesions that are deeper than 3 cm will have to be approached with a longer needle. The inner diameter of either needle is large enough to collect adequate cellular material for cytological analysis. When the needle is in alignment with the ultrasound beam, the entry of the needle

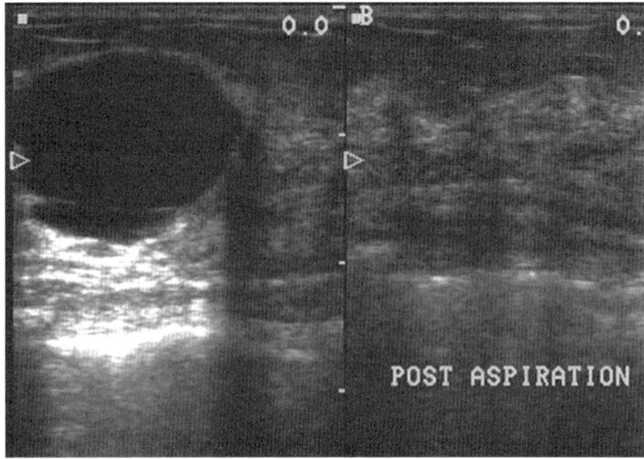

Fig. 6.2

into the mass is easily visualized/recognized. A pre-aspiration image should be saved electronically for inclusion in the electronic medical record, or alternatively printed for inclusion in a paper chart. If the mass is a cyst filled with fluid, gentle negative pressure applied to the barrel of the syringe will empty the cyst and the mass will no longer be visible because it is no longer present Fig. 6.2. Nontraumatic bloody cyst fluid is sent for cytologic analysis.

However, if gentle pressure does not yield fluid, then an aspirate is obtained for cytology. Gentle negative pressure is then applied to the barrel of the syringe, while the needle is directed into different areas of the solid mass to facilitate collection of an adequate aspirate sample. Prior to withdrawing the needle from the mass, for documentation purposes, another image is obtained then the negative pressure on the barrel of the syringe is released and the needle is withdrawn from the breast. Gentle pressure is applied to the breast while the aspirate is prepared.

The needle is separated from the syringe and the syringe is filled with air and reattached to the needle. The contents of the needle are then expelled on to a labeled clear glass microscope slide by advancing the plunger of the air-filled syringe while the needle is in close approximation to the slide. A second glass slide is then placed parallel in contact with the aspirate and drawn over the aspirate creating a smear. Both slides are immediately placed into a liquid preservative. The specimens are then sent to the laboratory for cytopathologic analysis. The time required to perform a fine-needle aspiration is usually less than 5 min.

Fine-needle aspiration biopsy can also be used to evaluate clinically suspicious axillary lymph nodes. Pathologic axillary nodes have a characteristic ultrasound appearance with a loss of normal architecture. Fine-needle aspiration of axillary lymph nodes is an office-based procedure that is performed under local anesthesia. Great care must be used in planning a fine-needle aspiration of an axillary mass, exercising care to avoid injury to the surrounding neurovascular structures. The principles for ultrasound guidance are identical to those described for fine-needle aspiration of breast masses.

Core Needle Biopsy

The use of percutaneous needle biopsy has been described for more than 100 years. The first core needle biopsy devices were hand operated and designed for single patient use. The device, rarely used in the twenty-first century, is composed of an inner and outer cannula. A sharp needle tip 2–3 mm in length is at the tip of the inner cannula to facilitate passage through dense breast tissue. The inner notch has a length of 15–20 mm and a diameter of approximately 1.5 mm. This notch serves as a sampling trough, which holds a core of tissue that is separated from the breast mass when the hollow outer cannula is manually advanced over the inner cannula. When the core needle is withdrawn from the breast, the outer cannula is retracted allowing manual retrieval of the cylindrical core of tissue in the sampling trough. The device can then be reinserted into the breast to obtain additional cores of tissue. The size of the core needle biopsy device ranges from 14- to 18-gauge. A 14-gauge core needle yields a cylindrical core of tissue approximately 1.5 mm in diameter. Precise pathological diagnosis can be obtained along with hormone receptor status and DNA analysis. Ultrasound core needle biopsy is applicable to palpable and nonpalpable breast masses.

The inherent variability in the density of breast tissue can create obstacles to the use of a hand-driven core needle biopsy device. Manual advancement of the core needle may be difficult and sometimes impossible, especially when encountering very dense breast tissue, leading to significant pain and patient discomfort. These barriers led to the development of automated devices. A single-use automated spring-loaded device was introduced in the early 1980s that, within a split second, deployed an inner sampling trough into the breast tissue followed immediately by the advancement of an outer cutting cannula, significantly reducing the patient discomfort associated with manual advancement. The efficiency of these devices was first demonstrated in stereotactic core needle breast biopsies. Core needle biopsy devices currently in use include completely disposable units that are spring activated, as well as reusable handheld units that utilize a disposable core needle biopsy holder device.

Core needle breast biopsy is an office-based procedure performed under local anesthesia. The supplies necessary to perform an ultrasound-guided core needle biopsy are listed in Table 6.2. Core needle devices were initially used to biopsy palpable breast masses. The use of ultrasound guidance has converted this "blind procedure" into an extremely accurate diagnostic procedure, as shown in Fig. 6.1, where the hyperechoic ultrasound signature of a biopsy needle can be seen passing through a solid breast mass.

Positioning of the patient and ultrasound-guided targeting techniques are identical to those described for fine-needle aspiration and biopsy.

However, when using an automated core needle biopsy device, one important concept must be kept in mind at all times: when the core needle biopsy device is activated, the inner core needle will instantly advance 15–22 mm from the prebiopsy position into the postbiopsy position as the biopsy needle passes into or through the targeted lesion. This advancement is known as the "throw" of the device. This throw

Table 6.2 Supplies for ultrasound-guided biopsy

Alcohol or Betadine swab
Automated or vacuum-assisted biopsy device
Sterile aperture drape
5 cm^3 syringe
27-gauge needle
18-gauge needle
#11 scalpel blade
1 % Xylocaine buffered with local anesthetic
Specimen container and formalin
Hemostat
Sterile gloves
Sterile gel
Sterile gauze
Tape
Mayo stand

varies with different devices depending on the manufacturer's specifications. Targeting of the lesion must therefore consider the structures immediately adjacent to the lesion. In addition, the targeting angle of the device must be kept in mind when considering the approach to the abnormality. The targeting angle is dependent upon the depth of the lesion, as well as the distance of the skin incision from the ultrasound transducer. If the incision is placed in close approximation to the transducer when a deep lesion is targeted, then the targeting angle will be very steep, placing vital structures deep to the lesion at risk for inadvertent puncture due to the throw of the device. This can lead to serious complications if the contiguous structure is the pleural interface, a breast implant, or a large blood vessel. Therefore, the operator must be aware of the throw of the device that is being used. A targeting angle that places the biopsy device parallel or nearly parallel to the long axis of the ultrasound transducer will not only avoid inadvertent puncture of structures deep to the lesion, it will also maximize the hyperechoic signature of the biopsy device during the procedure.

Another option for biopsy of a mass densities in the axilla or for masses that are in close proximity to the pectoralis muscle, or to a mammary implant is to prefire the needle biopsy device so that the sampling trough of the needle is inserted directly into the mass. After verifying the position of the trough, the outer cutting cannula is activated, resulting in a core needle tissue biopsy that does not result in a "throw" of the cutting device past the target. This technique can be useful when performing a biopsy of a solid density in a patient with "nearby" breast implants.

The transducer must be positioned to maximize the view of the targeted lesion. The projected path of the biopsy needle will follow the long axis of the transducer. The orientation of the transducer will determine if the course of the biopsy needle moves from right to left or left to right across the monitor screen. The transducer can be rotated to the position that best visualizes the target and optimizes the location of the 2–3 mm incision that is made to facilitate entry of the biopsy device into the breast. Considerations regarding the cosmesis of the biopsy scar and a

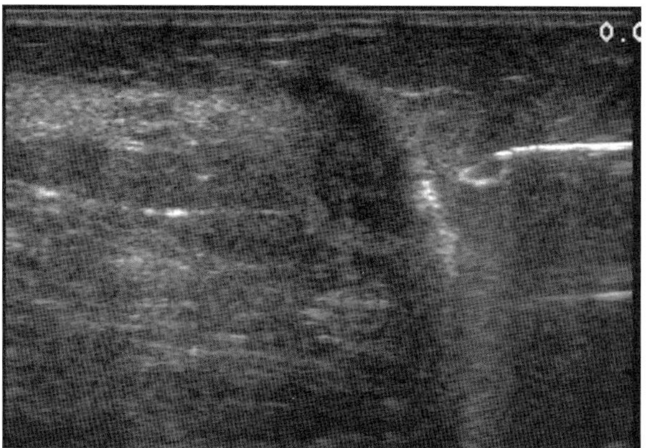

Fig. 6.3

future cancer operation should also be kept in mind when selecting the location for the incision.

Following preparation of the skin with a topical anesthetic, a sterile aperture drape is placed on the breast. Sterile gel is applied to the transducer and the lesion is targeted. Once the transducer is in the proper orientation, the operator must maintain the position of transducer in the same location for the duration of the procedure so that the lesion and the biopsy device are in view at all times. A skin wheal is made with local anesthetic and additional local anesthetic is infiltrated into the breast along the projected path of the core biopsy needle. A 3 mm skin incision is made with a scalpel blade and the skin edges are gently spread with a hemostat to ease the entry of the core needle into the breast. The core needle is inserted in exact alignment within the 1.5 mm beam of the ultrasound transducer so that the needle is always in view as it is advanced towards the lesion. This maneuver requires a high degree of eye-hand coordination. It is imperative that the needle be repositioned as necessary to maintain continuous visualization. Local anesthetic can be injected as necessary to maximize patient comfort. The tip of the needle is positioned with real-time imaging immediately adjacent to the lesion. Prior to performing the biopsy, imaging is obtained to document the position of the core biopsy device in relation to the target lesion (Fig. 6.3). The image is "unfrozen" and converted to real time. Prior to activating or firing the device the operator should pause and mentally review the projected throw of the core needle to ensure a safe trajectory. Prior to activating the biopsy device, the transducer can be moved parallel to the long axis of the device so that the operator can be sure that the biopsy device will be sampling the center of the mass.

The device is then activated and the needle can be seen passing into the lesion in real time. The transducer can then be rotated 90° directly over the lesion to demonstrate, in cross section, the hyperechoic signature of the biopsy needle within the lesion (Fig. 6.4).

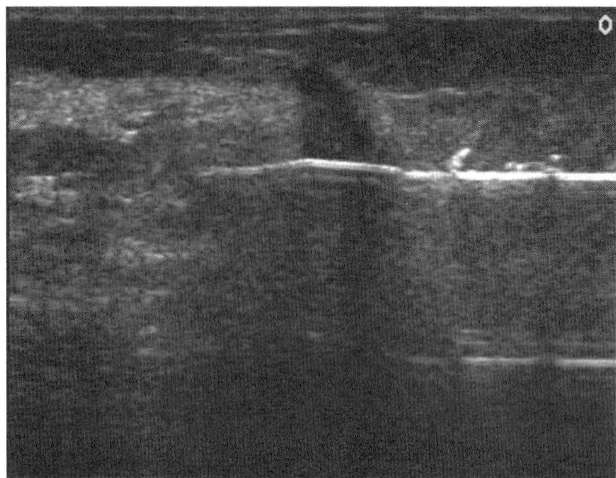

Fig. 6.4

Prior to withdrawing the biopsy device, imaging labeled "postbiopsy" should be obtained to document the position of the biopsy needle at completion of the biopsy. When the biopsy needle is withdrawn from the breast, the outer cannula is retracted to allow retrieval of the biopsy specimen. The core needle is then reloaded and reinserted into the breast through the same incision and advanced to the lesion with ultrasound guidance. The biopsy device must be kept in view at all times when it is within the breast. Each core of tissue should be inspected to verify the presence of solid tissue. The presence of only adipose tissue in the core sample of tissue should alert the operator that the suspected solid lesion has probably not been biopsied. A total of 3–5 cores of tissue are usually sufficient to obtain a diagnosis.

At the completion of the biopsy procedure a metal marking clip should be inserted into the biopsied lesion within the breast or axilla, and an ultrasound image obtained to document successful clip deployment (Fig. 6.5). An operative report should be dictated specifying the type of biopsy device for the medical record.

The biopsy cores are immediately placed into a labeled container filled with formalin. Solid cores of tissue will sink to the bottom of the specimen container, while adipose tissue will "float" on the surface of the liquid preservative. Following completion of the procedure gentle pressure is maintained at the biopsy site for approximately 3–5 min. A small sterile dressing is applied to the incision and the tissue samples are sent to pathology for histological evaluation. If a frozen section is planned, formalin should not be utilized and the cores of tissue should be placed into sterile saline solution and immediately delivered to pathology for processing. The time required to complete this procedure is usually 15–20 min. The patient should be assisted to the sitting position and observed for 5–10 min prior to leaving the office.

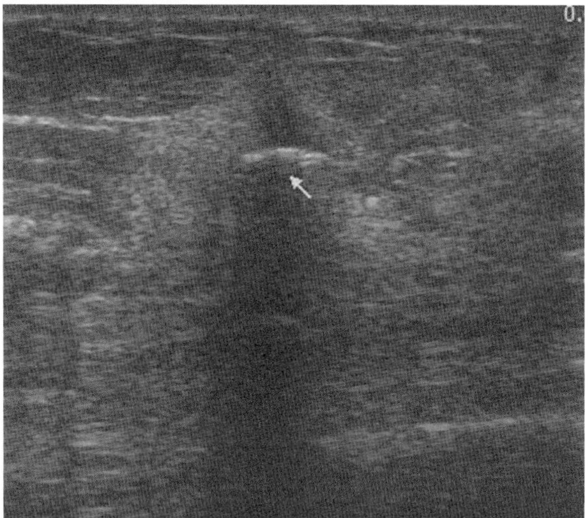

Fig. 6.5

Vacuum-Assisted Biopsy Devices

The first vacuum-assisted biopsy devices were developed for minimally invasive stereotactic image-guided breast biopsy. These devices have been modified to be held by hand and can be used with ultrasound guidance. The handheld biopsy devices are fully or partially disposable. The power source may be self-contained so that the device is truly disposable or the biopsy device may be tethered to a larger console that contains the machinery that "drives" the device.

Building upon the hollow core needle concept, these devices use a larger needle ranging in size from 8 to 14 gauge. A sampling trough is present near the distal portion of the device. When activated, a vacuum is automatically applied to the hollow needle that draws surrounding breast tissue into the sampling trough. An inner cannula is then advanced manually or automatically along the long axis of the needle effectively coring a cylinder of tissue from the lesion. The tissue samples are then automatically or manually delivered to a collection chamber or sample collection notch, which is a part of the biopsy device that is located outside of the breast. Additional cores of tissue can be obtained without removing and reinserting the biopsy device. The size of the biopsy probes range from 8 to 14 gauge. The cores of tissue removed during the biopsy can be visually inspected prior to placement in a specimen container.

Vacuum-assisted breast biopsy is an office-based procedure that is performed under local anesthesia. The imaging techniques are identical to those for fine-needle aspiration and the core needle biopsy. Following satisfactory ultrasound imaging of a mass density within the breast, a sterile tray is available stocked with the same supplies listed in Table 6.2. A topical antiseptic is applied to the breast along with sterile gel. After selecting the breast position for the ultrasound transducer and the planned incision, the ultrasound transducer is maintained in position directly over the mass density. Topical anesthesia and sterile gel are applied to the breast. A skin wheal is created with local anesthetic and additional local anesthetic is introduced into the breast in and around the mass density. The targeting angle is selected so that the sampling notch of the vacuum-assisted biopsy device will be positioned directly below/inferior to the mass or directly into the density. A 3 mm incision is made, the skin edges are separated with a hemostat, and the vacuum-assisted biopsy probe is inserted into the breast under continuous ultrasound guidance while the transducer is maintained in a fixed position. The size of these biopsy devices is such that they are readily visualized within the 1.5 mm width of the ultrasound beam. However, it is just as important that the entire length of the biopsy device be in view at all times when the device is within the breast. Image documentation is obtained before and after the procedure. The vacuum-assisted device can be activated by hand or by foot pedal. When the device is activated, the opening of the sampling notch and advancement of the cutting cannula can be observed with real-time ultrasound imaging. The biopsy probe must be kept in view at all times during the procedure. Lesions that are close to the pectoralis muscle can sometimes be displaced anteriorly away from the muscle by injecting sterile saline between the muscle and the lesion. This maneuver will create a space within which the probe can be located prior to activation. After completion of the procedure, the breast is maintained in gentle compression for 15 min. Prior to leaving the office, it is recommended that the patient be observed in the office an additional 15 min. An icepack for topical use can minimize postprocedure swelling and patient discomfort.

These vacuum-assisted core devices can theoretically remove an entire lesion; however, at the present time, the devices are approved for diagnostic purposes only.

Some vacuum-assisted core biopsy needles are designed to remove one core of tissue per insertion. As such, these devices require multiple reinsertions to retrieve multiple cores of tissue. Targeting techniques and surgical techniques with these devices are identical to those that have been previously prescribed.

Other biopsy devices utilize a radiofrequency (RF) tip to facilitate penetration of dense breast tissue. The procedure is performed in the office under local anesthesia. The device is inserted into the breast under ultrasound guidance, the RF tip is activated, and the device is manually advanced into and through the breast lesion. Prior to activating the biopsy process, the position of the device is verified within the lesion by rotating the transducer 90° and visualizing the probe in cross section within the lesion. Vacuum suction is activated, which draws a circumferential core of tissue into the long axis of the device. A circumferential rotary core cutter is advanced along the long axis of the probe that separates the core of tissue from the breast mass. The device is then removed from the breast and the core of tissue is retrieved. A total of 3–5 cores of tissue are usually sufficient for diagnosis.

Another minimally invasive breast biopsy device uses inert argon gas introduced through a needle tip to stick freeze the lesion prior to obtaining a vacuum-assisted core biopsy. This procedure is performed in the office under local anesthesia. The probe is inserted into the breast using ultrasound guidance and the needle tip of the device is inserted directly into the lesion. After confirming the insertion of the needle tip into the lesion with orthogonal ultrasound views with image documentation, the flow of argon gas is activated. The argon gas super cools the metal tip and freezes the surrounding tissue within the lesion to the needle tip. A circumferential cutting cannula is then automatically activated and advanced, which separates the core of tissue from the lesion. The biopsy device is then removed from the breast, and the core sample is separated from the needle tip. A total of three to five cores of tissue are usually adequate for diagnosis. Each tissue core can be evaluated when removed from the device to assess the adequacy of the specimen.

Ultrasound-Guided Needle Localization

Ultrasound-guided needle localization can be utilized when the decision is made to surgically remove a nonpalpable breast mass that is visible with ultrasound imaging. The localization procedure can be performed by the surgeon in the operating room or in the surgeon's office, depending upon the availability of ultrasound equipment. The technique for needle localization is similar to the technique described for fine-needle aspiration biopsy. Following preparation of the breast with a topical antiseptic, a sterile hollow core needle is introduced into the breast in alignment with the long axis of the transducer. The needle is kept in view at all times as it is guided into and, if possible, through the mass density. A sterile hook wire is then introduced through the inner core of the localizing needle and advanced until the tip of the wire can be seen exiting the hollow tip of the core needle. The hollow needle is then withdrawn from the breast, while the hook wire is maintained in position with the opposite hand. Care must be taken to avoid dislodgement of the hook wire during removal of the hollow needle. The skin of the breast is then prepped and draped in the usual sterile fashion and the excisional biopsy is performed. This technique can be used for excision of both benign and malignant nonpalpable masses. Intraoperative ultrasound, when available, can be used to scan the surgical specimen to verify that the density has been removed.

Ultrasound-guided topographic localization can also be used to identify the location of a nonpalpable breast mass. The procedure is most useful when the planned incision is directly over a nonmobile, nonpalpable mass. The exact location of the transducer can be outlined on the skin with a marking pen when the nonpalpable lesion is in the center of the viewing screen. The depth of the lesion below the skin is also noted. An incision within this "window" will be centered directly over the nonpalpable abnormality. When the breast is then prepped and draped in the usual sterile fashion, the incision is made and dissection is carried down to the previously noted depth. The lesion should be readily apparent. The ultrasound transducer can also be introduced into the surgical field if there is any question regarding the exact location of the mass.

Choice of Ultrasound-Guided Imaging Biopsy Device

Surgeons who embrace the concept of image-guided biopsy will be rewarded with the opportunity to use a wide array of accurate breast tissue sampling tools. The techniques for image-guided intervention have been reviewed for all of the devices described in this chapter. It should be apparent that the basic principles for ultrasound imaging remain the same for all of the devices that have been reviewed. What device or procedure should be used for biopsy?

The rationale for biopsy, therapeutic options, risks, and expectations must be discussed with the patient while obtaining informed surgical consent. The wishes of the patient are also an important consideration, as is the patient's physical condition. Anticoagulants and other medicines that are associated with increased bleeding such as non-steroidal anti-inflammatory medications and aspirin must be discontinued prior to the procedure. Specific guidelines for cessation/resumption of these medications should be followed. The surgeon must also assess the mental capacity of the patient to tolerate a minimally invasive image-guided breast biopsy in the office setting. Extremely anxious patients may not be suited to this type of procedure. It is also useful to question your patient regarding a history of fainting during other interventions such as dental procedures. Surgeons prefer to know ahead of time that their patient may pass out, so that other options for biopsy can be explored.

Ultrasound-guided fine-needle aspiration biopsy can be used for the evaluation of any type of palpable or nonpalpable abnormality, including breast cysts, intracystic masses, and solid masses. In the hands of an experienced cytopathologist, the sensitivity, specificity, and positive predictive value of a fine-needle aspiration biopsy of a suspicious breast lesion can approach 99 %. Fine-needle aspiration biopsy prior to neoadjuvant chemotherapy can diagnosis carcinoma in suspicious axillary lymph nodes. DNA gene expression arrays can be prepared from fine-needle aspirates of primary breast tumors before and after chemotherapy to identify those expression profiles that correlate with treatment response. Supplies for an ultrasound-guided biopsy are listed in Table 6.1.

An ultrasound-guided core needle biopsy or vacuum-assisted core needle biopsy can be utilized to obtain an exact tissue diagnosis for any palpable or nonpalpable breast mass. The surgeon must develop the highest level of proficiency with ultrasound imaging, eye-hand coordination, and ultrasound-guided biopsy techniques to utilize these devices effectively. Supplies for an ultrasound-guided biopsy are listed in Table 6.2.

The selection of a specific biopsy device depends upon the skill and experience level of the surgeon, as well as the surgeon's familiarity with the different biopsy devices. The costs associated with the automated vacuum-assisted biopsy devices are significantly higher than the costs associated with automated core needle biopsy. The equipment costs for these devices vary considerably. However, the costs associated with an open surgical biopsy are significantly higher. There is minimal cost associated with a fine-needle aspiration biopsy. The costs associated with a spring-loaded core needle biopsy device are slightly higher. The use of a vacuum-assisted biopsy device incurs two separate costs that can be significant: the cost of the capital equipment to drive these devices and the cost of the disposable vacuum-assisted biopsy devices. The surgeon should choose the device that offers the most cost-effective means of diagnosis.

As with any surgical procedure, there must be concordance between the ultrasonic characteristics of a mass and the final histology/cytology report. The core biopsy of a suspicious mass that yields a diagnosis of benign breast tissue is classified as a discordant biopsy which requires further investigation, including another image-guided biopsy procedure or perhaps an open surgical biopsy.

Ultrasound Characteristics of Benign and Malignant Lesions

The Breast Imaging Reporting and Data System (BIRADS) developed by the American College of Radiology in 1983 provides a framework for classification of mass densities that are discovered by mammographic Imaging. Surgeons should be familiar with the classification and management strategy for each category. A breast density must be visible in orthogonal views. A density that disappears when the transducer is rotated 90° is, by definition, not a mass. The utility of breast ultrasound is operator dependent, depending of course, on training and experience. An experienced breast surgeon has the ability to integrate risk assessment, clinical history, physical examination, and symptoms into the evaluation of an ultrasound image. All of this information is essential in making the decision to perform an image-guided breast biopsy.

A new, nonpalpable, ovoid, hypoechoic, nonshadowing density that is classified as probably benign (BIRADS 3) by radiology may require biopsy if the consulting surgeon has additional information such as a strong family history for breast cancer.

Benign breast masses include cystic and solid densities.

A cystic density can be described in terms of shape, echogenicity, shadowing, and enhancement. Cysts are usually well circumscribed and surrounded by a thin capsule. There is an absence of echoes within the structure, and due to the increased speed of the ultrasound beam through the liquid filled mass, there is enhancement, or brightening of the tissue posterior to the cyst, compared to the tissue adjacent to the cyst. Edge shadows, when present are usually thin. A trained eye can usually detect the presence of an intramural nodule in the wall of a cyst. An ultrasound-guided fine-needle aspiration is invaluable is obtaining a sample of such an intramural nodule, which can be solitary or multiple in number.

While the BIRADS classification ranges from BIRADS 0 to BIRADS 6, the surgeon can classify an imaged density into one of four categories, Simple (S)/complex cyst (CC), fibroadenoma, indeterminate mass, or suspicious for malignancy.

Simple cysts (Fig. 6.6) typically have smooth or sharp edges. There are no internal echoes within a cyst and are described as anechoic. The retrotumoral pattern is called enhancement, because the speed of the ultrasound traveling through a liquid medium is faster than the speed through solid tissue. As a result the returning echo travels back to the transducer at a faster rate of speed, resulting in a stronger sound signal (enhancement).

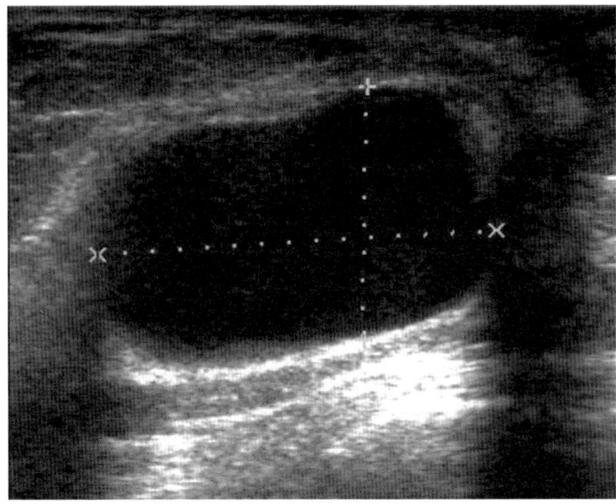

Fig. 6.6 Simple cyst

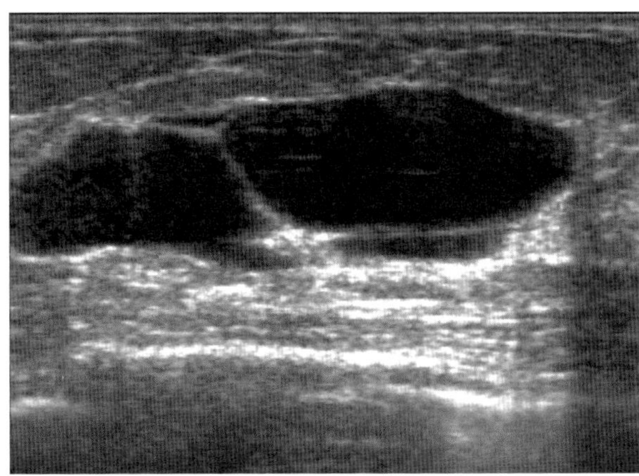

Fig. 6.7 Complicated cyst

Complex cysts (Fig. 6.7) may contain internal echoes due to the presence of crystals or thickened fluid. On occasion there may be internal septations within these cystic structures.

Solid densities are also described in terms of shape, echogenecity, and retro density characteristics of enhancement or shadowing. Benign solid masses such as a fibroadenoma (Fig. 6.8) are usually described as smooth, rounded, ovoid, or lobulated.

An indeterminate density (Fig. 6.9) may have characteristics of fibroadenoma and suspicious densities.

A mass that is suspicious for malignancy (Fig. 6.10) may have fuzzy or jagged edges, and an echo pattern that is hypoechoic or anechoic. The retrotumoral pattern of a suspicious density ranges from an irregular shadow to unilateral shadowing. Occasionally a suspicious mass will be nonshadowing.

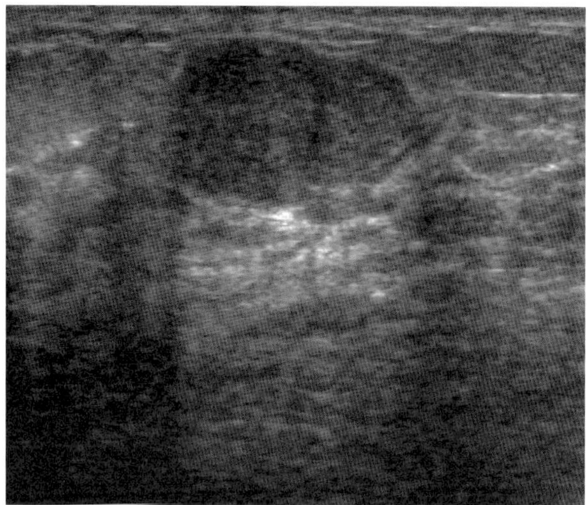

Fig. 6.8 Fibroadenoma

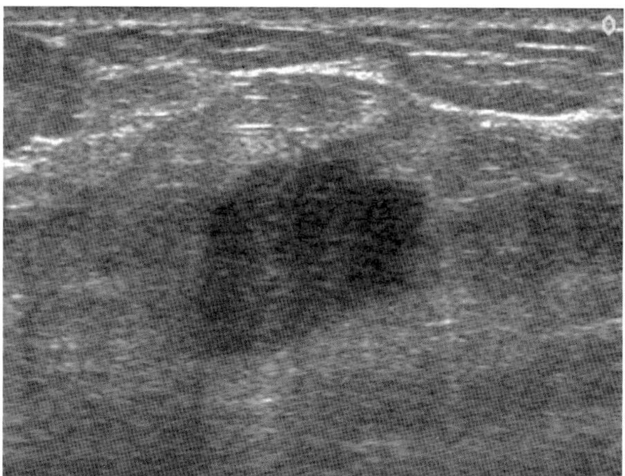

Fig. 6.9 Indeterminate mass

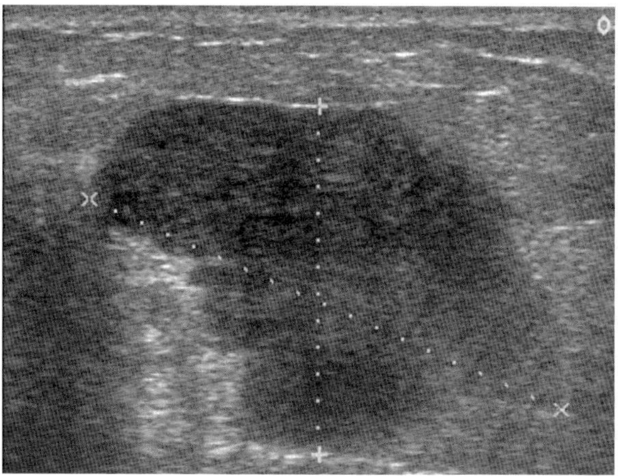

Fig. 6.10 Suspicious mass

An anechoic shadowing density is usually solid. However it is important to remember that a small percentage of benign appearing breast densities are malignant. Any newly detected or previously undescribed density must be classified, and if necessary, biopsied to make an accurate diagnosis.

Future Applications

The first Breast Ultrasound for Surgeons course was conducted in Chicago, Illinois, in 1994. During the past two decades, there has been increased awareness and utilization of minimally invasive surgery, as evidenced by the design and development of many minimally invasive ultrasound-guided breast biopsy devices and equipment platforms.

The common element that links many of these minimally invasive procedures is the prerequisite for advanced breast ultrasound imaging skills. These skills are essential for safe utilization of these diagnostic and therapeutic devices.

Newer image-guided therapies such as cryotherapy and laser ablation cryotherapy, for diagnostic and therapeutic procedures for benign lesions hold great promise for the future. Phase I clinical trials are now underway evaluating the efficacy of ultrasound-guided cryoablation of benign and malignant breast tumors and cryo-assisted lumpectomy (CAL).

Clinical trials are also underway evaluating the efficacy and safety of ultrasound-guided minimally invasive lumpectomy devices.

The transition from minimally invasive diagnostic procedures to minimally invasive therapeutic procedures is rapidly approaching. These therapies may soon be proven effective for treatment of early breast cancers. Surgeons who choose to ignore these technologies will find themselves watching from the sidelines as emerging minimally invasive therapies evolve into everyday treatment methods.

Suggested Reading

Staren ED, O'Neill TP. Breast ultrasound. Surg Clin North Am. 1998;78(2):219–35.

Parker SH, Jobe WE, Dennis MMAA, et al. Ultrasound-guided large core biopsy. Radiology. 1993;187:507–11.

Ariga R, Bloom K, Reddy VB, et al. Fine-Needle Aspirate of clinically suspicious palpable breast mass with histopathologic correlation. Am J Surg. 2002;184:410–3.

Sotiriou C, Powles TJ, Dowsett M, et al. Stereotactic breast biopsy with a breast biopsy gun. Radiology. 1990;176:741–7.

Lindgren PG. Percutaneous needle biopsy: a new technique. Acta Radiol. 1982;23:653–6.

Geller BM, Barlow WE, et al. Use of the American College of Radiology BI-RADS. Radiology. 2002;222:536–42.

Parker SH, Stavros AT. Interventional breast ultrasound; 1993.

Chapter 7
Role of Stereotaxis in Diagnosis and Treatment of Breast Tumors

Kambiz Dowlatshahi and Anna Katz

Historical Background

Breast stereotaxis developed by a Swedish radiologist and a Finish engineer was first deployed in early 1980s as a clinical tool in Karolinska Institute in Stockholm, Sweden [1]. Its emergence as a diagnostic device followed the popularization of screening mammography for early detection of breast cancer [2–4]. Women with mammographic abnormalities underwent wire localization and open biopsy for diagnosis of cancer when an abnormality was detected. Only 20 % of these shadows were proven to be malignant on subsequent histologic examination [5]. Thus four of five patients underwent stressful experience of unnecessary surgery and associated cost.

In 1985 the author (KD) travelled to Karolinska, evaluated the technology, and learned its application. The Swedish investigators reported on 2,594 patients whose breast lesions had been biopsied with a fine needle and noted suspicious lesions in 22.7 % of cases. Subsequent excisional biopsy proved the true positives to be 17.5 % [6]. The author then observed its utility by a gynecologist at the University of Kiel in West Germany who reported on 528 patients with an accuracy of 92 % [7]. The technology was then introduced into the United States at the University of Chicago.

The device was elegant and yet simple to operate (Fig. 7.1a). Its center piece consisted of a 20-gauged needle with a corkscrew stylet mounted on a manually operated module (Fig. 7.1b), which functioned on a polar principle in contrast to Cartesian system which formed the framework of another streotactic table at a later date. The coordinates of the lesion within the compressed immobilized breast were determined by measuring x- and y-dimensions on two images taken on a film in a single cassette by moving the X-ray arm 30° from right to left and exposing one half of the film at a

K. Dowlatshahi, M.D. (✉)
Department of General Surgery, Rush University Medical Center,
60 East Delaware Place, Suite 1400, Chicago, IL 60611, USA
e-mail: kdowlat@gmail.com

A. Katz, M.D.
Advocate Condell Medical Center, Libertyville, IL, USA

D.S. Francescatti and M.J. Silverstein (eds.), *Breast Cancer: A New Era in Management*, DOI 10.1007/978-1-4614-8063-1_7,

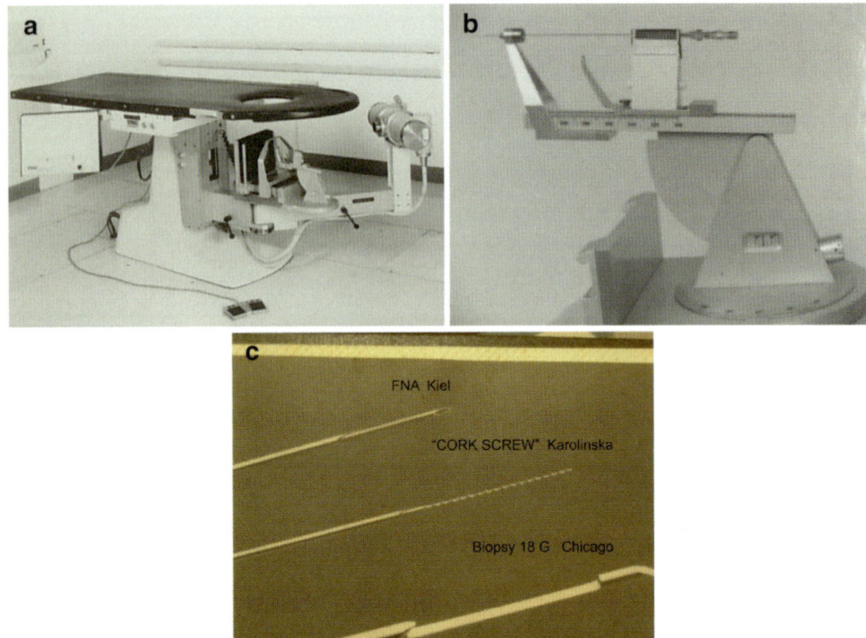

Fig. 7.1 (**a**) First stereotactic table imported into the United States in 1985. (**b**) The module on which the biopsy needle was positioned and manually operated. (**c**) Stereotactic breast biopsy needles used for sampling breast lesions. The two used at Karolinska and the University of Kiel, West Germany, retrieved cytologic samples. The 18-gauge needle was at that time used for renal biopsies and was adapted for breast lesions

time. The x,y,z-coordinates were determined by a calculator and the printed data was transferred to the needle holder module by the operator who would manually adjust the entry point of the needle into the breast. After preparing the skin with alcohol and local anesthetic, the needle was inserted into the breast and advanced to the border of the target. A second set of images was taken to confirm good positioning. Sampling consisted of "cork-screwing" the stylet of the needle into the breast lesion and then withdrawing it while leaving the needle in position for possible second or third attempts (Fig. 7.1c). The sample, a mixture of a sliver of tissue and cells, was smeared onto a sterile glass slide for immediate *cytologic* interpretation.

The accuracy of the test and the follow-up results were satisfactory provided an experienced cytopathologist was available, but was suboptimal otherwise [7]. The author then began taking core samples with a 20-gauged needle in a consecutive series of 250 patients who were scheduled to undergo open biopsy for suspicious mammograms. The results showed sensitivity of 71 %, specificity of 96 %, and insufficiency rate of 17 % [8]. Other investigators employed 14-gauged needles with improved results [9–11].

"Needle instead of knife" approach for diagnosis of mammographic abnormalities was presented to several local and national surgical meetings but it was not received with enthusiasm. Radiologists, on the other hand, accepted the technology immediately and began exploring its application on a large scale and dominating the field. A decade later general/breast surgeons appealed to the American College of Surgeons to organize training courses for stereotactic needle biopsy training, which started in 1998 in Chicago and presently continues at different sites by the American College of Breast Surgeons. Currently radiologists perform the majority of stereotactic needle biopsies nationally and consider the procedure as part of their specialty. A formal action was initiated through the Institute of Medicine, Congress, and FDA to block surgeons from performing this procedure. At the community level the executive health care committees hesitate to grant trained surgeons the priviledge of practicing the procedure. The issue is an ongoing dispute at this time.

Modern Stereotaxis

Since its inception in Sweden and introduction into the United States, stereotactic technology has undergone several major changes. The first one was the introduction of digital imaging [12, 13]. This change was incorporated in the stereotactic devices even before their application in routine mammography. The change facilitated the biopsy procedure significantly by shortening the operation time. Furthermore, the high resolution capability together with magnification and rapid image processing features enabled the operator to visualize minute parenchymal changes for sampling. The second development was computerization of the system which allowed rapid transfer of the data from the monitor screen to the mechanized platform. Third was the emergence of vacuum-assisted cutting probes which once appropriately positioned in the breast removed multiple samples from the targeted lesion with one instead of multiple passes as was the case with mechanized needles [14, 15]. Thus with the combination of high-resolution digital screening mammography resulting in detection of smaller cancers and larger needles removing 10–15 core samples, one is witnessing complete percutaneous removal of some breast tumors as documented on ensuing excisional biopsy.

Other Breast Stereotactic Technologies

In late 1980s Fischer Corporation based in Denver CO acquired the license and production rights of the stereotactic table in the United States. Soon afterwards LoRad/Hologic Corp. in Danbury CT introduced their version of breast stereotactic table whereby the biopsy unit including the X-ray arm could be rotated 180° around the breast, thus enabling the operator to biopsy the lesions from all directions. This was a technical advantage partially cancelled by slight disadvantage of the technology being based on Cartesian principle, meaning that the platform could be raised parallel with the table undersurface, limiting visualization of lesions in the far posterior 2–5 mm part of the breast close to the chest wall because the X-ray beam travels parallel with the undersurface of the table. This problem could in some cases be resolved, in rare occasions, by bringing the patient's arm through the table opening.

Both Fischer and LoRad tables have to be secured onto the floor although their "mobile" versions can be transported to a medical facility in an especially equipped truck on a prearranged date for performance of breast biopsies. In 2006, Siemens introduced yet another stereotactic table into clinical practice. This was an upright device which could be attached to a regular mammographic unit, thus lowering the cost and obviating the need for a dedicated space. The biopsy is done with the patient sitting upright, which is an advantage as lying prone on the traditional table for up to an hour causes neck discomfort in some patients. On the other hand the dedicated table allows the gravity to pull the breast away from the chest wall allowing access to the posterior targets. Additionally, patients are unlikely to faint in a prone position and the operating surgeon has a better sense of control.

Role of Ultrasound in Diagnosis of Breast Lesions

During the past decade there has been a dramatic improvement in the resolution of breast sonography. Soft tissue densities as small as 5 mm in diameter and even clusters of microcalcifications may be visualized by ultrasound. Miniaturization of the technology has made the device small enough to be portable and to be used in the office, at the bedside, as well as in the operating room. Ultrasound differentiates cystic from solid breast lesions. Its acoustic properties demonstrate homogeneity of the lesion, thus differentiating benign from malignant tumors. Additionally, color Doppler ultrasound demonstrates the vascularity of the suspected tumor.

Ultrasound has truly become the 21st-century stethoscope of the surgeon. In clinical practice ultrasound-guided needle biopsy has replaced most breast biopsies previously performed on a stereotactic table [16]. The emergence of three-dimensional ultrasound makes this breast imaging technology even more appealing.

Role of "Functional Imaging" in Diagnosis of Breast Lesions

1. Magnetic resonant imaging (MRI) is a technology which has come to play a significant role in breast imaging especially in dense breasts of younger women where mammography is not sensitive enough to detect small tumors at early phases of development [17–19]. In today's practice, MRI is deployed in patients with dense breasts to rule out multi-centricity as well as bilaterality once a focus of malignancy is documented in one breast. MR-guided breast biopsy is increasingly practiced in younger women with dense parenchyma and in patients with scars of previous interventions.
2. Positron emission mammography (PEM) is yet another emerging technology for detecting carcinoma in a dense breast and for surveillance of patients with known breast cancer [20].

Percutaneous Treatment of Breast Cancer on Stereotactic Table

Having established the ability to sample non-palpable lesions anywhere in the breast with a 2 mm accuracy, one could utilize the same technology for treatment. The breast tumor, either benign or malignant, may be removed mechanically with a probe such as Mammotome [21] or be ablated by heat using laser [22], radiofrequency [23], and high-intensity-focused ultrasound, or by freezing cryotherapy [24]. It is essential to determine the prognostic factors of the tumor on the needle core samples and to archive a segment of the tissue for future reference. The procedure is accomplished under local anesthesia in an outpatient setting with the patient lying prone on the stereotactic table and the breast compressed and immobilized. We have previously reported on a series of 54 patients whose laser-treated tumors were excised 1–8 weeks later for pathologic evaluation and two patients who were followed up with imaging and without excision [25].

In summary, we are witnessing a paradigm shift in treatment of breast tumors, both malignant and benign. *The shift is from tactile to visual.* The downward trend in the breast tumor size as a direct result of annual screening mammography and the emergence of related imaging technologies have enabled the physicians to offer less intrusive yet effective methods of treating breast tumors. The Internet access by the educated and informed women is forcing the health care providers to consider more aesthetically pleasing treatments. Equally significant is that these minimally invasive treatments are less painful and aesthetically superior and the recovery time for the patient is shorter. Finally, the overall cost is predicted to be lower as the operating room and general anesthesia expenses are reduced or eliminated.

References

1. Nordenstrom B, Zajicek J. Sterotaxic needle biopsy and preoperative indication of nonpalpable mammary lesions. Acta Cytol. 1977;21:350–1.
2. Moskowiz M. Mammographic screening: significance of minimal breast cancers. Am J Roentgenol. 1981;136:735–8.
3. Baker L. Breast cancer detection demonstration project: five-year summary report. CA Cancer J Clin. 1982;32(4):194–225.
4. Spivey G, Perry B, et al. Predicting the risk of cancer at the time of breast biopsy. Am Surg. 1982;48:326–32.
5. Bassett L, Liu TH, et al. The prevalence of carcinoma in palpable vs impalpable, mammographically detected lesions. Am J Roentgenol. 1991;157:21–4.
6. Azevado E, Svane G, et al. Stereotactic fine-needle biopsy in 2594 mammographically detected non-palpable lesions. Lancet. 1989;1:1033–6.
7. Dowlatshahi K, Gent H, et al. Nonpalpable breast tumors: diagnosis with stereotaxic localization and fine-needle aspiration. Radiology. 1989;170(2):427–33.
8. Dowlatashahi K, Yaremko ML, et al. Nonpalpable breast lesions: findings of stereotaxic needle-core biopsy and fine-needle aspiration cytology. Radiology. 1991;181(3):745–50.

9. Parker SH, Lovin JD, et al. Nonpalpable breast lesions: stereotactic automated large-core biopsies. Radiology. 1991;180:403–7.
10. Parker SH, Burbank F, et al. Percutaneous large-core breast biopsy: a multi-institutional study. Radiology. 1994;193:359–64.
11. Helbich TH, Rudas M, et al. Evaluation of needle size for breast biopsy: comparison of 14-, 16-, and 18-gauge biopsy needles. Am J Roentgenol. 1998;171:59–63.
12. Whitlock J, Evans A, et al. Digital imaging improves upright stereotactic core biopsy of mammographic microcalcifications. Clin Radiol. 2000;55(5):374–7.
13. Becker L, Taves D, et al. Stereotactic core biopsy of breast microcalcifications: comparison of film versus digital mammography, both using add-on unit. Am J Roentgenol. 2001;177: 1451–7.
14. Reynolds HE, Poon CM, et al. Biopsy of breast microcalcifications using an 11-guage directional vacuum assisted device. Am J Roentgenol. 1998;171:59–63.
15. Pfarl G, Helbich TH, et al. Stereotactic 11-gauge vacuum-assisted breast biopsy: a validation study. Am J Roentgenol. 2002;179:1503–7.
16. Helbich TH, Matzek W, et al. Stereotactic and ultrasound-guided breast biopsy. Eur Radiol. 2004;14:383–93.
17. Saslow D, Boetes C, et al. American Cancer Society guidelines for breast screening with MRI as an adjunct to mammography. CA Cancer J Clin. 2007;57:75–89.
18. Bkeicher RJ, Morrow M. MRI and breast cancer: role in detection, diagnosis, and staging. Oncology. 2007;21(12):1521–8.
19. Heywang-Kobrunner SH, Bick U, et al. International investigation of breast MRI: results of a multicentre study (11 sites) concerning diagnostic parameters for contrast-enhanced MRI based on 519 histopathalogically correlated lesions. Eur Radiol. 2001;11:531–46.
20. Berg WA, Madsen KS, et al. Breast cancer: comparative effectiveness of positron emission mammography and MR imaging in presurgical planning for the ipsilateral breast. Radiology. 2007;258(1):59–72.
21. Burbank F, Parker SH, et al. Stereotactic breast biopsy: improved tissue harvesting with the mammotome. Am Surg. 1996;62:738–44.
22. Dowlatshahi K, Francescatti DS, et al. Laser therapy for small breast cancers. Am J Surg. 2002;184:359–63.
23. Burak WE, Agnese DM, et al. Radiofrequency ablation of invasive breast carcinoma followed by delayed surgical excision. Cancer. 2003;98(7):1369–76.
24. Sabek MS, Kaufman CS, et al. Cryoablation of early-stage breast cancer: work-in-progress report of a multi-institutional trial. Ann Surg Oncol. 2004;11(5):542–9.
25. Bloom KJ, Dowlat K, et al. Pathalogic changes after interstitial laser therapy of infiltrating breast carcinoma. Am J Surg. 2001;182(4):384–8.

Chapter 8
Breast MR for Treatment Planning

Steven E. Harms

Introduction

Breast MR is the most sensitive imaging examination for the detection of breast cancer. Screening trials show that breast MR has about twofold to threefold the sensitivity of mammography [1–4]. Despite the higher cost compared to mammography, most cancer groups (American Cancer Society, National Comprehensive Cancer Network, British National Health Service, etc.) now recommend annual screening breast MR for women at increased risk for developing breast cancer [5–7]. Despite the success in screening applications, the use of breast MR for local staging has been increasingly criticized. This chapter reviews the current data and the controversies concerning the use of breast MR in patients with recently diagnosed breast cancer for pretreatment staging.

Arguments against the use of breast MR primarily center on the following objections: (1) mammography is the standard of care for staging women who are candidates for breast conservation, (2) use of breast MR increases the mastectomy rate, (3) the additional disease detected by breast MR is subclinical and is adequately treated with adjuvant therapy, (4) breast conservation has a low recurrence rate without breast MR and its use is unlikely to lower the recurrence rate, and (5) breast MR does not reduce the re-excision rate. We will evaluate the evidence as it applies to each of these arguments. There are several potential benefits for breast MR

S.E. Harms, M.D., F.A.C.R. (✉)
Department of Radiology, The Breast Center of Northwest Arkansas,
University of Arkansas for Medical Sciences, 55 Sunbridge, Fayetteville, AR 72703, USA
e-mail: seharms@earthlink.net

D.S. Francescatti and M.J. Silverstein (eds.), *Breast Cancer: A New Era in Management*,
DOI 10.1007/978-1-4614-8063-1_8,

staging: (1) reduced local recurrence rate, (2) reduced positive margin rate, (3) more appropriate treatment management, (4) detection of contralateral occult disease, and (5) detection of occult invasive disease in women with DCIS. While survival is often discussed, it is very difficult to control in a study because of the variability in treatment subsequent to the imaging study. Most of the MR trials only look at the diagnostic performance relative to other imaging studies. While one may infer that treatment may improve with more reliable diagnosis, very little information is available to show an actual benefit for MR in lowering recurrence rates. Surrogate endpoints, however, point to the potential for significant improvements in patient management in some situations.

Mammography Is a Poor Standard

Mammography is currently accepted as the standard imaging method for the local staging of breast cancer in most of the industrialized world. Its use for breast conservation, however, was never validated. The NSABP B6 trial did not require mammography [8].

It is often falsely stated that the mammographic sensitivity of 85–90 % is sufficient to determine the local extent of disease. No clinical trial validates mammographic sensitivity in that range. The major mammographic screening trials using follow-up as a gold standard show the sensitivity to be only about 70 % at best [9]. The average sensitivity is about 50 % [9–11]. As we will see when a better gold standard, breast MR, is available for comparison, the true mammographic sensitivity is much lower.

International screening trials were performed comparing breast MR to mammography and/or ultrasound for the screening of women with increased risk of developing breast cancer. These data consistently show significant improvements in sensitivity. MR sensitivity is in the 71–100 % range compared to mammographic sensitivity in the 13–40 % range (Table 8.1). The studies that reported MR misses were mostly DCIS that could not be seen on the low-resolution MR scans that were

Table 8.1 MR screening of high-risk women

Source	Number of patients	Additional cancer yield of MR (%)	MR sensitivity (%)	MR specificity (%)	Mammographic sensitivity (%)
Kriege	1,909	2.4	71.1	89.8	33
Warner	236	9.3	85	93	36
MARIBS	649	2.9	77	81	40
Kuhl	192	3.0	100	75	33
Lehman	367	1.1	100	94	25
Podo	105	4.8	100	99	13

generated at that time. The increased cancer detection rate over mammography varies from 1 to 9 %. Most experts predicted breast MR to improve sensitivity, but the concern was that the higher false [12] positive rate could outweigh the benefits of the new test. The clinical trials, however, consistently show positive predictive values for MR that meet or exceed commonly accepted performance for mammographic screening [1, 2, 13, 14]. It is surprising that a test with 40 % sensitivity is uniformly accepted while the test with 71–100 % sensitivity is questioned.

Dense Breasts

Mammography performs poorly in women with dense breasts [15]. This problem led some health care organizations to recommend against screening mammography in women under 50 [16, 17].

There is evidence in the non-MR literature that indicates impaired staging in women with dense breasts. Women with dense breasts are more likely to fail breast conservation due to occult disease. A study showed that 10-year local recurrence rate for women with dense breasts was 21 % compared to 5 % for low density (hazard ratio of 5.7). This difference was greater in women who did not receive radiotherapy with recurrences in 40 % of the dense breast group compared to none with less than 25 % density [18]. Another study from UCSF showed similar findings. Women with dense breasts (greater than 75 % density) had a hazard ratio of 4.3 for local recurrence compared to low-density women (less than 25 % density) [19]. Morrow's group recently translated this experience to actual practice where they showed that women with radiographically dense breasts are more likely to be treated with mastectomy (61 %) compared with women with lesser density (43 %). Failure of breast conservation was due to luminal A tumors, lobular histology, multicentricity, and occult tumors [20]. Patients where the original tumor was mammographically occult are more likely to have diffuse histology and more difficult to follow [21].

A recent study from Canada comparing mammographic and MR screening in high-risk women showed mammographic sensitivity in women with greater than 50 % breast density to only be 12 %, compared with MR sensitivity in the same group of 75 %. However, even in women with the lowest breast density (less than 10 % density) mammographic sensitivity only improved to 31 %, compared to 92 % sensitivity for MR [22]. An example of an incidentally detected cancer on MR in a woman with extensive fibrocystic changes is shown in Fig. 8.1.

The poor diagnostic performance of mammography in women with dense breasts has prompted several states to pass laws requiring breast imaging centers to inform women if their mammogram shows increased breast density. Breast density is in itself a risk factor amounting to a cumulative lifetime risk of about 20 % [23]. This observation will likely lead to increased use of breast MR for the screening and diagnostic management of women with dense breasts (Fig. 8.1).

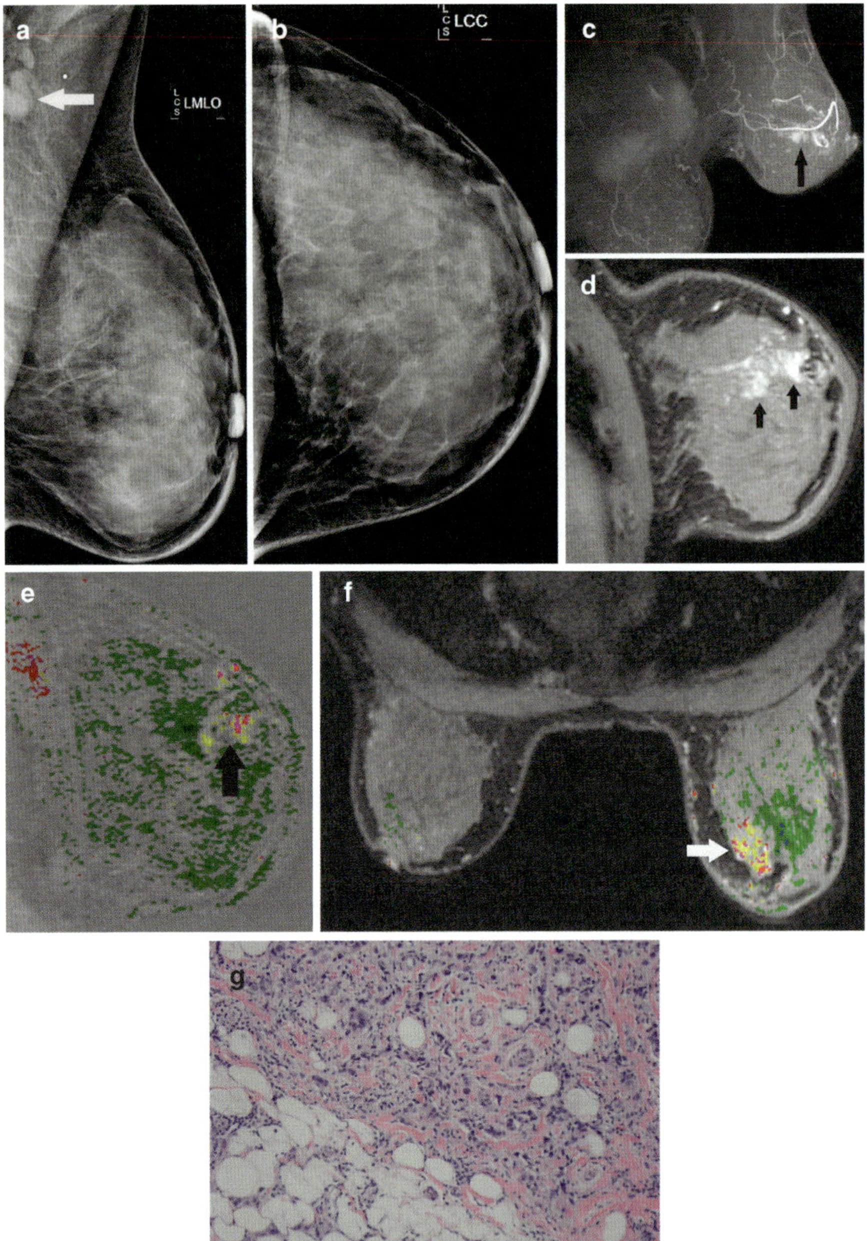

Fig. 8.1 Radiographically dense breasts and axillary adenopathy. This 45-year-old woman presented with a left axillary mass. Workup with diagnostic mammography and ultrasound fail to show any primary. The MLO (**a**) and CC (**b**) mammographic views show the enlarged axillary lymph node (*arrow*) but no abnormality in the breast. She has radiographically dense breasts that are known to impair mammographic sensitivity. Breast MR demonstrates extensive disease in the left breast. The oblique projection maximum intensity projection (MIP) (**c**) shows extensive enhancement in the left breast (*arrow*). The oblique sagittal slice (**d**) depicts the intensive enhancement extending within the ductal ray (*arrows*). Washout (*red*) intermixed with persistent (*yellow*) dynamics is seen with the area of abnormal enhancement (*arrow*) on the sagittal (**e**) and axial (**f**) subtractions with computer-aided detection (CAD). Biopsy of the MR finding shows a Bloom–Richardson grade III/III infiltrating ductal carcinoma (**g**)

High-Risk Histology

Certain benign histologies such as LCIS, atypical ductal hyperplasia, atypical lobular hyperplasia, and peripheral papillomas are considered markers for and increased risk of malignancy. Needle biopsies that result in high-risk histology present management challenges. Excisional biopsy is often recommended due to the frequency of upgrade to malignancy. The upgrade to malignancy for excisional biopsy after a needle biopsy for LCIS ranges from 14 to 50 % [24]. The cancer upgrades are largely attributed to sampling errors that are reduced when larger volumes of tissue are removed with an excisional biopsy. The upgrade rate typically decreases with use of larger bore needles, but a 38 % upgrade rate has been reported with 9-gauge needles [25]. So larger needles is not the whole solution. Atypia has an upgrade rate to malignancy that is generally less than LCIS (10–35 %).

These high-risk lesions reflect an increased risk of malignancy in all the breast tissue, not just the biopsy site. One paper states that the cancer is three times more likely to develop in the ipsilateral breast [26]. Other papers show a preference for the contralateral breast [27]. Three studies have shown a benefit for breast MR screening in patients with high-risk histology (Table 8.2) [27–29]. The cancer detection rate of 3.8–4 % is consistent with the detection rates in the high-risk screening trials. One screening trial only included BRCA patients resulting in about a 9.3 % yield [14]. Most of the other trials were less than the 4 % yield for the high-risk histology trials [2, 7]. The higher biopsy rates for high-risk histology are attributed to the tendency for these patients to have more substantial background enhancement. The American Cancer Society guidelines discussed the potential for including high-risk histology as an indication but cited a lack of clinical trial data [7]. The more recent NCCN guidelines include an indication for breast MR for LCIS [6]. A breast MR will likely be beneficial in the pre-surgical evaluation of women with high-risk histology on needle biopsy prior to surgical excision. The MR may identify occult ipsilateral and contralateral disease that could be missed on excision (Fig. 8.2).

New MR techniques are particularly well suited for the accurate diagnosis and treatment of intraductal papillomas. Intraductal papilloma is the most common neoplasm associated with unilateral, spontaneous bloody or serous nipple discharge (31–78 %). Yet, malignancy may be seen in 5–18 % of cases [30]. High-contrast, high-resolution breast MR using positive- and negative-scale subtractions provide excellent definition of intraductal lesions, but can also depict malignancies that may be missed with conventional imaging, including galactography (Fig. 8.3). This improved definition may facilitate the correct identification and biopsy of

Table 8.2 MR screening in women with high-risk histology

Study	Cancer rate	PPV	Biopsy rate
Port (LCIS, ADH)	4 % (5/135)	9.2 % (5/46)	25 % (46/182)
Friedlander (LCIS)	3.8 % (5/133)	18.5 % (5/27)	18.8 % (25/133)
Sung (LCIS)	4 % (10/220)	20 % (12/60)	27 % (59/220)
High-risk genetics studies	1.1–9.3 %	7.1–63 %	2.9–15.8 %

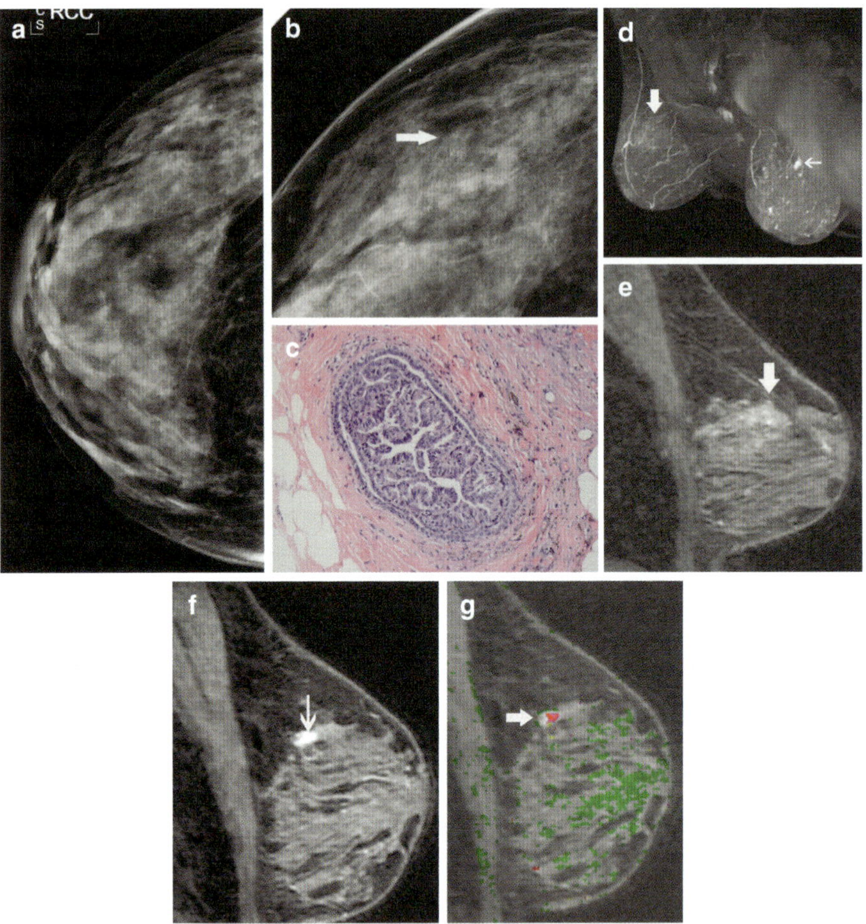

Fig. 8.2 Occult infiltrating carcinoma in a patient with a recent needle biopsy showing atypical ductal hyperplasia. This 59-year-old woman was recalled from screening mammography for a cluster of heterogeneous calcifications in the right breast. The CC (**a**) and magnification CC (**b**) mammographic views show the calcifications (*arrow*). No abnormality was seen in the left breast. A stereotactic biopsy was performed which showed atypical ductal hyperplasia (**c**). As our routine for all patients with recently diagnosed high-risk histology, a breast MR was performed to evaluate for possible occult disease. Breast MR shows no occult disease in the right breast, but does show a spiculated mass in the left breast that could not be seen on mammography or ultrasound even in retrospect. The MIP of the immediate post-contrast series (**d**) shows low-level diffuse enhancement from the biopsy site on the right (*large arrow*) and an intensely enhancing mass (*small arrow*) on the left. The reformatted sagittal image (**e**) of the biopsy site on the right shows low-level enhancement typical of post-biopsy change, but no evidence of malignancy. The reformatted sagittal image (**f**) of the left breast shows intense irregular enhancement typical of infiltrating carcinoma. Washout (*red*) is depicted on the sagittal subtraction with computer-aided detection (**g**). Biopsy on the left revealed an infiltrating ductal carcinoma

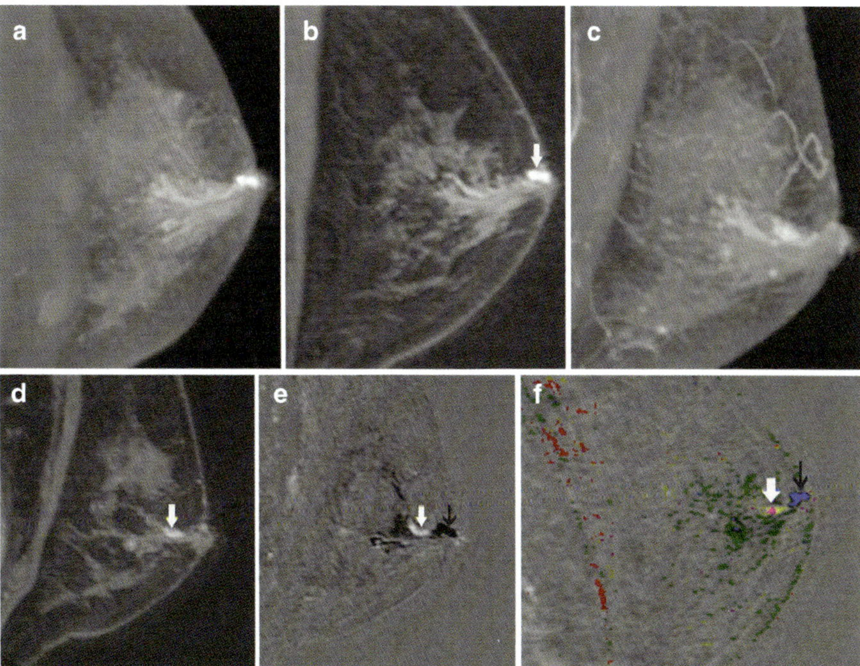

Fig. 8.3 Intraductal papilloma shown with positive- and negative-scale subtracted MR imaging. This 57-year-old patient presented with a spontaneous, unilateral, bloody nipple discharge on the left. The sagittal, pre-contrast, non-spoiled (T2 weighted) maximum intensity projection (MIP) image (**a**) shows dilated ducts in the subareolar region. A 700-μm oblique slice calculated along the duct from the same pre-contrast acquisition (**b**) shows hyperintense fluid in a dilated duct (*arrow*). The sagittal, post-contrast, spoiled (T2 weighting reduced) MIP image (**c**) shows continued increased signal from dilated ducts due to hemorrhagic fluid shortening the T1. The intraductal mass is not well seen. The 700-μm slice along the duct from the post-contrast acquisition (**d**) shows a small enhancing lesion (*arrow*). The relationship to the ducts, however, is not clear. When the pre-contrast, non-spoiled images are subtracted from the post-contrast, spoiled images, the positive- and negative-scale subtracted images (**e**) provide optimal contrast between enhancing lesions (*bright scale*) and the fluid-filled ducts (*dark scale*). The enhancing mass (*white arrow*) is clearly within the duct (*black arrow*). This is a typical appearance for an intraductal papilloma. The computer-aided detection (CAD) image (**f**) shows a *magenta mass* depicting plateau enhancement (*white arrow*) within the dilated duct shown with CAD to be fluid containing, depicted as *blue* (*black arrow*). The mass was removed with vacuum-assisted biopsy in its entirety and no surgery was required

malignancies. Solitary intraductal papillomas are not commonly associated with malignancy. Lesions that have a characteristic appearance of an intraductal papilloma on MR may be removed in their entirety with vacuum-assisted biopsy, sparing unnecessary excision [31, 32].

Choice of Mastectomy vs. Lumpectomy

Some argue that the use of breast MR needlessly increases the mastectomy rate due to the detection of incidental lesions not seen by conventional imaging [33]. A paper from the Mayo Clinic showed that the breast conservation therapy rate was 54 % in women without MR staging compared with 36 % for those with MR staging. They concluded that MR converted some patients to mastectomy. The women, however, were not randomized and it is likely (by the authors' admission) that the MR cohort had some additional clinical features such as dense breasts, young age, and positive pathologic margins among others that lead to the MR examination. The non-MR cohort had a higher mastectomy rate than historical controls indicating that there is an overall shift to mastectomy from breast conservation [34].

Bleicher reported similar findings with the mastectomy rate increasing by 1.8 when controlled for T stage. However, there is strong evidence for selection bias in this trial with 130/577 patients having been referred for breast MR. One presumes that the breast MR group was selected for a reason that may predispose to a decision towards mastectomy such as young age, dense breasts, and positive margins. One-third of the MR patients had already undergone one excision before the study. It was not mentioned how many of this group had positive margins. The MR group was younger than the non-MR group. The greater prevalence of dense breasts in younger women that may impair diagnosis on MR due to the more likely presence of signifificant background enhancement [35] .

The biggest problem with most of the breast conservation to mastectomy measurements is that they assume that the conversion is only one way (Fig. 8.4). How can you measure the total effect on management without looking at the potential for conversion from mastectomy to lumpectomy? Hollingsworth evaluated this effect and found that indeed some women were converted to mastectomy, but even more were converted the other way from mastectomy to breast conservation. The net effect was that more patients were having breast conservation (60 %) when compared to historical controls before breast MR (48 %). If the women who elect to have mastectomy but qualified for lumpectomy based upon MR extent are excluded, the breast conservation rate increased to 65 %. Hollingsworth concludes that some women who were leaning towards a choice for mastectomy are in fact reassured by the breast MR and elect for breast conservation. To substantiate this impression, the women who had falsely positive MR (false-positive rate 8.4 %) and subsequently had a benign biopsy had an even higher breast conservation rate (70 %) than the study as a whole (60 %) [36]. A similar paper from Mann et al. that evaluated MR staging for lobular carcinoma showed a nonsignificant trend towards conversion from mastectomy to breast conservation in patients who had a breast MR examination [37]. An example of an MR examination where the improved demonstration of disease extent improved surgical management and probably sparing the patient multiple surgeries or mastectomy is shown in Fig. 8.4.

In some cases, where mastectomy is indicated on the basis of clinical or conventional imaging information, MR provides additional information that may alter the mastectomy, convert to patient to breast-conserving surgery, or modify adjuvant

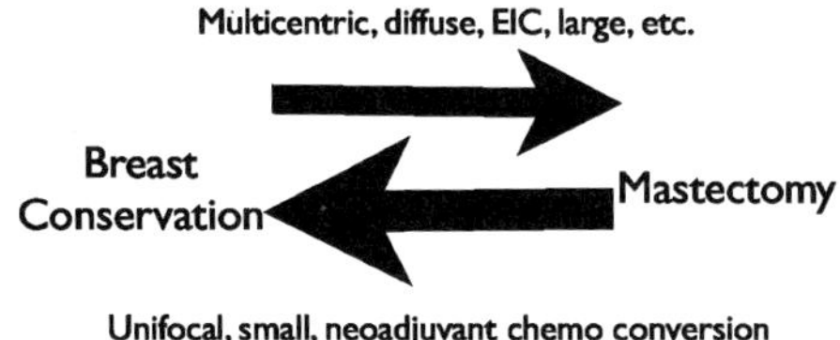

Fig. 8.4 The surgery choice is a two-way street. A number of factors affect the decision for surgical treatment. Information that may affect the decision in favor of mastectomy includes multicentric or diffuse disease, extensive intraductal component, a large tumor size, etc. In some cases, the appearance of the image may favor breast-conserving surgery such as unifocal disease and small size. The addition of neoadjuvant chemotherapy may change an appearance that favors mastectomy towards more localized disease on the post-chemotherapy image. The problem with many of the papers reporting a conversion of treatment decision to mastectomy after MR is that only the situation depicted by the *top arrow* is considered. Some have reported that if both sides of the street are considered, that MR can result in a net gain for breast conservation

therapy. More extensive disease on MR does not necessarily lead to mastectomy. A common situation in our practice is a patient who on the basis of MR extent may be treated with neoadjuvant chemotherapy (Fig. 8.5). MR after neoadjuvant chemotherapy can demonstrate a small residual that could be effectively treated with breast conservation. The mastectomy itself may be modified by the presence of chest wall disease, nipple involvement, and/or skin involvement (Fig. 8.6). MR is very effective in the diagnosis of internal mammary nodal disease. Routine whole breast and partial breast irradiation does not typically treat internal mammary nodes. Radiation therapy may be modified based upon the MR information to include the internal mammary nodes.

Reducing Positive Margins in Breast Conservation Candidates

It is recognized that some women who opt for breast conservation therapy may ultimately be converted to mastectomy due to positive pathologic margins. Huston advocates taking additional margins to reduce the need to re-excision. Taking 4–6 additional margins reduced the re-excision rate from 38.7 to 17.7 % [38]. Re-excision of margins is associated with an increased potential for recurrence. Menes showed the recurrence rate for a single excision to be 4 %, but for 1 and 2 re-excisions the recurrence rate was 7 and 17 %, respectively [39]. O'Sullivan showed a 10-year recurrence rate of 5.6 % if the lumpectomy had clear margins on the first excision, but the recurrence rate increased to 10 % if 2 or more excisions were needed to establish clear margins. The average re-excision rate in the study was 60 % [40]. A large study of 2,206 women reported a single re-excision rate of 22.9 %, two re-excisions 9.4 %, 1.4 % three re-excisions, and ultimate conversions to mastectomy 8.5 % [41]. Unsurprisingly, this is about the same number of conversions to mastectomy with MR information (Fig. 8.7). MR may identify the patients who will

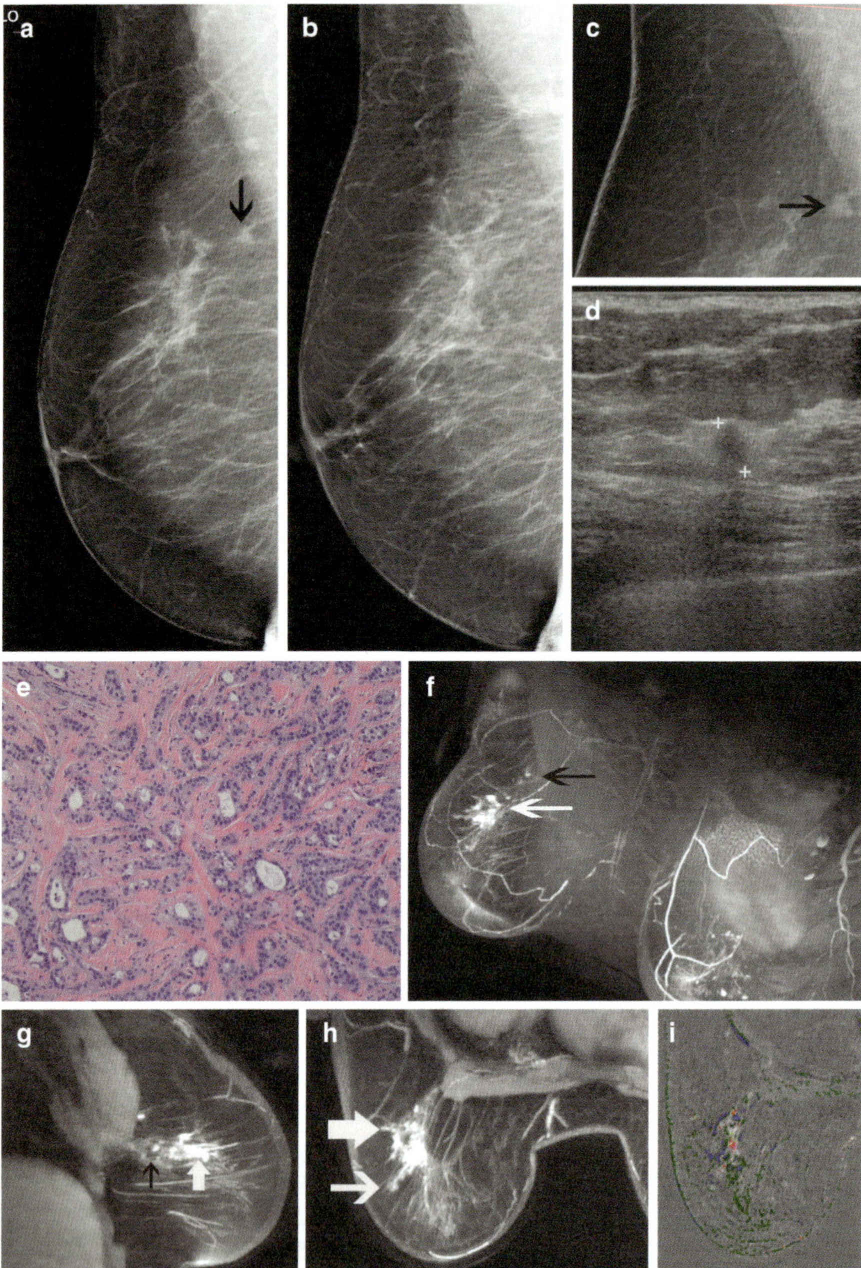

Fig. 8.5 Additional disease seen on MR affects surgery. This 65-year-old patient was recalled from screening mammography for a new irregular mass seen at the 10 o'clock position in the right breast. A small mass (*arrow*) is shown on the current MLO view (**a**). The MLO mammographic view (**b**) from the year before shows no mass. The irregular mass (*arrow*) is better seen on the magnification view (**c**). The ultrasound (**d**) shows a focal hypoechoic 7 mm mass with posterior

likely fail breast conservation surgery due to positive pathologic margins and avoid the unnecessary attempted lumpectomy procedures (Fig. 8.8).

Clearly, the establishment of clear margins on the first excision is the goal. However, the rate of positive pathologic margins is high. An acceptable positive margin rate is 25–40 %. Morrow's group reported a positive margin rate from 1987 to 2006 that varied from 67 to 50 % per year. The ability to establish clear margins did not seem to vary over time. Since the studies were limited to women who had successful breast conservation, the number of women who were ultimately converted to mastectomy is not included. The real positive margin rate was likely much higher [40].

There are other ill effects from positive margins besides the higher recurrence rate. Additional surgeries contribute higher health care costs and morbidity. The location of the excisions may impair the cosmetic result should the patient ultimately opt for breast reconstruction after mastectomy. Decisions regarding adjuvant therapy may be compromised due to the incorrect assessment of tumor size.

Can the improved sensitivity of breast MR be used to reduce positive pathologic margins? Or will the high false-positive rate of breast MR outweigh the possible benefits? There have been two randomized trials that sought to answer if MR could reduce the positive margin rate breast conservation candidates: the COMICE trial in the UK and the MONET trial in the Netherlands [42, 43]. Both of these studies showed that MR provided no benefit.

The COMICE trial was designed to reduce the re-operative rate to below 10 % and was limited to patients scheduled for a wide local excision. Of the 5,496 patients that were eligible, only 1,623 (816 with MR and 807 without MR) were included in the analysis. The re-excision rate for the MR group was 16.3 and 18.7 % for the group without MR (no statistical difference) although they reported a higher mastectomy rate in the MR group (7 %) compared to the control group that was the only

Fig. 8.5 (continued) acoustic shadowing that is highly suspicious for malignancy. No other lesions could be seen in either breast with conventional imaging. A vacuum-assisted biopsy was obtained showing Bloom–Richardson grade I/III infiltrating ductal carcinoma (**e**). This would be an example that some might say could be treated with lumpectomy and spared the need for a breast MR. However, the MR shows more extensive non-mass-like enhancement more typical of DCIS. The post-contrast MIP (**f**) shows a large area of non-mass-like enhancement (*white arrow*) anterior to the biopsy site (*dark arrow*) within the same ductal ray. This is better seen on the sagittal oblique thick slice (**g**) calculated from the immediate post-contrast series. The dark plus-shaped area (*black arrow*) identifies the artifact from the clip marker at the biopsy site. Non-mass-like enhancement representing occult DCIS extends in the same ductal ray anterior to the biopsy site (*white arrow*). The axial oblique slice (**h**) calculated from the post-contrast series shows the extent of the occult DCIS (*large arrow*). A small projection can be seen extending towards the skin (*small arrow*). Washout (*red*) is identified within the mass on the axial subtracted image with computer-aided detection (**i**). A small lumpectomy would likely have resulted in positive pathologic margins requiring either re-excision or mastectomy. The inability to achieve clear margins may have led to conversion to mastectomy. Using the MR information, the initial surgery was modified so that clear margins could be achieved without the need for re-excision or mastectomy

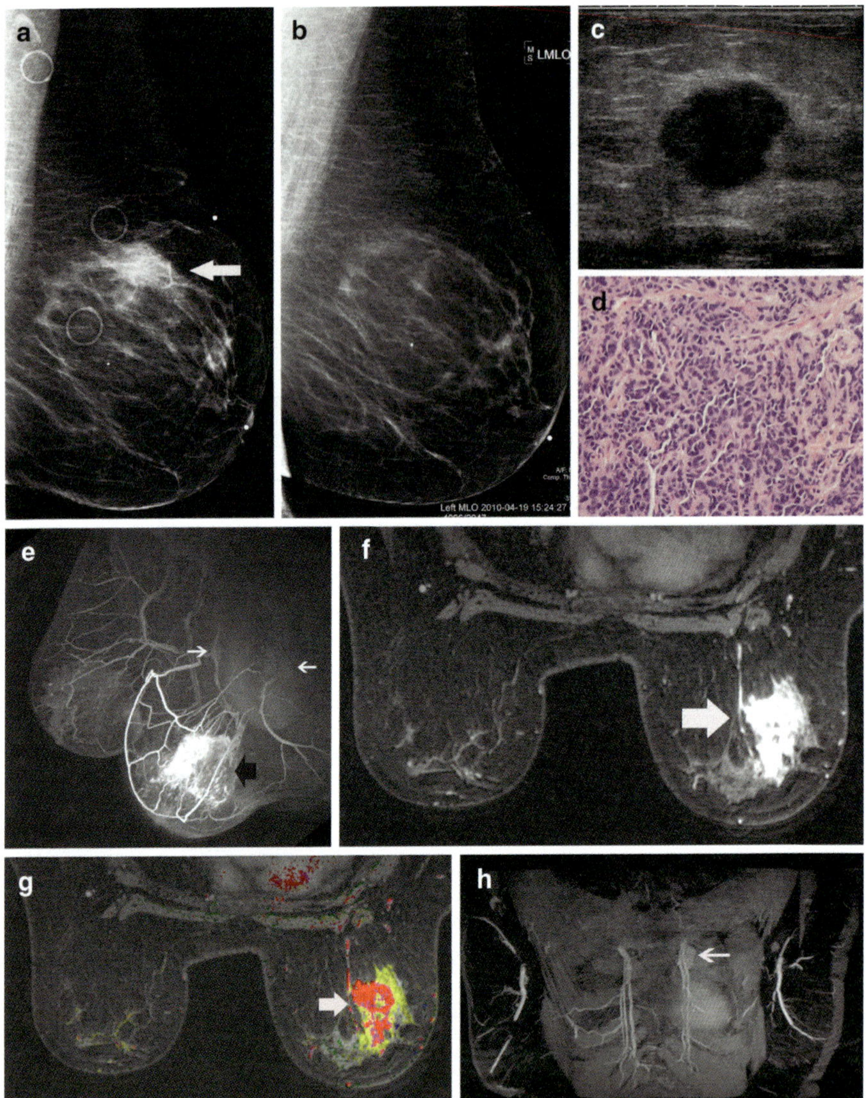

Fig. 8.6 MR findings alter treatment. This 52-year-old woman was recalled from screening mammography for an asymmetric density in the superior left breast. The MLO mammographic view (**a**) shows the density in the superior left breast that has developed since the prior study a year before (**b**). The ultrasound (**c**) performed at an outside institution was originally thought to be cystic. A cyst aspiration was attempted but failed. Subsequent core needle biopsy showed a Bloom–Richardson grade II/III infiltrating ductal carcinoma (**d**). Based upon the mammograms and ultrasound, a lumpectomy might have been attempted. The MR information significantly changed management. The oblique projection (**e**) generated from the immediate post-contrast series shows a large, enhancing mass with spiculated and irregular margins (*dark arrow*). Also on the projection notice the enlarged axillary and internal mammary (*white arrows*) nodes. The axial immediate post-contrast image (**f**) shows the spiculation of the mass (*arrow*) highly indicative of an infiltrating carcinoma.

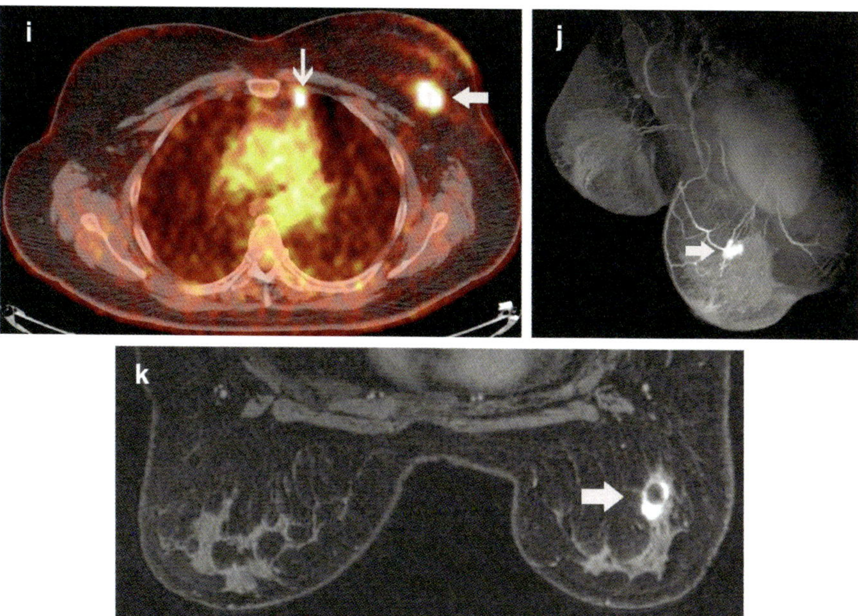

Fig. 8.6 (continued) The axial CAD image (**g**) shows a predominate mass with washout (*red*). Washout is associated with highly malignant lesions. The surrounding *yellow* areas (persistent enhancement) indicate spread of disease into the surrounding tissue. The highly suspicious internal mammary node (*arrow*) is well demonstrated on the oblique, thick slice image (**h**) calculated from the immediate post-contrast series. This was confirmed on a PET-CT (**i**) where the mass (*large arrow*) and the internal mammary nodal metastasis (*small arrow*) are shown. If a lumpectomy had been attempted, it is likely that positive margins would have resulted. Re-excision or mastectomy likely would have resulted. Based upon the MR information, the patient had neo-adjuvant chemotherapy. The projection from the immediate post-contrast series (**j**) performed after chemotherapy shows a concentric response to chemotherapy. Only a small residual remains (*arrow*). This is better seen on the axial image from the immediate post-contrast series (**k**). On this image the central low-signal area within the mass (*arrow*) represents the clip marker surrounded by enhancing residual disease. Based upon the MR information, the patient was able to have successful breast-conserving surgery without the need for re-excision. The radiation therapy was modified to include the internal mammary nodes

possible outcome. Since mastectomy candidates were not evaluated, the conversion of mastectomy to breast conservation by MR could not be observed. Subsequent analysis of the mastectomy specimens demonstrated that in 5 % of the patients mastectomies were justified by demonstration of malignancy outside the lumpectomy site. Biopsy of the incidental MR lesions was not required. Only three multicentric lesions were subjected to biopsy. Only routine pathology analysis of the mastectomy specimens was preformed. So, it is likely that the 2 % "false positives" may have been pathology-missed lesions rather than MR overcalls [42].

The study design emphasized a generalizable (average user) approach rather than optimized to centers of excellence. The ability of a surgeon to exploit the

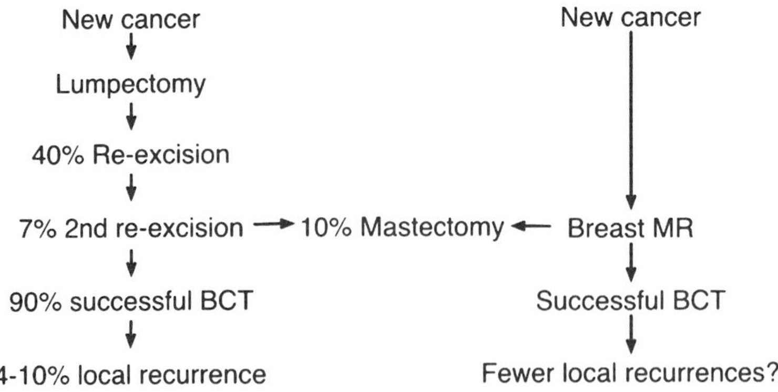

Fig. 8.7 MR may reduce positive margins and identify patients better suited to mastectomy before surgery. Breast conservation candidates may need one or two re-excisions in order to establish clear margins. About 10 % ultimately fail all attempts for clear margins and require mastectomy. MR has two potential benefits: the reduction of positive pathologic margins and the upfront identification of patients best suited for mastectomy. Ultimately, better staging should lead to lower recurrences, but this has not been scientifically established to date

information gleaned from a breast MR takes experience. Yet it appears that most of the surgeons lacked experience in not only breast MR but also breast surgery. 107 surgeons at 45 sites participated in the COMICE study. The 86 % of surgeons that were deemed "high accrual" performed an average of only two or more breast surgeries per year between the years of 2002 and 2007. The adequacy of the margin was left to the surgeon. Probably the biggest criticism of the COMICE study is the lack of quality MR images. The study protocol used 4 mm section thickness coronal slices with no fat suppression. This protocol would be insufficient to pass accreditation and would not even meet the first ACR guidelines issued over a decade ago. The lack of any demonstrated benefit in this study may not mean that breast MR could not succeed in another setting.

The MONET trial in the Netherlands also examined the potential for MR to reduce positive margins with a randomized trial of 418 patients (207 with MR and 211 without). There was no difference in the breast conservation rate or mastectomy rates between the two groups. This study showed a significantly increased re-excision rate of 34 % in the MR group compared to 21 % in the group without MR. It would appear that imaging protocol was more modern than the COMICE. The instrument was a 3 T Philips using dynamic 2 mm section thickness with fat suppression. However, the performance of the breast MR raises some concern. About half the cancers in this study were non-palpable DCIS. Yet, the reported MR sensitivity was only 51 % for DCIS. This is remarkably low compared with other MR trials. The NCI 6883 showed sensitivity for DCIS of 73 %. More modern methods should have sensitivity for DCIS of 80–95 %. The inability to accurately define the margins of DCIS could account for the problems in establishing clear margins in the MR cohort [43].

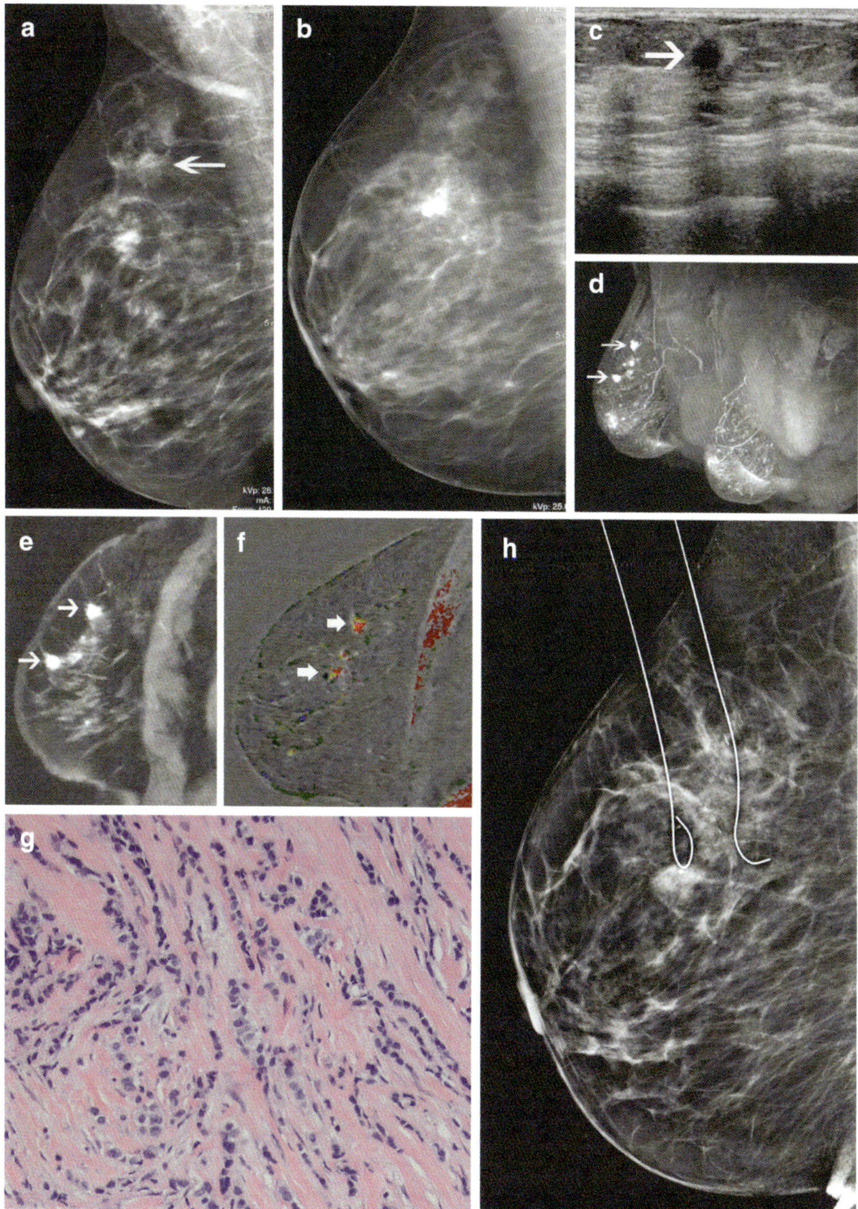

Fig. 8.8 Multifocal lobular carcinoma. This 68-year-old woman was recalled from screening mammography for a subtle increasing focal asymmetry (*arrow*) in the right breast (**a**) when compared with the screening mammogram the year before (**b**). Ultrasound (**c**) confirmed a hypoechoic mass (*arrow*) suspicious for malignancy. Because of the subtle findings on mammography, a breast MR was performed which showed additional occult lesions within the same ductal ray. These are well seen on the MIP (**d**) and the thick oblique sagittal slice (**e**) both calculated from the immediate post-contrast series. The abnormal enhancement extends over a 6 cm length (*arrows*) along a ductal ray. The sagittal subtraction with CAD (**f**) displays washout enhancement (*red*) within the lesions (*arrows*). Biopsy reveals lobular carcinoma (**g**). The patient desired breast-conserving surgery. Since the disease was confined to a long, but narrow ray of tissue, a tailored lumpectomy was performed with MR guidance (**h**). A cigar-shaped piece of tissue was removed that had clear pathologic margins. Without MR, this patient would likely have had multiple re-excisions in an attempt to get clear margins. Because of the disease extent and lobular histology, this patient likely would have ended her surgical treatment with a mastectomy

Other non-randomized studies point to a possible explanation for the COMICE and MONET failures. Hollingsworth reported great success using MR to reduce positive margin rates. The positive margin rate was only 9 % when MR was used compared with historical controls in prior years of 25–40 % [36]. Pengel showed no difference in the positive margin rates with MR or without MR for all cancers, but did find a significant improvement in the MR cohort for invasive cancer [44]. Mann showed a significant improvement in patients with lobular carcinoma, consistent with the known difficulty in establishing accurate local staging of lobular carcinomas with conventional breast imaging [37]. Bleicher did not show a slightly increased re-excision rate in the MR cohort (21.6 %) compared to the non-MR cohort (13.8 %). These findings can be explained by the fact that MR performs best with the identification of infiltrating cancers, but most have difficulty with DCIS [35]. Hollingsworth used a dedicated breast MR with high-contrast, high-resolution images and saw only slightly lower performance (13 % positive margin rate) compared to infiltrating cancer [36].

Other studies point to technical and interpretative differences that may account for the widely varied success when employing breast MR staging. A recent study performed by the American College of Radiology using a high-contrast, high-resolution technique on a dedicated breast MR demonstrated substantially higher diagnostic performance when compared to other studies using whole body approaches. This instrument uses spiral acquisitions to produce 700-μm-resolution isotropic images. The RODEO pulse sequence provides water excitation (not fat suppression as usually performed with whole body) and fibroglandular tissue suppression. This allows lesion discrimination from background without the need for subtraction [45]. The major limitation of MR in diagnostic studies is negative predictive value. The NCI 6883 trial showed an NPV of 85 %. This paper stated that an NPV of 85 % was insufficient to use MRI as an alternative to biopsy for suspicious lesions [46]. The recent study using the dedicated high-resolution system showed an NPV of 98.9 %. This NPV exceeded the American College of Radiology definition for a BIRADS 3 lesion, or less than 2 % chance of malignancy. Therefore, the improved NPV of the dedicated machine can be used to avoid biopsy in some circumstances to reduce the number of unnecessary benign biopsies. False positives are a common problem with breast MR. The false-positive rate for screening trials varies from 5 to 29 % [1, 3, 4, 13]. In the NCI 6884 trial, incidental lesions were identified for biopsy in 24 % of cases [4]. The recall rate for MR was three times that of mammography in the MARIBS trial [3]. In the German trial, 18 % of patients were recalled for follow-up [13]. The false-positive rate for diagnostic studies varies from 32 to 41 % [46–48]. The false-positive rate for the dedicated instrument was 4.7 % for the screening cohort and 11 % for the diagnostic cohort [45]. 27 % of the false positives reported in this study were high-risk histology for which excision or chemoprevention is often recommended. Probably the best measure for imaging studies is the area (A_z) under the receiver operator characteristic (ROC) curves

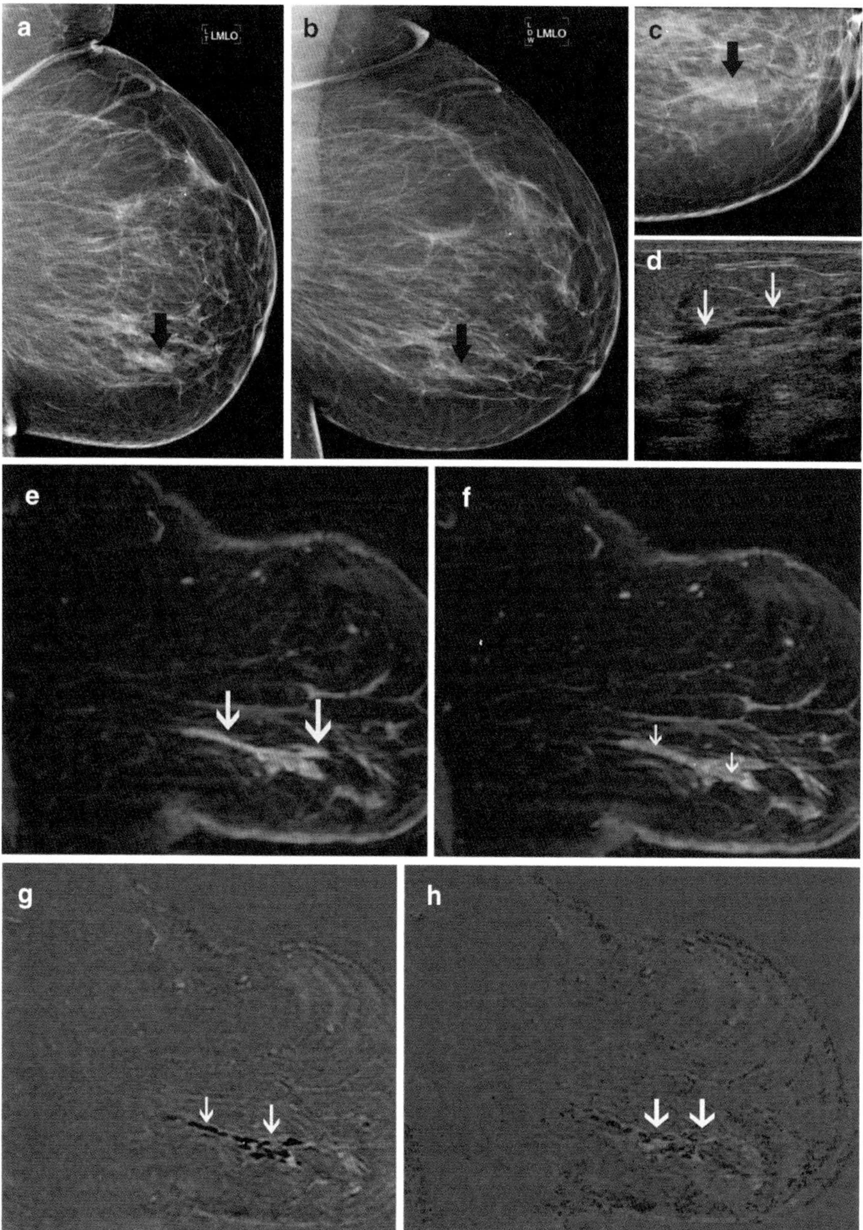

Fig. 8.9 High-contrast, high-resolution MR depiction of micropapillary DCIS. This 55-year-old patient was recalled from screening mammography for a subtle increased density in the inferior left breast on mammography. The current MLO mammogram (**a**) when compared to the MLO mammogram from the prior year (**b**) shows slightly more density (*arrow*). The diagnostic mammogram with magnification views (**c**) confirms a density (*arrow*) in the inferior left breast. Evaluation with ultrasound (**d**) shows some prominent ducts (*arrows*). Because of the inconclusive mammographic

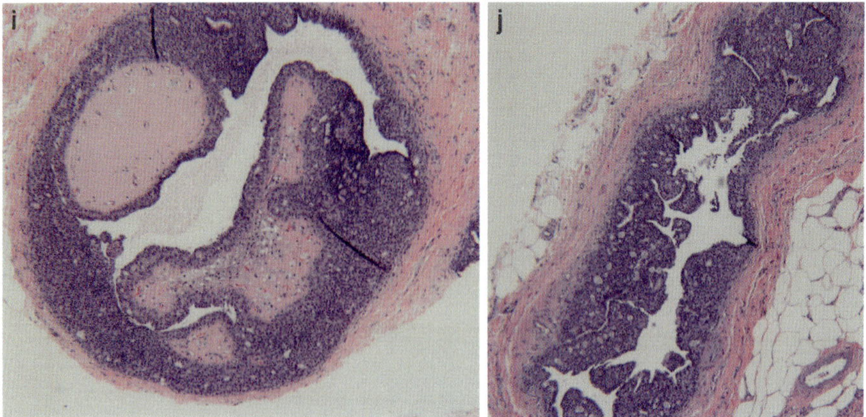

Fig. 8.9 (continued) and ultrasound findings, a breast MR was performed. An asymmetric area of non-mass-like enhancement (*arrow*) was seen on the projection image (**e**). Separating benign proliferative change from DCIS is often difficult on MR—leading to more false positives and false negatives. Insight into differentiation comes with the use of high-contrast, high-resolution images and positive/negative-scale subtractions. Comparing the pre-contrast (**f**) to the immediate post-contrast (**g**) image shows only subtle enhancement (*arrows*). Looking more closely at the post-contrast images, notice the thin dark line that is etched in white (*arrows*). This dark, distended duct outlined by enhancement (*arrows*) can be seen much better on the subtraction image (**h**). The subtracted image with CAD (**h**) depicts the blue (pure fluid on CAD) surrounded by yellow (persistent enhancement) typical of DCIS. Biopsy of this area shows micropapillary DCIS (**i**, **j**). When cut in cross section (**i**) the distended duct outlined by enhancement looks like a donut. A longitudinal section (**j**) depicts the tram-track effect where the distended duct is bordered on either side by DCIS. Both of these microscopic appearances can be seen with high-resolution, high-contrast breast MR

where the contributions of both sensitivity and specificity are considered. An A_z of 1 is a perfect test. An A_z of 0.5 is random. The NCI 6883 trial had an A_z of 0.88 when multivariate criteria (morphology and enhancement dynamics) were considered. If univariate features were used, the A_z was 0.78–0.54. The worst performance was non-mass-like enhancement, the typical appearance of DCIS [49]. The A_z for the dedicated breast MR was substantially better, 0.942 [45]. A more recent study using a whole-body instrument showed an A_z of 0.9 for irregular masses but decreased to 0.64 for non-mass-like enhancement [50]. The performance of the dedicated instrument is even more impressive when it is considered that 23 % of the cases were DCIS [45]. An example of how improved spatial and contrast resolution can improve the interpretation of breast MR is shown in Fig. 8.9.

In summary, the experience for use of breast MR to reduce positive margins in breast conservation candidates is mixed (Table 8.2). Since many infiltrating cancers also have associated DCIS within the specimen, the inability of low-resolution

MR protocols to visualize DCIS may impair staging of many cancers, in situ and infiltrating. The best chances for success depend upon the experience of the surgeon in using MR information and the use of high-resolution, high-contrast imaging protocols that are capable of accurately depicting DCIS.

Multifocal and Multicentric Disease

Occult disease present at the time of the initial diagnosis can reduce treatment effectiveness. The NSABP B-6 multicenter trial that validated breast conservation treatment showed significantly higher recurrences (39.2 %) when radiation was not used compared with the lumpectomy with radiation cohort (14.3 %) due to the treatment of subclinical disease by radiation [8]. Some argue that the detection of otherwise occult disease by MR may not have any benefit for treatment since adjuvant therapy seems to adequately address the problem [33, 51–53]. However, the presence of multiple lesions has been shown to carry a significantly worse prognosis. Two separate pathology papers using serial pathologic sectioning showed that multifocal or diffuse cancers comprise about 60 % of breast cancers [54, 55]. Tot showed that unifocal disease is present in about 40 % of cases irrespective of tumor size. About 20 % of multifocal or diffuse cancers were confined to an area of less than 4 cm, a size that could conceivably be removed with lumpectomy. About 40 % of multifocal or diffuse breast cancers extended over an area larger than 4 cm. The presence of multiple lesions was associated with lymphovascular invasion or lymph node metastases at about twice the rate of unifocal disease. This aggressive tendency of multifocal disease compared to unifocal disease was consistent across all size cohorts from less than 1 cm to over 4 cm [55]. Clinical data from Weissenbacher indicates the significantly worse prognosis for multifocal/multicentric disease that justifies an independent risk factor. The demonstration of additional cancers by MR clearly should be beneficial in determining prognosis [56].

The increasing complexity of breast cancer management has increased the need for better demonstration of disease extent. The NSABP B-6 showed a 39.2 % recurrence rate in women not treated with radiation. However, 60.8 % in that cohort did not recur, indicating that many women do not benefit from radiation [8]. Subsequently, several studies have proven that subgroups of women with better prognoses may be spared whole-breast irradiation. Hughes showed that radiation might be spared in women over 70 for invasive T1N0 tumors [57]. The Van Nuys criteria were developed to select a group of low risk DCIS lesions that could be treated with lumpectomy alone. Achieving good surgical margins is a critical of the Van Nuys criteria [58, 59]. Partial breast irradiation is now a successful alternative to whole-breast irradiation [60, 61]. Oncoplastic surgery can be used to improve the cosmetic outcome for breast conservation surgery [61]. Neoadjuvant chemotherapy can be used to improve the success of breast conservation surgery by reducing

Table 8.3 Effect of breast MR staging on positive margin rate

Study	With MR	Without MR
Hollingsworth	9 % (13 % DCIS)	25–40 % (historical)
Pengel (all cancers)	13.8 %	19.4 %
Pengel (invasive only)	1.6 %	8.1 %
Mann (lobular only)	9 %	27 %
Bleicher	21.6 %	13.8 %
COMICE	16.3 %	18.7 %
MONET	34 %	12 %

disease burden [62]. All of these alternatives to traditional breast conservation are affected by the extent of disease. Accurate definition of disease extent by breast MR may be useful in these patients.

If breast MR improves the management of breast conservation therapy a measurable endpoint might be the local recurrence rate. Three published studies that attempted to answer this question provided mixed results (Table 8.3). Fisher reported a significantly lower recurrence rate using MR [63]. Solin and Hwang did not see any difference [64, 65]. All of the studies were retrospective. There is significant potential for selection bias. For example, in the Solin study over half of the MR cohort participants were scanned after an attempted excision. MR performs poorly in postoperative patients [64]. Why was the MR performed on this group compared to the non-MR group—positive margins, extensive intraductal component, dense breasts, etc.? The lack of scientific rigor in these studies does not permit a conclusion to the question. Without clear scientific evidence, we will have to rely on surrogate endpoints such as positive margin rate and contralateral disease to determine a benefit for preoperative staging.

Contralateral Disease

Breast-conserving surgery trials have demonstrated the need for adjuvant radiation to treat subclinical disease in the affected breast. What about occult disease that may occur in the other breast? The opposite breast is not treated with radiation. Is adjuvant hormonal therapy and chemotherapy adequate? If systemic therapy is inadequate for the ipsilateral breast how can it be adequate for the opposite breast? We have some answers from treatment trial data. A large retrospective study from MD Anderson compared a subset of 8,902 women who had preventive contralateral mastectomy to the remainder of the 107,106 patients who were treated with mastectomy during the period from 1998 to 2003 (before the routine use of breast MR). The patients electing for contralateral preventive mastectomy had an improved adjusted breast cancer survival of 4.8 % [66]. Another retrospective study evaluated 194 patients with bilateral breast cancer (80 synchronous and 114 metachronous) and compared outcomes with 2,237 patients with unilateral breast cancer. The

Table 8.4 Effect of staging breast MR on local recurrence rates

Study	Recurrence rate with MR % (number)	Recurrence rate without MR % (number)
Fisher et al.	1.2 % (86)	6.8 % (122)
Solin et al.	3 % (215)	4 % (541)
Hwang et al.	1.8 % (127)	2.5 % (345)

15-year survival was 65.5, 52.3, and 37.2 % for unilateral, metachronous bilateral, and synchronous bilateral, respectively. The survival after 5 years was the same for metachronous as unilateral, but synchronous carcinoma was associated with a significantly worse prognosis. They concluded that synchronous breast cancer should be an independent risk factor for mortality [67].

The use of MR for detecting contralateral disease is very consistent having about a 3–5 % detection rate (Table 8.4) [36, 68–70]. This is very similar to the difference in recurrence rates reported in the MD Anderson trial. The Brennan study was a meta-analysis using other trial data. This paper stated that the PPV for MR of 48 % is too low. Yet the commonly accepted PPV for mammography by the American College of Radiology is 20 %—less than half what is reported for MR [69]. The Solin paper which primarily studied recurrence rates also reported no difference in the 8-year rates of contralateral disease in women who had or did not have a breast MR. This paper is often cited as evidence that MR detection of contralateral disease makes no clinical difference. Unfortunately, the data for the paper was obtained at a time when the University of Pennsylvania used only unilateral MR acquisitions. To image both breasts two MR sessions would have been required on separate days. There was no information in the paper to indicate how many, if any, of the patients actually had the opposite breast examined. Unfortunately, the misinterpretation of the information was used to write a lay article in Time magazine questioning the benefit of preoperative breast MR. Some evidence that the opposite breast may not have been examined lies in the statement that the 6 % contralateral recurrence rates in the contralateral breast were the same for both groups. If MR were performed, then about 4 % of the cancers should have been detected which would have shown up as an event-free period in the MR cohort [64].

Hollingsworth showed that half of all contralateral cancers detected incidentally with MR were at the same stage or higher than the known cancer. It is clear that synchronous cancers should not be dismissed as insignificant disease (Fig. 8.10).

DCIS-Specific Issues

Pure DCIS can represent up to 40 % of mammographically screened breast cancers. There is often an association of DCIS with infiltrating cancer. Patients with infiltrating cancer are often treated with chemotherapy, while pure DCIS patients are usually spared chemotherapy. Missing the infiltrating disease in a patient with a presumed diagnosis of pure DCIS may lead to undertreatment. Mammography will

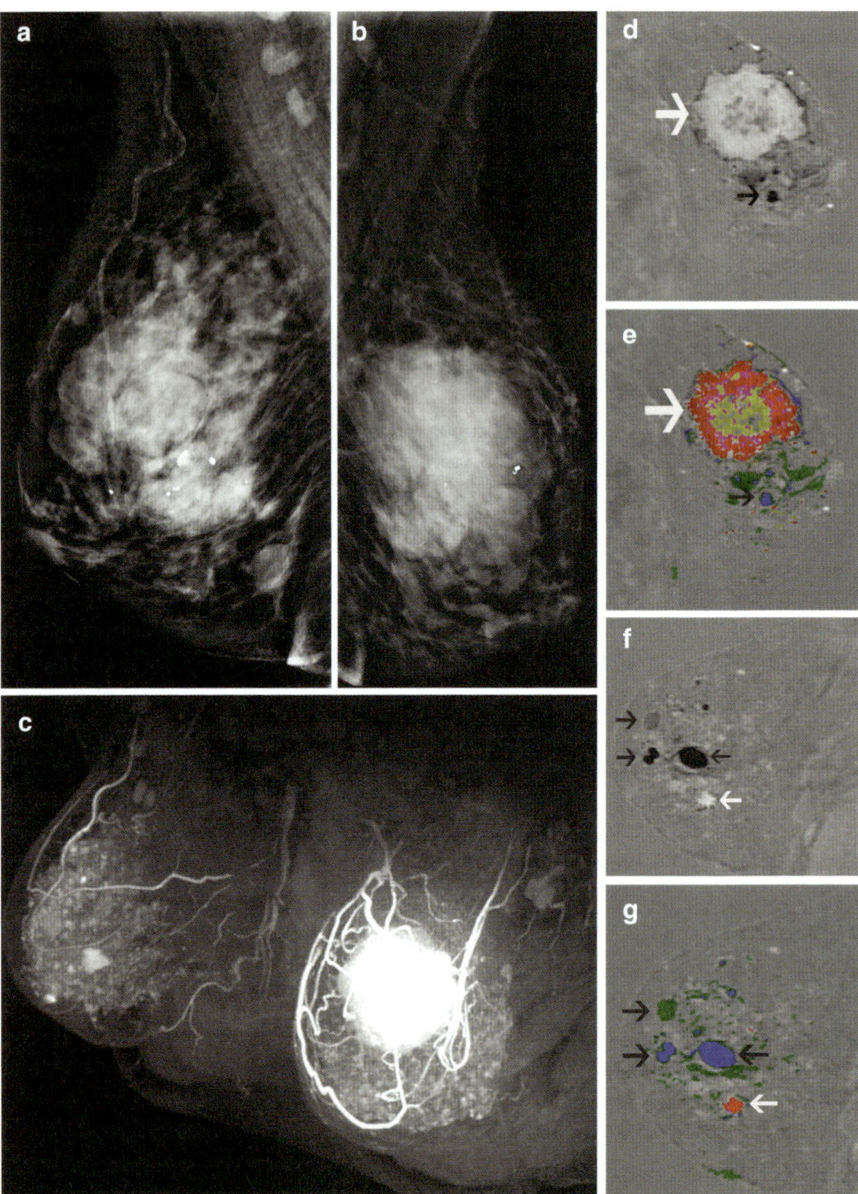

Fig. 8.10 Bilateral infiltrating ductal carcinoma. This patient presented with a palpable mass on the left. A needle biopsy was performed revealing low-grade infiltrating ductal carcinoma. The MLO views on the right (**a**) and left (**b**) show a large left breast mass with a clip marker. Multiple other masses are seen in both breasts due to her extensive fibrocystic change. Ultrasound demonstrated extensive pure fluid and complex cysts in both breasts in addition to the large solid mass representing cancer on the left. The immediate post-contrast projection MIP (**c**) shows the large mass on the left. The interpretation is complex because of the extensive cysts in both breasts. This interpretation is made easier with positive- and negative-scale subtraction images where the

often show the microcalcifications produced by DCIS, but miss intermixed areas of invasive disease that do not produce calcification. Breast MR may be helpful in identifying invasive components within known DCIS that are not histologically sampled or visualizing occult invasive disease elsewhere in either breast (Fig. 8.11).

The argument that adjuvant therapy can address occult invasive disease can be refuted with strong clinical evidence. A study from MD Anderson in 799 patients with DCIS showed with a median follow-up of 2.9 years that 5.6 % (45 patients) had a second event. The cumulative incidence of recurrence at 5 years was 6.6 %. Of these recurrent cancers, 31 % (14) were in situ and 69 % (31) were invasive. The majority of second events (63 %) occurred in the opposite breast. The overall survival was 97.4 %, but the survival for women with second events dropped to 76.1 %. They concluded that second events after DCIS have a negative impact on survival [71]. This information was gathered before breast MR became common. The rapid recurrence time indicates that the disease likely was present at the time of the diagnosis and likely would have been detected with breast MR.

Other Issues

Local staging involves more than just extent within the breast. Patients who will likely be treated with mastectomy may still benefit from breast MR. The location of disease relative to the pectoralis muscle and chest wall may affect the surgical approach [72]. This is anatomy that is not available on conventional imaging. MR is highly sensitive to muscle involvement. Removal of some muscle may be necessary to achieve an adequate margin (Fig. 8.12). MR can determine the extent of chest wall disease to determine if it is resectable. This may be particularly advantageous in patients with extra-abdominal fibromatosis or desmoid tumor. The proximity of the tumor to the nipple will have implications in patients who desire nipple-preserving reconstruction. The differentiation of skin edema from tumor involvement is helpful in determining which portions of the skin may need to be removed. The identification of nodal metastases involving internal mammary, subpectoral, Rotter's nodes, and mediastinal nodes can be done very effectively with breast MR.

Fig. 8.10 (continued) enhancing mass (*white arrow*) can be distinguished from *black* cysts (*black arrow*) as seen on the sagittal image from the left breast (**d**). When CAD is added to the subtraction (**e**), the mass has a periphery of washout (*red*) and central persistent enhancement (*yellow*). The pure fluid cyst is encoded as *blue* (*black arrow*). The sagittal positive and negative subtraction image on the right (**f**) shows an enhancing, spiculated mass (*white arrow*) and multiple cysts (*black arrows*). The cysts vary in protein content. The pure fluid cysts are black and the proteinaceous cysts are gray. The sagittal subtraction with CAD (**g**) on the right shows intense washout enhancement from the mass (*white arrow*). This occult cancer seen only on MR was an infiltrating ductal carcinoma of higher grade than the large mass on the left. The pure fluid cysts are encoded *blue* and the proteinaceous cysts are encoded *green* with CAD (*black arrows*)

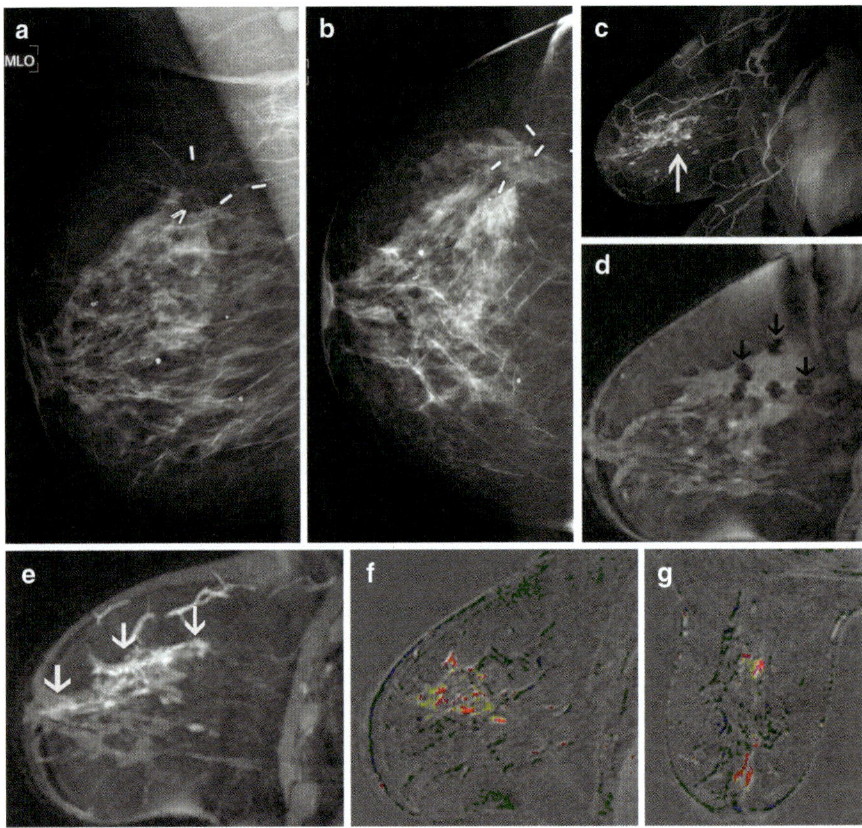

Fig. 8.11 Undetected infiltrating lobular carcinoma. This patient initially presented 6 months earlier with a cluster of microcalcifications in the upper outer quadrant of the right breast. This was excised at another institution and found to be low-grade DCIS. Pathology revealed clear margins. Because of her age, low-grade disease, and clear margins, she was treated with excision alone. She then presented with the symptom of diffuse fullness in the same breast. Her physical examination and mammogram showed no evidence of recurrence. The MLO (**a**) and CC (**b**) mammographic views performed at the time demonstrated the lumpectomy site with multiple clips but no suspicious calcifications or masses. She sought a second opinion at our institution where a breast MR was performed. The oblique MIP (**c**) from the immediate post-contrast series shows a large area of enhancement (*arrow*) in the upper inner quadrant. A thick sagittal slice (**d**) from the same series depicts multiple low-intensity clips (*black arrows*) identifying the operative site. Non-enhancing bland scar is seen at the lumpectomy site. A sagittal thick slice from the same data set in the medial breast shows extensive enhancement (*white arrows*) extending along a ductal ray towards the nipple. The sagittal (**e**) and axial (**f**) subtractions with CAD show washout enhancement (*red*) within this enhancing area. MR-directed biopsy of the most suspicious area showed infiltrating lobular carcinoma. No MR was performed during the initial staging. The short time period between the recurrence and the initial presentation suggests that the disease was likely present at the time of the initial surgery

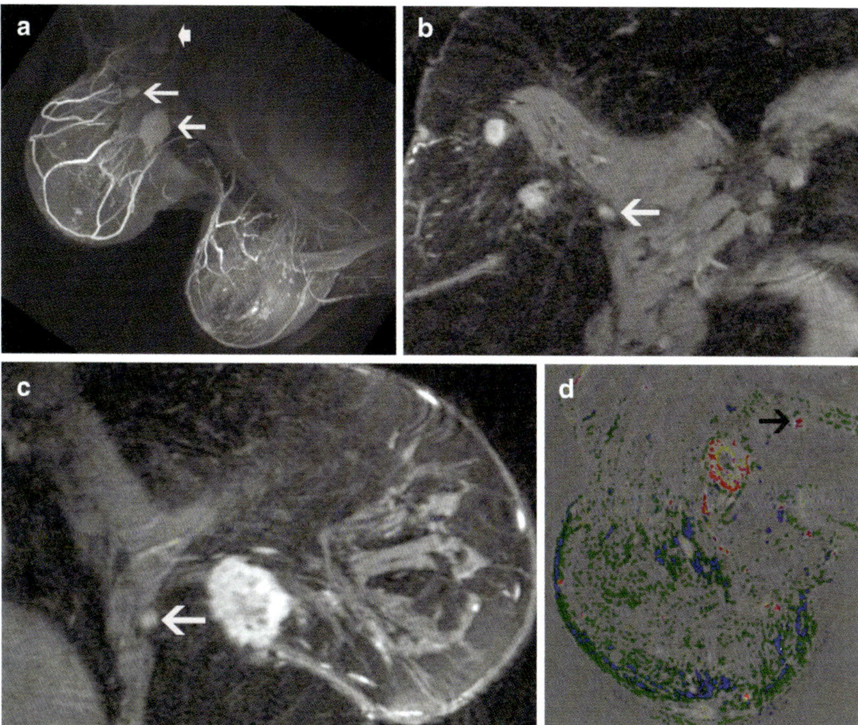

Fig. 8.12 Mastectomy surgery modified to include disease near the chest wall. The MIP of the (**a**) immediate post-contrast image set shows two enhancing lesions (*thin arrows*) in the right breast and an enlarged right axillary lymph node (*thick arrow*) that were identified on prior conventional imaging. The patient was scheduled for a mastectomy, but had breast MR for local staging. Many would argue that MR would not be needed since any additional disease found on MR would likely be included in the mastectomy. An additional lesion was identified on the MR just beneath the edge of the pectoralis major muscle near the chest wall. The lesion (*arrow*) is well seen on the reformatted oblique coronal (**b**) and the oblique sagittal (**c**) images generated from the immediate post-contrast series. An axial subtraction with CAD (**d**) shows washout (*arrow*) typical of invasive disease. This lesion could have been left behind if the usual mastectomy surgery was performed. Instead the resection was changed to include tissue deep to this small focus of infiltrating disease

Summary

Despite the widespread success of breast MR screening, results remain mixed for the implementation of breast MR in the management of patients with recently diagnosed breast cancer. How can a method that has two to three times the sensitivity of

Table 8.5 Detection of occult contralateral breast cancer using MR

Study	% Contralateral	% DCIS	% Invasive
Lehman (ACRIN 6667)	3.1	40	60
Hollingsworth	3.7	32	68
Liberman	5	50	50
Brennan	4.1	35	65

mammography not be helpful? Failures are likely due to several factors: lack of surgical experience using the information and low-quality breast MR technique and interpretation. Many centers do not have the MR integrated with other breast imaging methods. This leads to time delays and potential for misinterpretation. The interpretation of breast MR by radiologists who do not have access to all the mammographic and sonographic information is a setup for failure. Significant management changes such as conversion from lumpectomy to mastectomy should typically be made on the basis of histologic confirmation of findings rather than imaging information alone. When breast MR is part of the breast center the imaging workup can integrate MR just as easily as breast ultrasound. The use of MR need not delay treatment when approached in this way. When done well, breast MR should result in a lower re-excision rate, detection of contralateral occult disease (Table 8.5), detection of occult invasive disease in women with DCIS, and overall better treatment management. Complex decisions such as the use of neoadjuvant chemotherapy, oncoplastic surgery, and partial breast irradiation are all better determined with accurate staging information. As with many complex medical approaches, difficulties will likely be worked out with more experience over time.

References

1. Kriege M, et al. Efficacy of MRI and mammography for breast-cancer screening in women with a familial or genetic predisposition. N Engl J Med. 2004;351(5):427–37.
2. Lehman CD, et al. Screening women at high risk for breast cancer with mammography and magnetic resonance imaging. Cancer. 2005;103(9):1898–905.
3. Leach MO, et al. Screening with magnetic resonance imaging and mammography of a UK population at high familial risk of breast cancer: a prospective multicentre cohort study (MARIBS). Lancet. 2005;365(9473):1769–78.
4. Lehman CD, et al. Cancer yield of mammography, MR, and US in high-risk women: prospective multi-institution breast cancer screening study. Radiology. 2007;244(2):381–8.
5. Familial breast cancer: the classification and care of women at risk of familial breast cancer in primary, secondary and tertiary care, in NICE clinical guideline 412006.
6. NCCN clinical practice guidelines in oncology: breast cancer, in http://www.nccn.org/professionals/physician_gls/pdf/breast.pdf2012.
7. Saslow D, et al. American Cancer Society guidelines for breast screening with MRI as an adjunct to mammography. CA Cancer J Clin. 2007;57(2):75–89.
8. Fisher B, et al. Twenty-year follow-up of a randomized trial comparing total mastectomy, lumpectomy, and lumpectomy plus irradiation for the treatment of invasive breast cancer. N Engl J Med. 2002;347(16):1233–41.

9. Pisano ED, et al. Diagnostic performance of digital versus film mammography for breast-cancer screening. N Engl J Med. 2005;353(17):1773–83.
10. Tabar L, et al. Swedish two-county trial: impact of mammographic screening on breast cancer mortality during 3 decades. Radiology. 2011;260(3):658–63.
11. Pisano ED, et al. American College of Radiology Imaging Network digital mammographic imaging screening trial: objectives and methodology. Radiology. 2005;236(2):404–12.
12. Podo F, et al. The Italian multi-centre project on evaluation of MRI and other imaging modalities in early detection of breast cancer in subjects at high genetic risk. J Exp Clin Cancer Res. 2002;21(3 Suppl):115–24.
13. Kuhl CK, et al. Breast MR imaging screening in 192 women proved or suspected to be carriers of a breast cancer susceptibility gene: preliminary results. Radiology. 2000;215(1):267–79.
14. Warner E, et al. Surveillance of BRCA1 and BRCA2 mutation carriers with magnetic resonance imaging, ultrasound, mammography, and clinical breast examination. JAMA. 2004;292(11):1317–25.
15. Sardanelli F, et al. Sensitivity of MRI versus mammography for detecting foci of multifocal, multicentric breast cancer in fatty and dense breasts using the whole-breast pathologic examination as a gold standard. AJR Am J Roentgenol. 2004;183(4):1149–57.
16. Miller AB, et al. Canadian National Breast Screening Study: 2. Breast cancer detection and death rates among women aged 50 to 59 years. CMAJ. 1992;147(10):1477–88.
17. Miller AB, et al. Canadian National Breast Screening Study: 1. Breast cancer detection and death rates among women aged 40 to 49 years. CMAJ. 1992;147(10):1459–76.
18. Cil T, et al. Mammographic density and the risk of breast cancer recurrence after breast-conserving surgery. Cancer. 2009;115(24):5780–7.
19. Park CC, et al. High mammographic breast density is independent predictor of local but not distant recurrence after lumpectomy and radiotherapy for invasive breast cancer. Int J Radiat Oncol Biol Phys. 2009;73(1):75–9.
20. Arora N, et al. Impact of breast density on the presenting features of malignancy. Ann Surg Oncol. 2010;17 Suppl 3:211–8.
21. Hollingsworth AB, Taylor LD, Rhodes DC. Establishing a histologic basis for false-negative mammograms. Am J Surg. 1993;166(6):643–7. discussion 647–8.
22. Bigenwald RZ, et al. Is mammography adequate for screening women with inherited BRCA mutations and low breast density? Cancer Epidemiol Biomarkers Prev. 2008;17(3):706–11.
23. Boyd NF, et al. Mammographic density and the risk and detection of breast cancer. N Engl J Med. 2007;356(3):227–36.
24. Georgian-Smith D, Lawton TJ. Controversies on the management of high-risk lesions at core biopsy from a radiology/pathology perspective. Radiol Clin North Am. 2010;48(5):999–1012.
25. Liberman L, et al. Underestimation of atypical ductal hyperplasia at MRI-guided 9-gauge vacuum-assisted breast biopsy. AJR Am J Roentgenol. 2007;188(3):684–90.
26. Arpino G, Laucirica R, Elledge RM. Premalignant and in situ breast disease: biology and clinical implications. Ann Intern Med. 2005;143(6):446–57.
27. Sung JS, et al. Screening breast MR imaging in women with a history of lobular carcinoma in situ. Radiology. 2011;261(2):414–20.
28. Friedlander LC, Roth SO, Gavenonis SC. Results of MR imaging screening for breast cancer in high-risk patients with lobular carcinoma in situ. Radiology. 2011;261(2):421–7.
29. Port ER, et al. Results of MRI screening for breast cancer in high-risk patients with LCIS and atypical hyperplasia. Ann Surg Oncol. 2007;14(3):1051–7.
30. Tabar L, Dean PB, Pentek Z. Galactography: the diagnostic procedure of choice for nipple discharge. Radiology. 1983;149(1):31–8.
31. Dennis MA, et al. Incidental treatment of nipple discharge caused by benign intraductal papilloma through diagnostic Mammotome biopsy. AJR Am J Roentgenol. 2000;174(5):1263–8.
32. Liberman L, et al. Percutaneous large-core biopsy of papillary breast lesions. AJR Am J Roentgenol. 1999;172(2):331–7.
33. Morrow M. Magnetic resonance imaging in breast cancer: one step forward, two steps back? JAMA. 2004;292(22):2779–80.

34. Katipamula R, et al. Trends in mastectomy rates at the Mayo Clinic Rochester: effect of surgical year and preoperative magnetic resonance imaging. J Clin Oncol. 2009;27(25):4082–8.
35. Bleicher RJ, et al. Association of routine pretreatment magnetic resonance imaging with time to surgery, mastectomy rate, and margin status. J Am Coll Surg. 2009;209(2):180–7. quiz 294–5.
36. Hollingsworth AB, et al. Breast magnetic resonance imaging for preoperative locoregional staging. Am J Surg. 2008;196(3):389–97.
37. Mann RM, et al. The impact of preoperative breast MRI on the re-excision rate in invasive lobular carcinoma of the breast. Breast Cancer Res Treat. 2010;119(2):415–22.
38. Huston TL, et al. The influence of additional surgical margins on the total specimen volume excised and the reoperative rate after breast-conserving surgery. Am J Surg. 2006;192(4):509–12.
39. Menes TS, et al. The consequence of multiple re-excisions to obtain clear lumpectomy margins in breast cancer patients. Ann Surg Oncol. 2005;12(11):881–5.
40. O'Sullivan MJ, et al. The effect of multiple reexcisions on the risk of local recurrence after breast conserving surgery. Ann Surg Oncol. 2007;14(11):3133–40.
41. McCahill LE, et al. Variability in reexcision following breast conservation surgery. JAMA. 2012;307(5):467–75.
42. Turnbull L, et al. Comparative effectiveness of MRI in breast cancer (COMICE) trial: a randomised controlled trial. Lancet. 2010;375(9714):563–71.
43. Peters NH, et al. Preoperative MRI and surgical management in patients with nonpalpable breast cancer: the MONET – randomised controlled trial. Eur J Cancer. 2011;47(6):879–86.
44. Pengel KE, et al. The impact of preoperative MRI on breast-conserving surgery of invasive cancer: a comparative cohort study. Breast Cancer Res Treat. 2009;116(1):161–9.
45. Hillman B, Harms SE, Stevens G, Stough R, Hollingsworth A, Kozlowski K, Moss LJ. Diagnostic performance of a dedicated 1.5T breast MRI system. Radiology. 2012; 265:51–58.
46. Bluemke DA, et al. Magnetic resonance imaging of the breast prior to biopsy. JAMA. 2004;292(22):2735–42.
47. Teifke A, et al. Undetected malignancies of the breast: dynamic contrast-enhanced MR imaging at 1.0 T. Radiology. 2002;224(3):881–8.
48. Fischer U, Kopka L, Grabbe E. Breast carcinoma: effect of preoperative contrast-enhanced MR imaging on the therapeutic approach. Radiology. 1999;213(3):881–8.
49. Schnall MD, et al. Diagnostic architectural and dynamic features at breast MR imaging: multicenter study. Radiology. 2006;238(1):42–53.
50. Wedegartner U, et al. Differentiation between benign and malignant findings on MR-mammography: usefulness of morphological criteria. Eur Radiol. 2001;11(9):1645–50.
51. Morrow M. Magnetic resonance imaging in the preoperative evaluation of breast cancer: primum non nocere. J Am Coll Surg. 2004;198(2):240–1.
52. Morrow M. Magnetic resonance imaging in the breast cancer patient: curb your enthusiasm. J Clin Oncol. 2008;26(3):352–3.
53. Morrow M. Should routine breast cancer staging include MRI? Nat Clin Pract Oncol. 2009;6(2):72–3.
54. Holland R, et al. Histologic multifocality of Tis, T1-2 breast carcinomas. Implications for clinical trials of breast-conserving surgery. Cancer. 1985;56(5):979–90.
55. Tot T. The metastatic capacity of multifocal breast carcinomas: extensive tumors versus tumors of limited extent. Hum Pathol. 2009;40(2):199–205.
56. Weissenbacher TM, et al. Multicentric and multifocal versus unifocal breast cancer: is the tumor-node-metastasis classification justified? Breast Cancer Res Treat. 2010;122(1): 27–34.
57. Hughes KS, et al. Lumpectomy plus tamoxifen with or without irradiation in women 70 years of age or older with early breast cancer. N Engl J Med. 2004;351(10):971–7.
58. Silverstein MJ, et al. A prognostic index for ductal carcinoma in situ of the breast. Cancer. 1996;77(11):2267–74.
59. Silverstein MJ, et al. Prognostic classification of breast ductal carcinoma-in-situ. Lancet. 1995;345(8958):1154–7.

60. Vicini F, et al. A phase I/II trial to evaluate three-dimensional conformal radiation therapy confined to the region of the lumpectomy cavity for Stage I/II breast carcinoma: initial report of feasibility and reproducibility of Radiation Therapy Oncology Group (RTOG) Study 0319. Int J Radiat Oncol Biol Phys. 2005;63(5):1531–7.
61. Vicini F, et al. Initial efficacy results of RTOG 0319: three-dimensional conformal radiation therapy (3D-CRT) confined to the region of the lumpectomy cavity for stage I/II breast carcinoma. Int J Radiat Oncol Biol Phys. 2010;77(4):1120–7.
62. Fisher B, et al. Effect of preoperative chemotherapy on local-regional disease in women with operable breast cancer: findings from National Surgical Adjuvant Breast and Bowel Project B-18. J Clin Oncol. 1997;15(7):2483–93.
63. Fischer U, et al. The influence of preoperative MRI of the breasts on recurrence rate in patients with breast cancer. Eur Radiol. 2004;14(10):1725–31.
64. Solin LJ, et al. Relationship of breast magnetic resonance imaging to outcome after breast-conservation treatment with radiation for women with early-stage invasive breast carcinoma or ductal carcinoma in situ. J Clin Oncol. 2008;26(3):386–91.
65. Hwang N, et al. Magnetic resonance imaging in the planning of initial lumpectomy for invasive breast carcinoma: its effect on ipsilateral breast tumor recurrence after breast-conservation therapy. Ann Surg Oncol. 2009;16(11):3000–9.
66. Bedrosian I, Hu CY, Chang GJ. Population-based study of contralateral prophylactic mastectomy and survival outcomes of breast cancer patients. J Natl Cancer Inst. 2010;102(6):401–9.
67. Vuoto HD, et al. Bilateral breast carcinoma: clinical characteristics and its impact on survival. Breast J. 2010;16(6):625–32.
68. Lehman CD, et al. MRI evaluation of the contralateral breast in women with recently diagnosed breast cancer. N Engl J Med. 2007;356(13):1295–303.
69. Brennan ME, et al. Magnetic resonance imaging screening of the contralateral breast in women with newly diagnosed breast cancer: systematic review and meta-analysis of incremental cancer detection and impact on surgical management. J Clin Oncol. 2009;27(33):5640–9.
70. Liberman L, et al. MR imaging findings in the contralateral breast of women with recently diagnosed breast cancer. AJR Am J Roentgenol. 2003;180(2):333–41.
71. Dawood S, et al. Development of new cancers in patients with DCIS: the M.D. Anderson experience. Ann Surg Oncol. 2008;15(1):244–9.
72. Morris EA, et al. Evaluation of pectoralis major muscle in patients with posterior breast tumors on breast MR images: early experience. Radiology. 2000;214(1):67–72.

Chapter 9
Digital Breast Tomosynthesis

Gary Levine and January Lopez

Screening mammography remains the gold standard for the early detection of breast cancer and it alone has proven, through randomized clinical trials, to reduce the mortality from breast cancer [1]. There has been significant advancement in mammographic technology since the widespread deployment of screening began in the 1970s. Industrial film mammography gave way to xeromammography, then film-screen mammography and eventually modern digital mammography. The penetration of digital mammography in the US market has recently reached 85 %.

Utilization of screening mammography has dramatically altered the clinical presentation of breast cancer. Approximately 25 % of breast carcinoma is now being discovered when still confined to the ducts (in situ) whereas invasive breast carcinomas are often being found when still small and non-palpable. Breast cancer is no longer a disease diagnosed through visual inspection and manual palpation; instead, diagnosis now essentially always involves imaging. The median size of breast cancer at time of diagnosis is currently approximately 15 mm and continues to fall. This trend toward earlier diagnosis through screening has resulted in markedly improved breast cancer survival rates [2].

There remains, however, a subset of breast cancer (accounting for approximately 15–20 %), which is not detectable with even modern digital 2D mammography. This is generally seen in women with radiographically dense breasts in whom mammographic sensitivity for breast cancer falls to just 50 % [3]. This can lead to the development of advanced cancers even in women who undergo regular mammographic screening. Normal parenchymal elements that lie outside the plane of interest can obscure an abnormality, leading to false-negative results and decreasing sensitivity. The native dense-breast parenchyma effectively hides the developing

G. Levine, M.D. (✉)
Hoag Breast Care Center, One Hoag Drive, Newport Beach, CA 92658, USA
e-mail: stratgml@aol.com

J. Lopez, M.D.
Department of Radiology, Hoag Breast Care Center, Newport Beach, CA, USA

D.S. Francescatti and M.J. Silverstein (eds.), *Breast Cancer: A New Era in Management*,
DOI 10.1007/978-1-4614-8063-1_9,

breast cancer. Conversely, superimposed tissue elements may give the appearance of a breast abnormality when none exists and thus lead to false-positive results. This limitation in both sensitivity and specificity has been a frequent source of criticism of 2D mammography.

Unfortunately, according to a recent study in the Journal of the National Cancer Institute, these women with dense breast tissue, in whom conventional 2D mammography is limited, are actually at a higher risk for developing breast cancer [4]. The study found that women with ≥50 % breast density on mammographic study had triple the risk of breast cancer compared with women who had <10 % density. Breast density is not based on family history and cannot be determined by the look and feel of the breast. Approximately 75 % of women in their 1940s have dense breasts. This percentage typically decreases with age; however, even elderly women can continue to have dense breasts.

Digital Breast Tomosynthesis

Digital breast tomosynthesis (DBT), commonly called 3D mammography, is essentially a tomographic application of digital mammography. The physical principles of this technology have been described [5]. Tomosynthesis acquisition mimics conventional mammography with regard to breast positioning, but unlike conventional mammography, the X-ray tube arcs over the breast taking multiple low-dose "projection" images during an exposure that lasts several seconds. The resulting digital data set is reconstructed by a computer algorithm into 1 mm thick tomographic sections through the breast. The 3D reconstruction of this limited scan leads to excellent in-plane resolution. Coarser *Z*-axis resolution (1 mm thick slices) still provides enough separation of normal overlapping tissue to detect cancer that may otherwise be obscured.

DBT allows radiologists to examine breast tissue one layer at a time, at a thickness of only 1 mm. The images can be reviewed individually or played back in a cine loop. Fine details become more visible and are no longer hidden by superimposed dense breast tissue. Primarily by resolving the issue of tissue superimposition, 3D mammography provides radiologists measurable improvements in sensitivity and specificity when compared to conventional full field digital mammography (FFDM) alone, increasing the accuracy of mammography.

To date, only one vendor's DBT system has been approved for marketing in the USA, but others have been approved for use in Europe and still other vendors' tomosynthesis systems remain in development. DBT is presently performed in the USA as a combination 2D+3D exam. The 2D portion of the exam is utilized primarily for comparison with prior exams to assess interval change and for the detection and analysis of microcalcifications. The 3D tomosynthesis portion of the exam addresses the issue of tissue superimposition and best demonstrates masses and architectural distortion. Tomosynthesis images can be obtained in any of the standard radiographic orientations including, but not limited to, craniocaudal (CC), mediolateral oblique (MLO), and true mediolateral (ML).

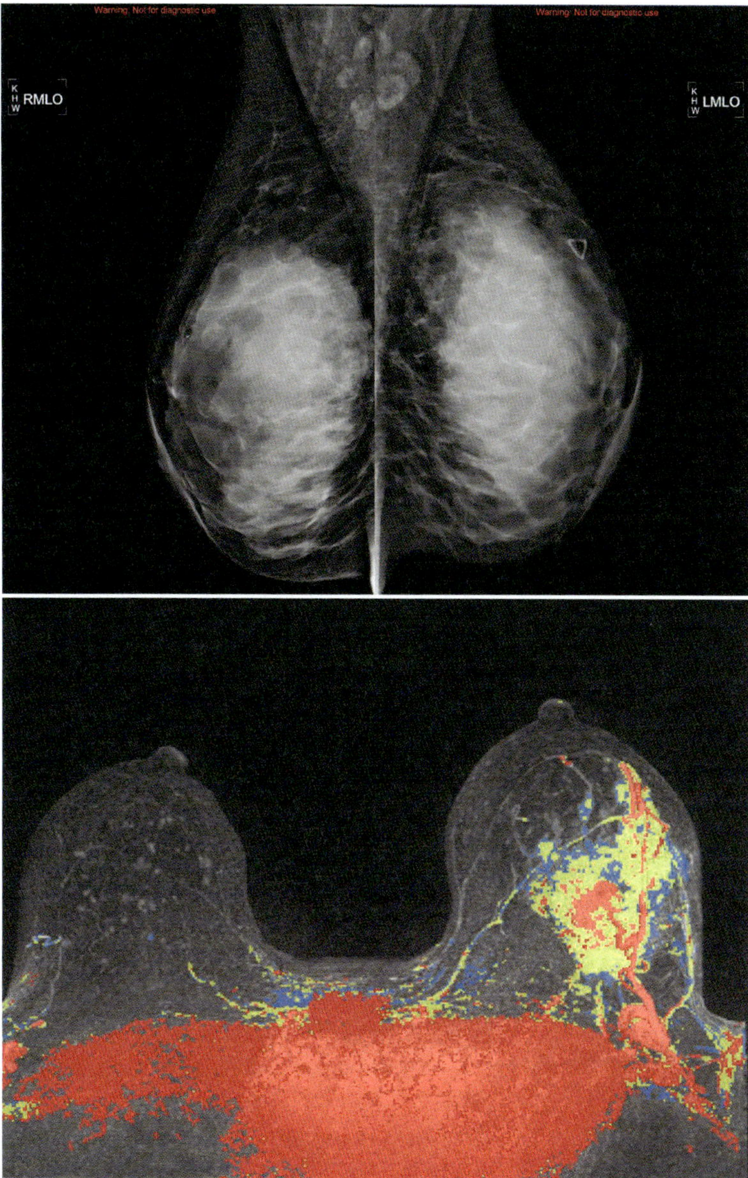

Fig. 9.1 A large 10cm IDC is occult on 2D mammography but well demonstrated on CEMRI imaging in this woman with dense breasts

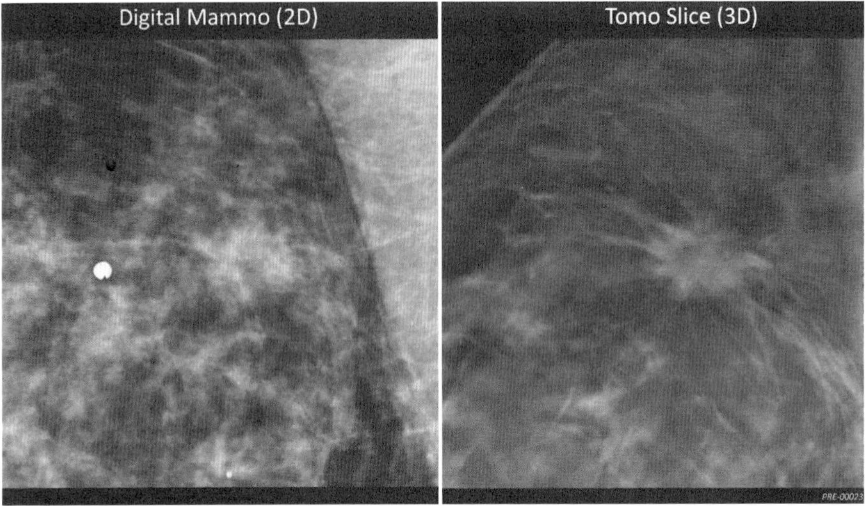

Fig. 9.2 A 2cm. spiculated IDC is partially obscured (by overlying parenchyma) on 2D mammography but is discretely seen on 3D Tomosynthesis

Evidence of Efficacy

DBT has the potential to improve both mammographic sensitivity and specificity in the detection of breast cancer. The current published literature on this emerging technology predominately includes smaller pilot and retrospective studies with enriched data sets. However, at least two large-scale prospective, population-based screening trials are currently underway in Sweden and Norway, with projected completion dates in 2014 and 2015, respectively.

The literature to date shows that the addition of DBT to standard FFDM significantly improves diagnostic accuracy compared to FFDM alone. A recent study by Rafferty et al. comparing FFDM alone to FFDM combined with DBT in 293 cases with dense breast tissue showed that the combined modalities performed significantly better for both calcification cases and non-calcification cases, increasing cancer detection rate and decreasing non-cancer recall rate (Area under the receiver operating conditions (ROC) curve (AUC) equaling 0.94 for 2D + 3D vs. 0.857 for 2D alone [$p < 0.0001$]) [6]. Similarly, Gur and colleagues found a 16 % improvement in performance for the detection, localization, and characterization of cancer with the addition of DBT to FFDM alone in a study of 125 cancer enriched cases [7]. Early data from a population-based screening study in Norway examining 3,356 cases demonstrated a 47 % increase in cancer detection with DBT in combination with either conventional or synthetic FFDM (created from DBT) compared to FFDM alone [8].

Studies comparing the efficacy of DBT head-to-head with FFDM also suggest superior diagnostic accuracy with two-view DBT. A recently published study by Wallis et al. comparing the two modalities in 130 women, both symptomatic and asymptomatic, found significantly greater accuracy with two-view DBT compared with FFDM, with AUC values of 0.851 and 0.772, respectively [$p=0.021$] [9]. Preliminary data from a population-based screening trial in Sweden also suggests higher diagnostic precision of DBT compared with DM [10].

With regards to single-view DBT, prospective studies have shown it is comparable to standard two-view FFDM with regards to diagnostic accuracy [9, 11].

Calcifications

A potential concern with regards to the utilization of DBT in lieu of FFDM for screening purposes relates to both the detection and analysis of microcalcifications. There is limited data on the performance of DBT compared to DM specifically with regards to calcifications. An early investigation by Poplack et al. found that image quality of DBT was inferior to DM in the characterization of calcifications [12]. However, a recent study by Kopans and colleagues found that in 92 % of cases, the clarity of calcifications was felt to be equivalent or better (50.4 % and 41.6 %, respectively) with single-view DBT vs. standard CC and MLO FFDM [13]. Spangler et al. investigated the performance of DBT vs. FFDM with regards to detection and classification of calcifications and found that although FFDM was slightly more sensitive than two-view DBT in detecting calcifications (0.84 % vs. 0.75 %), the diagnostic performance as measured by the AUC was not statistically different (0.76 for DM vs. 0.72 for DBT [$p=0.1277$]) [14].

Recall Rate Reduction

In addition to improved breast cancer detection, an additional potential benefit of DBT is a reduction in screening recall rate for non-cancer cases. Current studies indicate that the addition of DBT to FFDM results in a significant reduction in non-cancer recall rate ranging between 28 and 40 % [6, 12, 15], while DBT alone results in a 9.5–11 % reduction vs. DM alone [9, 15]. It should be noted that most of this recall data is derived from retrospective studies with enriched case sets and may not reflect the true performance of DBT in a screening population setting. However, promising preliminary data by Gur et al. from the first 120 patients of a prospective breast cancer screening trial shows a 28 % reduction in recall rate with the addition of DBT to FFDM [16].

DBT Compared to Additional Diagnostic Mammographic Views

Studies comparing DBT to additional diagnostic mammographic views indicate that DBT is comparable in accuracy [17, 18], and equivalent or superior in subjective image quality in 81–89 % of cases [12, 19]. These results suggest that the use of DBT in the diagnostic mammographic workup of patients will result in improved accuracy and workflow efficiency.

Radiation Risk

Modern mammography utilizes very low dose X-ray and even most critics of mammography have stopped using radiation exposure as a reason to avoid mammography. However, as previously described, the current practice in the USA is to utilize DBT in conjunction with 2D FFDM for optimal diagnostic accuracy, which does expose a patient to approximately twice the radiation dose of a 2D FFDM study alone and warrants some consideration.

The FDA mandated MQSA dose limit for mammography is based on the dose delivered to an ACR phantom and is presently 3 mGy. Modern 2D digital mammography units deliver a phantom dose of approximately 1.3 mGy. A combination 2D+3D tomosynthesis exam delivers a phantom dose of approximately 2.7 mGy, less than the FDA MQSA regulatory limit of 3 mGy for a single 2D exposure but roughly double the dose of a FFDM alone.

The effective dose (measured in milliSieverts) is defined as the dose to the breast normalized to whole body exposure. The effective dose of 2D mammography is approximately 0.5 mSv. A 2D+3D combination study delivers an effective dose of 1.0 mSv. To put this in perspective, the average annual background effective dose from solar and background radiation is 3 mSv or three times the effective dose from the combination 2D+3D Tomosynthesis exam. Moving to Denver Colorado from sea level results in an additional 1 mSv of annual background radiation exposure, i.e., twice the dose from a DBT exam. According to the Health Physics Society, "estimation of health risk associated with radiation doses that are of similar magnitude as those received from natural sources should be strictly qualitative and encompass a range of hypothetical health outcomes, including the possibility of no adverse health effects at such low levels [20]."

The mortality risk estimates of the additional radiation exposure associated with DBT are based on worst case (linear no threshold) extrapolations from the known risk at the high doses associated with the nuclear Hiroshima blast. Over the course of their lives, about 375 women out of 3,000 will develop naturally occurring breast cancer. Of these, 125 will prove fatal. At worst, based on the BEIR VII data, annual breast screening from age 40–80 would hypothetically increase breast cancer mortality by about 1 % to 126 for 2D and 127 for 2D plus 3D. This risk is far outweighed by the apparent benefit of digital breast tomosynthesis in diagnosing additional early stage breast cancer and saving lives.

Despite this data on radiation risk, the increased dose associated with a combination 2D+3D DBT exam has been a source of criticism of the technology. One vendor has now developed a synthetic 2D mammogram, which is created from the 3D projection images. This "synthetic view" obviates the need for the 2D portion of the present combination exam. The dose of the DBT exam is then similar to a present 2D FFDM exam. The synthetic view is presently being utilized on Digital Breast Tomosynthesis systems in Europe, Asia, and Australia and is awaiting FDA approval in the USA.

Challenges with DBT

Image Storage

Tomosynthesis exams are large data sets and require greater storage capacity than conventional full field digital mammograms. It is important to engage your IT department early during planning of tomosynthesis deployment in order to ensure adequate storage capacity and optimal imaging archiving and retrieval. A DBT study is a significantly larger file size when compared to a standard four view 2D mammogram. For example, the currently commercially available DBT system in the USA produces approximately 1GB of data for a 4-view DBT exam. This is stored at a 4:1 lossless compression, meaning the study requires 250 MB of storage space. Currently, the DBT images can be stored on PACS, but in order to be reviewed must be sent to a proprietary workstation. It is expected that this issue will be resolved shortly.

Interpretation Time

While a standard 2-view screening mammogram consists of four total images, a 2-view DBT exam with, for example, a breast that compresses to 4 cm consists of 160 images to review. The amount of time required to interpret a DBT exam as compared to a conventional 2D digital mammogram is therefore receiving significant attention.

A study by Kopans et al. found a mean reading time for DBT of just 35 s [21]. However, Good et al. found a mean reading time of 2.72 min (±1.44 min) compared to FFDM 1.58 min (±1.07 min) [22]. In a third study, readers required 1.2 min to interpret FFDM, 2 min to interpret DBT and 2.4 min to interpret a combination 2D+3D exam [15].

It is our experience that the combination 2D+3D study that exists presently in clinical practice initially requires significantly more time to interpret than a 2D FFDM alone. However, there is a steep learning curve with DBT and speed of interpretation rapidly improves. The transition is somewhat analogous to the transition from film-screen mammography to FFDM.

The professional interpretation of DBT exams presently requires 8 h of specialized training. Training programs for DBT are readily accessible to the industry and can provide the needed information to streamline reading digital breast tomosynthesis.

Artifacts

DBT is associated with several characteristic artifacts that a reader quickly becomes familiar with. The limited number of projections and the typically narrow angular range often cause high contrast objects like macrocalcifications, surgical clips and even tissue markers to cause a characteristic ghosting artifact.

Breast Compression

According to the US Centers for Disease Control and Prevention, just 67 % of American women age 40 and above had a mammogram in the past 2 years [23]. The major reason given for avoiding a mammogram is the discomfort caused by compression of the breast during the exam. The ability of DBT to resolve to great extent the issue of tissue superimposition has led many researches to consider whether DBT could allow less compression applied to the breast during mammography while preserving its accuracy.

Two significant studies have been done to date. Saunders et al. utilized an anthropomorphic breast phantom to analyze the conspicuity of masses and calcifications with varied compression [24]. They concluded that "reduced compression would have a minimal effect on radiologists' performance," suggesting that there may be justification for a measured reduction of breast compression during DBT, improving the comfort of women undergoing mammography.

A second study compared image quality in 45 women undergoing DBT utilizing full compression versus half compression [25]. Three radiologists evaluated the images and concluded that DBT "may be performed with substantially less compression force compared with 2D mammography."

Although additional clinical studies need to be performed, the proposition of performing mammography with less, little or even no compression is compelling. Certainly more women could be convinced to undergo regular screening mammography, which would translate into more lives saved.

Future Applications

Digital Breast Tomosynthesis has only recently been incorporated into clinical practice and already there is extensive clinical research being done. It is expected that many of the forthcoming developments in mammography will be based on the DBT platform.

Contrast Enhanced DBT (CE-DBT) by utilizing the angiogenesis associated with malignant breast lesions has the potential to improve the visibility of malignant breast lesions. Chen et al. studied the effectiveness of contrast enhanced DBT, comparing it to FFDM, ultrasound, and magnetic resonance imaging (MRI) [26].

The recent development of functional breast imaging systems such as positron emission tomography (PET) and breast specific gamma imaging (BSGI) have led some to suggest combined functional–anatomic imaging as a way to improve both sensitivity and specificity. Pilot studies have been published describing Dual Modality Breast Tomosynthesis combining DBT and technetium 99 m sestamibi scanning [27] and DBT and optical imaging [28].

Conclusion

Digital Breast Tomosynthesis is a new, FDA-approved 3D imaging technology designed to address the major limitation of conventional 2D mammography, the issue of tissue superimposition. Potential benefits of DBT include higher cancer detection rates (sensitivity), fewer unnecessary screening recalls (specificity), higher positive predictive value for a biopsy recommendation, and improved overall radiologist confidence. Research presently underway will help shape the manner in which DBT is incorporated into clinical practice.

References

1. Tabar L, Yen M, Vitak B, et al. Mammography service screening and mortality in breast cancer patients: 20-year follow-up before and after introduction of screening. Lancet. 2003;361:1405–10.
2. Cady B, Stone MD, Schuler JG, Thakur R, Wanner MA, Lavin PT. The new era in breast cancer: invasion, size and nodal involvement dramatically decreasing as a result of mammographic screening. Arch Surg. 1996;131:301–8.
3. Carney PA, Miglioretti DL, Yankaskas BC, et al. Individual and combined effects of age, breast density, and hormone replacement therapy use on the accuracy of screening mammography. Ann Intern Med. 2003;138:168–75.
4. Yaghjyan L et al. Mammographic breast density and subsequent risk of breast cancer in postmenopausal women according to tumor characteristics. J Natl Cancer Inst. 2011;103(15):1179–89.
5. Niklason LT, Christian BT, Niklason LE, et al. Digital tomosynthesis in breast imaging. Radiology. 1997;205:399–406.
6. Rafferty E, Niklason L. FFDM vs. FFDM with tomosynthesis for women with radiographically dense breasts: an Enriched Retrospective Reader Study. Presented at Radiological Society of North America 2011 scientific assembly and annual meeting, Chicago, IL. rsna2011.rsna.org/search/event_display.cfm?am_id=2&em_id=11016626&printmode=Y&autoprint=N.
7. Gur D, Bandos AI, Rockette HE, et al. Localized detection and classification of abnormalities on FFDM and tomosynthesis examinations rated under an FROC paradigm. AJR Am J Roentgenol. 2011;096:737–41.

8. Skaane P, Gullien R, Eben E, et al. Reading time of FFDM and tomosynthesis in a population-based screening program (abstr). Presented at Radiological Society of North America 2011 scientific assembly and annual meeting, Chicago, IL. rsna2011.rsna.org/search/event_display.cfm?am_id=2&em_id=11011027&printmode=Y&autoprint=N
9. Wallis MG, Moa E, Zanca F, et al. Two-view and single-view tomosynthesis versus full-field digital mammography: high resolution X-Ray Imaging Observer Study. Radiology. 2012;262(3):788–96. doi:10.1148/radiol.11103514. 103514; Published online January 24, 2012.
10. Tingberg A, Förnvik D, Mattsson S, et al. Breast cancer screening with tomosynthesis – initial experiences. Radiat Prot Dosimetry. 2011;147(1–2):180–3.
11. Gennaro G, Toledano A, di Maggio C, et al. Digital breast tomosynthesis versus digital mammography: a clinical performance study. Eur Radiol. 2010;20:1545–53.
12. Poplack SP, Tosteson TD, Kogel CA, et al. Digital breast tomosynthesis: initial experience in 98 women with abnormal digital screening mammography. AJR Am J Roentgenol. 2007;189:616–23.
13. Kopans D, Gavenonis S, Halpern E, et al. Calcifications in the breast and digital breast tomosynthesis. Breast J. 2011;17:638–44.
14. Spangler ML, Zuley ML, Sumkin JH, et al. Detection and classification of calcifications on digital breast tomosynthesis and 2D digital mammography: a comparison. AJR Am J Roentgenol. 2011;196:320–4.
15. Gur D, Abrams GS, Chough DM, et al. Digital breast tomosynthesis: observer performance study. AJR Am J Roentgenol. 2009;193:586–91.
16. Gur D, Sumkin J, Zuley M, et al. Recall rate reduction with tomosynthesis during baseline examinations: preliminary assessment from a prospective screening trial. Presented at Radiological Society of North America 2011 scientific assembly and annual meeting, Chicago, IL. rsna2011.rsna.org/search/event_display.cfm?am_id=2&em_id=11004417&printmode=Y&autoprint=N
17. Noroozian M, Hadjiiski L, Rahnama-Moghadam S, et al. Digital breast tomosynthesis is comparable to mammographic spot views for mass characterization. Radiology. 2012;262:61–8.
18. Tagliafico A, Astengo D, Cavagnetto F, et al. One-to-one comparison between digital spot compression view and digital breast tomosynthesis. Eur Radiol. 2012;22(3):539–44.
19. Hakim CM, Chough DM, Ganott MA, et al. Digital breast tomosynthesis in the diagnostic environment: a subjective side-by-side review. AJR Am J Roentgenol. 2010;195:172–6.
20. Position Statement of the Health Physics Society—Radiation Risk in Perspective. 2010.
21. Kopans D, Moore R. Digital breast tomosynthesis (DBT) NCI 3000-Women Trial. Presented at the 95th scientific assembly and annual meeting of the Radiological Society of North America, Chicago, IL, 30 Nov 2009. Abstract SSE01-01.
22. Good WJ, Abrams GS, Catullo VJ, et al. Digital breast tomosynthesis: a pilot observer study. AJR Am J Roentgenol. 2008;190:865–9.
23. National Center for Health Statistics. Health, United States, 2011: with special feature on socioeconomic status and health. Hyattsville, MD: National Center for Health Statistics; 2012.
24. Saunders RS, Samei E, Lo JY, et al. Can compression be reduced for breast tomosynthesis? Monte Carlo Study on mass and microcalcification conspicuity in tomosynthesis. Radiology. 2009;251:673–82.
25. Förnvik D, Andersson I, Svahn T, et al. The effect of reduced breast compression in breast tomosynthesis: human observer study using clinical cases. Radiat Prot Dosimetry. 2010;139(1–3):118–23.
26. Chen SC, Carton AK, Albert M, et al. Initial clinical experience with contrast-enhanced digital breast tomosynthesis. Acad Radiol. 2007;14:229–38.
27. Williams MB, Judy PG, Gunn S, et al. Dual-modality breast tomosynthesis. Radiology. 2010;255:191–8.
28. Fang Q, Selb J, Carp SA, et al. Combined optical and X-ray tomosynthesis breast imaging. Radiology. 2011;258:89–97.

Part III
Ablative Surgical Techniques

Chapter 10
Interstitial Laser Therapy (ILT) of Breast Tumors

Kambiz Dowlatshahi and Rosalinda Alvarado

Introduction

The widespread practice of screening mammography in the USA and Europe has resulted in detection of smaller breast cancers and reduction in mortality [1]. However, the surgical management of the primary cancer has not kept pace with the diagnostic advances. The concept of in situ ablation of breast cancer with a non-cutting technique appeals to patients, provided it is safe and efficacious. Several in situ techniques, either by heat (laser, radiofrequency, focused ultrasound, and microwave) or by cold (cryotherapy), are emerging as alternatives to lumpectomy [2].

Interstitial laser therapy (ILT) as a minimally invasive technique used for treatment of benign and malignant breast tumors is the subject of this chapter.

LASER stands for Light Amplification by Stimulated Emission of Radiation. Lasers are high-intensity monochromatic lights, which were introduced into medical practice in the 1960's for palliative treatment of advanced tumors of gastrointestinal, bronchial, and urinary tracts [3–6]. Recanalization of the obstructed lumens of the esophagus and the bronchus was achieved using a non-contact high-power Nd:YAG laser, which vaporized the tumor [7, 8]. In contrast to the high power (40–60 W) and short exposure times to vaporize obstructing tumors, much lower powers (1–2 W) and longer exposure times of several minutes were employed for local ablation of tumors. The laser light, in the infrared wave range of 800–1,034 nm, given continuously through an optic fiber, heats the tissue and causes a zone of necrosis measuring 1.5–2 cm (Figs.10.1 and 10.2). The treated area undergoes resorption by phagocytosis and is repaired by fibrosis (Fig. 10.3). In the case of mammographically detected breast cancers, this in situ ablation of tumors may obviate the need for surgical excision in selected cases.

K. Dowlatshahi, M.D. (✉)
Department of General Surgery, Rush University Medical Center,
60 East Delaware Place, Suite 1400, Chicago, IL 60611, USA
e-mail: kdowlat@gmail.com

R. Alvarado, M.D.
Department of Surgery, Rush University Medical Center, 1725 West Harrison, Chicago, IL 60612, USA

D.S. Francescatti and M.J. Silverstein (eds.), *Breast Cancer: A New Era in Management*,
DOI 10.1007/978-1-4614-8063-1_10, © Springer Science+Business Media New York 2014

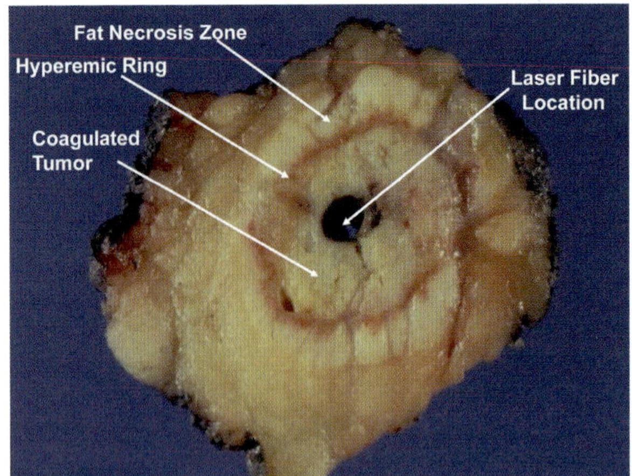

Fig. 10.1 Post-lumpectomy section of a laser treated breast cancer showing concentric zones of coagulated tumor, hyperemic ring, and zone of fat necrosis around the laser fiber

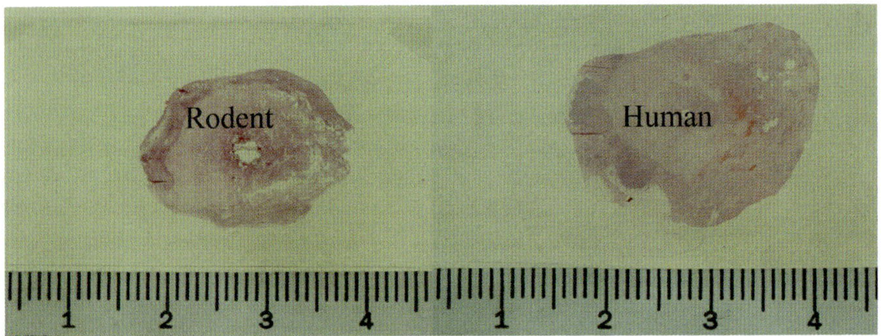

Fig. 10.2 Gross histology of laser treated tumors in a rodent tumor model and in a patient demonstrating 15–20 mm tissue necrosis caused by laser energy

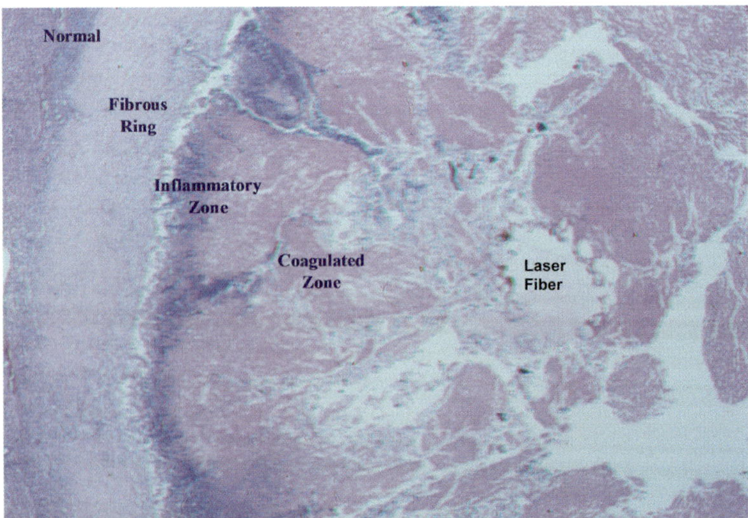

Fig. 10.3 Microscopic appearance of laser treated tumor at 1 month showing clearance of the coagulated tissue by inflammatory cells and formation of a fibrous ring

Experimental Basis for ILT

Mathewson et al. were probably the first to show the coagulation effect of Nd:YAG laser light delivered within a normal rat liver [9]. Employing low power (0.5–2.0 W) and long exposures of 1–40 min, they observed well-defined highly reproducible necrotic lesions of up to 16 mm in diameter consistent with tissue damage by a purely thermal effect. Radiological examination of the treated tissue in which arterial tree had been filled with a radio-opaque polymer demonstrated loss of all small and some larger vessels. These investigators, however, noted tissue charring around the fiber tip with higher (>2 W) power settings and corresponding fall in the laser light transmission. To overcome this problem and to shorten the operation time, Dachman et al. were able to show the coagulative necrosis of the pig liver by ultrasound-guided Nd:YAG laser at power setting of less than 5-W over 6–10 min duration [10].

In 1988, the author developed a technique which allowed the delivery of laser energy into tumors at higher powers (5–10 W) and in shorter time [11, 12]. Thus, a typical 1-cm tumor could be ablated in 10–15 min. This goal was achieved by dripping normal saline at 1–2 cm^3/min para-axially to the laser fiber into the tumor. The small pool of fluid in front of the fiber tip prevents the heated tissue sticking to and defacing the fiber tip. This allows laser light transmission to a distance of 5–8 mm into the target tissue for coagulation. The volume of the normal saline dripped into the tissue during the treatment time is about 15–20 cm^3; small enough to be easily absorbed by the body. The temperature at the point of the laser light emission is continuously monitored with a thermocouple soldered to the laser needle (Fig. 10.4). By adjusting the laser power and the rate of the saline drip, this temperature is not allowed to exceed 100 °C. The temperature at the periphery of the tumor is monitored with a second multi-sensor thermal needle inserted parallel to the laser needle and 1 cm away from it. Experimental observation on rodent mammary tumors treated with laser (unpublished data) revealed that when the peripheral temperature reaches 60 °C, 100 % tumor necrosis occurs.

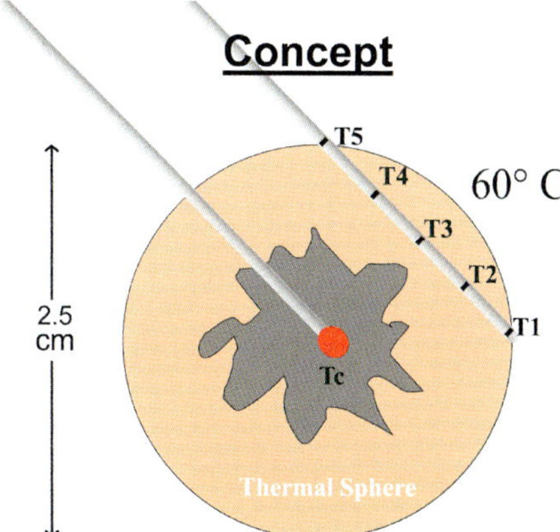

Fig. 10.4 A sketch of the laser probe tip in the center of the tumor and an adjacent multi-sensor thermal probe to continuously monitor the heating of the tumor

Clinical Experience with ILT

Liver Tumors

Most published reports related to clinical application of interstitial laser therapy are from investigators who treated primary or metastatic liver tumors with this technique. Hashimoto et al. first reported successful treatment of patients with hepatocellular and metastatic carcinoma of the liver treated intraoperatively with Nd:YAG laser given through a quartz fiber inserted into the tumor with ultrasound guidance [13]. There were no procedure-related complications. Schroder et al. reported similar experience in treating patients with liver tumors [14]. Nolsoe et al. reported successful interstitial laser treatment in 11 of 12 patients [15]. They employed multiple laser fibers with diffuser tips, sonographically guided into the center of tumors at 5 mm intervals through a template. Nd:YAG laser at power setting of 4–8 W was used. The periphery temperature reaching 60 °C during treatment was measured by micro-thermocouples. The treated tumors were noted to become hyperechoic. Follow-up ultrasound examination showed central cyst formation and needle biopsy revealed necrotic material. Patients experienced minor pain, transient pyrexia, and in one case pleural effusion which resolved spontaneously. Amin et al. reported on interstitial laser photocoagulation of 21 patients with 55 liver metastases using Nd:YAG laser at 2-W through a 200 μm bare-tipped fiber [16]. 100 % necrosis was achieved in 38 % of tumors as judged by ultrasound and CT scan. Their success rate was higher in tumors smaller than 4 cm in diameter. There were four cases of subcapsular hematoma and six cases of pleural effusion. The author treated 26 patients with primary and metastatic liver cancers, either as a sole treatment or in conjunction with surgical resection of the liver disease. It was concluded that ILT can successfully ablate tumors up to 25 mm. in diameter [17].

Malignant Breast Tumors

Harries et al. reported on interstitial laser photocoagulation of 44 patients with breast cancer treated with diode laser under local anesthesia [18]. Tumors measured 1–5 cm in diameter, were treated with ultrasound guidance in 42 cases and with CT in two cases. The investigators observed that greater tumor necrosis was achieved when there was tissue carbonization around the laser fiber tip and they confirmed the advantage of this effect by pre-charring the laser tip. There was no attempt at dosimetry or thermometry of the tumor during treatment. Real-time monitoring by ultrasound did not appear to predict the size of necrosis. Mumtaz et al. reported on 20 patients with breast cancer and noted that gadolinium-enhanced magnetic resonance imaging defined the extent of laser-induced necrosis and residual tumor after laser photocoagulation therapy [19]. Milne et al. measured the temperature changes in porcine tissue models using thermocouples inserted at various distances from the

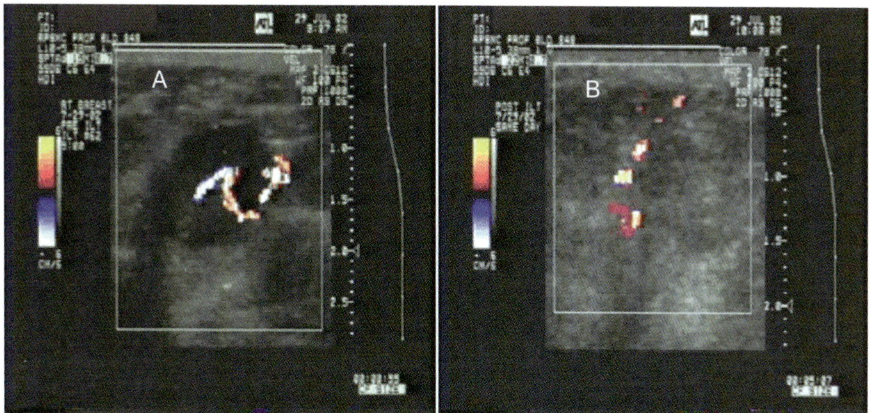

Fig. 10.5 Color Doppler ultrasound of a breast cancer treated with ILT showing a small vessel traversing the tumor before (**a**) and its disappearance due to thrombosis afterwards (**b**)

laser probe [20]. They concluded that interstitial laser thermotherapy produces symmetrical and predictable volumetric temperature increases.

The author's experience at Rush University consists of two phases:

1. From 1994 to 2001, the feasibility, efficacy and safety of ILT was tested in 54 patients with small (T1) breast cancers and periodically reported [11, 21, 22]. Patients underwent surgical excision of the laser treated tumors as part of the standard treatment of their breast cancers. All 54 patients underwent wire localization, surgical excision of the tumor and removal of the regional lymph nodes 1–8 weeks later. The blood flow to the tumor was redetermined with color Doppler ultrasound prior to excision (Fig. 10.5a, b). The overall success rate of the procedure including the learning phase and technical changes was 71 %. Under optimal operating conditions, total tumor necrosis was achieved in two series of 13 of 14 and 14 of 14 consecutive cases (96 %) [23].
2. Having gained technical proficiency and established the parameters for adequate treatment, the author treated selected patients, on volunteer basis, with laser and without excision. Over the next 4 years, ten patients with mammographically detected invasive breast cancers were treated with ILT without excision. The laser-treated tumors were monitored with imaging (ultrasound, mammography and MRI in one patient) and needle biopsy from marked areas at 1 month post-treatment (Fig. 10.6).

The mean tumor diameter as measured on mammogram and ultrasound was 11 (range: 7–21) mm. Patients required minimal oral analgesics and experienced no adverse systemic effects over a period of 1–12 years. Laser treated tumors became non-palpable after 3–6 months. Color Doppler ultrasound demonstrated loss of blood flow in the ablated zone and needle biopsies showed fibrosis. In three patients the laser- treated tumor became cystic (Fig. 10.7) and the aspirated fluid showed no malignant cells. In one patient, a 2 mm × 2 mm island of cancer, adjacent to an

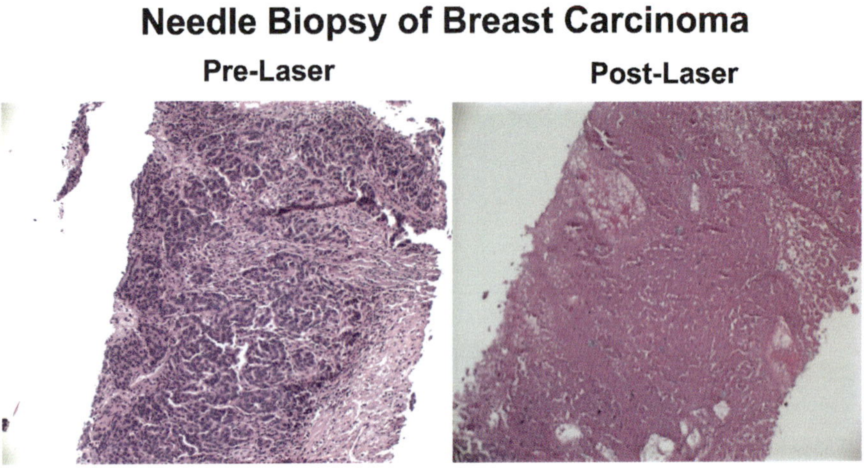

Needle Biopsy of Breast Carcinoma

Pre-Laser Post-Laser

Fig. 10.6 Histologic appearance of needle biopsies of a breast cancer taken before and after treatment with laser

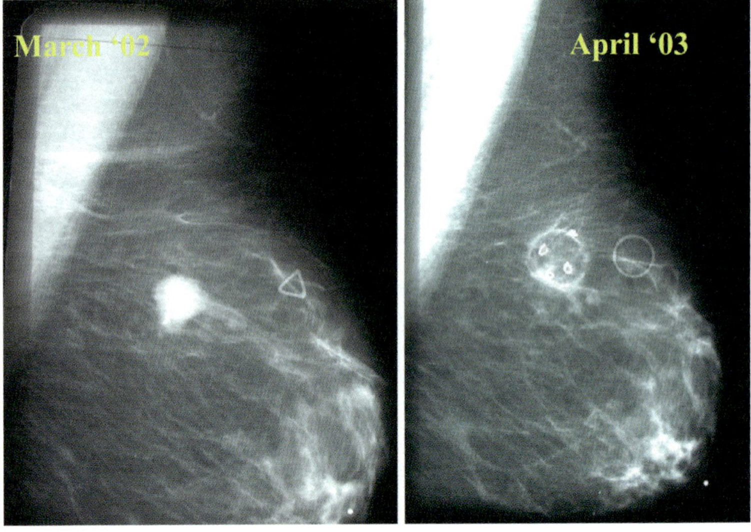

Fig. 10.7 Mammographic appearance of a breast cancer 1 year after laser therapy demonstrating conversion of the tumor into a cyst

artery, was detected by ultrasound and confirmed by histological examination of the excised tumor (Fig. 10.8). This was deemed to be due to the heat-sink effect of the vessel. A multi-site prospective clinical trial to duplicate this experience is planned to commence in the near future.

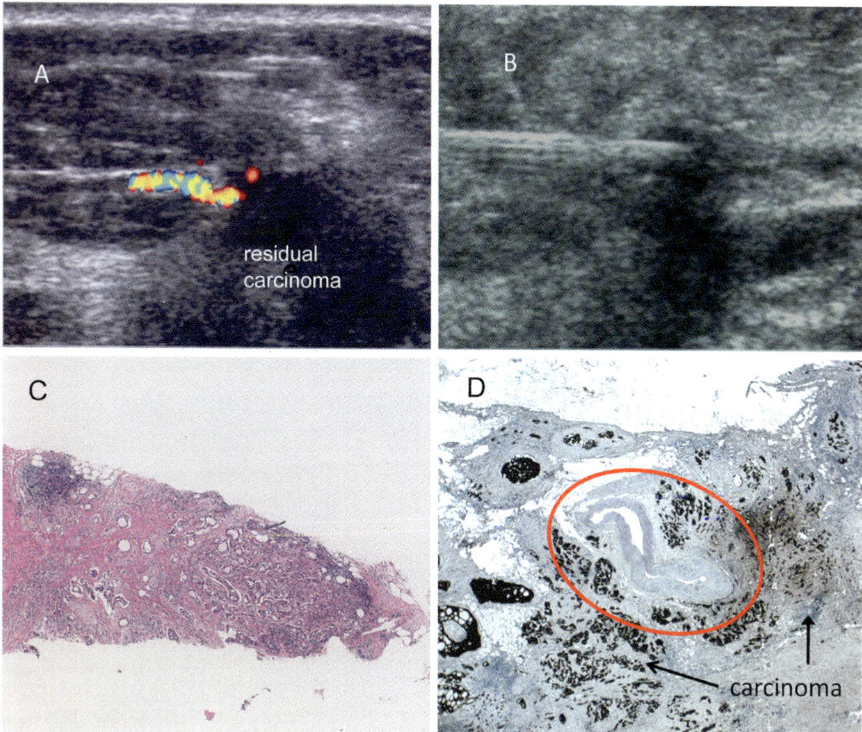

Fig. 10.8 Detection of residual carcinoma: (**a**) Color Doppler ultrasound at 1 month after ILT. (**b**) US guided needle biopsy. (**c**) Needle core biopsy showing coagulated carcinoma on the left and residual malignancy on the right. (**d**) Malignant tissue seen surrounding the artery (*circled*)

It is emphasized that laser therapy of mammographically detected breast cancers is only to replace lumpectomy. All other components of the treatment, i.e., sentinel node/axillary node biopsy, radiation therapy to the breast and whenever indicated chemo-hormonal therapy is given per current standard of care.

Patient Selection

The following criteria are suggested for treatment of breast cancers with ILT:

1. Clearly visualized masses or clusters of micro-calcifications detected by mammography (Fig. 10.9).
2. Tumor size: Up to 15 mm as determined by ultrasound and MRI.
3. A distance of 1 cm should separate the tumor from the skin or the chest wall.
4. Definitive needle core diagnosis of the tumor indicating: in situ or invasive cancer and determination of prognostic factors on the samples.

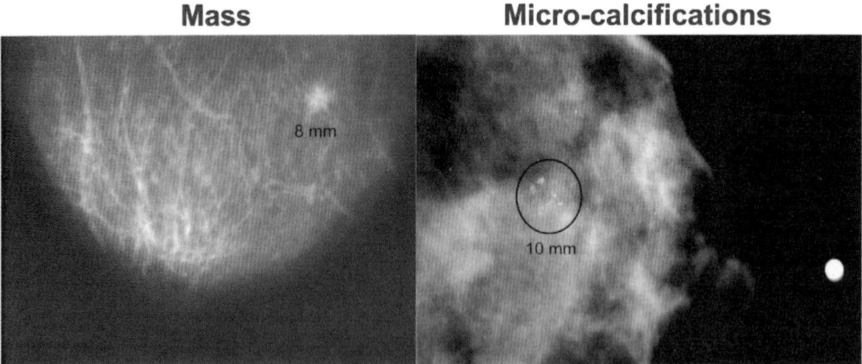

Fig. 10.9 Mammographically detected breast cancer as a mass or a cluster of micro-calcifications

Pretreatment Evaluation

Imaging work up of the breast should include diagnostic mammography, grey scale and color Doppler ultrasound as well as contrast enhanced MRI. High resolution US provides very precise measurements of the tumor dimensions. Color Doppler US evaluates the blood flow in and around the tumor prior to intervention [11]. MRI excludes any secondary focus of cancer before laser therapy as well as any residual malignancy afterwards.

On the day of treatment, the tumor images are reviewed and its boundaries with all its visible extensions plus 0.5 cm of normal appearing tissue are marked on the films. This approach is also applicable to clustered microcalcifications associated with tissue densities. The volume of the tumor and 0.5 cm of the adjacent surrounding zone are calculated by $V=4/3\cdot R3$, R being the radius of the therapeutic sphere. Based upon the previous experimental data, the amount of laser energy needed for 100 % tumor coagulation is 1,400 J per cubic centimeter of the calculated tissue (tumor + surrounding breast parenchyma). Thus, for a typical 1.0 cm. tumor + 0.5 cm rim of surrounding parenchyma, the volume is 4.0 cubic cm and the laser energy for its complete destruction is 5,600 J. In practice, the treatment endpoint is reached when the thermal sensors on the needle adjacent to the tumor display 60 °C. The tumor blood flow is also assessed by contrast enhanced color Doppler ultrasound. This test is repeated after laser therapy.

Treatment on Stereotactic Table

The patient is positioned on a stereotactic table and the shortest skin-to-tumor route, avoiding any intervening vessels, is chosen. Additional needle core samples are taken from the tumor and archived. Field anesthesia around the tumor is achieved

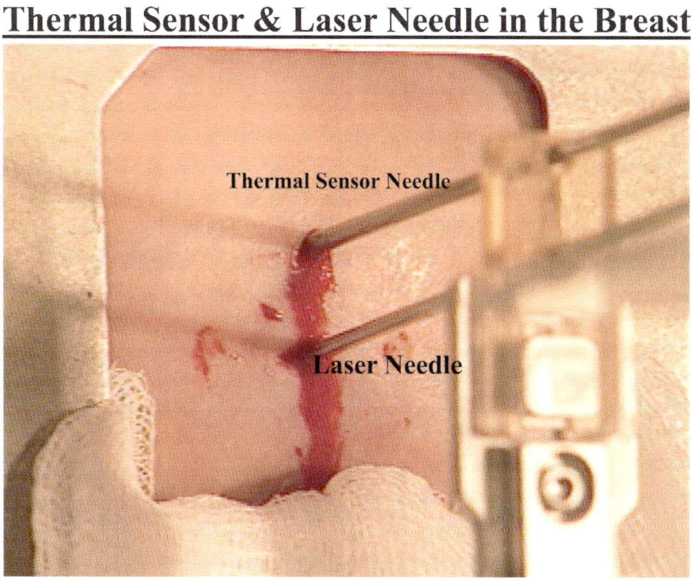

Thermal Sensor & Laser Needle in the Breast

Fig. 10.10 External appearance of an immobilized breast of a patient on a stereotactic table with laser and thermal probes inserted to a predetermined depth into the breast

with approximately 50 cm^3 of 0.25 % bupivacaine. Four metal markers are inserted around the tumor at positions 3, 6, 9, and 12 o'clock for future reference. The laser needle is inserted into the center of the tumor through a 2 mm skin incision and a multi-sensor thermal needle through a second incision, 1 cm away and parallel with the laser needle, to a predetermined length so that its tip is 1 cm in front of the laser needle (Fig. 10.10). Stereoimages are taken to confirm proper positions (Fig. 10.11). The laser needle stylet is replaced with an optic fiber held by a y-connector, the second arm of which is connected to a fluid pump delivering normal saline up to 2.0 cm^3/min.

Typically the treatment is commenced by starting the fluid pump at 1.0 cm^3/min and the laser power at 5.0 W. The central temperature rises within a few seconds and the peripheral temperatures rise within a minute when the heat generated by the laser from the center of the tumor reaches them. When all thermal sensors record 60 °C, the treatment is stopped. Patient's vital signs are monitored during treatment. Stereotactic images are taken during and at the completion of the procedure to document satisfactory needle alignment. Additional interstitial anesthesia is given if the patient experiences pain higher than 3 on a scale of 0–10. The skin overlying the tumor is sprayed with a coolant fluid when the tumor is close to 1 cm from the skin. At the completion of the treatment, the needles are removed, the breast is decompressed, light dressing is applied, and after 1 h of observation, the patient is discharged home with oral analgesics and ice pack on the breast.

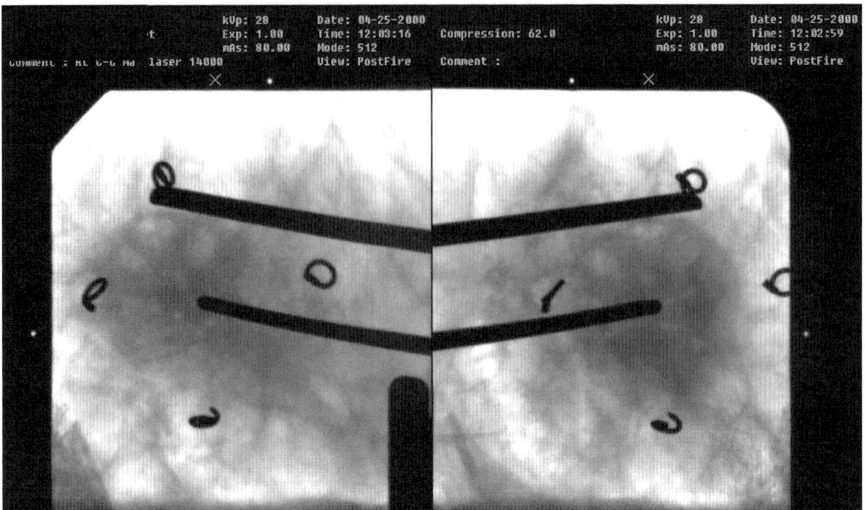

Fig. 10.11 Stereotactic images of laser and thermal sensor needles taken prior to the start of treatment. Four metal clips mark the periphery of the tumor for future reference

Benign Breast Tumors

Majority of benign breast tumors suitable for laser therapy are fibroadenomas although occasional cases of papilloma or lipoma may be treated with ILT.

Fibroadenoma (FA) is a benign tumor of the breast commonly seen in teenagers and young women as a palpable breast mass and in older females as a mass reported on the baseline mammogram. In the USA, fibroadenoma is as common as breast cancer with a life time incidence of one in eight, primarily affecting younger women in contrast to cancer which is a disease of older women. The diagnosis is made by a combination of physical findings, a rubbery, mobile mass, usually non-tender, with sonographic features of smooth borders, homogeneous interior and finally by needle core biopsy. The current treatment options of surgical removal or observation are suboptimal; especially to a teenager who dislikes a scar on her breast and finds it worrisome if not embarrassing to live with the lump. Percutaneous laser ablation of FA is a new option which makes the breast tumor non-palpable and leaves two needle marks on the skin. It is clinically and aesthetically superior to the current management of this condition. The treatment was approved by the FDA in 2007 and a Registry was set up to monitor the outcome. This presentation describes the experience on 28 patients treated with ILT under local anesthesia in an outpatient setting.

The diagnosis of fibroadenoma is primarily clinical, i.e., a self-discovered, palpable, discrete, mobile mass of 1–3 cm in diameter, usually non-tender which may be lobulated, multiple, and bilateral. The sonographic appearance is that of a hypoechoic mass with discrete borders and homogeneous interior casting a posterior enhancing shadow (Fig. 10.12). The definitive diagnosis is made by image-guided

Ultrasound of a Breast Fibroadenoma

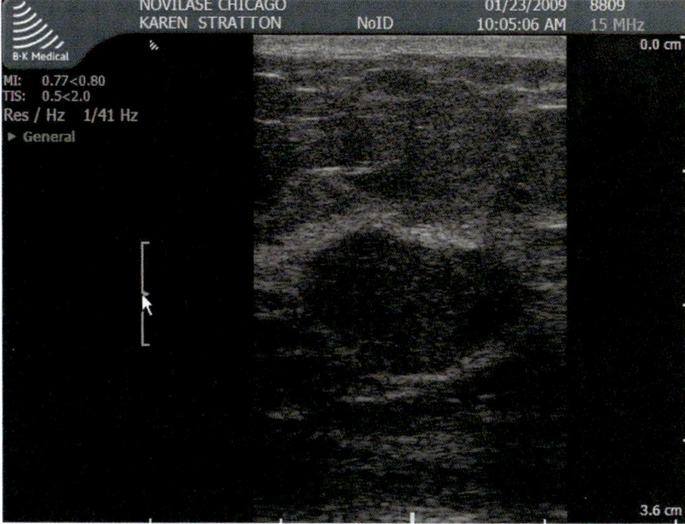

Fig. 10.12 Typical sonographic appearance of a breast fibroadenoma treated with ILT

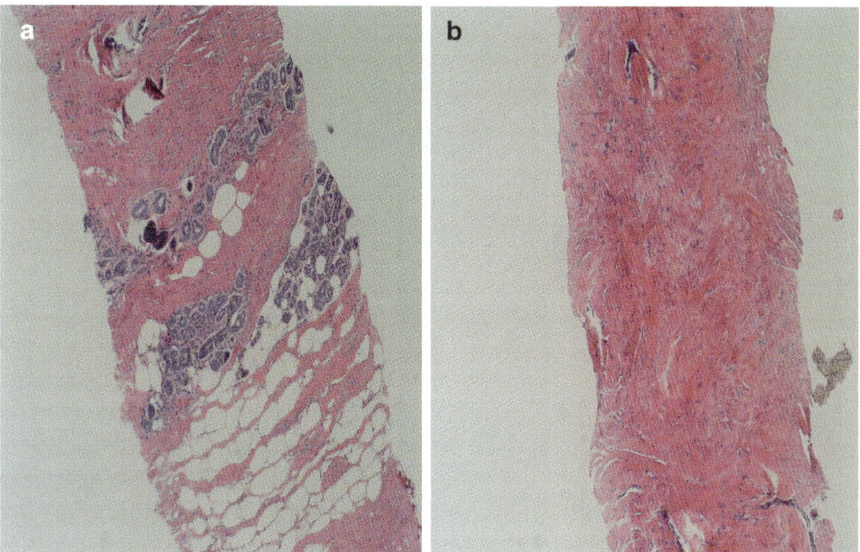

Fig. 10.13 Low power histologic appearance of needle core biopsies taken from a breast fibroadenoma (**a**) before and (**b**) 3 months after ILT

needle core biopsy under local anesthesia. Histologically, fibro-glandular elements interspersed with supportive collagen and fibroblasts are typical of fibroadenoma (Fig. 10.13) which must be differentiated from its rarer malignant variety: cystosarcoma phyllodes.

In this chapter the authors describe their early experience with percutaneous treatment of fibroadenoma in a group of patients deploying infrared laser previously reported on patients with breast cancer [23].

Treatment

Initially patients were treated on a stereotactic table, which immobilizes the breast and to some degree the tumor within it. But soon it became apparent that ultrasound was the preferred technology because the majority of patients were young with dense parenchyma and the tumors could be better visualized by ultrasound. Accurate probe placement and treatment monitoring in real time are additional advantages. Furthermore, ultrasound is less expensive and a more available device. The treatment was given under local anesthesia, in an outpatient setting, through a needle probe either stereotactically or sonographically guided to the target. The latter was a preferred option because the operator observes the laser heat effect on the ultrasound screen in addition to the displayed rise in tissue temperature transmitted by the thermal probe shown on its monitor.

Procedure Details

The skin at the two puncture points is anesthetized with 1 % Lidocaine using a 27 G needle. Subcutaneous tissue between the skin and the superficial surface of the tumor is also infiltrated with 1 % Lidocaine. If the tumor is in a subcutaneous location, this maneuver pushes it away from the skin; thus preventing thermal injury during the treatment. Using a spinal needle, guided by US, the parenchyma surrounding the tumor is anesthetized with 20–30 cm^3 of ½% Marcaine. Two 3 mm long incisions, 1 cm apart, are made with a #11 blade on the skin approximately 3 cm from the tumor. Guided by ultrasound the laser probe (Novilase Corp) is inserted through the skin into the tumor and the stylet is replaced with the optic fiber. Next, the thermal probe with five sensors at 5 mm intervals from its tip is inserted through a second puncture site 1 cm away and 1.5 cm deeper than the laser probe. The distance between the probes is fixed with a clip which secures their spatial relationship.

Laser goggles are worn by the patient and the attendants. The fluid pump starts at 0.5 cm^3/min and the bolus arrival into the tissue is seen on the ultrasound monitor. Continuous wave diode laser starts at 3 W and its effect on the tissue as mini-bubble formation is observed and monitored. The central temperature (T_c) begins to rise within seconds. If delayed, the fluid is stopped until the T_c reaches 90 °C. The five peripheral temperatures (T1–T5) begin to rise in a bell-shaped formation until they reach 60 °C. During the following 15 min the heated tumor gradually opacifies (Fig. 10.14). Approximately 3,000 J of laser energy is needed to ablate a

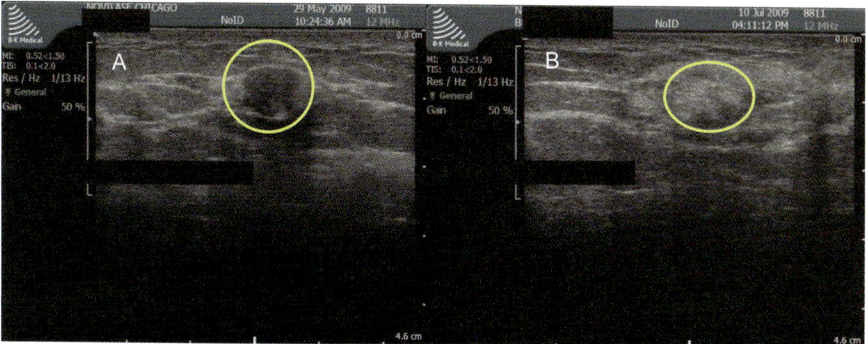

Fig. 10.14 Ultrasound images of a breast fibroadenoma. (**a**) Before laser therapy, (**b**) 6 weeks afterwards displaying opacification of the tumor

fibroadenoma measuring 1 cm in diameter in 15 min. The laser power setting and the saline flow may be adjusted to maintain the central temperature between 90 and 100 °C. During the treatment, the operator ensures that the patient's pain level does not exceed 3 on a scale of 0–10 by either reducing the laser power or by increasing the saline flow rate. Additional local anesthesia may be infused or the skin may be cooled with methylene chloride spray. Infrequently the procedure may be interrupted if one or a combination of the above steps is not effective.

Comments

The current surgical management of breast cancer is not in line with rapid advances in imaging technology. Lumpectomy was designed for surgical removal of a palpable breast mass. The image-detected (by mammogram or MRI) in situ and invasive breast cancer is beyond the tactile appreciation, even at times, intra-operatively. In an attempt to remove the lesion, the surgeon excises a large portion of the breast tissue. An image-guided, less invasive local therapy should be considered for such small well defined cancers. Two decades ago "knife was replaced with needle" for diagnosis of mammographically detected breast cancers. Clearly image guided therapy of breast cancer is at its infancy and has to be tested in prospective randomized trials before it can be accepted for clinical application in selective cases. However, the main obstacle to the acceptance of this technique by breast surgeons is the lack of information on the tumor margins. Up to 20–70 % of lumpectomies for breast carcinoma have been reported with positive resection margins [24]. In a comprehensive review of the subject, Singletary reported that it was the gross presence of the malignant cells and not the width of the clear margin which dictated the risk of local recurrence. Thus the margin width of 1 mm versus 2–3 mm versus 10 mm does not appear to influence the rate of local recurrence of 3–5 % in 5 years [25]. As illustrated by the cases described above, the laser therapy ablates 2.5–3.0 cm^3 of breast

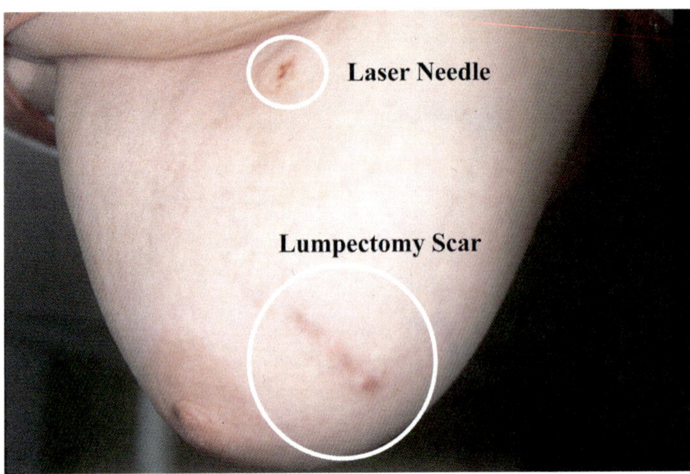

Fig. 10.15 Cosmetic appearance of a patient's breast showing the past lumpectomy scar and a just completed ILT needle site

tissue. With the precision of the stereotactic technology it is possible to guide the needle to the center of the tumor and deliver the ablative laser energy. The high resolution US plays a pivotal role in the surveillance of this paradigm shift. With the introduction of magnetic resonance spectroscopy (functional MRI), which differentiates malignant from benign tissue [26], it may become possible to determine the total tumor ablation by imaging [27].

In summary, diagnosis and determination of the prognostic factors of breast cancer may be made by image-guided needle biopsy. Employing existing technology, surgeons may be trained to treat selected breast cancers with laser energy percutaneously. Experimental and clinical reports to date indicate the technique to be safe. High resolution ultrasound, mammography, MRI, and needle biopsy, when necessary, will confirm the tumor ablation. Newer imaging modalities, such as positron emission mammography [28, 29] will further support the rationale for a less disfiguring approach to the treatment of image-detected breast cancers (Fig 10.15).

References

1. Nelson HD, Tyne K, Naik A, et al. Screening for breast cancer: an update for the U.S. Preventive Services Task Force. Ann Intern Med. 2009;151:727–37. W737–742.
2. Huston TL, Simmons RM. Ablative therapies for the treatment of malignant diseases of the breast. Am J Surg. 2005;189:694–701.
3. Mantovani G, Astara G, Manca G, et al. Endoscopic laser ablation as palliative treatment of endobronchial, nonresectable, or recurrent lung cancer: assessment of its impact on quality of life. Clin Lung Cancer. 2000;1:277–85. discussion 286.
4. Fleischer D, Sivak MV. Endoscopic Nd:YAG laser therapy as palliative treatment for advanced adenocarcinoma of the gastric cardia. Gastroenterology. 1984;87:815–20.

5. Rao SK, Srinivasan B, Sitalakshmi G, et al. Photorefractive keratectomy versus laser in situ keratomileusis to prevent keratectasia after corneal ablation. J Cataract Refract Surg. 2004;30: 2623–8.
6. Bader MJ, Sroka R, Gratzke C, et al. Laser therapy for upper urinary tract transitional cell carcinoma: indications and management. Eur Urol. 2009;56:65–71.
7. Hetzel MR, Nixon C, Edmondstone WM, et al. Laser therapy in 100 tracheobronchial tumours. Thorax. 1985;40:341–5.
8. Swain CP, Bown SG, Edwards DA, et al. Laser recanalization of obstructing foregut cancer. Br J Surg. 1984;71:112–5.
9. Matthewson K, Coleridge-Smith P, O'Sullivan JP, et al. Biological effects of intrahepatic neodymium:yttrium–aluminum–garnet laser photocoagulation in rats. Gastroenterology. 1987;93:550–7.
10. Dachman AH, McGehee JA, Beam TE, et al. US-guided percutaneous laser ablation of liver tissue in a chronic pig model. Radiology. 1990;176:129–33.
11. Dowlatshahi K, Fan M, Gould VE, et al. Stereotactically guided laser therapy of occult breast tumors: work-in-progress report. Arch Surg. 2000;135:1345–52.
12. Dowlatshahi K, Francescatti DS, Bloom KJ. Laser therapy for small breast cancers. Am J Surg. 2002;184:359–63.
13. Hashimoto D, Takami M, Ideezuli Y. In depth radiation therapy by Nd:YAG laser for malignant tumors of the liver under ultrasonic imaging. Gastroenterology. 1985;88:1663.
14. Hahl J, Haapiainen R, Ovaska J, et al. Laser-Induced hyperthermia in the treatment of liver tumors. Lasers Surg Med. 1990;10:319–21.
15. Nolsoe CP, Torp-Pedersen S, Burcharth F, et al. Interstitial hyperthermia of colorectal liver metastases with a US-guided Nd-YAG laser with a diffuser tip: a pilot clinical study. Radiology. 1993;187:333–7.
16. Amin Z, Donald JJ, Masters A, et al. Hepatic metastases: interstitial laser photocoagulation with real-time US monitoring and dynamic CT evaluation of treatment. Radiology. 1993;187:339–47.
17. Dowlatshahi K, Bhattacharya AK, Silver B, Matalon T, Williams JW. Percutaneous interstitial laser therapy of a patient with recurrent hepatoma in a transplanted liver. Surgery. 1992; 112(3):603–606.
18. Harries SA, Amin Z, Smith ME, et al. Interstitial laser photocoagulation as a treatment for breast cancer. Br J Surg. 1994;81:1617–9.
19. Mumtaz H, Hall-Craggs MA, Wotherspoon A, et al. Laser therapy for breast cancer: MR imaging and histopathologic correlation. Radiology. 1996;200:651–8.
20. Milne PJ, Parel JM, Manns F, et al. Development of stereotactically guided laser interstitial thermotherapy of breast cancer: in situ measurement and analysis of the temperature field in ex vivo and in vivo adipose tissue. Lasers Surg Med. 2000;26:67–75.
21. Dowlatshahi K, Fan M. Interstitial laser therapy (ILT) with diode laser: correlation of laser energy and tumor coagulation. Lasers Surg Med. 1995;Suppl 7.
22. Dowlatshahi K, Fan M, Shekarloo M. Stereotactic interstitial laser therapy of early-stage breast cancer. Breast J. 1996;2:304–11.
23. Dowlatshahi K, Wadhwani S, Alvarado R, et al. Interstitial laser therapy of breast fibroadenomas with 6 and 8 year follow-up. Breast J. 2010;16:73–6.
24. Jacobs L. Positive margins: the challenge continues for breast surgeons. Ann Surg Oncol. 2008;15:1271–2.
25. Singletary SE. Surgical margins in patients with early-stage breast cancer treated with breast conservation therapy. Am J Surg. 2002;184:383–93.
26. Glunde K, Jacobs MA, Pathak AP, et al. Molecular and functional imaging of breast cancer. NMR Biomed. 2009;22:92–103.
27. Vilar VS, Goldman SM, Ricci MD, et al. Analysis by MRI of residual tumor after radiofrequency ablation for early stage breast cancer. AJR Am J Roentgenol. 2012;198:W285–91.
28. Tafra L, Cheng Z, Uddo J, et al. Pilot clinical trial of 18F-fluorodeoxyglucose positron-emission mammography in the surgical management of breast cancer. Am J Surg. 2005;190:628–32.
29. Berg WA, Weinberg IN, Narayanan D, et al. High-resolution fluorodeoxyglucose positron emission tomography with compression ("positron emission mammography") is highly accurate in depicting primary breast cancer. Breast J. 2006;12(4):309–23.

Chapter 11
Cryoablation for Breast Cancer

Deanna Attai

Cryoablation, or the destruction of lesions with extreme cold, has generated significant interest as a potential alternative to surgical therapy for early-stage breast cancer. Technology has advanced to the point where the procedure is able to be performed in the office setting under local anesthesia and with minimal recovery, especially when compared to surgery. Freezing produces a predictable volume of necrosis and is easily observed and controlled during treatment [1]. In addition, cryoablation of breast tumors has been shown in animal models to generate a tumor-specific immune response that can eradicate systemic micrometastases and improve outcomes compared with surgical excision [2].

Background

Cryoablation for breast cancer was described by Rand in 1985 [3]. Additional case reports followed, suggesting that this was a viable method for breast cancer treatment. There are several case reports describing the natural history of ablated cancers, but the majority of series involve resection of the ablated lesion. Sabel [4] reported the results of 29 patients treated by cryoablation using a single treatment probe. Tumor destruction was complete in cancers less than 1.0 cm in size. For tumors between 1.0 and 1.5 cm, this success rate was achieved only in patients with invasive ductal (as opposed to invasive lobular) carcinoma without a significant ductal carcinoma in situ (DCIS) component. Unselected tumors greater than 1.5 cm, as well as with patients with noncalcified DCIS not appreciated on pretreatment imaging were the cause of most cryoablation failures. Littrup [5] reported successful ablation of larger tumors or multiple tumor foci using more than one probe.

D. Attai, M.D., F.A.C.S. (✉)
Center for Breast Care, Inc, 191 S. Buena Vista #415, Burbank, CA 91505, USA
e-mail: dattaimd@cfbci.com

D.S. Francescatti and M.J. Silverstein (eds.), *Breast Cancer: A New Era in Management*, DOI 10.1007/978-1-4614-8063-1_11, © Springer Science+Business Media New York 2014

Mechanism of Action

Cryoablation causes cell death by three mechanisms: (1) intracellular ice formation, (2) extracellular osmotic imbalance with cell lysis upon thawing, and (3) vascular disruption and ischemia. Tissue temperature varies depending on the distance from the probe. Tumor cells closest to the probe, where the temperature is the lowest, undergo intracellular ice formation, cell membrane disruption, and cell death. At a greater distance from the probe, extracellular ice crystal formation occurs, which results in an increase in the extracellular osmotic gradient. To regain osmotic equilibrium water exits the cell, and upon thawing, cell rehydration usually expands beyond the surrounding membrane resulting in cell lysis. Additional tissue necrosis following cryoablation is a result of destruction of blood vessel endothelial cells, which leads to platelet aggregation and vascular stasis resulting in vascular occlusion and tissue ischemia. In the hours and days following cryoablation, ischemic sequelae continue to occur throughout the previously treated tissue [6]. Multiple studies have shown that breast cells as well as cells of various other organs which are exposed to –40 °C during two subsequent freeze–thaw cycles will be uniformly ablated [1].

Technique

The procedure and equipment have evolved to the point where it is feasible for a breast surgeon to incorporate this technique into clinical practice. The anterior aspect of the iceball is visible under ultrasound, and cold acts as a natural anesthetic. These two properties make cryoablation of breast cancer a procedure well-suited to the office environment. Initial experience used argon gas as a coolant, and helium as a warming agent, and required the use of large industrial tanks for storage of the gas. Currently, liquid nitrogen is more commonly used for cooling, which is readily available and easily stored. The control console is similar in size to those used for vacuum-assisted biopsy (see Fig. 11.1).

Importantly, since ablation will result in tissue destruction, it is essential that a core biopsy be performed prior to treatment. Sufficient tissue should be obtained for diagnosis, assessment of estrogen and progesterone receptors, HER2/neu status, and for genomic profiling studies.

Cryoablation treatment protocols have been developed, all involving at least two freeze cycles. The most commonly used algorithm now involves a rapid freeze–thaw–rapid freeze protocol. Regardless of the technique used, it is imperative that the entire lesion is engulfed by the iceball which is easily demonstrated under ultrasound by scanning in multiple planes. The current generation of commercially available cryoablation devices utilizes liquid nitrogen circulating through a hollow, closed-end probe. The probe is placed in the center of the tumor under ultrasound guidance and positioning is confirmed by scanning in multiple planes (see Figs. 11.2, 11.3 and 11.4). The probe is insulated with the exception of the active tip so that

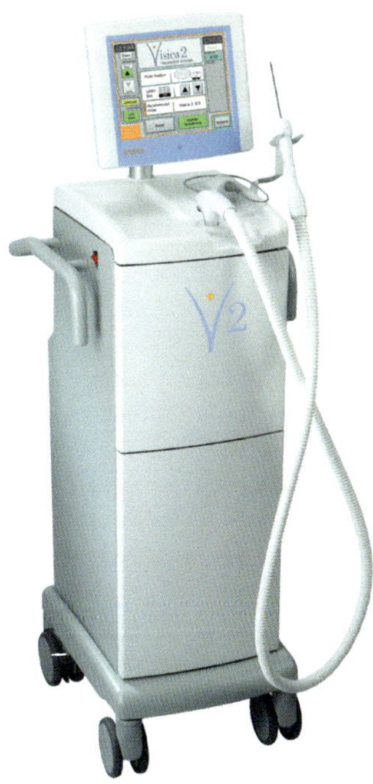

Fig. 11.1 Cryoablation console and probe

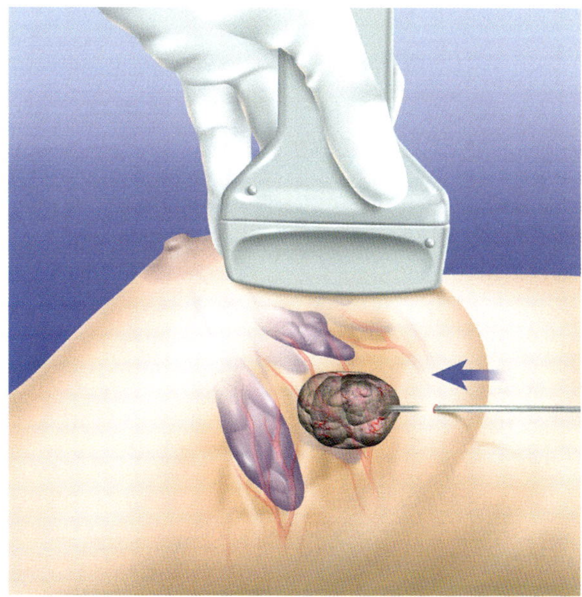

Fig. 11.2 Cryoprobe placement

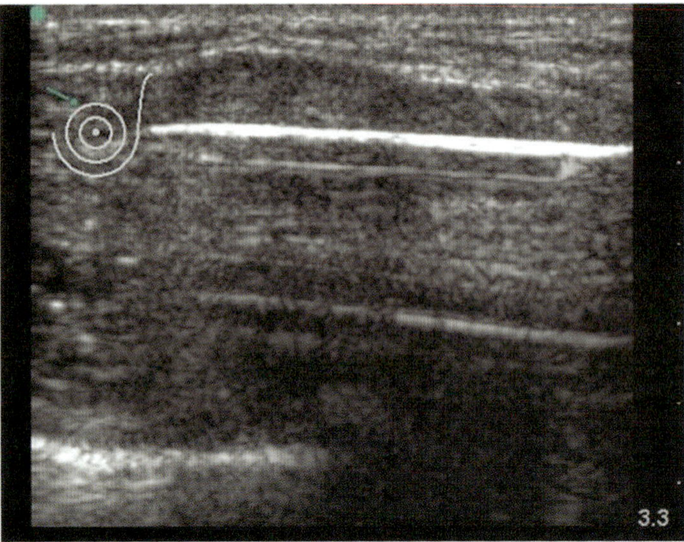

Fig. 11.3 Cryoprobe placement under ultrasound—longitudinal view

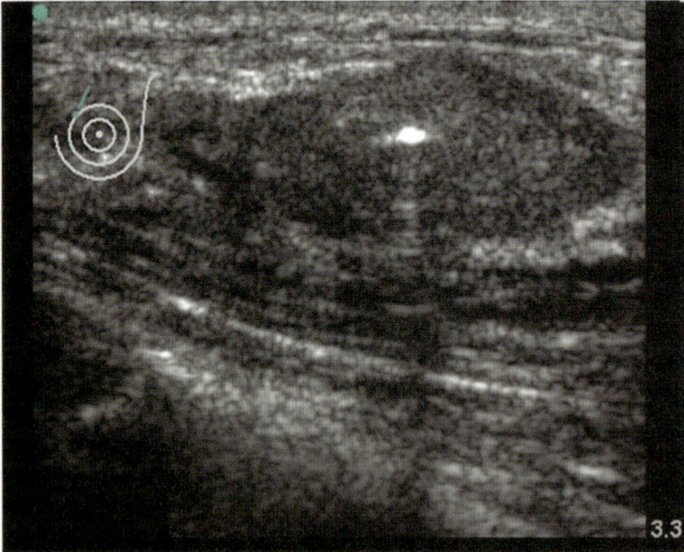

Fig. 11.4 Cryoprobe placement under ultrasound—transverse view

there is no risk of cold injury to the skin at the insertion site. The tumor is approached through its long axis, but due to the length of the probe, the incision can often be placed in the lateral, inframammary, or periareolar location to optimize cosmesis. Usually no more than 10–20 cm^3 of local anesthetic is required. Saline solution is

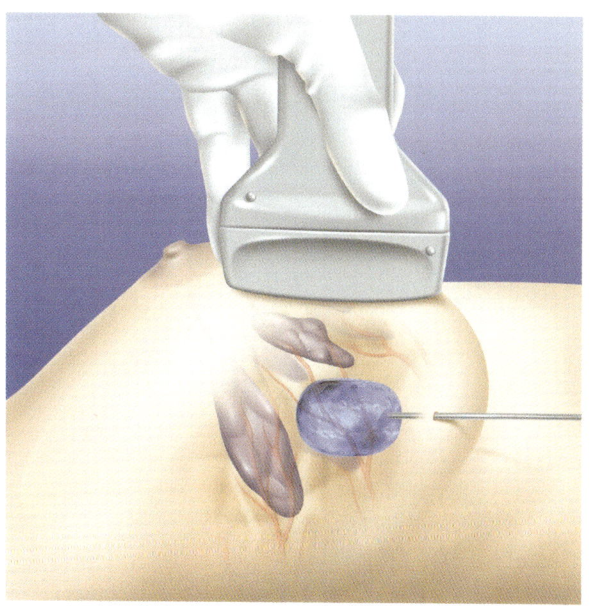

Fig. 11.5 Iceball formation

used to "lift" a lesion away from the pectoralis major muscle, or to "float" a lesion away from the skin surface to avoid cold injury to the muscle or skin. The size of the lesion dictates the duration of the procedure which then determines the size of the iceball that is generated. Unlike cryoablation of a benign fibroadenoma in which the goal is treatment of the lesion while minimizing ablation of the surrounding tissue, current cancer treatment protocols require treating the lesion and a surrounding 1 cm margin of normal tissue. All current devices are able to manually increase the treatment zone intraprodecurally if the lesion is not fully engulfed (see Figs. 11.5 and 11.6).

After the procedure, the patient should be counseled that there may be a palpable mass. The degree of palpability and the size of the resulting mass will depend on the depth and size of the initial lesion. A modest inflammatory response and induration develops over the first few days after the procedure and some bruising is common. Most patients tolerate the procedure very well and discomfort can usually be managed using nonsteroidal anti-inflammatory agents. Within 1–2 weeks of the procedure the initial inflammation and induration begins to resolve, and if surgical excision is not performed, the patient will notice a gradual decrease in the size of the lesion. Resolution of the inflammatory response can be documented by a combination of physical examination and ultrasound (see Figs. 11.7 and 11.8). In the case of ablation for malignant disease, magnetic resonance imaging (MRI) is proving to be very useful for evaluating the initial tumor response to treatment as well as for follow up in those patients who do not undergo surgical excision. The expected MRI appearance will be that of a non-enhancing zone surrounded by a variably enhancing rim (see Figs. 11.9 and 11.10). If surgical excision is not

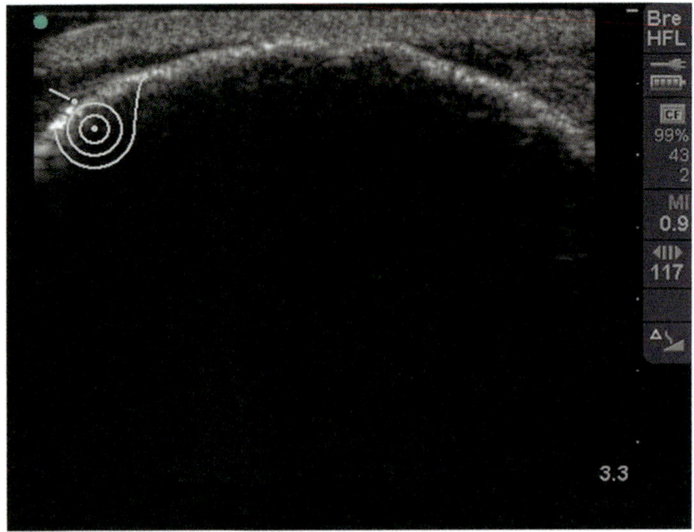

Fig. 11.6 Ultrasound image of iceball formation

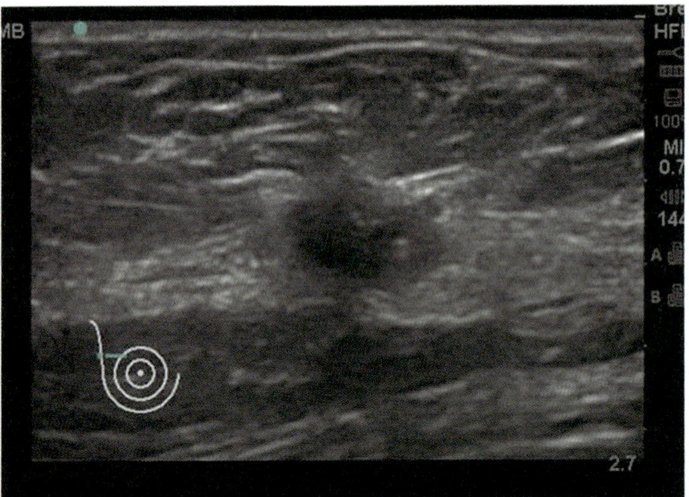

Fig. 11.7 Ultrasound image of cancer prior to ablation

performed, it is expected that the ablation margin will decrease in size over time. Based on experience with fibroadenoma cryoablation in which the ablated lesion is generally not removed, there has not been difficulty interpreting subsequent mammogram and ultrasound imaging studies [8].

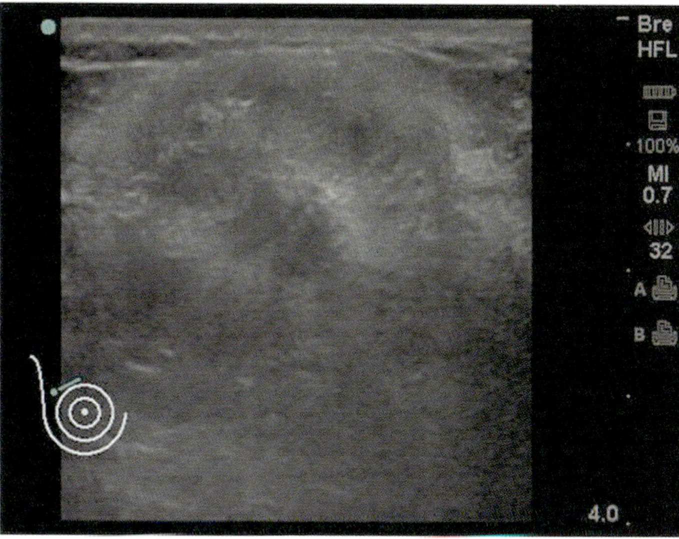

Fig. 11.8 Ultrasound image of cancer 4 weeks after ablation with clear demarcation of ablation zone

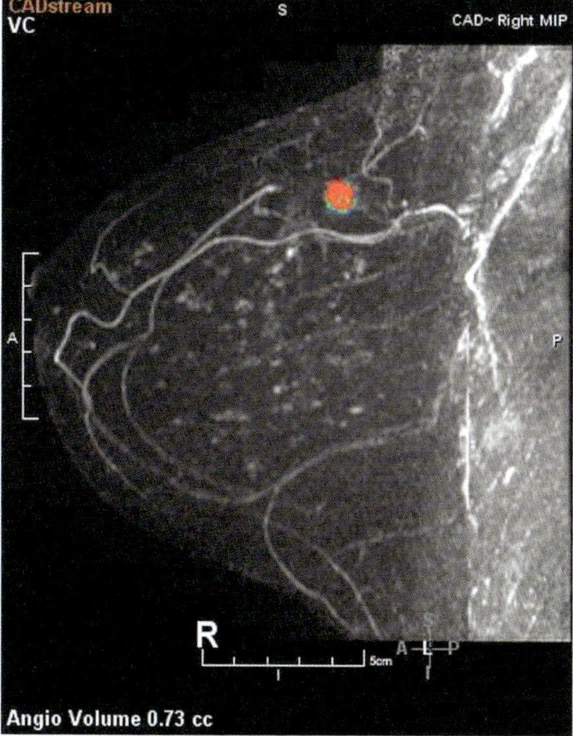

Fig. 11.9 MRI image of cancer prior to ablation

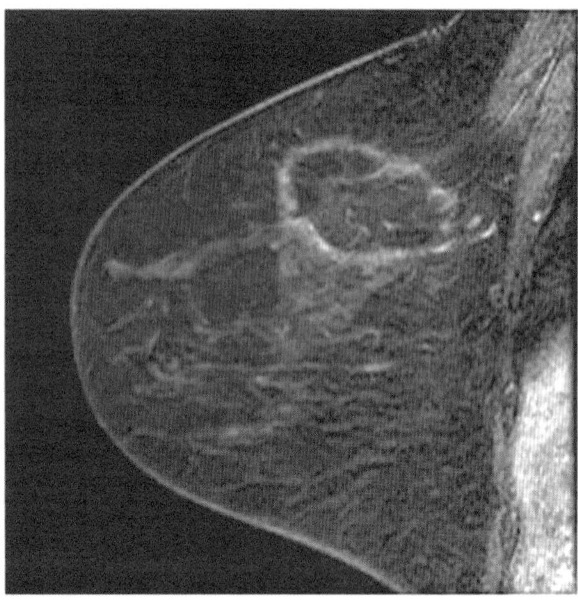

Fig. 11.10 MRI image 4 weeks after ablation with clear demonstration of ablation zone

Immune Response

In addition to potentially avoiding surgical resection in those patients with a diagnosis of early-stage breast cancer, studies have shown that there is a potential immunologic benefit because of an immune response generated by the residual nonviable tumorous protein material after cryoablation that may inhibit the growth of tumor foci distant from the primary tumor. Tanaka treated 49 patients with advanced or recurrent breast cancer with cryosurgery, reporting not only alleviation of pain, control of hemorrhage, and reduction of tumor bulk, but also a 5-year survival of 44.4 % in this group of "incurable" patients [4]. Sabel more recently demonstrated that a tumor-specific immune response is generated in response to cryoablation which can eradicate systemic micrometastases and improve outcomes in mice, and that the rate of freeze is an additional factor that will alter the immune response [2]. Ongoing research will continue to examine whether cryoablation of early-stage breast cancer will stimulate a clinically relevant immune response in women with breast cancer.

Unanswered Questions and Concerns

The American College of Surgeons Oncology Group has recently conducted a clinical trial (ACOSOG Z1072) assessing the safety and efficacy of cryoablation for early-stage breast cancer, as well as the predictive value of post-ablation MRI in assessing tumor response. Serum samples to assess immune response were also collected. It is hoped that this important trial will provide confirmation of earlier smaller studies. All patients enrolled in the trial underwent surgical resection after post-ablation MRI was performed. Data analysis from this trial is pending.

Detection and treatment of associated in situ carcinoma is a concern. Studies to date have shown that the majority of residual disease at the margin of resection has been DCIS that is not detected by preoperative imaging. In the ACOSOG Z1072 trial, patients were excluded who had an extensive intraductal component (greater than 25 % of tumor volume) on initial core biopsy. Because breast cancers are heterogeneous and the extent of associated DCIS is not always accurately predicted by core biopsy or preoperative imaging, this lack of histological certainty at the bonder of an identifiable and proven cancerous. Lesion is an important issue to be resolved if nonoperative ablation is to become an alternative method of therapy to surgical excision.

A transition from excisional to ablative therapy of breast carcinoma is accompanied by the question of treatment of the axilla. While surgical therapy has transitioned from a level I/II axillary dissection to a less invasive sentinel lymph node dissection for early stage breast cancer, the presence or absence of axillary nodal involvement remains an important factor in determining the need for adjuvant chemotherapy and may also influence radiation therapy fields. Recent studies have demonstrated no advantage in overall survival, disease-free survival, or axillary recurrence in women with positive sentinel nodes treated with sentinel lymph node dissection followed by chemotherapy and radiation therapy [7]. Using commercially available genomic profiling assays, the biologic behavior of a cancer may be predicted. This information, combined with imaging studies, may provide the essential information needed to safely ablate a breast cancer in the absence of lymph node sampling. In addition, the benefit of a possible immune response to the ablation may also influence adjuvant therapy decisions.

The Future

Breast cancer treatment has evolved rapidly, particularly in the past 15–20 years. Although lumpectomy is generally performed as an outpatient surgery, it requires a surgical procedure with tissue resection, anesthesia, postoperative pain, and the potential for less than ideal cosmetic results. Improvements in imaging allow for the detection of ever smaller cancers, and surgical research continues to prove that more aggressive surgery does not translate into improved clinical outcomes. Molecular techniques can predict the behavior of an individual patient's tumor and are being used to direct adjuvant therapy. The nonsurgical ablative treatment of breast cancer is an important transitional step in the truly minimally invasive approach to the treatment of breast cancer.

References

1. Whitworth PW, Rewcastle JC. Cryoablation and cryolocalization in the management of breast disease. J Surg Oncol. 2005;90:1–9.
2. Sabel MS, Su G, Griffith KA, Chang AE. Rate of freeze alters the immunologic response after cryoablation of breast cancer. J Surg Oncol. 2005;17:1187–93.
3. Huston TL, Simmons RM. Ablative therapies for the treatment of malignant diseases of the breast. Am J Surg. 2005;189:694–701.
4. Sabel MS, Kaufman CS, Whitworth P, Chang H, Stocks LH, Simmons R, Schultz M. Cryoablation of early-stage breast cancer: work-in-progress report of a multi-institutional trial. Ann Surg Oncol. 2004;11(5):542–9.
5. Littrup PJ, Jallad B, Chandiwala-Mody P, D'Agostini M, Adam BA, Bouwman D. Cryotherapy for breast cancer: a feasibility study without excision. J Vasc Interv Radiol. 2009;20:1329–41.
6. Tatli S, Acar M, Tuncali K, Morrison PR, Silverman S. Percutaneous cryoablation techniques and clinical applications. Diagn Interv Radiol. 2010;16:90–5.
7. Giuliano AE, Hunt KK, Ballman KV, Beitsch PD, Whitworth PW, Blumencranz PW, Leitch AM, Saha S, McCall LM, Morrow M. Axillary dissection vs no axillary dissection in women with invasive breast cancer and sentinel node metastasis—a randomized clinical trial. JAMA. 2011;305(6):569–75.
8. Kaufman CS, Rewcastle JC. Cryosurgery for breast cancer. Technol Cancer Res Treat. 2004; 3(2):165–75.

Chapter 12
RF Therapy

Preya Ananthakrishnan and Sheldon Marc Feldman

The use of heat to cause local tissue damage in patients with breast cancer dates back to over 1,000 years ago in ancient India, and is based on the principle that tumor cells are more susceptible to heat than normal cells. Historically, metallic or clay insulated electrodes were placed into locally advanced breast cancers in order to palliate symptoms as well as shrink tumors [1]. Radiofrequency ablation (RFA) is a technology based on the principle of heating tumors or tumor margins to destroy tumor cells with heat. The RFA procedure was initially used for ablation of aberrant conduction pathways to treat cardiac arrythymias as well as to treat chronic neuropathy syndromes [2]. It has evolved into use for ablation of solid tumors, since it causes a reproducible pattern of cell death in a predictable volume of tissue. For solid tumors, it was initially used for ablation of unresectable tumors (primarily in the liver and lung). Technical advances in RFA have led to increased ablation volumes, which has led to use of RFA for primary tumor ablation in the breast, liver, lung, bone, kidney, pancreas, prostate, and adrenal glands [3].

Since RFA is a localized procedure, it does not produce any systemic side effects. It can be performed under imaging guidance in percutaneous, laparoscopic, or open surgical procedure settings. A small needle is guided into the tumor, and radiofrequency energy is transmitted into the target tissue where it produces heat which either shrinks or kills tumor cells depending on the size of the tumor. Following RFA, the ablated tissue shrinks and forms an internal scar. The treatment can be repeated as often as needed. While most studies related to RFA and breast cancer involve ablation followed by surgical resection, some studies have investigated the safety of ablation only in patients who are poor surgical candidates since RFA can be done under local anesthesia.

P. Ananthakrishnan, M.D. • S.M. Feldman, M.D., F.A.C.S. (✉)
Division of Breast Surgery, Columbia University College of Physicians and Surgeons, 161 Fort Washington Avenue, 10th Floor, Suite 1005, New York, NY 10032, USA
e-mail: Sf2388@columbia.edu

D.S. Francescatti and M.J. Silverstein (eds.), *Breast Cancer: A New Era in Management*, DOI 10.1007/978-1-4614-8063-1_12,

How Does RFA Work?

RFA converts radiofrequency waves into heat by ionic vibration. The ionic vibration is created by passing a high frequency alternating current from an electrode into surrounding tissues, which causes ions to vibrate as they attempt to follow the change in the alternating current. This vibration generates frictional heat. The higher the current, the higher the temperature reached since the motion of the ions is more vigorous. The heat causes coagulation necrosis and cell death in the tissue [4]. The ability to accurately perform ablation depends on the energy balance between the heat conduction of localized RF energy and the heat convection from circulation of blood, lymph, intracellular fluid, and extracellular fluid [5].

Description of the Procedure

The procedure is performed by placing the RF probe (which is connected to a generator) into the center of a tumor or the tumor bed under ultrasound guidance. The RF probe itself contains a small electrode, and a larger electrode pad is placed on the patient's hip or thigh. Under imaging guidance (usually ultrasound or MRI), small prongs or tines are deployed around the RF probe which enter the breast tissue to a depth of 1 cm. The zone of ablation depends on the size and shape of the probe, and can extend up to 7 cm.

Different manufacturers use different strategies to obtain larger ablation zones, with the goal of obtaining uniform temperatures throughout the tumor. There are three manufacturers of RFA devices in the USA (Boston Scientific, Angiodynamics, and Valleylab), while one additional manufacturer is present in Europe (Celos.) [6] Boston Scientific and Angiodynamics use multipronged electrodes, so that the prongs increase the surface area and volume of tissue heating. These involve an incremental deployment of the prongs, with ablation performed at each position until the target temperature is reached to enable ablation of the entire target volume. Valleylab and Celon use a single needle probe with internal electrode cooling with circulating water or saline, to cool the tissue surrounding the electrode. This effectively "pushes" the zone of maximal temperature further into the tissue, leading to a larger zone of ablation [6]. A recent comparative review found no significant differences between the two systems, as both types are designed to avoid charring and prevent rises in tissue impedance [7].

The actual ablation involves activating the probe over at least 5 min to a target temperature of 100 °C for 15 min [8]. There is a 1 min cool-down period before the probe is removed. Some protocols allow for repeat RFA if the cool down is too rapid. Temperature is monitored by sensors during the entire ablation. RFA causes thermal destruction and cell death by coagulation necrosis in the tumor. Thermal injury begins at temperatures above 42 °C. Actual cell necrosis is identified at temperatures above 46 °C. Irreversible cell death occurs above 60 °C with denaturing of intracellular proteins and melting of the lipid bilayer, which finally interrupts cell replication [6].

Imaging to monitor the ablation continues to be optimized. The ablation zone is most frequently visualized with ultrasonography with spectral Doppler. Nahirnyak [9] demonstrated Doppler ultrasound signals can detect the creation of gas bubbles from tissue boiling. Doppler ultrasound is used to monitor the progression of heat radially into the treated tissue. Doppler has the ability to record and visualize the "outgassing" of microbubbles that occurs when the tissue is heated by the RFA to 100 °C. Projected on a monitor, the operator can monitor the radial penetration of heat during the ablation and guard against the potential of skin burns. Real time adjustment of the RFA probe location or angulation can be performed with feedback from the Doppler signal. Doppler ultrasound is used to determine the width and depth of ablation as well as to make sure that the skin is not injured. The RF probe should be maintained 1 cm away from any structure that is to be protected from ablation (skin or chest wall.) For percutaneous ablations, a solution of 5 % glucose can be injected between the skin and tumor or tumor and chest wall in order to achieve this 1 cm distance [10]. The skin is kept away from the probe so that steam from the ablation does not burn the skin. If the ablation is done intraoperatively, stay sutures and a retractor can be placed to separate the skin from the RF probe. A step ablation, overlapping contiguous regions, can be performed for tumor beds that are larger than what can be achieved with a single ablation. Once the ablation is complete, the RF probe is removed (after a cool-down period). If the ablation is intraoperative in a lumpectomy cavity, the cavity is irrigated, hemostasis is obtained, and the cavity is closed. After ablation, a hyperechoic area may be seen on ultrasound corresponding to a gross yellow-white appearance with red rim of the ablated tissue.

It is difficult to monitor the effects of heat on the breast tissue with ultrasound alone. The visualized cancers are usually hypoechoic with clear margins prior to ablation, and as the ablation progresses the tissue becomes hyperechoic. This makes it difficult to differentiate between the ablated tissue and residual breast tumor. No definitive conclusions can be drawn about the size or completeness of the ablation zone, since US cannot accurately assess the zone of coagulative necrosis. Three-dimensional properties of a tumor are difficult to visualize well with ultrasound, making it difficult to match the zone of ablation to the tumor shape [11].

As an alternative to RF ablation under US guidance, two studies describe RF ablation under MRI guidance. MRI is quite sensitive to temperature changes which is ideal for assessing zone of ablation; however, MRI compatible RF probes are expensive. Van der Bosch et al. treated three patients, and monitored four distinct areas during the procedure [12]. These areas included the actual tumor undergoing ablation, normal tissue away from the ablation site, retromammary fascia along the chest wall, and subcutaneous tissue along the tract of the probe. This study achieved complete ablation in only one of the three patients; however, the authors did demonstrate that MRI allows monitoring of different regions during the actual ablation.

Yamamoto used MRI guidance for RFA in a pilot study of 26 patients. In this study, 92 % of patients had complete ablation of the tumor on histopathologic analysis. He also used a shorter ablation time with higher temperatures. Complications reported included burns on the breast and in the area of the grounding pad in three patients, and a fourth patient had a reaction in the breast similar to a granulomatous mastitis. One concern about performing RFA under MRI guidance is that the RFA device is usually operating at a frequency up to 500 kHz, which may cause imaging artifact with MRI [13].

In addition to RF under ultrasound guidance, there is one case report that describes stereotactic guided RFA followed by delayed surgical resection. This achieved complete tumor ablation, with no residual tumor seen on the surgical specimen 4 weeks after ablation [14].

Studies to Date

Published studies of RFA for breast cancer involve RF for ablation of the tumor followed by either immediate or delayed surgical resection, or ablation of the primary tumor with clinical follow-up only. Some centers have performed RF and followed it with percutaneous biopsy techniques. Application of RF has also extended into ablation of the lumpectomy cavity at the time of surgical resection of a tumor in order to extend the margins achieved with resection alone while limiting volume of tissue resected.

The first clinical study regarding RFA of breast tumors was published in 1999 by Jeffrey et al., and consisted of five patients with locally advanced breast cancer (T3 lesions) who underwent RFA prior to mastectomy [15]. Patients were under general anesthesia, and an RF ablation was performed on a portion of the tumor under sonographic guidance prior to excision. Only a portion of the tumor was treated, in order to evaluate the zone of RF ablation and the margin between ablated and nonablated tissue. Cell death was measured by NADH-diaphorase cell viability stains. The ablated areas measured between 0.8 and 1.8 cm diameter. All tumors showed some cell death, with four out of five having complete destruction. The fifth patient had a single focus of <1 mm remaining. This study was the first to demonstrate that RF ablation caused invasive breast cancer cell death.

The next studies were small pilot series involving 10–50 patients, and investigated surgical ablation followed by resection of cancers (Table 11.1) [8, 15–24]. Endpoints were either extent of ablation of target zone, which ranged from 90 to 96 %, or extent of cell necrosis, which ranged from 61 to 100 %. These studies demonstrated that in appropriately selected patients, RF ablation could be done safely with minimal side effects. The patients with residual tumor cells at the tumor site were noted to have preoperative underestimation of tumor size on imaging studies.

Success of RF is governed by patient selection, with optimal patients having small well-defined unifocal lesions whose borders are clearly visible on US. RF is contraindicated in patients with multifocal or multicentric tumors, as well as DCIS and lobular cancers. MRI is useful to evaluate for mammographically occult multicentric disease or multifocal disease, since these patients are not optimal RF candidates. Again, a 1 cm distance from the skin or chest wall is also necessary. Other options for preoperative imaging include ultrasound and PET. Neoadjuvant chemotherapy is considered to be a contraindication for RFA, since it may produce nonhomogenous responses in the tumor bed [17].

Table 11.1 Trials of percutaneous RFA followed by surgical resection in patients with breast cancer

Trial	Year	Disease	*N*	Treatment	Complete ablation	Complications
Jeffrey et al. [15]	1999	T3–T4 breast cancer or tumors >5 cm	5	Intraoperative RFA—mastectomy	80 %	None
Izzo et al. [16]	2001	T1–T2	26	US guided RFA (margin >5 mm)	96 % Coagulative necrosis	One full thickness skin burn
Singletary et al. [17]	2002	T2	30	Intraoperative RFA—excision	87 %	None
Burak et al. [18]	2003	≤2 cm	10	RFA—surgery 1–3 weeks later		Breast ecchymosis
Hayashi et al. [19]	2003	≤3 cm	10	RFA—surgery 1–2 weeks later	86 % Coagulative necrosis	Skin burn, mild discomfort
Fornage et al. [20]	2004	≤2 cm	21	RFA—surgery	95 % Coagulative necrosis	None
Noguchi et al. [21]	2006	≤2 cm	10	RFA—surgery	100 %	None
Earashi et al. [22]	2007	≤2 cm	24	RFA—surgery	100 %	None
Manenti et al. [23]	2009	≤2 cm	34	RFA—surgery 4 weeks later	97 % Coagulative necrosis	Hyperpigmentation/skin burn
Wiksell et al. [24]	2010	≤1.6 cm	31	RFA—surgery	84 % Complete necrosis	One skin burn, three chest wall burns, one pneumothorax
Kinoshita et al. [10]	2011	≤3 cm	50	RFA—surgery	61 % Complete ablation (83 % in tumors <2 cm)	Two skin burns, three muscle burns
Klimberg et al. [8]	2011	≤1.5 cm	15	Percutaneous excision (stereotactic or vacuum assisted device), percutaneous RFA, then surgery	100 %	None

It appears that efficacy of tumor ablation may be dependent on tumor size, with RFA more likely to completely ablate tumors <2 cm than in larger tumors over 2 cm. Kinoshita et al. demonstrated a complete ablation rate of 86 % in tumors less than 2 cm, and only 30 % in tumors over 2 cm [10]. This study also demonstrated the extensive intraductal component (EIC) makes it difficult to achieve complete ablation, as the rate of success was 39 % in those with EIC and 85 % in those with EIC. Interestingly, the authors suggest preoperative MRI/US to try and determine which patients have extensive EIC prior to proceeding with RFA [10].

Several studies involving RFA of small breast cancers without resection have been performed in Japan and France (Table 11.2) [25–30]. These studies are primarily in patients who are poor surgical candidates, and some include postprocedure radiation. After ablation, the cavity is subsequently percutaneously biopsied to follow the patient for recurrence. In Japan, Tamaki et al. performed RFA on 100 patients with a mean follow-up of 12 months. US guided FNA was done on the ablated lesions to assess for residual disease. Cosmesis was described as excellent in 83 % of cases, good in 12 %, and fair in 6 % [30].

The above studies noted that a hard lump may persist in the breast at the site of ablation for several months [25–30]. The majority of ablated tumors had shrunk considerably after 6 months, and within a year became occult on physical exam and ultrasound. One proposed option for tumors that persisted on mammography and ultrasound post ablation was excision via percutaneous biopsy devices (such as vacuum assisted devices).

Across most of the studies, increased tumor impedance (caused by increased fat content of tumors due to the high electrical resistance of fat) reduces the effectiveness of RFA. Since older patients have breast atrophy leading to a lower fat content of tumors compared to younger women, RFA may be more successful in older age groups due to reduced resistance to thermal energy. Again, this reinforces that RFA may be ideal for tumor ablation in the frail elderly population who are not good operative candidates [17, 31].

Issues Yet to Be Addressed

Optimal imaging follow-up for patients after ablation is controversial. Potential modalities include mammography, US, MRI, and PET scan. While MRI is useful for preprocedure patient selection, accuracy post-ablation has not yet been determined. Burak et al. used MRI for assessment of the tumor before and after ablation [18]. Before ablation, 90 % of patients had MRI enhancement. After ablation, no residual disease was seen in 89 % of patients on MRI. The ten patients in the study were taken to surgery 1–3 weeks after ablation, and the one patient with residual disease on MRI also had residual disease on final pathology. Imaging combined with biopsies of the region is most frequently used for surveillance if the tumor has not been resected.

Table 11.2 Trials of percutaneous RFA without resection (with or without radiation) and periodic biopsy of cavity

Trial	*N*	Assessment of ablated lesion	Length of follow-up	Outcome	Complications
Oura et al. [25]	52	FNA biopsy	15 months	One local recurrence	One skin burn
Brkljacic et al. [26]	6	Routine (patients very ill)	9–49 months	Two deaths from other causes	One infection
Susini et al. [27]	3	Core	18 months	No local recurrence	None
Earashi et al. [20]	6	Mammotome	4 months	No local recurrence	None
Marcy et al. [28]	4	Core needle biopsy	29 months	One local recurrence	One abscess
Yamamoto et al. [29]	29	Vacuum-assisted core biopsy	1 month	No local recurrence, no viable tumor in 24/26 patients	None
Tamaki et al. [30]	100	FNA biopsy	12 months	One local recurrence, one death from distant metastases	None

After RFA, there is no reliable method to ensure complete ablation of the lesion. Cellular sampling with percutaneous biopsies or surgical excision provides a way to evaluate cellular destruction with standard hematoxylin and eosin staining. Cell viability can also be assessed with nicotinamide adenine dinucleotide-diaphorase (NADPH) staining. Proliferating cell nuclear antigen (PCNA) stains enable detection of actively replicating DNA, so that absence of PCNA staining confirms cell death. All these pathologic methods require tissue for evaluation of residual disease, whether through needle biopsy or surgical excision.

Another criticism of RF as a tool for primary ablation of a breast cancer is that the final pathologic margin status is unknown following ablation of a tumor. Percutaneous biopsy techniques can demonstrate whether residual tumor cells are present, but they do not provide complete assessment of an entire cavity margin. Standard pathologic sampling techniques might not provide an accurate assessment of an entire margin after RFA.

The other drawback to minimally invasive ablative techniques is that there is a lack of ability to bank tissue for further study, including genetic and proteomic testing. In order to obtain this tissue while still providing the benefits of ablative therapy to open surgical resection, percutaneous excision of tumors followed by RFA for sterilization of the margins has been proposed by Klimberg's group [8]. In a pilot feasibility study, patients diagnosed by percutaneous biopsy with tumors <1.5 cm, >1 cm from the skin, and with <1 cm residual disease and no multicentric disease on MRI were selected. US guided ablation followed by immediate surgical resection was performed. Of the 15 patients who received RFA, seven showed no residual tumor and eight showed residual dead tumor only at the biopsy site with clear margins. This study demonstrated the feasibility of percutaneous excision of lesions followed by RFA for breast cancers in a manner that allow for removal of the lesion with full histopathologic evaluation and potential for tissue banking, as well as margin ablation.

Finally, since surgical lymph node staging still remains standard of care for both prognostic and therapeutic reasons, a cancer patient still has to undergo surgery for lymph node evaluation. Published studies on RFA differ in their approach to the sentinel node, with some groups performing it pre and post RFA, while other groups routinely performed axillary dissection. Several studies did not describe nodal evaluation. There is little benefit to ablating the primary tumor if the patient has to undergo surgery for lymph node evaluation. Therefore, use of RF has expanded from ablation of the primary tumor to intraoperative ablation of lumpectomy cavity margins after resection, in order to extend the margins while limiting volume of tissue resected.

The role of RFA for benign lesions has not been well studied. In benign lesions, issues including margins or incomplete ablation are not as concerning and therefore RFA may be a good alternative to surgical excision. The drawback is that a hard lump may be present for several months after the procedure, which may be psychologically disturbing to the patient after treatment of a lesion.

Future of RFA

The ABLATE (RFA after Breast Lumpectomy Added To Extend intraoperative margins in the treatment of breast cancer) trial is currently accruing patients, and involves assessing whether intracavitary RFA can decrease surgical reexcision rates by extending the final margin after lumpectomy. Primary goals are to estimate reexcision rate for close or positive margins, and to decrease local recurrence rates. Secondary goals of the trial include assessment of cosmesis and quality of life, monitoring the peri-cavitary zone of Doppler enhancement, monitoring complications and side effects, and monitoring ablation effects on postoperative imaging. Dr. Klimberg is the P.I. for is a multicenter trial which will accrue 250 patients in which the intraoperative RFA is performed using an optimized standard protocol. An intraoperative video which details this technique is accepted for publication (Ann Surg Onc; Mackey et al.). Inclusion criteria are patients over 50 years old with <3 cm unicentric/unilateral tumors that do not involve the skin, with DCIS or grade I–III hormone receptor positive IDC. Exclusion criteria include invasive lobular carcinoma, bilateral malignancy, clinically positive lymph nodes, and neoadjuvant chemotherapy.

Other potential benefits of RFA may be to obviate the need for postoperative radiation in the setting of breast conservation. In an abstract presented at the 2009 SSO meeting, Klimberg's group performed RFA on 94 patients after lumpectomy. After RFA, 24 patients had inadequate margins (≤2 mm) including 8 grossly positive and four focally positive margins. Eight patients underwent reresection and were excluded. With a mean follow-up of 23 months ± 15 months (6–67 months) no LRs in the tumor bed were seen. There were four elsewhere recurrences—3 ipsilateral and 1 contralateral. Cosmesis was scored in 56 patients rating 26 excellent, 22 good, and 8 fair. In a more recent series (Klimberg-personal correspondence), sixty patients (mean age of 68.7 ± 11.4 years) with invasive cancer who had an average tumor size of 1.1 cm underwent excision followed by radiofrequency ablation. After follow-up for 44 (12–84) months, one patient (1.7 %) developed an tumor bed recurrence. There was one recurrence at another site. Average cosmesis rating was good to excellent. They concluded that RFA could potentially decrease local recurrence without the side effects/complications of radiation.

There is some suggestion that RFA may have beneficial immunomodulatory effects [32]. In an experimental model of rat breast tumors treated with RFA, Todorova et al. demonstrated that circulatory regulatory T cells were reduced. The reduction was not as pronounced as in those rats who had undergone surgical excision of the primary tumor. RFA may also influence expression of heat shock protein expression, which can affect the immunogenicity of tumor cells [33].

Ongoing studies are underway to determine the safety, local failure rates, cosmesis, and patient satisfaction with RFA. As breast cancer care has evolved from radical mastectomy to breast conservation, ablative therapies represent the future direction of local therapy. Studies to date demonstrate the RFA achieves reasonable complete ablation rates while improving cosmesis by minimizing breast scarring and deformity. We look forward to continued improvement in breast screening that will allow even earlier breast cancer diagnosis. Small favorable breast cancers appear ideally suited for ablative local therapy with RFA. More wide spread application of this approach is extremely promising. Additionally it is conceivable that small biologically favorable tumors may be treated with local therapy including RFA. This may obviate the need for radiation and expand breast conservation for patients worldwide who are unable to access radiation therapy facilities.

References

1. Breasted JH. The Edwin Smith surgical papyrus, vol. 54. Chicago, IL: Chicago University Press; 1930.
2. Friedman M, Mikityansky I, Kam A, Libutti SK, McClellan MW, Neeman Z, Locklin JK, Wood BJ. Radiofrequency ablation of cancer. Cardiovasc Intervent Radiol. 2004;27(5):427–34.
3. Mirza AN, Fornage BD, Sneige N, Kuerer HM, Newman LA, Ames FC, Singletary SE. Radiofrequency ablation of solid tumors. Cancer J. 2001;7:95–102.
4. Singletary SE. Applications of radiofrequency ablation in the treatment of breast cancer. Breast Cancer Online. 2005;8(9):e48.
5. Scudamore C. Volumetric radiofrequency ablation: technical consideration. Cancer J. 2000;6:316–8.
6. Cepeda MFJ, Vera A, Leija L. Electromagnetic hyperthermia ablation devices for breast cancer: State of the art and challenges for the future. 2009. Pan American Health Care Exchanges – PAHCE. Conference, Workshops, and Exhibits, 16–20 March, 2009.
7. Hung WK, Mak KL, Ying M, Chan M. Radiofrequency ablation of breast cancer: a comparative study of two needle designs. Breast Cancer. 2011;18(2):124–8.
8. Klimberg VS, Boneti C, Adkins LL, Smith M, Siegel E, Zharov V, Ferguson S, Henry-Tillman R, Badgwell B, Korourian S. Feasibility of percutaneous excision followed by ablation for local control in breast cancer. Ann Surg Oncol. 2011;18:3079–87.
9. Nahirnyak VM, Moros EG, Novak P, Klimberg S, Shaferstein G. Doppler signals observed during high temperature thermal ablation are the result of boiling. Int J Hyperthermia. 2010;26(6):586–93.
10. Kinoshita T, Iwamoto E, Tsuda H, Seki K. Radiofrequency ablation as local therapy for early breast carcinomas. Breast Cancer. 2011;18:10–7.
11. Noguchi M. Is radiofrequency ablation treatment for small breast cancer ready for "prime time"? Breast Cancer Res Treat. 2007;106:307–14.
12. Van der Bosch M, Daniel B, Rieke V, Butts-Pauly K, Kermit E, Jeffery S. MRI guided radiofrequency ablation of breast cancer: preliminary clinical experience. J Magn Reson Imaging. 2008;27:204–8.
13. Yamamoto N, Fujimoto H, Nakamura R, Arai M, Yoshi A, Kaji S, Itami M. Pilot study of radiofrequency ablation of therapy without surgical excision for T1 breast cancer: evaluation with MRI and vacuum assisted core needle biopsies and safety management. Breast Cancer. 2011;18(11):3079–87.
14. Elliott RL, Rice PB, Suits JA, Ostrowe AJ, Head JF. Radiofrequency ablation of a stereotactically localized nonpalpable breast carcinoma. Am Surg. 2002;68:1–5.
15. Jeffrey SS, Birdwell RL, Ikeda DM, Daniel BL, Nowels KW, Dirbas FM, Griffey SM. Radiofrequency ablation of breast cancer: first report of an emerging technology. Arch Surg. 1999;134:1064–8.
16. Izzo F, Thomas R, Delrio P, et al. Radiofrequency ablation in patients with primary breast carcinoma: a pilot study in 26 patients. Cancer. 2001;92(8):2036–44.

17. Singletary SE, Fornage BD, Sneige N, et al. Radiofrequency of early-stage invasive breast cancers: an overview. Cancer. 2002;8:177–80.
18. Burak Jr WE, Agnese DM, Povoski SP, et al. Radiofrequency ablation of invasive breast carcinoma followed by delayed surgical excision. Cancer. 2003;98:1369–76.
19. Hayashi AH, Silver SF, Van der Westhuizen NG, et al. Treatment of invasive breast carcinoma with ultrasound-guided radiofrequency ablation. Am J Surg. 2003;185:429–35.
20. Fornage BD, Sneige N, Ross MI, Mirza AN, Kuerer HM, Edeiken BS, Ames FC, Newman LA, Babiera GV, Singletary SE. Small (<2 cm) breast cancer treated with US-guided radiofrequency ablation: feasibility study. Radiology. 2004;231(1):215–24.
21. Noguchi M, Earashi M, Fujii H, Yokoyama K, Harade K, Tsuneyama K. Radiofrequency ablation of small breast cancer followed by surgical resection. J Surg Oncol. 2006;93:120–8.
22. Earashi M, Noguchi M, Motoyoshi A, Fujii H. Radiofrequency ablation therapy for small breast cancer followed by immediate surgical resection or delayed mammotome excision. Breast Cancer. 2007;14:39–47.
23. Manenti G, Bolacchi F, Perretta T, et al. Small breast cancers: in vivo percutaneous US-guided radiofrequency ablation with dedicated cool-tip radiofrequency system. Radiology. 2009;251:339–46.
24. Wiksell H, Lofgren L, Schassburger KU, et al. Feasibility study on the treatment of small breast carcinoma using percutaneous US-guided preferential radiofrequency ablation (PRFA). Breast. 2010;19:219–25.
25. Oura S, Tamaki T, Hirai I, et al. Radiofrequency ablation therapy in patients with breast cancers two centimeters or less in size. Breast Cancer. 2007;14:48–54.
26. Brkljacic B, Cikara I, Ivanac G, et al. Ultrasound guided bilpolar radiofrequency ablation of breast cancer in inoperable patients: a pilot study. Ultraschall Med. 2010;31:156–62.
27. Susini T, Nori J, Olivieri S, et al. Radiofrequency ablation for minimally invasive treatment of breast carcinoma: a pilot study in elderly inoperable patients. Gynecol Oncol. 2007;104(2):304–10.
28. Marcy PY, Magne N, Castadot P, et al. Ultrasound-guided percutaneous radiofrequency ablation in elderly breast cancer patients: preliminary institutional experience. Br J Radiol. 2007;80(952):267–73.
29. Yamamoto N, Fujimoto H, Nakamura R, et al. Pilot study of radiofrequency ablation therapy without surgical excision for T1 breast cancer: evaluation with MRI and vacuum-assisted core needle biopsy and safety management. Breast Cancer. 2011;18:3–9.
30. Tamaki T, Oura S, Yoshimatsu T, Ohta F, Shimizu Y, Okamura Y. Radiofrequency ablation therapy in 100 patients: its safety and short-term outcome (abstract in Japanese). J Jpn Surg. 2009;Assoc 67 Suppl:305.
31. Soukup B, Bismohun S, Reefy S, Mokbel K. The evolving role of radiofrequency ablation therapy of breast lesions. Anticancer Res. 2010;30(9):3693–7.
32. Todorova VK, Klimberg VS, Hennings L, Kieber-Emmons T, Pashov A. Immunomodulatory effects of radiofrequency ablation in a breast cancer model. Immunol Invest. 2010;39(1):74–92.
33. Teng LS, Jin KT, Han N, Cao J. Radiofrequency ablation, heat shock protein 70 and potential anti-tumor immunity in hepatic and pancreatic cancers: a minireview. Hepatobiliary Pancreat Dis Int. 2010;9(4):361–5.

Chapter 13
HiFrequency Ultrasound

David Brenin

Modalities for in-situ tumor ablation utilize various energy forms including radiofrequency ablation, laser ablation, cryoablation, microwave thermotherapy, and focused ultrasound ablation (FUSA). Of the aforementioned techniques, only FUSA is truly noninvasive. Gradient-echo MRI techniques for temperature monitoring based on the temperature sensitivity of the proton chemical shift can be used to monitor the temperature of the ablation zone in real time, requiring no incision or penetration into the breast [1]. Radiofrequency ablation, laser ablation, and cryoablation all require the transcutaneous insertion of a treatment probe into the tumor. Microwave thermotherapy is controlled by a thermistor probe that must be inserted into the breast. The noninvasive nature of FUSA combined with the ability to plan, guide, measure ablation zone temperature, and control the treatment in real time via MRI imaging result in FUSA being the front-runner of ablative breast cancer therapies.

How Does FUSA Work?

Standard diagnostic ultrasound typically utilizes frequencies between 1 and 20 MHz. Ultrasound waves propagate through the tissue causing alternating waves of pressure resulting in compression and rarefaction of the tissue. In diagnostic ultrasound, the waves are reflected back to the probe resulting in information that can be used to synthesize an image of the tissue under interrogation. Devices designed for FUSA use higher power ultrasound waves at lower frequencies, between 0.8 and 3.5 MHz. The ultrasound beam is focused at a selected point, passing innocuously through the skin and underlying tissues to the focal point, where alternating waves of compression and rarefaction rapidly heat and physically disrupt the target tissue (Fig. 13.1).

D. Brenin, M.D. (✉)
Division of Surgical Oncology, Department of Surgery, University of Virginia, P.O. Box 800709, Charlottesville, VA 22908-0709, USA
e-mail: DRB8X@hscmail.mcc.virginia.edu

D.S. Francescatti and M.J. Silverstein (eds.), *Breast Cancer: A New Era in Management*, DOI 10.1007/978-1-4614-8063-1_13, © Springer Science+Business Media New York 2014

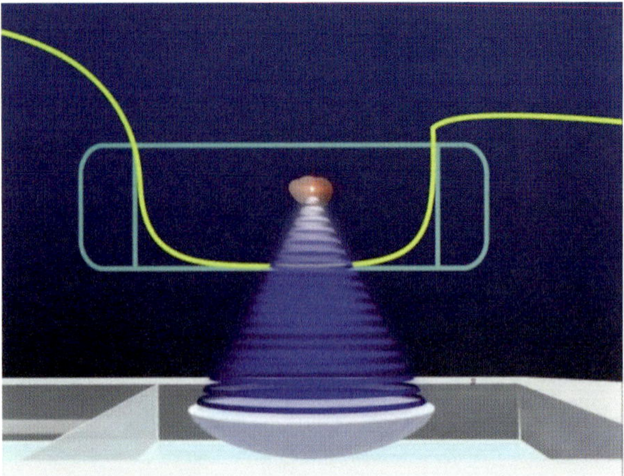

Fig. 13.1 Depiction of path of ultrasound waves from transducer to focal point with heating of target breast tissue in sonication zone

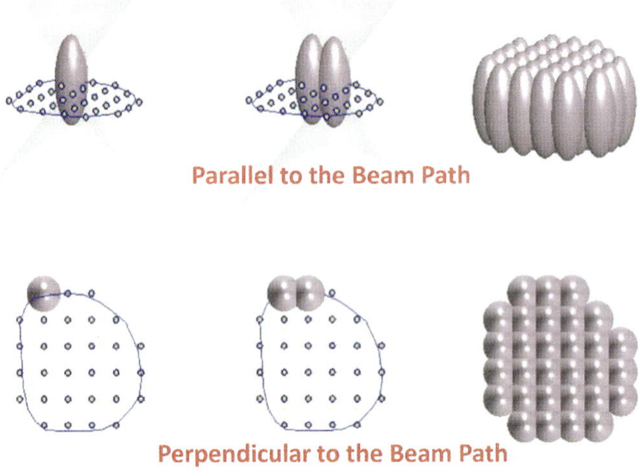

Fig. 13.2 Depiction of "cigar" shaped sonication zones arrayed side by side covering an entire tumor (*blue circle*) and small zone of surrounding tissue

The energy is typically delivered to a small cigar-shaped target volume measuring up to 3 mm × 15 mm. The treatment zone is precisely controlled, leaving the surrounding tissue unaffected. In order to treat a larger volume of tissue, multiple cigar-shaped sonification zones are arrayed side by side, in the manner of individual pixels, to cover the entire tumor and a small zone of surrounding tissue (Fig. 13.2).

The tissue in the FUSA treatment zone is subjected to two lethal forces: thermal energy, and mechanical stress. Over a few seconds, focused ultrasound ablation can raise the temperature of the cigar-shaped target volume to over 80 °C [2]. The rate of change, as well as the final target temperature, can be closely controlled. Maintenance of tissue temperature over 56 °C for more than one second is generally accepted to result in cell death. In addition to thermal energy, the rapidly cycling waves of rarefaction and compression at the target zone create micro-bubbles. The bubbles form and collapse many times a second, resulting in intracellular mechanical disruption. The end-result of these two forces is a precisely controlled zone of coagulative necrosis [3].

Focused ultrasound ablation can be guided via MRI or diagnostic ultrasound imaging. As mentioned above, MRI guidance allows for temperature monitoring of the ablation zone in real time using gradient-echo MRI techniques. The measurement of ablation zone temperature during ultrasound guided FUSA requires thermistor probe placement through the skin into the breast. In most studies of ultrasound guided FUSA, ablation zone temperatures were not measured [4, 5].

Description of the Procedure

Appropriate patient selection is essential. Successful MRI guided FUSA (MRgFUSA) requires that the tumor be visible on MRI and clearly delineated from the surrounding tissue. The location of the tumor must be at least 1 cm from the skin, and not adjacent to the chest wall.

The patient is positioned prone on a specially designed MRI table in which the treatment device is embedded (Fig. 13.3). The breast is positioned in the center of the MRgFUSA surface coil and an emergency stop button is placed in the patient's hand. The breast and surface coil are lowered into a tub that contains the ultrasound transducer. The tub is filled with degassed water to ensure acoustic coupling to the transducer. During the procedure, the degassed water is maintained at 20 °C and circulated around the breast to provide active cooling of the skin. Conscious sedation is typically maintained throughout the procedure through the use of an intravenous anxiolytic/analgesic cocktail.

Contrast enhanced MRI images are then obtained of the breast. The tumor is identified and the treatment volume is determined (Fig. 13.4). The treatment is then delivered as a series of interlaced elliptical sonication zones delivered within the prescribed treatment area comprised of the tumor and a rim of surrounding normal tissue. Each prescribed sonication zone is individually treated and monitored, raising the temperature within it to between 50 and 90 °C. The total treatment duration is a function of the number of individual sonification zones required to treat the volume in the prescribed treatment region. Each sonification cycle requires 18–74 s, with typical total treatment time ranging between 35 and 150 min [6, 7].

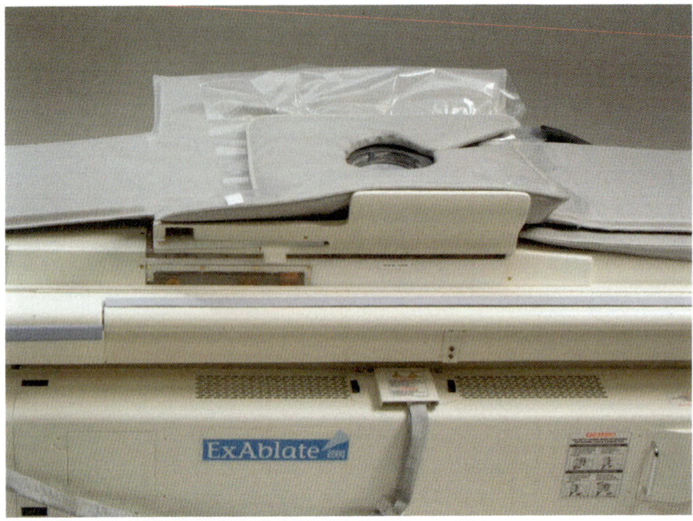

Fig. 13.3 The MRgFUSA device embedded in the MRI table (ExAblate 2000, InSightec, Ltd, Haifa Israel)

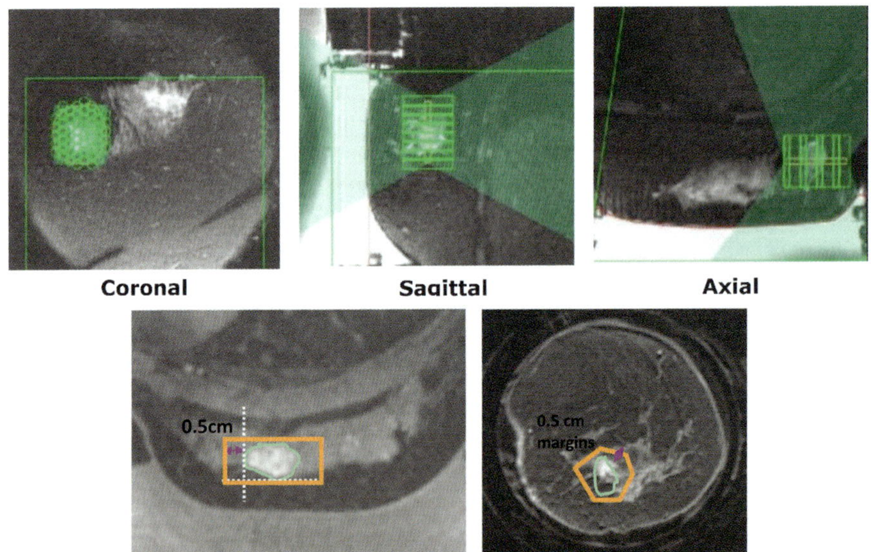

Fig. 13.4 MRgFUSA breast treatment plan (ExAblate 2000, InSightec, Ltd, Haifa Israel). The treatment is provided as a series of interlaced elliptical sonication zones delivered within the prescribed treatment area comprising of the tumor and rim of surrounding tissue. Photos courtesy of Dr. Furusawa at Breastopia, Namba Hospital, Miyazaki, Japan

Ultrasound Guided FUSA

Again, appropriate patient selection is essential. Ultrasound guided FUSA (USgFUSA) requires that the tumor be clearly visible on ultrasound. The location of the tumor must be at least 0.5 cm from the skin, or chest wall. Most studies of USgFUSA required that the tumor be more than 2 cm from the nipple [4, 5].

The patient is positioned prone on a table in which the treatment device is embedded. The breast is positioned in a tub filled with degassed water to ensure acoustic coupling to the transducer/imaging device. Conscious sedation or general anesthesia is typically maintained.

The transducer/imaging device consists of a 3.5–5.0 MHz ultrasound imaging probe situated in the center of a 12 cm therapeutic ultrasound transducer. This configuration allows for near real-time ultrasound guidance during the procedure. The transducer/imaging device is mounted to an arm that can be moved via servo motors in six dimensions.

The transducer/imaging device is used to obtain images of the breast. The tumor is identified and the treatment volume is determined. The treatment is then delivered to the tumor and a rim of surrounding normal tissue, in a similar fashion as described above for MRgFUSA. However, sonification zone temperature is not measured during USgFUSA. Typical total treatment time ranges between 45 and 180 min [4, 5].

Studies to Date

To date, there have been seven published trials evaluating MRgFUSA for the treatment of breast cancer [4, 8–13]. All but two can best be described as small feasibility studies. Gianfelice and coworkers were the first to describe a series of patients who underwent MRgFUSA followed by resection in a study completed in 2001 [6]. Twelve patients with invasive breast cancers less than 3.5 cm in greatest dimension underwent MRgFUSA of a volume of breast tissue which included the tumor and an estimated normal margin of 0.5 cm. Within 24 days of MRgFUSA, all patients underwent routine segmental resection. All patients had a minimum distance of 1 cm between the tumor and the skin or ribs. The resected specimen was evaluated with mapping of the tumor and treatment zone using three-dimensional macroscopic and microscopic histopathologic measurements combined with standard hematoxylin–eosin staining in 5 μm sections. The results from the first three patients treated in this study were not ideal, with a mean of 43.3 % of the tumor necrosis. Subsequent improvements in the targeting system used on the final nine patients in this series resulted in 88.3 % mean tumor volume necrosis. Two of the final nine patients had no residual viable tumor. Two patients in this series suffered from second-degree skin burns, both under 2.3 cm in size. Four patients reported slight discomfort, and eight reported moderate discomfort on a three point scale (slight, moderate, intolerable). Based on their initial feasibility study, Gianfelice and coworkers concluded that MRgFUSA held significant promise in terms of patient tolerability, but that the observation of residual tumor at the margins of the treatment zone suggested that refinements in tumor imaging and targeting were required.

Furusawa and colleagues reported on a study of 30 women with invasive breast cancer less than 3.5 cm in greatest diameter treated by MRgFUSA [11]. The tumor and "at least a 5-mm safety margin of normal tissue" were treated, followed 5–23 days later by routine breast conserving surgery or mastectomy. All tumors were greater than 1 cm from the skin or ribs. Histopathologic analysis of the specimens was conducted in a similar fashion to the previously mentioned study by Gianfelice and coworkers [6]. There were five protocol violations resulting in 25 evaluable patients. Mean tumor necrosis was 98 % by volume (range 90-100 %). One hundred percent necrosis was observed in 15 patients (60 %), and only one patient had less than 95 % necrosis of her tumor. One patient suffered a skin burn which was excised at the time of surgery. Two patients reported mild to moderate breast pain during sonication. Furusawa and coworkers concluded that MRgFUSA was well tolerated and effective, and that in well-selected patients, it had the potential to replace lumpectomy [11].

The use of MRgFUSA as the primary treatment of breast cancer without excision was first reported by Gianfelice et al, when he described a series of 24 patients with estrogen receptor positive, non-metastatic breast cancers. Mean tumor size was 1.5 cm (range 0.6–2.5 cm) [7]. All patients in the study had refused surgery or were considered to be "at too high a risk to undergo surgery." After consent was obtained, all patients underwent MRgFUSA followed by or concurrent with tamoxifen therapy. Patients did not undergo tumor excision. Following MRgFUSA, breast MRI's were obtained at 10 days, 1, 3, and 6 months. Following the MRI at 6 months, image-guided core biopsies (4–8 cores) were obtained from the area of the previously treated cancer. In the event that residual tumor was identified on biopsy, a second session of MRgFUSA was provided. Fourteen of 24 patients (58 %) had no residual disease identified on core biopsy 6 months following MRgFUSA. Ten patients with positive post-ablation biopsies were retreated with MRgFUSA, and five of the 10 were core biopsy negative 1 month later. The final success rate, defined as core biopsy negative, 7 months after initial MRgFUSA treatment was 19 of 24 patients (79 %). Mean follow-up was 20.2 months (range 12–39 months). One complication, in the form of a second-degree skin burn resolving with local wound care, was reported (4 %). The treatment was well tolerated, with ten patients reporting mild pain and 14 reporting moderate pain. Pain control was thought to be satisfactory with conscious intravenous sedation. The authors of the study concluded that MRgFUSA combined with adjuvant systemic treatment was well tolerated, had low-morbidity, and was an effective treatment for small breast cancers in selected patients.

In 2010, Dr. Furusawa reported on the most recent experience in Japan with MRgFUSA for the treatment of patients with breast cancer at the Second International Symposium on MR-guided Focused Ultrasound [14]. At that time, Furusawa and colleagues had enrolled 47 patients in a prospective single arm trial of MRgFUSA followed by routine whole breast radiation therapy with no excision. All patients had a single well-demarcated tumor equal to or less than 1.5 cm in greatest dimension, well visualized on MRI, with a skin-to-tumor distance of 1.0 cm or greater.

MR-G HIFU ABLATION OF BREAST CANCER, EXCISIONLESS STUDY

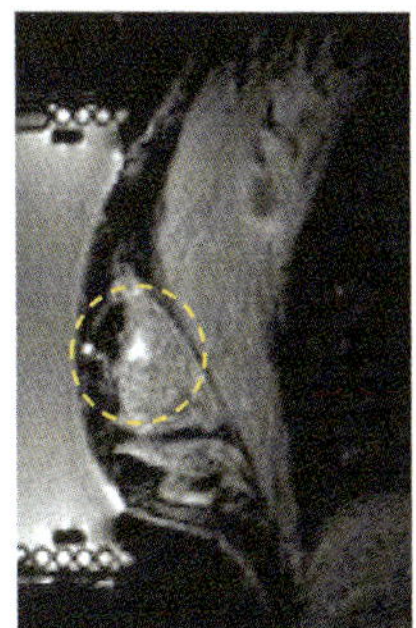
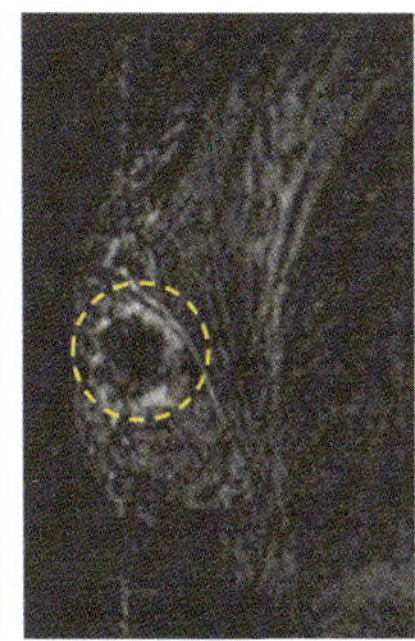
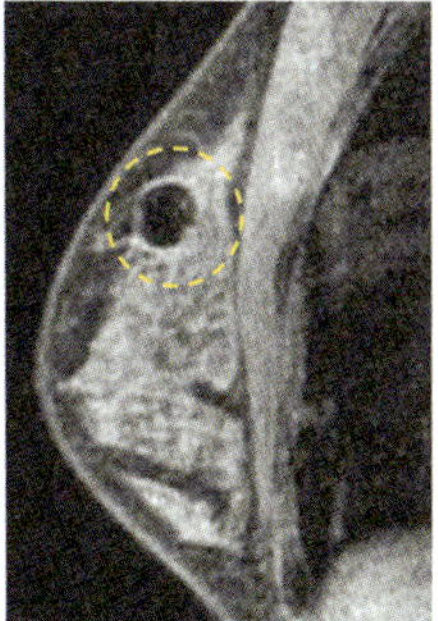
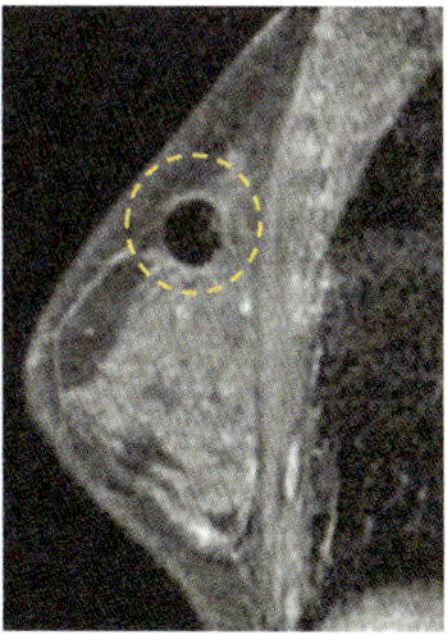

Fig. 13.5 Serial breast MRIs of a breast cancer patient treated by MRgFUSA and no excision. The *broken circle* identifies the area where the treated tumor was present, not the treatment zone. Photos courtesy of Dr. Furusawa at Breastopia, Namba Hospital, Miyazaki, Japan

Prior to treatment, patients underwent definitive diagnosis by core biopsy and were found to be node negative by sentinel node biopsy. Patients underwent ultrasound guided core needle biopsy of the tumor site 3 weeks after completion of MRgFUSA. If no viable tumor was identified, patients received routine whole breast radiation therapy and were followed with mammography and breast MRI every 6 months (Fig. 13.5). As of October 2010, 47 patients with mean tumor size of 1.1 cm had been treated. The mean treatment duration was 108 min (range 65–209 min). Mean follow-up was 43 months, with no local recurrences or significant adverse events reported.

To date, all studies of MRgFUSA have been performed outside of the USA. ACRIN 6674 is a proposed phase II, multicenter single arm study of patients with clinical T_1N_0 breast cancer to be conducted in the USA. In the initial phase of the study, 30 breast cancer patients will undergo MRgFUSA of their tumor followed by MRI tumor viability assessment at 10–14 days. All patients will then undergo excision and standard therapy. The volume of ablated tumor in the specimen will be compared to the preoperative viability assessment by MRI. Patient safety and treatment efficacy will also be evaluated. This study is in its final stages of preparation for FDA approval (M. Schnall, personal communication, May 20, 2011).

Ultrasound guided focused ultrasound ablation of breast tumors has been evaluated in China by Dr. Feng Wu and coworkers, who have published three studies describing the evolution of the technique [3, 4, 15].

The first study, published in 2003, described 48 women with T_{1-2}, N_{0-2}, M_0 breast cancers located more than 0.5 cm from the skin, or chest wall, and more than 2 cm from the nipple [4]. These patients were randomized to undergo modified radical mastectomy or USgFUSA followed within 14 days by modified radical mastectomy. Twenty-three patients were randomized to the USgFUSA arm and completed the protocol. Four patients received intravenous sedation, and 19 patients underwent general anesthesia during treatment. The ablation zone included the tumor and a margin of "1.5–2.0 cm" around the tumor. Pathologic evaluation of the ablation zone after mastectomy revealed "homogeneous coagulative necrosis, including the [tumor] and normal breast tissue within the target region." No further statistical evaluation of the treatment zone was provided. One of 23 patients (4 %) suffered a "minimal" skin burn. Treatment time ranged from 45 to 150 min (mean 1.3 h). Dr. Wu and coworkers concluded that "USgFUSA is effective, safe, and feasible in the treatment of localized breast cancer," but that additional studies were required.

The same group of investigators also described the use of USgFUSA as the primary treatment of breast cancer without excision in a series of 22 patients [5]. These stage I–IV patients had tumors ranging from 2 to 4.8 cm (mean 3.4 cm) measured on ultrasound. Eight patients received intravenous sedation, and 14 patients underwent general anesthesia during the treatment. All patients received a combination of chemotherapy, radiation therapy, and tamoxifen following USgFUSA. After ablation, patients underwent diagnostic ultrasound evaluation every 3–6 months, and ultrasound guided biopsies at 2 weeks, 3 months, 6 months, and 1 year. All patients were reported to tolerate the treatment well and no complications were observed. No viable tumor was identified on the core biopsies preformed within the first year of treatment. Median follow-up was 54.8 months (range 36–72 months). Two of 22 patients developed local recurrence in the treated area, one at 18 months and the other at 22 months after ablation.

Issues Yet to Be Addressed

Even if MRgFUSA is shown to be equivalent to breast-preserving surgery in the treatment of patients with small breast cancers, there are currently three significant obstacles to its clinical implementation: long duration of treatment, uncertainty of margin status, and the persistence of a breast mass after ablation in some patients. To date, these issues, along with a paucity of data, have prevented the widespread adoption of ablative treatments of breast cancer.

Long Treatment Time

The most recently presented data on MRgFUSA reported a median treatment duration of 108 min (range 65–209 min) [12]. There is no doubt that treatment time must be reduced before MRgFUSA can compare favorably to the operative time of lumpectomy. The lengthy treatment times required by current devices are unlikely to remain a significant problem. Advances in technology will likely result in reduced treatment times. The most commonly used MRgFUSA device for breast cancer treatment and research, the ExAblate 2000 (InSightec, Ltd, Haifa Israel), is only somewhat specialized. Most of its components are utilized to treat a variety of organs including the uterus, breast, prostate, brain, and bone. If studies demonstrate that MRgFUSA is equivalent to breast-preserving surgery in the treatment of patients with small breast cancers, then it is likely that specialized multi-transducer breast specific treatment devices will be developed with the potential to substantially reduce treatment times.

Uncertainty of Margin Status

The idea that excellent margin control is vital to the prevention of local recurrence in cancer patients treated with standard breast preserving surgery is well-founded and should be closely adhered to. However, it has long been established that a small amount of residual tumor remains behind in the conserved breast in a substantial proportion of patients [16]. This residual tumor is typically undetectable on breast imaging, nor predicted by pathologic margin evaluation. Adjuvant radiation therapy is an integral component of breast preserving surgery, as it is intended to treat residual tumor assumed to remain in the breast.

The excellent local control observed to date in the limited number of patients enrolled in FUSA without excision studies is likely due to multi-modality care. Routine whole breast radiation therapy and adjuvant systemic treatment has been part of these protocols. Hopefully, these excellent results will prove durable on longer term follow-up and in future studies. If so, then the uncertainty of margin status should not prove to be a significant obstacle to the clinical implementation of FUSA.

Persistent Breast Mass After Ablation

Fat necrosis, resulting in persistent palpable masses, can occur in a minority of patients following ablative therapy. Luckily, this is usually a self-limiting problem, typically slowly resolving over the course of a year [17]. A breast mass in a patient after breast preservation is problematic as it can be anxiety provoking to both the patient and her surgeon, and has the potential to obscure locally recurrent disease. Consistent use of various breast imaging modalities can minimize the likelihood of a missed local recurrence. However, there is little doubt that patients and surgeons will be intolerant of persistent palpable breast masses in cancer patients. Fat necrosis following ablative treatment of breast cancer may prove to be a significant challenge to the widespread adoption of the technique. However, the prevention and management of persistent palpable masses after ablation is an area that has yet to be investigated and may be amenable to systemic or local pharmacologic therapy. In the worst case, the small minority of patients who develop a persistent, problematic post-ablation breast mass could simply undergo surgical excision.

Future of FUSA

Magnetic resonance guided focused ultrasound ablation has been studied in several small trials. To date, these studies have proven MRgFUSA to be safe, but efficacy has ranged widely from 43 % to 100 % in the treatment followed by excision trials [4, 6, 8, 9]. In Japan, the ongoing Furusawa "excisionless" MRgFUSA only trial has reported no recurrences in 47 carefully selected patients with mean follow-up of 43 months [12]. The results of this study have aided in the development of proper treatment guidelines and the standardization of the procedure. A large prospective "treat and excise" study conducted in the USA, such as ACRIN 6674, is the next logical step in the determination of the efficacy of this technique.

To date, all studies evaluating the use of USgFUSA to treat patients with breast cancer have been conducted by a single group. The nature of these studies is best described as exploratory, thus the data on USgFUSA remains incomplete. Future more rigorous studies may result in a better understanding of the ability of USgFUSA to effectively treat breast tumors.

Focused ultrasound ablation has the potential to be a "disruptive technology," taking the primary treatment of patients with early stage breast cancer out of the hands of surgeons. However, surgeons should not feel imperiled. We already work closely with our breast imaging colleagues to provide outstanding multidisciplinary breast cancer care. The same multidisciplinary team will be required to develop and refine ablative techniques. There is no doubt that collaboration is the best way to assure that we continue to actively participate in the treatment of patients with early stage breast cancer.

Breast conserving surgery combined with radiation therapy has been extensively studied and is the "gold standard" for the treatment of patients with small breast cancers [18, 19]. In comparison, FUSA is a relatively new technique with minimal data, requiring complex technology with very limited availability. Much work remains to be completed before FUSA can be directly compared to breast preserving surgery. Studies of FUSA addressing local failure rates, cosmesis, cost-effectiveness, and long-term patient satisfaction are ongoing [12].

References

1. Graham SJ, Chen L, Leitch M, Peters RD, Bronskill MJ, Foster FS, Henkelman RM, Plewes DB. Quantifying tissue damage due to focused ultrasound heating observed by MRI. Magn Reson Med. 1999;41:321–8.
2. Hill CR, ter Haar GR. High intensity focused ultrasound: potential for cancer treatment. Br J Radiol. 1995;68:1296–303.
3. Wu F, et al. Pathological changes in human malignant carcinoma treated with high-intensity focused ultrasound. Ultrasound Med Biol. 2001;27:1099–106.
4. Wu F, Wang Z-B, Cao Y-D, Chen W-Z, Bai J, Zou J-Z, Zhu H. A randomized clinical trial of high-intensity focused ultrasound ablation for the treatment of patients with localised breast cancer. Br J Cancer. 2003;89:2227–33.

5. Wu F, Wang Z-B, Zhu H, Chen W-Z, Zou J-Z, Bai J, Li K-Q, Jin C-B, Xie F-L, Su H-B. Extracorporeal high intensity focused ultrasound treatment for patients with breast cancer. Breast Cancer Res Treat. 2005;92:51–60.
6. Furusawa H, Namba K, Thomsen S, Akiyama F, Bendet A, Tanaka C, Yasuda Y, Nakahara H. Magnetic resonance-guided focused ultrasound surgery of breast cancer: reliability and effectiveness. J Am Coll Surg. 2006;203:54–63.
7. Gambos EC, Kacher DF, Furusawa H, Namba K. Breast focused ultrasound surgery with magnetic resonance guidance. Top Magn Reson Imaging. 2006;17:181–8.
8. Gianfelice D, Khiat A, Amara M, Belblidia A, Boulanger Y. MR imaging-guided focused US ablation of breast cancer: histopathologic assessment of effectiveness-initial experience. Radiology. 2003;227:849–55.
9. Gianfelice D, Khait A, Boulanger Y, Amara M, Beblidia A. Feasibility of magnetic resonance imaging-guided focused ultrasound surgery as an adjunct to tamoxifen therapy in high-risk surgical patients with breast carcinoma. J Vasc Interv Radiol. 2003;14:1275–82.
10. Gianfelice D, Khiat A, Amara M, Belblindia A, Boulanger Y. MR imaging-guided focused ultrasound surgery of breast cancer: correlation of dynamic contrast-enhanced MRI with histopathological findings. Breast Cancer Res Treat. 2003;82:93–101.
11. Zippel DB, Papa MZ. The use of MR imaging guided focused ultrasound in breast cancer patients; a preliminary phase one study and review. Breast Cancer. 2005;12:32–8.
12. Khiat A, Gianfelice D, Amara M, Boulanger Y. Influence of post treatment delay on the evaluation of the response to focused ultrasound surgery of breast cancer by dynamic contrast enhanced MRI. Br J Radiol. 2006;79:308–14.
13. Furusawa H, Namba K, Nakahara H, Tanaka C, Yasuda Y, Hirabara E, Imahariyama M, Komaki K. The evolving non-surgical ablation of breast cancer: MR guided focused ultrasound (MRgFUS). Breast Cancer. 2007;14:55–8.
14. Furusawa H. Treatment of Breast Cancer. Plenary session presented at the second International Symposium on MR-guided Focused Ultrasound, October 2010, Washington, DC.
15. Wu F, Wang Z-B, Cao Y-D, Zhu X-Q, Zhy H, Chen W-Z, Zou J-Z. Wide local ablation of localized breast cancer using high intensity focused ultrasound. J Surg Oncol. 2007;96:130–6.
16. Holland R, Veling SHJ, Mravunac M, Hendriks JHCL. Histologic multifocality of Tis, T 1–2 breast carcinomas: implications for clinical trials of breast-conserving surgery. Cancer. 1985;56:979–90.
17. Bland KL, Gass J, Klimberg VS. Radiofrequency, cryoablation, and other modalities for breast cancer ablation. Surg Clin N Am. 2007;87:539–50.
18. Fisher B, Anderson S, Bryant J, Margolese RG, Deutsch M, Fisher ER, Jeong JH, Wolmark N. Twenty-year follow-up of a randomized trial comparing total mastectomy, lumpectomy, and lumpectomy plus irradiation for the treatment of invasive breast cancer. N Engl J Med. 2002;347:1233–41.
19. Veronesi U, Cascinelli N, Mariani L, Greco M, Saccozzi R, Luini A, Agular M, Marubini E. Twenty-year follow-up of a randomized study comparing breast-conserving surgery with radical mastectomy for early breast cancer. N Engl J Med. 2002;347:1227–32.

Part IV
Surgical Management of the Breast

Chapter 14
High Risk Lesions

Jill R. Dietz

Introduction

There is a remarkably varied spectrum of noncancerous breast lesions that can be identified by screening mammography since the advent of improved imaging techniques. The variety and volume of such lesions has increased dramatically over the last decade. The physicians who are responsible for the care of these patients are challenged with the interpretation of the results with minute amounts of tissue from minimally invasive biopsies. It is essential for the multidisciplinary breast team to evaluate the concordance of each biopsy in relation to histology, imaging, history and physical examination. This is most easily accomplished with a concordance conference attended by all of the involved specialists including pathologists, breast imagers, as well as surgeons. In some institutions, this is done by whoever performs the biopsy, which is usually the radiologist or surgeon.

Evaluation of these lesions not only has immediate implications in terms of potential upgrading to atypia or frank carcinoma upon excision, but also, the long term potential for the future development of cancer in these patients. The risk associated with the pathologic diagnosis, combined with patient factors such as, family history and breast density, need to be considered on an individual basis in order to be able to plan appropriate screening, evaluation and intervention. Underestimation of malignancy and radiologic–pathologic discordance are two main reasons for excisional biopsy after benign core biopsy [1].

Minimally invasive biopsy is conclusive in most cases of abnormal mammogram requiring biopsy. This should be the preferred method of diagnosis rather than needle localization excisional biopsy. NCCN guidelines emphasize the benefits of minimally invasive biopsy including avoidance of surgery in a substantial number of

J.R. Dietz, M.D., F.A.C.S. (✉)
Cleveland Clinic Foundation, 9500 Euclid Ave, Cleveland, OH 44195, USA
e-mail: dietzj3@ccf.org

D.S. Francescatti and M.J. Silverstein (eds.), *Breast Cancer: A New Era in Management*,
DOI 10.1007/978-1-4614-8063-1_14,

Table 14.1 Relative risk of developing cancer associated with benign proliferative lesions of the breast

Lesion	Relative risk
Usual ductal hyperplasia	2.0
Subareolar papilloma	2.0
Radial scar	1.8
Multiple papillomas	3.1
Papilloma with atypia	5.1
Radial scar with atypia	5.8
Papillomatosis with atypia	7.0
LCIS	8–10

cases, overall decrease in the amount of tissue removed, and if malignancy is found, increased sentinel node identification rates [2].

This chapter serves to discuss the diagnosis and implications of high risk breast lesions found on core biopsy, as incidental lesions in a specimen, or on excision. We focus on the histologic findings, appropriate surgical therapy, and the potential for upgrading upon excisional biopsy. The lesions discussed in this chapter will be grouped based on the relative risk of developing cancer. Finally, we will discuss the management of patients diagnosed with these high risk lesions. Table 14.1 lists the relative risks of the benign high risk lesions that will be discussed in this chapter. Bear in mind that a patient's individual risk factors such as age, hereditary and environmental factors, hormonal exposure, breast density, and obesity can greatly impact these relative risks (Table 14.1).

Benign Proliferative Lesions (Relative Risk 1.5–3×)

Women who have a clinical symptom or imaging abnormality resulting in biopsy have an increased risk of developing breast cancer in the future about twice that of asymptomatic women with normal imaging and no risk factors [3]. In this chapter, we will discuss the benign proliferative lesions that increase a woman's risk for developing breast cancer.

Usual Ductal Hyperplasia

Usual hyperplasia is often seen on pathology reports after biopsy for imaging abnormalities or after excisional biopsy of a mass or thickening. In of itself, there is no direct imaging corollary. It is often found in association with sclerosing adenosis, apocrine metaplasia, and psuedoangiomatous stromal hyperplasia [4].

Ductal hyperplasia is defined as the ducts or lobular units having more than two cell layers of thickness above the basement membrane. Hyperplasia may be further subdivided by the number of cell layers present. Mild and moderate hyperplasia has

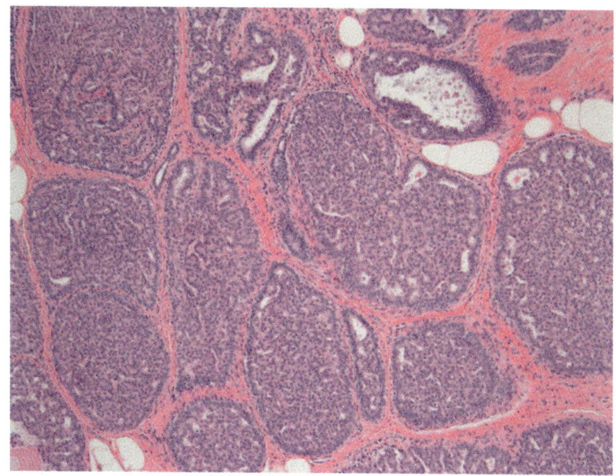

Fig. 14.1 Histologic appearance of usual ductal hyperplasia (10×)

a few identifiable cell layers. The transition to severe or florid hyperplasia is not well defined. As the level of hyperplasia increases, cellularity increases such that the entire lumen may be filled with cells. The cells have reduced cytoplasmic volume compared to normal ductal cells, although mitotic figure are rare [5] (see Fig. 14.1).

While ductal hyperplasia is considered a proliferative lesion, the cells are not associated with atypia, and therefore, are not premalignant. The risk of subsequent cancer, for usual hyperplasia without atypia varies from 1 to 8.6 % in the literature. The lesion is generally considered to double a patient's risk. The relative risk of this lesion is dependent on the degree of hyperplasia and other risk factors, such as family history [6].

Identification of this incidental finding on core needle biopsy or excision does not warrant further intervention. Patients found to have ductal hyperplasia are encouraged to continue annual screening mammography and are referred for high risk evaluation only if other patient risk factors are present.

Solitary Papilloma

Symptomatic papillomas are often identified on clinical examination of a patient presenting with nipple discharge. In fact, a papilloma is the most common cause of pathologic nipple discharge [7, 8]. Central papillomas more often present with discharge (86 %) compared to peripheral papillomas (29 %) [9].

Ultrasound imaging of central papillomas can identify a hypoechoic mass within a dilated duct. Peripheral papillomas, which are usually asymptomatic, are often larger and are found on screening imaging studies. They may manifest in imaging as calcifications, nodules, or masses. They may also be multiple and form a mass like effect on clinical examination [10].

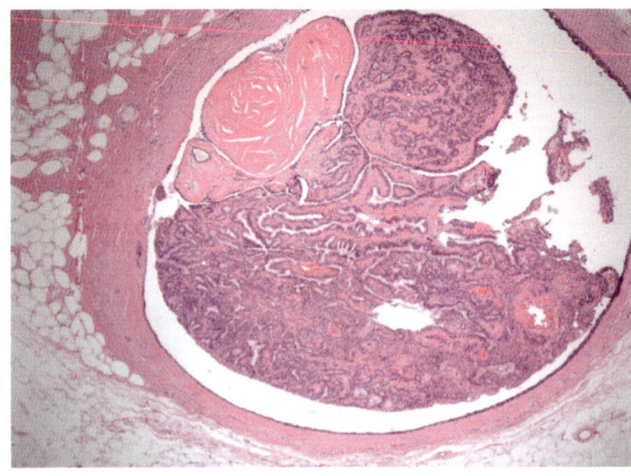

Fig. 14.2 Histologic appearance of excised papilloma

Papillary lesions are proliferative ductal lesions with a fibroepithelial core and are often described as "frond" like. They range in size from a few millimeters to a centimeter or more. Evidence of necrosis and or hemorrhage is common. Fragmented specimens obtained by core needles may be difficult for pathologists to interpret [11]. The concern with core needle biopsy for diagnosis of a papilloma is the potential of missing a well differentiated papillary carcinoma [12]. Excisional biopsy provides the pathologists with the entire lesion which is helpful in making the diagnosis (see Fig. 14.2).

The excisional upgrade rate of a core biopsy diagnosed benign papillary lesion to atypia or carcinoma is widely varied. Large vacuum assisted core biopsies that remove more of the visible lesion have lower upgrade rates. Without atypia in the core specimen, the upgrade rate to malignancy is reported to be from 5 to 25 %. Peripheral lesions are more often found to harbor malignancy (rates up to 30 %) than central lesions. Subareolar papillomas have less than a 10 % risk of associated malignancy on excision [13]. The risk of malignancy in patients with a papilloma, increases with patient age, palpability, abnormal imaging, and peripheral location [14].

The risk of in situ or invasive carcinoma upon excision with an atypical papillary lesion diagnosed by core biopsy is reported as high as 29 % [15]. Another study reviewed 345 patients with intraductal papilloma (IDP) on core biopsy. Among those patients with a benign IDP who subsequently underwent a surgical biopsy, 14 % upgraded to atypical ductal hyperplasia while 10.5 % upgraded to ductal carcinoma in situ (DCIS). If the core biopsy also showed atypia, 22.2 % upgraded to DCIS [16].

There is literature to support imaging follow up for papillary lesions that are concordant when the entire imaging abnormality has been removed [12]. This should be institution dependent based on upgrade rates and size of needle used for biopsy. In general, symptomatic papillomas identified by clinical examination and peripheral papillomas identified by imaging studies, should be surgically removed to avoid the risk of pathologic upgrade to malignancy.

Symptomatic papillomas often present as pathologic nipple discharge (PND). These patients present with single duct, spontaneous, often bloody or serous discharge. If mammography shows no mass or calicfications, and the lesion is not palpable, the chance that this clinical presentation results in a diagnosis of malignancy is less than 10 %. Unfortunately, there is no test, including guaiac testing, smear cytology, ductography, or even ultrasound core biopsy, which can exclude malignancy. The combination of symptoms and risk of malignancy warrant excisional biopsy [17].

Directed-duct excision for patients with PND will yield a benign proliferative lesion up to 90 % of cases. The more directed the excision, the higher the yield. Ductogram with needle localization or ductoscopy-directed duct excision provide the highest proliferative lesion rates. Fibrocystic change and duct ectasia are not true causes of PND and a pathology report showing these non-proliferative findings likely mean that the lesion was not within the specimen or at least not identified by the pathologist. Proliferative lesion rates are much lower for nondirected central duct excisions. Recurrent discharge can be found in patients undergoing major duct excision without localization. Many of these lesions are within the nipple itself. Ductogram and ductoscopy can identify these lesions within the nipple. Second deeper lesions can be visualized and excised in 25 % of cases when using ductoscopy [8, 18].

An additional benefit of ductoscopy directed duct excision, besides direct visualization of the abnormality and detection of additional lesions, is removal of only the abnormal ductal system. This accomplishes lesion removal with lower volume of tissue resected.

It should be noted, if cannulation of the duct at the nipple is not possible, then major duct excision should be carried out because there is a higher chance of malignancy associated with duct obliteration [19] (see Fig. 14.3a–d).

The risk of future development of malignancy is dependent on associated pathology, the number of papillomas, location of papilloma, and other risk factors. As evidenced by Lewis et al, the relative risk of breast cancer in a patient with a history of solitary papilloma without atypia is 2.04. In the same study, the relative risk increases to 5.11 if the patient had a solitary papilloma with associated atypia. However, the presence of a solitary papilloma with atypical hyperplasia does not significantly elevate the risk of future carcinoma above the level attributable to the atypical hyperplasia itself [14]. Like all breast lesions, the risk of malignancy is multifactorial and affected by other patient risk factors.

Radial Scar/Complex Sclerosing Lesions

Radial scars are most often identified incidentally upon biopsy for other abnormalities on physical examination or imaging studies. They may be found on imaging as a spiculated mass with or without microcalcifications. Radio graphically described as having the appearance of a "black star," they may have linear radiating spicules with a radiolucent black center [20]. Incidence rates for radial scars are estimated to be from

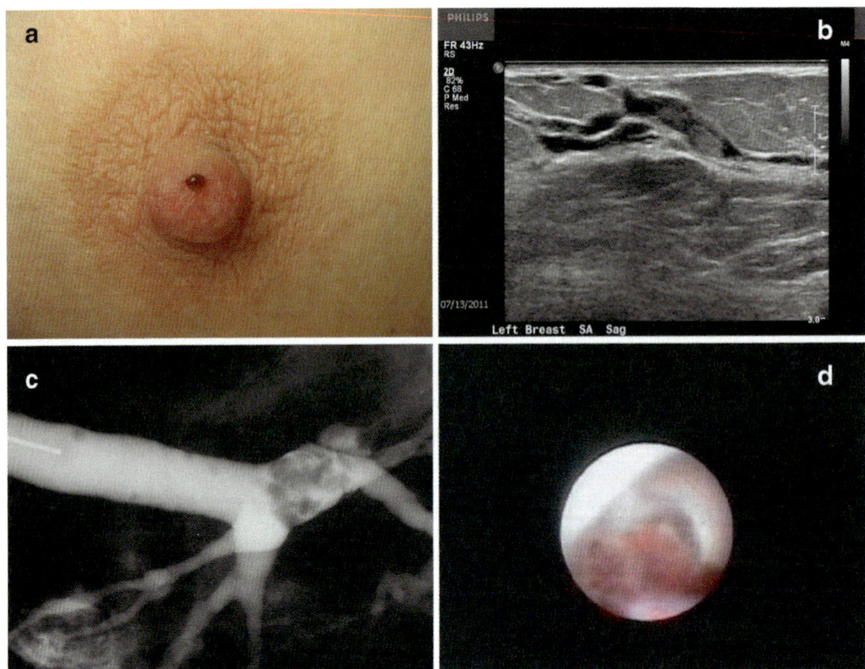

Fig. 14.3 (**a**) Classic appearance of pathologic nipple discharge. (**b**) Ultrasound image of intraductal mass. (**c**) Ductogram showing an intraductal filling defect. (**d**) Mammary ductoscopy image of an intraductal papillary lesion

0.6 to 0.9 per 1,000 women screened [21, 22]. A radial scar is considered a complex sclerosing lesion if the radial scar is greater than 1 cm in diameter [1] (see Fig. 14.4a).

On gross pathology, a tumor with a retracted center may be seen, mimicking a carcinoma. These lesions, microscopically, have a central fibroelastic core containing entrapped glandular elements and ducts that radiate from the lesions center. The periphery of the lesion appears to be drawn inward toward the central core. Epithelial elements entrapped within the fibrous stroma may simulate an invasive carcinoma [23] (see Fig. 14.4b).

Despite their ominous appearance on imaging and pathology, these lesions are benign and no further treatment is needed for benign radial scars found on excisional biopsy. Radiologic–pathologic concordance is often difficult to establish when the biopsy is performed for a mammographically detected lesion. Due to the frequently discordant nature of the pathology, radial scars are often excised on that basis alone. Linda, et al. found that the mammographic and sonographic features of the radial scar were not helpful in determining which harbored malignancy [24]. Because of the significant risk of upgrading to a more advanced histology, excision is usually recommended when a core biopsy demonstrates a radial scar or complex sclerosing lesion.

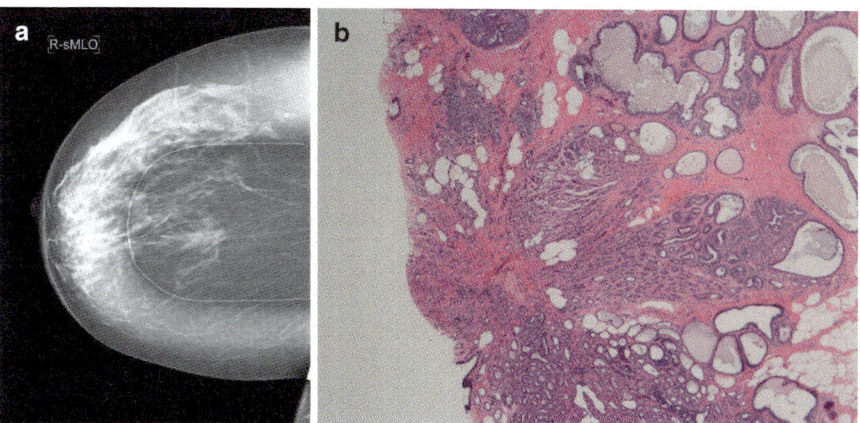

Fig. 14.4 (**a**) Mammographic appearance of a radial scar with linear radiating spicules. (**b**) Histologic appearance of a radial scar

Pathologic upgrade rates upon surgical excision to a high risk lesion or carcinoma for radial scars without atypia on core biopsy range from 0 to 28 %. If they are found to harbor atypia on core biopsy, the range increases dramatically, from 28 to 44 % [25]. In these and other reviews, increasing age, postmenopausal status and increasing lesion size are suggested as risk factors for higher upgrade rates [26].

The relative risk of cancer developing in women with a previous radial scar is 1.8 without associated atypia. In those women with atypia, the relative risk increases to 5.8 [27]. As is the case with women diagnosed with papillomas, the risk of cancer development in patients with radial scars and complex sclerosing lesions is dependent on the risk potential of the associated histology, not the lesion itself.

Mucocele-Like Lesions

Initially described by Rosen in 1986, these lesions appear as mucin containing ducts or cysts that may discharge the mucin into the surrounding stroma. There are varying degrees of epithelial cells within the stroma, some completely acellular. Inflammatory cells may also be found. Mucinous or colloid carcinoma is in the differential when evaluating mucocele-like lesions (MLL) [28].

Mucocele-like lesions typically present as indeterminate calcifications on mammography. In a study from 2011, 27 of 44(61 %) patients presented with calcifications alone while an additional seven (16 %) had microcalcifications associated with a mass [29]. Others may present as a mass lesion on sonography or exam or incidentally upon biopsy for other reasons. Imaging characteristics have been described to differentiate benign from malignant MLL. The malignant MLL or those with associated atypia are more likely to have concerning microcalcifications or complex cystic structures [30].

Recent review from Carkaci reports the conversion from a MLL with atypia on core biopsy to DCIS upon excision in 3 of their 16 patients (19 %). None of their patients without atypia had DCIS upon excision [29]. Conversely, Liebmanns study found patients with a benign mucocele-like lesion on core needle biopsy, 25 % upgraded to an indraductal carcinoma when excised. In addition, those with associated atypia were found to harbor it 75 % of the time [31]. Although some authors advocate observation in those patients with complete removal of the imaging abnormality with the core biopsy procedure, concern for potential upgrading of the pathology as well as the misdiagnosis of a mucinous carcinoma is significant enough to warrant excision of mucocele-like lesions found on core biopsy [32, 33].

Mild Risk Lesions (Relative Risk 2–3×)

Papillomatosis (Epitheliosis)

These lesions are found either as a mammographic density or calcifications, and may present as pathologic nipple discharge. If multiple or large, papillomatosis can present as a palpable abnormality on examination. The majority of cases of multiple papillomas are found in the peripheral terminal ductal lobular units [13]. Papillomatosis is most consistent with micropapillary ductal hyperplasia rather than "multiple papillomas." Gendler defines papillomatosis as at least five papillomas in the same quadrant, or in at least two consecutive pathology tissue blocks [34].

The use of MRI for preoperative planning for the extent of disease in papillomatosis is controversial because of the high sensitivity of MRI for papillary lesions. The problem is that it is difficult to distinguish papillomatosis from malignancy on MRI. A large portion of the breast may enhance which cannot be surgically removed without significant deformity. For this reason, many surgeons prefer to forgo MRI when the diagnosis is papillomatosis, concentrating on removing the portion of the lesion that is clinically symptomatic, or mammographically abnormal [35] (see Fig. 14.5).

Papillomatosis is a mild to moderate risk lesion that differs both histologically and in its risk from solitary papilloma. It is at times not possible to completely excise, although the most mammographically evident or palpable portion should be removed to rule out associated malignancy. As with other proliferative lesions, the risk of subsequent malignancy is multifactorial and associated with other patient risk factors.

There is a higher risk of associated cancer (especially DCIS) with papillomatosis than with solitary papillomas. Ohuchi reported that 6/16 patients with peripheral papillomas originating in the terminal ductal lobular unit harbored carcinoma, whereas, none of the nine central papilloma patients had malignancy [13]. In the review of patients in the SEER database, it was demonstrated that the relative risk of cancer development in patients with multiple papillomas was 3.01 without atypia and 7.01 with atypia. This is in contrast to patients with solitary papillomas whose relative risk was 2.04 with and 5.11 without atypia [14].

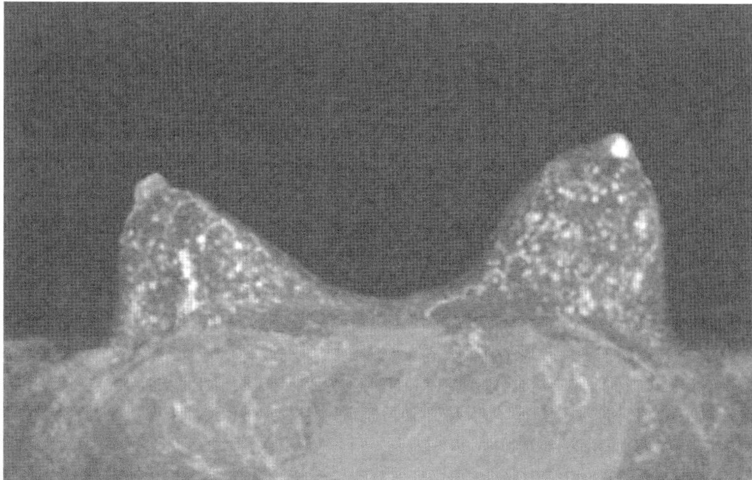

Fig. 14.5 MRI findings of a patient with a negative mammogram and pathologic nipple discharge. She has diffuse papillomatosis which can be difficult to differentiate from malignancy on MRI

Moderate Risk Lesions (Relative Risk 4–6×)

Atypical Ductal Hyperplasia (ADH)

Like many of the other high risk lesions atypical ductal hyperplasia, ADH is found incidentally or upon biopsy of indeterminate or suspicious microcalcifications. One study found that 9 % rate of ADH for all of the stereotactic biopsies performed for BIRAD's category 4 or higher mammographic abnormalities [36]. ADH is defined as an intraductal proliferation showing the features of low grade ductal carcinoma in situ (DCIS), but in less than two duct spaces or less than 2 mm in diameter [37]. The cells in ADH have distinct borders, increased nuclear to cytoplasmic ratio, nuclear enlargement, and irregular chromatin/nucleoli. The difference between ADH and DCIS is a measure of degrees, or magnitude of the cellular change. Therefore, there is significant intraobserver variability when making the diagnosis (see Fig. 14.6).

Because the diagnosis of ADH or DCIS is dependent on a multitude of factors, the upgrade rate to carcinoma upon excisional biopsy varies. As an example, when large bore vacuum assisted breast biopsy is used for diagnosis, upgrade rates can be as low as 10 % [38]. Not surprisingly, when using a 14 gauge needle, upgrade rates have been reported as high as 87 % [25]. The extent of ADH within the specimen, the type of microcalcifications biopsied, and the pattern of the ADH ,with micropapillary having a higher risk, have all been determined to play a role in increasing the upgrade rate [39].

Atypical ductal hyperplasia is associated with increased risk of developing future breast cancer with a relative risk (4.5–5×) or even higher if the patient is

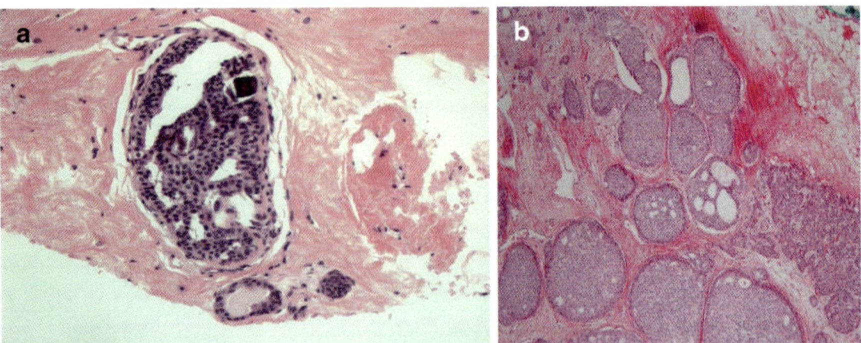

Fig. 14.6 ADH and DCIS are similar in characteristics but differ in the degree of abnormality present. (**a**) Histologic appearance of atypical ductal hyperplasia. (**b**) Histologic appearance of ductal carcinoma in situ

premenopausal or has a family history of breast cancer. The risk is for bilateral breast cancer which suggests that ADH may be a marker for breast cancer instead of a direct precursor [37].

Due to the risk of finding concomitant carcinoma in the specimens, and significant intraobserver variability of the diagnosis, excisional biopsy should be done for all patients with core biopsy diagnosed ADH. Upgrade rates vary in the literature and average around 25 %. They are never lower than 10 %, however, even when large bore vacuum-assisted biopsies are performed [40]. Once excision has been performed, patients diagnosed with ADH should be referred to a high risk screening program or assessed for other risk factors.

Atypical Lobular Hyperplasia

Much of the literature does not differentiate lobular carcinoma in situ (LCIS) from atypical lobular hyperplasia (ALH), but instead uses the term lobular neoplasia (LN) to encompass both entities. Although lobular neoplasia is often found incidentally with core needle biopsy or excisional biopsy of imaging abnormalities, it may be associated with microcalcifications or a mass on imaging [1]. More recently, two studies have found LN associated with microcalcifications in notable numbers of their reported core biopsies suggesting that it can be associated with imaging abnormalities [41, 42].

Both ALH and LCIS are a proliferative growth of a monotonous cell population. The difference lies in the percentage of the terminal duct-lobular unit (TDLU) that is occupied by the cells. If the acini are greater than 50 % filled, it is considered LCIS. If less than 50 % filled, it is considered ALH [43]. Mitoses, calcifications and necrosis are rarely found in cases of ADH. As is the case with ADH and DCIS, there may be much observer variability in making the distinction (see Fig. 14.7).

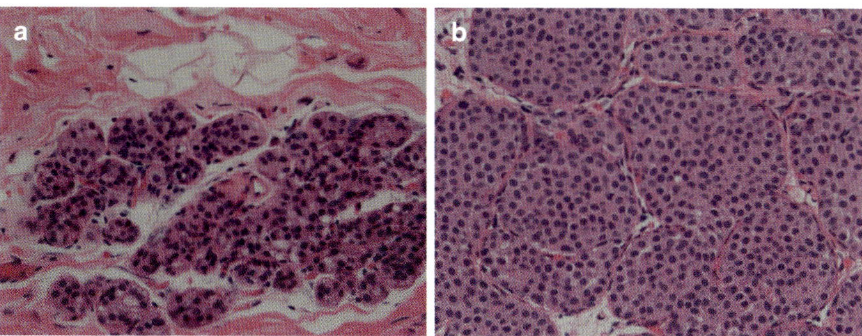

Fig. 14.7 ALH and LCIS are similar in characteristics but differ in the degree of abnormality present. (**a**) Histologic appearance of atypical lobular hyperplasia. (**b**) Histologic appearance of lobular carcinoma in situ

Upgrade rates for ALH to cancer on core needle biopsy is generally lower than it is for ADH and LCIS. Many studies do not separate the lobular neoplasias. However, the upgrade rate for ALH is still substantial enough (over 10 % in most series) to warrant excisional biopsy for women with ALH found on core needle biopsy [39].

Multiple studies over the years have shown an increased risk of development of carcinoma (both ipsilateral and contralateral) in patients that have ALH. The subsequent ipsilateral cancer is most often at the site of the original lesion [44]. Relative risk for the development of carcinoma in a patient with the diagnosis of ALH is 4–5 times the general population. As with other high risk lesions, the patient's individual risk factors influence their overall risk [43, 45].

High Risk Lesions (Relative Risk 8–10×)

Lobular Carcinoma In Situ

LCIS is found incidentally in benign breast biopsy specimens in .5–3.8 % of the cases reviewed [46]. In 2002, Li et al. reported the incidence of LCIS to be 3.19/100,000 person-years [47]. LCIS is often an incidental finding associated with histologic lesions identified in pathology reports for mammographic abnormalities or excisional breast biopsy for symptomatic breast disease.

If the acini of the TDLU are greater than 50 % filled, it is considered LCIS. As with the distinction between ADH and DCIS, there may be significant intraobserver variability in making the diagnosis. Histologically, LCIS often has neoplastic cells with scant cytoplasm and small, round, bland nuclei. The great majority of LCIS is lacking E-cadherin expression, although this is not universal [48]. Mitoses, calcifications and necrosis are rarely found. The basement membrane remains intact and there is no evidence of invasion [49]. Lobular carcinoma in situ is frequently multicentric and bilateral [50].

As with other high risk breast lesions, there is controversy and variation in the literature regarding the upgrade rates and subsequent need for excision. Most series suggest the chance of finding cancer on excision after CNB showing LCIS is around 13–20 %. Again, in most circumstances, excisional biopsy is recommended to rule out malignancy [39].

Women who are diagnosed with LCIS on CNB or excision have the highest relative risk of developing breast cancer in the future; 8–10 times that of the average woman.

In patients with biopsy proven LCIS, reports cite the risk of developing ipsilateral breast cancer varies between 7 and 17 % at 10 years [45, 51, 52]. Contra lateral risk is also significantly increased. Ten year estimate was found to be 13.9 % in this series [53]. Individual patient risk factors such as family history can be additive to this risk.

Pleomorphic LCIS

Pleomorphic LCIS is a variant of LCIS that has recently been recognized as distinct from LCIS. Studies show that in the past, this lesion was in many cases lumped in with the diagnosis of DCIS. Pleomorphic LCIS is more frequently associated necrosis and microcalcifications on pathology or mammography [54].

When CNB or excisional biopsy results in a diagnosis of LCIS, surgeons are more often than not treating these lesions like DCIS. Pleomorphic LCIS can behave clinically like DCIS with high rates of local recurrence. Consideration is given to obtaining clear margins and consult to radiation oncology is contemplated [55, 56]. Histologically, pleomorphic LCIS can easily be distinguished from DCIS with a negative e-cadherin stain (see Fig. 14.8).

Management of High Risk Patients

There are two basic methods to identify a patient at high risk for developing breast cancer; hereditary and environmental factors and intrinsic breast disease. Certainly a thorough personal and family history may detail hereditary or environmental risk factors that predispose patients to an elevated risk. There are many risk models available that attempt to quantify a patient's risk for developing breast cancer. These are designed to help decipher which patient may benefit from a more comprehensive evaluation. These include the Gail model, the Tyrer–Cuzick model, the Clause model and tables, the Bodeciea model, and the BRCAPRO to name a few. Each of these has strengths and weaknesses in its inherent design. Care must be taken when counseling patients about the results of their risk based on these models because there are varying opinions about the validity of each model reported in the literature.

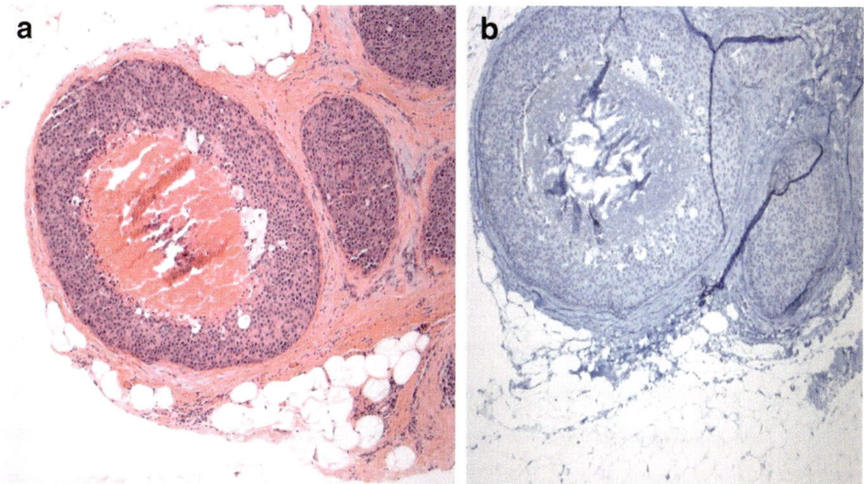

Fig. 14.8 Histologic appearance of lobular carcinoma in situ. The negative E-cadherin stain differentiates this lesion from DCIS. (**a**) Histologic appearance of pleomorphic LCIS. (**b**) Negative E-cadherin stain

Some more detailed examples of the most commonly used risk assessment tools include:

The Gail model which was first designed in 1989 and since has been modified twice. It can easily be found on the National Cancer Institute Web site. This model is very assessable, quick to perform and probably the most widely used risk assessment model by nongenetic counseling providers. This assessment includes age, prior biopsies, with or without atypia and first degree relatives with breast cancer [57, 58]. There are some limitations that have been identified by several validation studies including underestimation of risk in women with an extensive family history (as the GAIL model only uses information about first degree relative), and also women with atypia [59–62].

The Claus model focuses on family history and is useful for patients with a more extensive breast cancer family tree. The Claus model however does not include nonfamilial risk factors such as hormonal or reproductive history [59, 63].

The Tyrer–Cuzick Model, also called the IBIS model for the International Breast Cancer Intervention Study, incorporates family history, gene abnormalities, and estrogen exposure among other factors [64]. It is more thorough but can be cumbersome and time-consuming to use. This model does include benign breast disease in its calculation. One study showed that this model was one of the most accurate [65, 66].

Many women will seek evaluation for risk assessment with their breast surgeon and thus the decision to initiate a consultation with a genetics counselor will often fall upon the surgeon caring for the patient. It is important for physicians to recognize patients at high risk and address or make appropriate referrals. Genetic testing may also be considered for those deemed high enough risk. Table 14.2 lists the risk

Table 14.2 Risk factors included in commonly used risk assessment models

Risk factor	Risk assessment tool			
	GAIL	Claus	T-C (IBIS)	BRCAPRO
Age	+	+	+	+
First degree relative	+	+	+	+
Extended family Hx	–	+	+	+
Other cancers	–	–	+	+
Hormonal	+	–	+	–
Reproductive	+	–	+	–
Biopsy with atypia	+	–	+	–

factors that are assessed by the more commonly used risk assessment tools being used in nongenetic clinics and may assist with choosing the best risk assessment tool for a particular patient (see Table 14.2).

The other method of establishing increased risk in a patient is identification of pathologic lesions such as those mentioned in this chapter. In most cases, upgrade rates of premalignant lesions are significant enough to warrant excision if found on core needle biopsy. If found on excisional biopsy, these lesions do not require further surgical intervention, and similarly do not require reexcision to clear margins except perhaps for the entity pleomorphic lobular carcinoma in situ.

Patients with these moderate to high risk lesions such as ADH, ALH, and LCIS are considered to be at high risk for developing breast cancer, even with no family history. A first degree relative or strong family history increases the magnitude of the relative risk in these women. Identification of atypia in a patient at increased risk for breast cancer due to hereditary or environmental factors can help stratify this group into those at higher and more immediate risk.

Large studies of nipple aspirate fluid (NAF) have been done on thousands of women with hereditary risk factors with over 10 years of follow up. NAF can be obtained applying n aspiration device to the end of the nipple and applying suction. Fluid that comes to the surface of the nipple can be collected in a capillary tube and analyzed under the microscope for cellular content. Findings show that the ability to obtain NAF increases the chance of a women developing cancer by 1.8 times. Women with increased cellularity (hyperplasia) had a 2.5 time risk and patients with atypia had a 4.9 time risk. These findings are similar to the risks of women with the same lesions identified on excisional biopsy [67].

Ductal lavage uses a similar technique of obtaining NAF. After massage of the breast, a small catheter is inserted into any duct that produces secretions. 10–15 cm^3 of sterile saline is injected into the duct via the micro catheter and breast compression is used to collect he ductal fluid in the micro catheter. The process is repeated several times for each NAF producing duct. The fluid is placed in CyloLyt and the ducts lavaged are marked on a grid. The cells are interpreted based on NCI consensus criteria for breast FNA biopsy [68].

Ductal lavage identifies more cells and more cellular atypia in high risk women then the NAF procedure (Fig. 14.9). One study showed an atypia rate of 24 % in the

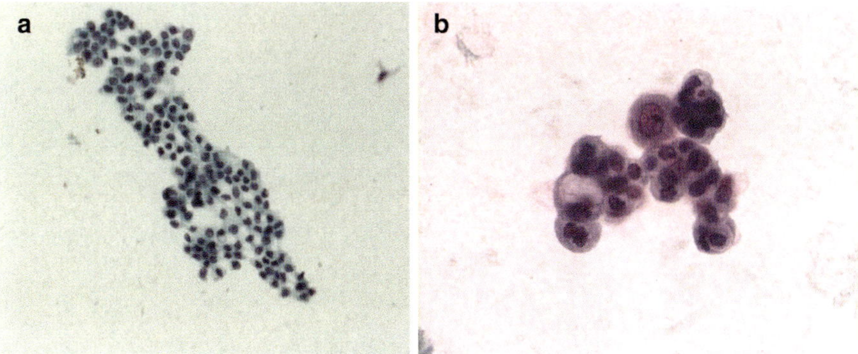

Fig. 14.9 Ductal lavage washings can produce ductal cells that are benign, atypical or malignant. (**a**) Benign cytology from ductal washing. (**b**) Malignant cytology form ductal washing

group, which is similar to the 21 % incidence of atypia in random FNA of high risk women [69, 70].

Patients found to have atypia by any of the above mentioned means or LCIS should be counseled as to their increased risk of developing breast cancer. However, telling a patient of their relative risk may not be helpful. Carol Fabian did a study in patients with a family history of breast cancer where she performed random peri-areolar fine needle aspirations (FNA). Two groups were followed, those with and without atypia. At 3 years, 15 % of patients with atypia had developed breast cancer, whereas, only 4 % of those without atypia developed cancer. I like to quote this study as it gives some perspective for the patient as to their actual risk over the near term [70].

There are two basic strategies for management of patients that are at high risk for the development of breast cancer; prevention and early detection. Screening regimens as formulated by the American Cancer Society guidelines are adequate for most normal risk patients. Higher risk patients may be better served by alternating mammography with bilateral breast MRI. Some of the screening may be limited by insurance carrier funding, although many insurance carriers follow national guidelines. Current American Cancer Society guidelines for breast cancer screening do not include atypia in and of itself as an indication for MRI screening. Atypia does factor into most high risk calculations such as the Gail or Clause models. MRI is indicated in patients where life time risk is greater than or equal to 20 %, according to ACS guidelines [71]. Unfortunately, none of the existing high risk models accurately assess risk in patients with atypia. The Tyrer–Cuzick model overestimates breast cancer risk in women with atypia and the Gail model significantly underestimates breast cancer risk in women with atypia [72].

Once a patient has been identified at increased risk for developing breast cancer, options for prevention may be discussed in addition to increased surveillance. Although the topic of chemoprevention is beyond the scope of this chapter, studies have shown that patients at high risk of developing cancer have a 50–75 % reduction in their risk by taking Tamoxifen [73]. The NSABP P1 Breast Cancer Prevention Trial was a pivotal study of Tamoxifen use in women with ADH. It showed an 86 % reduction in the risk of invasive breast cancer in women treated with Tamoxifen compared with controls [74].

Many women choose not to use chemoprevention for fear of side effects, such as the increased risk of uterine cancer, increased risk of thromboembolic events, as well as the symptoms of menopause [75]. Women with atypia however are the group most likely to benefit from chemoprevention [76]. Studies have shown most women at risk for developing cancer increase use of Tamoxifen from 0 % if they do not have atypia to 50 % if atypia is identified on biopsy [77].

Patients at highest risk for developing breast cancer because of atypia or LCIS and a strong family history of breast cancer may want to consider prophylactic surgery. While this is more commonly reserved for gene positive patients, advances in nipple sparing prophylactic surgery and reconstruction techniques make prophylactic surgery a more palatable consideration.

In summary, patients at increased risk for developing breast cancer can be a strongly motivated and educated group of women who clearly understand their options. Other women overestimate their risk and have an unwarranted fear of developing breast cancer based on an emotional response to a personal tragedy. The process of sorting out the magnitude of risk often falls to the surgeon caring for these women. A multidisciplinary approach using the services of advanced imaging specialists, genetic counseling and pathology experts will be needed to accurately manage this group of patients. In the future, this task may become easier as advanced imaging techniques and risk assessment with biomolecular analysis of tissue become more mainstream.

References

1. Georgian-Smith D, Lawton T. Controversies on the management of high-risk lesions at core biopsy from a radiology/pathology perspective. Radiol Clin N Am. 2010;48:999–1012.
2. National Comprehensive Cancer Network. Guidelines for treatment of cancer by site. http://www.nccn.org/professionals/physician_gls/f_guidelines.asp. Accessed 30 Jun 2012.
3. Hartmann L, Sellers T, Frost M, et al. Benign breast disease and the risk of breast cancer. N Engl J Med. 2005;353:229–37.
4. Boecker W, Moll R, Dervan P, et al. Usual ductal hyperplasia of the breast is a committed stem (progenitor) cell lesion distinct from atypical ductal hyperplasia and ductal carcinoma in situ. J Pathol. 2002;198:458–67.
5. Rosen PP. Rosen's breast pathology. 3rd ed. Philadelphia, PA: Lippincott Williams & Wilkins; 2009. p. 232.
6. Fitzgibbons PL, Henson DE, Hutter RVP. Benign breast changes and the risk for subsequent breast cancer: an update of the 1985 consensus statement. Arch Pathol Lab Med. 1998;122:1053–5.
7. Nelson R, Hoehn JL. Twenty-year outcome following central duct resection for bloody nipple discharge. Ann Surg. 2006;243:522–4.
8. Dietz JR, Crowe JP, Grundfest S, Arrigain S, Kim JA. Directed duct excision by using mammary ductoscopy in patients with pathologic nipple discharge. Surgery. 2002;132:582–8.

9. Cardenosa G, Eklund G. Benign papillary neoplasms of the breast: mammographic findings. Radiology. 1991;181:751–5.
10. Brookes M, Bourke A. Radiological appearances of papillary breast lesions. Clin Radiol. 2008;63:1265–73.
11. Rosen PP. Rosen's breast pathology. 3rd ed. Philadelphia, PA: Lippincott Williams & Wilkins; 2009. p. 76–87.
12. Bennett LE, Ghate SV, Bentley R, Baker JA. Is surgical excision of core biopsy proven benign papillomas of the breast necessary? Acad Radiol. 2010;17(5):553–7.
13. Ohuchi N, Abe R, Kasai M. Possible cancerous change of intraductal pappilloma of the breast. Cancer. 1984;54:605–11.
14. Lewis JT, Hartmann LC, Vierkant RA, et al. An analysis of breast cancer risk in women with single, multiple, and atypical papilloma. Am J Surg Pathol. 2006;30(6):665–72.
15. Valdes EK, Tartter PI, Genelus-Dominique E, Guilbaud DA, Rosenbaum-Smith S, Estabook A. Significance of papillary lesions at percutaneous breast biopsy. Ann Surg Oncol. 2006;13(4):480–2.
16. Rizzo M, Lund MJ, Oprea G, Schniederjan M, Wood WC, Mosunjac M. Surgical follow-up and clinical presentation of 142 breast papillary lesions diagnosed by ultrasound-guided core-needle biopsy. Ann Surg Oncol. 2008;15(4):1040–7.
17. Fisher CS, Margenthaler JA. A look into the ductoscope: it's role in pathologic nipple discharge. Ann Surg Oncol. 2011;18:3187–91.
18. Cabioglu N, Hunt K, Singletary SE. Surgical decision making and factors determining a diagnosis of breast carcinoma in women presenting with nipple discharge. J Am Coll Surg. 2003;196(3):354–64.
19. Sharma R, Dietz JR, Wright H, Crowe J, DiNunzio A, Woletz J, Kim J. Comparative analysis of minimally invasive microductectomy versus major duct excision in patients with pathologic nipple discharge. Surgery. 2005;138(4):591–7.
20. Alleva DQ, Smetherman DH, Farr Jr GH, Cederbom GJ. Radial scar of the breast: radiologic–pathologic correlation in 22 cases. Radiographics. 1999;19 suppl 1:S27–35.
21. Cawson JN, Malara F, Kavanagh A, Hill P, Balasubramanium G, Henderson M. Fourteen-gauge needle core biopsy of mammographically evident radial scars: is excision necessary? Cancer. 2003;97(2):345–51.
22. Burnett SJ, Ng YY, Perry NM, et al. Benign biopsies in the prevalent round of breast screening: a review of 137 cases. Clin Radiol. 1995;50(4):254–8.
23. Rosen PP. Rosen's breast pathology. 3rd ed. Philadelphia, PA: Lippincott Williams & Wilkins; 2009. p. 87–94.
24. Linda A, Zuiani C, Furlan A, et al. Radial scars without atypia diagnosed at imaging-guided needle biopsy: how often is associated malignancy found at subsequent surgical excision, and do mammography and sonography predict which lesions are malignant? Am J Roentgenol. 2010;194(4):1146–51.
25. Krishnamurthy S, Bevers T, Kuerer H, Yang WT. Multidisciplinary considerations in the management of high-risk breast lesions. Am J Roentgenol. 2012;198(2):W132–40.
26. Andacoglu O, Kanbour-Shakir A, Teh YC, et al. Rationale of excisional biopsy after the diagnosis of benign radial scar on core biopsy: a single institutional outcome analysis. Am J Clin Oncol. 2013;36(1):7–11.
27. Jacobs TW, Byrne C, Colditz G, Connolly JL, Schnitt SJ. Radial scars in benign breast-biopsy specimens and the risk of breast cancer. N Engl J Med. 1999;340(6):430–6.
28. Rosen PP. Mucocele-like tumors of the breast. Am J Surg Pathol. 1986;10(7):464–9.
29. Carkaci S, Lane DL, Gilcrease MZ, et al. Do all mucocele-like lesions of the breast require surgery? Clin Imaging. 2011;35(2):94–101.
30. Kim SM, Kim HH, Kang DK, et al. Mucocele-like tumors of the breast as cystic lesions: sonographic–pathologic correlation. Am J Roentgenol. 2011;196(6):1424–30.
31. Leibman AJ, Staeger CN, Charney DA. Mucocelelike lesions of the breast: mammographic findings with pathologic correlation. Am J Roentgenol. 2006;186(5):1356–60.

32. Jaffer Ş, Bleiweiss IJ, Nagi CS. Benign mucocele-like lesions of the breast: revisited. Mod Pathol. 2011;24(5):683–7.
33. Ohi Y, Umekita Y, Rai Y, et al. Mucocele-like lesions of the breast: a long-term follow-up study. Diagn Pathol. 2011;6:29.
34. Gendler LS, Feldman SM, Balassanian R, et al. Association of breast cancer with papillary lesions identified at percutaneous image-guided breast biopsy. Am J Surg. 2004;188(4):365–70.
35. Iglesias A, Arias M, Santiago P, Rodríguez M, Mañas J, Saborido C. Benign breast lesions that simulate malignancy: magnetic resonance imaging with radiologic–pathologic correlation. Curr Probl Diagn Radiol. 2007;36(2):66–82.
36. Liberman L, Cohen N, Dershaw D, Abramson A, Hann L, Rosen PP. Atypical ductal hyperplasia diagnosed at stereotaxic core biopsy of breast lesions: an indication for surgical biopsy. Am J Roentgenol. 1995;164(5):1111–3.
37. Ellis IO. Intraductal proliferative lesions of the breast: morphology, associated risk and molecular biology. Mod Pathol. 2010;23:S1–7.
38. Cangiarella J, Guth A, Axelrod D, et al. Is surgical excision necessary for the management of atypical lobular hyperplasia and lobular carcinoma in situ diagnosed on core needle biopsy? A report of 38 cases and review of the literature. Arch Pathol Lab Med. 2008;132(6):979–83.
39. Margenthaler JA, Duke D, Monsees BS, Barton PT, Clark C, Dietz JR. Correlation between core biopsy and excisional biopsy in breast high-risk lesions. Am J Surg. 2006;192(4):534–7.
40. Jain RK, Mehta R, Dimitrov R, et al. Atypical ductal hyperplasia: interobserver and intraobserver variability. Mod Pathol. 2011;24:917–23.
41. Arpino G, Allred DC, Mohsin SK, Weiss HL, Conrow D, Elledge RM. Lobular neoplasia on core-needle biopsy – clinical significance. Cancer. 2004;101(2):242–50.
42. Crisi GM, Mandavilli S, Cronin E, Ricci Jr A. Invasive mammary carcinoma after immediate and short-term follow-up for lobular neoplasia on core biopsy. Am J Surg Pathol. 2003;27(3): 325–33.
43. Page DL, Dupont WD, Rogers LW, Rados MS. Atypical hyperplastic lesions of the female breast: a long-term follow-up study. Cancer. 1985;55(11):2698–708.
44. Fisher ER, Land SR, Fisher B, Mamounas E, Gilarski L, Wolmark N. Pathologic findings from the national surgical adjuvant breast and bowel project: twelve-year observations concerning lobular carcinoma in situ. Cancer. 2004;100(2):238–44.
45. Page DL, Kidd Jr TE, Dupont WD, Simpson JF, Rogers LW. Lobular neoplasia of the breast: higher risk for subsequent invasive cancer predicted by more extensive disease. Hum Pathol. 1991;22(12):1232–9.
46. Kuerer HM. Kuerer's breast surgical oncology. 1st ed. New York, NY: McGraw-Hill; 2010.
47. Li CI, Anderson BO, Daling JR, Moe RE. Changing incidence of lobular carcinoma in situ of the breast. Breast Cancer Res Treat. 2002;75(3):259–68.
48. Da Silva L, Parry S, Reid L, et al. Aberrant expression of E-cadherin in lobular carcinomas of the breast. Am J Surg Pathol. 2008;32(5):773–83.
49. Venkitaraman R. Lobular neoplasia of the breast. Breast J. 2010;16(5):519–28.
50. Beute BJ, Kalisher L, Hutter RV. Lobular carcinoma in situ of the breast: clinical, pathologic, and mammographic features. Am J Roentgenol. 1991;157(2):257–65.
51. Chuba PJ, Hamre MR, Yap J, et al. Bilateral risk for subsequent breast cancer after lobular carcinoma-in-situ: analysis of surveillance, epidemiology, and end results data. J Clin Oncol. 2005;23(24):5534–41.
52. Andersen JA. Lobular carcinoma in situ of the breast: an approach to rational treatment. Cancer. 2006;39(6):2597–602.
53. Bland K. William hunter harridge lecture: contemporary management of pre-invasive and early breast cancer. Am J Surg. 2011;201(3):279–89.
54. Monhollen L, Morrison C, Ademuyiwa FO, Chandrasekhar R, Khoury T. Pleomorphic lobular carcinoma: a distinctive clinical and molecular breast cancer type. Histopathology. 2012;61(3): 365–77.
55. Murray L, Reintgen M, Akman K. Pleomorphic lobular carcinoma in situ: treatment options for a new pathologic entity. Clin Breast Cancer. 2012;12(1):76–9.

56. Downs-Kelly E, Bell D, Perkins GH, Sneige N, Middleton LP. Clinical implications of margin involvement by pleomorphic lobular carcinoma in situ. Arch Pathol Lab Med. 2011;135(6): 737–43.
57. Gail MH, Brinton LA, Byar DP, et al. Projecting individualized probabilities of developing breast cancer for white females who are being examined annually. J Natl Cancer Inst. 1989;81:1879–86.
58. Costantino JP, Gail MH, Pee D, et al. Validation studies for models projecting the risk of invasive and total breast cancer incidence. J Natl Cancer Inst. 1999;91:1541–8.
59. Amir E, Freedman OC, Seruga B, Evans DG. Assessing women at high risk of breast cancer: a review of risk assessment models. J Natl Cancer Inst. 2010;102(10):680–91.
60. Pankratz V. Assessment of the accuracy of the Gail model in women with atypical hyperplasia. J Clin Oncol. 2008;26:5374–9.
61. Rockhill B, Spiegelman D, Byrne C, Hunter DJ, Colditz GA. Validation of the Gail et al. Model of breast cancer risk prediction and implications for chemoprevention. J Natl Cancer Inst. 2001;93:358–66.
62. Euhus DM, Leitch AM, Huth JF, Peters GN. Limitations of the Gail model in the specialized breast cancer risk assessment clinic. Breast. 2002;8(1):23–7.
63. Claus EB, Risch N, Thompson WD. Genetic analysis of breast cancer in the cancer and steroid hormone study. Am J Hum Genet. 1991;48(2):232–42.
64. Tyrer J, Duffy SW, Cuzick J. A breast cancer prediction model incorporating familial and personal risk factors. Stat Med. 2004;23(7):1111–30.
65. Amir E, Evans DG, Shenton A, et al. Evaluation of breast cancer risk assessment packages in the family history evaluation and screening programme. J Med Genet. 2003;40(11):807–14.
66. Bondy ML, Lustbader ED, Halabi S, Ross E, Vogel VG. Validation of a breast cancer risk assessment model in women with a positive family history. J Natl Cancer Inst. 1994;86(8):620–5.
67. Wrensch MR, Petrakis NL, King EB, et al. Breast cancer incidence in women with abnormal cytology in nipple aspirates of breast fluid. Am J Epidemiol. 1992;135(2):130–41.
68. The uniform approach to breast fine-needle aspiration biopsy. NIH Consensus Development Conference. Am J Surg 1997;174(4):371–85.
69. Dooley WC, Ljung BM, Veronesi U, et al. Ductal lavage for detection of cellular atypia in women at high risk for breast cancer. J Natl Cancer Inst. 2001;93(21):1624–32.
70. Fabian CJ, Kimler BF, Zalles CM, et al. Short-term breast cancer prediction by random periareolar fine-needle aspiration cytology and the Gail risk model. J Natl Cancer Inst. 2000;92(15): 1217–27.
71. Saslow D, Boetes C, Burke W, et al. American cancer society guidelines for breast screening with MRI as an adjunct to mammography. CA Cancer J Clin. 2007;57(2):75–89.
72. Boughey JC, Hartmann LC, Anderson SS, et al. Evaluation of the tyrer-cuzick (international breast cancer intervention study) model for breast cancer risk prediction in women with atypical hyperplasia. J Clin Oncol. 2010;28(22):3591–6.
73. Fisher ER, Land SR, Fisher B, et al. Pathologic findings from the national surgical adjuvant breast and bowel project: twelve-year observations concerning lobular carcinoma in situ. Cancer. 2003;100(2):238–44.
74. Fisher B, Costantino JP, Wickerham DL, et al. Tamoxifen for prevention of breast cancer: report of the national surgical adjuvant breast and bowel project P-1 study. J Natl Cancer Inst. 1998;90:1371–88.
75. Gail MH, Costantino JP, Bryant J, et al. Weighing the risks and benefits of tamoxifen treatment for preventing breast cancer. J Natl Cancer Inst. 1999;91:1829–46.
76. Coopey SB, Mazzola E, Buckley JM, et al. The role of chemoprevention in modifying the risk of breast cancer in women with atypical breast lesions. Breast Cancer Res Treat. 2012;136(3):627–33.
77. Goldenberg VK, Seewaldt VL, Scott V, et al. Atypia in random periareolar fine-needle aspiration affects the decision of women at high risk to take tamoxifen for breast cancer chemoprevention. Cancer Epidemiol Biomarkers Prev. 2007;16(5):1032–4.

Chapter 15
Ductal Carcinoma In Situ of the Breast

Melvin J. Silverstein and Michael D. Lagios

Introduction

Ductal carcinoma in situ (DCIS) of the breast is a heterogeneous group of lesions with diverse malignant potential and a range of treatment options. It is the most rapidly growing subgroup in the breast cancer family of disease with more than 65,000 new cases diagnosed in the USA during 2013 [1]. Most new cases (>90 %) are nonpalpable and discovered mammographically.

It is now well appreciated that DCIS is a stage in the neoplastic continuum in which most of the molecular changes that characterize invasive breast cancer are already present [2]. All that remains on the way to invasion are quantitative changes in the expression of genes that have already been altered. Genes that may play a role in invasion control a number of functions, including angiogenesis, adhesion, cell motility, the composition of extracellular-matrix, and more. To date, genes that are uniquely associated with invasion have not been identified. DCIS is clearly the precursor lesion for most invasive breast cancers but not all DCIS lesions have the time or the genetic ability to progress to become invasive breast cancer [3–5].

Therapy for DCIS ranges from simple excision to various forms of wider excision (segmental resection, quadrant resection, oncoplastic resection using various forms of breast reduction, etc.), all of which may or may not be followed by radiation therapy. When breast preservation is not feasible, total mastectomy (often skin and nipple-areola-sparing), generally with immediate reconstruction is performed.

M.J. Silverstein, M.D. (✉)
Hoag Breast Program, Hoag Memorial Hospital Presbyterian, One Hoag Drive, Newport Beach, CA 92658, USA

Keck School of Medicine, University of Southern California, Los Angeles, CA, USA
e-mail: melsilver9@gmail.com

M.D. Lagios, M.D.
Breast Cancer Consultation Service, Tiburon, CA, USA

Stanford University School of Medicine, Stanford, CA, USA

D.S. Francescatti and M.J. Silverstein (eds.), *Breast Cancer: A New Era in Management*,
DOI 10.1007/978-1-4614-8063-1_15, © Springer Science+Business Media New York 2014

Since DCIS is a heterogeneous group of lesions rather than a single entity [6, 7] and because patients have a wide range of personal needs that must be considered during treatment selection, it is clear that no single approach will be appropriate for all forms of the disease or for all patients. At the current time, treatment decisions are based upon a variety of measurable parameters (tumor extent, margin width, nuclear grade, the presence or absence of comedonecrosis, age, etc.), physician experience and bias, and upon randomized clinical trial data, which suggest that all conservatively treated patients should be managed with post-excisional radiation therapy and tamoxifen.

The Changing Nature of Ductal Carcinoma In Situ

There have been dramatic changes in the past 20 years that have affected DCIS. Before mammography was common, DCIS was rare, representing less than 1 % of all breast cancer [8]. Today, DCIS is common, representing 20 % of all newly diagnosed cases and as much as 30–50 % of cases of breast cancer diagnosed by mammography [1, 9–13].

Previously, most patients with DCIS presented with clinical symptoms, such as breast mass, bloody nipple discharge, or Paget's disease [14, 15]. Today, most lesions are nonpalpable and generally detected by imaging alone.

Until approximately 20 years ago, the treatment for most patients with DCIS was mastectomy. Today, almost 75 % of newly diagnosed patients with DCIS are treated with breast preservation [16]. In the past, when mastectomy was common, reconstruction was uncommon; if it was performed, it was generally done as a delayed procedure. Today, reconstruction for patients with DCIS treated by mastectomy is common; when it is performed, it is generally done immediately, at the time of mastectomy. In the past, when a mastectomy was performed, large amounts of skin were discarded. Today, it is considered perfectly safe to perform a skin-sparing mastectomy for DCIS and in many instances, nipple-areola sparing-mastectomy.

In the past, there was little confusion. All breast cancers were considered essentially the same and mastectomy was the only treatment. Today, all breast cancers are different and there is a range of acceptable treatments for every lesion. For those that chose breast conservation, there continues to be a debate as to whether radiation therapy is necessary in every case. These changes were brought about by a number of factors. Most important were increased mammographic utilization and the acceptance of breast-conservation therapy for invasive breast cancer.

The widespread use of mammography changed the way DCIS was detected. In addition, it changed the nature of the disease detected by allowing us to enter the neoplastic continuum at an earlier time. It is interesting to note the impact that mammography had on The Breast Center in Van Nuys, California in terms of the number of DCIS cases diagnosed and the way they were diagnosed [17].

From 1979 to 1981, the Van Nuys Group treated a total of only 15 patients with DCIS, five per year. Only two lesions (13 %) were nonpalpable and detected by mammography. In other words, 13 patients (87 %) presented with clinically apparent disease, detected by the old-fashioned methods of observation and palpation. Two state-of-the-art mammography units and a full-time experienced radiologist were added in 1982 and the number of new DCIS cases dramatically increased to more than 30 per year, most of them nonpalpable. When a third and fourth machine were added, the number of new cases increased to more than 50 per year.

The DCIS patients discussed in this chapter were accrued at Van Nuys from 1979 to 1998, at the University of Southern California, Norris Comprehensive Cancer Center from 1998 to 2008, and at the Hoag Memorial Hospital Presbyterian from 2008 to 2011. Analysis of the entire series of 1,585 patients through 2011 shows that 1,402 lesions (89 %) were nonpalpable (subclinical). If we look at only those diagnosed during the last 5 years at the USC/Norris Cancer Center, 95 % were nonpalpable. At Hoag, from 2008 through 2011, 93 % were nonpalpable.

The second factor that changed how we think about DCIS was the acceptance of breast conservation therapy (lumpectomy, axillary node dissection, and radiation therapy) for patients with invasive breast cancer. Until 1981, the treatment for most patients with any form of breast cancer was generally mastectomy. Since that time, numerous prospective randomized trials have shown an equivalent rate of survival for selected patients with invasive breast cancer treated with breast conservation therapy [18–23]. Based on these results, it made little sense to continue treating a lesser disease (DCIS) with mastectomy while treating more aggressive invasive breast cancer with breast preservation.

Current data suggest that many patients with DCIS can be successfully treated with breast preservation, with or without radiation therapy. This chapter will show how easily available data can be used to help in the complex treatment selection process.

Pathology

Classification

Although there is no universally accepted histopathologic classification, most pathologists have traditionally divided DCIS into five major architectural subtypes (papillary, micropapillary, cribriform, solid, and comedo), often comparing the first four (noncomedo) with comedo [6, 13, 24]. Comedo DCIS is frequently associated with high nuclear grade [6, 13, 24, 25] aneuploidy, a higher proliferation rate [26], HER2/neu gene amplification or protein overexpression [27–31], and clinically more aggressive behavior [32–35]. Noncomedo lesions tend to be just the opposite.

The division by architecture alone, comedo versus noncomedo, is an oversimplification and does not work if the purpose of the division is to sort patients into those with a high risk of local recurrence versus those with a low risk. It is not uncommon for high nuclear grade noncomedo lesions to express markers similar to those of high-grade comedo lesions and to have a risk of local recurrence similar to comedo

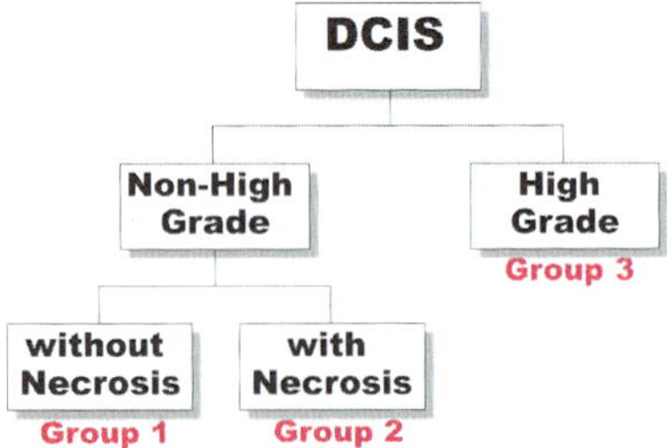

Fig. 15.1 Van Nuys DCIS Classification. DCIS patients are separated in high nuclear grade (grade 3) and non-high nuclear grade (grades 1 and 2). Non-high nuclear grade cases are then separated by the presence or absence of necrosis. Lesions in group 3 (high nuclear grade) may or may not show necrosis

lesions. Adding to the confusion is the fact that mixtures of various architectural subtypes within a single biopsy specimen are common. In our series of patients, more than 73 % of all lesions had significant amounts of two or more architectural subtypes, making division into a predominant architectural subtype problematic.

Regarding comedo DCIS, there is no uniform agreement among pathologists of exactly how much comedo DCIS needs to be present to consider the lesion a comedo DCIS. Although it is clear that lesions exhibiting a predominant high-grade comedo DCIS pattern are generally more aggressive and more likely to recur if treated conservatively than low-grade noncomedo lesions, architectural subtyping does not reflect current biologic thinking. Rather, it is the concept of nuclear grading that has assumed importance. Nuclear grade is a better biologic predictor than architecture, and therefore, has emerged as a key histopathologic factor for identifying aggressive behavior [32, 35–39]. In 1995, the Van Nuys Group introduced a new pathologic DCIS classification [40] based on the presence or absence of high nuclear grade and comedo-type necrosis (the Van Nuys Classification).

The Van Nuys Group chose high nuclear grade as the most important factor in their classification because there was general agreement that patients with high nuclear grade lesions were more likely to recur at a higher rate and in a shorter time period after breast conservation than patients with low nuclear grade lesions [32, 35, 38, 41–43]. Comedo-type necrosis was chosen because its presence also suggests a poorer prognosis [44, 45] and it is easy to recognize [46].

To use the Van Nuys DCIS Classification, the pathologist, using standardized criteria as noted below, first determines whether the lesion is high nuclear grade (nuclear grade 3) or non-high nuclear grade (nuclear grades I or II). Then, the presence or absence of necrosis is assessed in the non-high-grade lesions. This results in three groups (Fig. 15.1).

Nuclear grade is scored by previously described methods [32, 38, 40]. Essentially, low-grade nuclei (grade 1) are defined as nuclei 1–1.5 red blood cells in diameter with diffuse chromatin and unapparent nucleoli. Intermediate nuclei (grade 2) are defined as nuclei 1–2 red blood cells in diameter with coarse chromatin and infrequent nucleoli. High-grade nuclei (grade 3) are defined as nuclei with a diameter

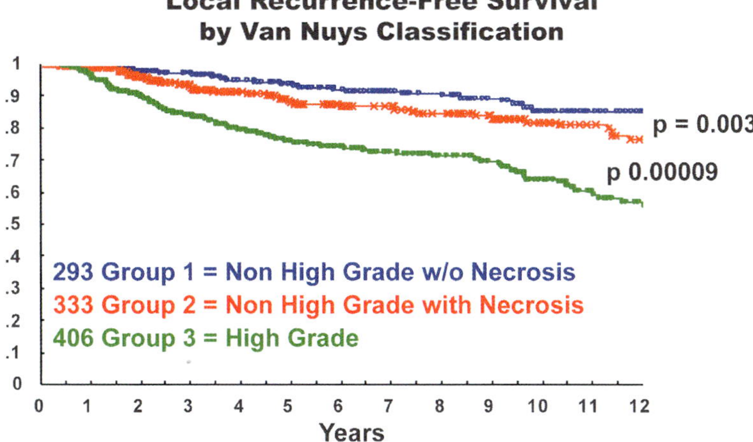

Fig. 15.2 Probability of local recurrence-free survival for 1,046 breast conservation patients using Van Nuys DCIS pathologic classification

greater than two red blood cells, with vesicular chromatin, and one or more nucleoli. Mitotic activity is usually identifiable in high grade DCIS, but infrequently in lower grades I and II.

In the Van Nuys classification, no requirement is made for a minimum or specific amount of high nuclear grade DCIS, nor is any requirement made for a minimum amount of comedo-type necrosis. Occasional desquamated or individually necrotic cells are ignored and are not scored as comedo-type necrosis.

The most difficult part of most classifications is nuclear grading, particularly the intermediate grade lesions. The subtleties of the intermediate grade lesion are not important to the Van Nuys classification; only nuclear grade 3 need be recognized. The cells must be large and pleomorphic, lack architectural differentiation and polarity, have prominent nucleoli and coarse clumped chromatin, and generally show mitoses [32, 40, 44].

The Van Nuys classification is useful because it divides DCIS into three different biologic groups with different risks of local recurrence after breast conservation therapy (Fig. 15.2). This pathologic classification, when combined with tumor size, age, and margin status, is an integral part of the USC/Van Nuys Prognostic Index (USC/VNPI), a system that will be discussed in detail.

Progression to Invasive Breast Cancer

Which DCIS lesions will become invasive and when will that happen? These are the most important questions in the DCIS field today. Currently, there is intense molecular biologic study regarding the progression of genetic changes in normal breast epithelium to DCIS and then to invasive breast cancer. Most of the genetic and epigenetic changes present in invasive breast cancer are already present in DCIS. To date, no genes uniquely associated with invasive cancer have been identified. As DCIS progresses to invasive breast cancer, quantitative changes in the expression of genes related to angiogenesis, adhesion, cell motility, and the composition of the extracellular-matrix may occur [2, 16].

Immunohistochemical and Molecular Phenotypes in DCIS

It has been recognized for some time that there is a substantial concordance between the grade of a DCIS and its associated invasive carcinoma, such that low grade lesions, regardless of the classification scheme used, are largely associated with lower grade invasive carcinomas while high grade DCIS are associated with higher grade invasive carcinomas. Additionally the frequency of specific biomarkers in DCIS varies with the grade of the lesion: estrogen and progesterone receptors are usually expressed in DCIS, but less so in high grade DCIS, while HER-2 and elevated proliferative markers such as Ki-67 are features of high grade DCIS. More recently surrogate molecular phenotypes defined by immunohistochemistry have identified DCIS phenotypes corresponding to luminal A, luminal B, Her-2 and triple negative/basal phenotypes in invasive breast cancer. Luminal A and B DCIS phenotypes are more frequent in the low = intermediate grade lesions, where HER-2, triple negative and basal phenotypes are more common among high grade DCIS [47, 48].

Currently gene expression profiling for invasive carcinomas can segregate carcinomas at significantly different risks of distant relapse (10 years) and indicate the likelihood of a benefit from chemotherapy. Hannemann et al. were able to segregate DCIS with and without invasive carcinomas by a group of 35 genes, and stratify DCIS by another 43 gene classifer into well differentiated vs. poorly differentiated (high grade) subtypes [49]. Additionally these authors confirmed the association of ER expression in low-intermediate DCIS and HER-2 in high grade DCIS.

Solin et al. presented a new DCIS gene signature RT-PCR assay which can separate out three risk groups based on their gene expression profiles [50]. The genes were selected from the existing Oncotype DX assay and the ECOG 5194 registration trial archived tissue was used for validation. The ECOG trial examined the frequencies of local recurrences in DCIS patients treated by excision alone with minimum 3 mm margins. Low to intermediate grade DCIS had to be 25 mm or less in greatest extent, while high grade DCIS could not exceed 10 mm.

All patients entered into the trial had to have specimens examined by a serial sequential tissue protocol which permits reproducible determination of size (extent), margin widths and excludes microinvasive foci. Cases which did not meet these criteria were excluded. Specimens examined by less rigorous means cannot be reliably evaluated by the assay, e.g., the DCIS may exceed the size limit or exhibit margins which are suboptimal and the RS reported may not be valid for the case submitted. By way of contrast two recent nomograms designed to predict recurrence following breast conservation therapy for DCIS were based on archival materials which were not processed in the serial sequential method and for which data on size and margins was frequently missing. Kerlikowski et al. evaluated specimens which were generated from many institutions without a common protocol, and without accurately determined size or margin status [51]. Rudloff et al. developed a nomogram which was obtained from a single institution but without a single protocol and not examined by the serial subgross technique [52].

The ECOG study dichotomized DCIS into low intermediate vs. high grade and only required a 3 mm margin. It will remain to be seen whether reanalysis of the pathology data will permit greater separation of subsets of DCIS comparable to what can be achieved in the USC/VNPI.

Because most patients with DCIS had been treated with mastectomy, knowledge of the natural history of this disease is relatively recent. The studies of Page et al. [53, 54] and Rosen et al. [55] provide information regarding the outcome of low grade DCIS without treatment. In these studies, patients with noncomedo DCIS, the majority, incidental foci in diagnostic excision biopsies for palpable disease, were initially misdiagnosed as benign lesions and therefore went untreated, aside from initial biopsy. Subsequently, approximately 25–35 % of these patients developed invasive breast cancer, generally within 10 years [53, 54]. Had the lesions been high-grade comedo DCIS, the invasive breast cancer rate likely would have been higher than 35 % and the time to invasive recurrence shorter. With few exceptions, in both of these studies, the invasive breast carcinoma was of the ductal type and located at the site of the original DCIS. These findings suggest that not all DCIS lesions progress to invasive breast cancer or become clinically significant [56]

Page and associates updated their series in 2002 and 2005 [53, 54, 57]. Of 28 women with low-grade DCIS misdiagnosed as benign lesions and treated only by biopsy between 1950 and 1968, 11 patients have recurred locally with invasive breast cancer (39 %). Eight patients developed recurrence within the first 12 years. The remaining three were diagnosed over 23–42 years. Five patients developed metastatic breast cancer (18 %) and died from the disease within 7 years of developing invasive breast cancer. These recurrence and mortality rates, at first glance, seem alarmingly high. However, they are only slightly worse than what can be expected with long-term follow-up of patients with lobular carcinoma in situ, a disease that most clinicians are willing to treat with careful clinical follow-up. In addition, these patients were treated with biopsy only. No attempt was made to excise these lesions with a clear surgical margin. The natural history of low-grade DCIS can extend over 40 years and is markedly different from that of high-grade DCIS.

Microinvasion

The incidence of microinvasion is difficult to quantitate because until 1997 there was no formal and universally accepted definition of exactly what constitutes microinvasion. The fifth edition of *The Manual for Cancer Staging* carried the first official definition of what is now classified as pT1mic and read as follows: "Microinvasion is the extension of cancer cells beyond the basement membrane into adjacent tissues with no focus more than 0.1 cm in greatest dimension. When there are multiple foci of microinvasion the size of only the largest focus is used to classify the microinvasion (do not use the sum of all individual foci). The presence of multiple foci of microinvasion should be noted, as it is with multiple larger invasive carcinomas."

The reported incidence of occult invasion (invasive disease at mastectomy in patients with a biopsy diagnosis of DCIS) varies greatly, ranging from as little as 2 % to as much as 21 % [58]. This problem was addressed in the investigations of Lagios et al. [32, 38].

Lagios et al. performed a meticulous serial subgross dissection correlated with specimen radiography. Occult invasion was found in 13 of 111 mastectomy specimens from patients who had initially undergone excisional biopsy of DCIS. All occult invasive cancers were associated with DCIS greater than 45 mm in extent; the incidence of occult invasion approached 50 % for DCIS greater than 55 mm. In the study of Gump et al. [59], foci of occult invasion were found in 11 % of patients with palpable DCIS but in no patients with clinically occult DCIS. These results suggest a correlation between the size of the DCIS lesion and the incidence of occult invasion. Clearly, as the size of the DCIS lesion increases, microinvasion and occult invasion become more likely.

If even the smallest amount of invasion is found, the lesion should not be classified as DCIS. It is a T1mic (if the largest invasive component is 1 mm or less) with an extensive intraductal component (EIC). If the invasive component is 1.1 mm to 5 mm, it is a T1a lesion with EIC. If there is only a single focus of invasion, these patients do quite well. When there are many tiny foci of invasion, these patients have a poorer prognosis than expected [10]. Unfortunately, the TNM staging system does not have a T category that fully reflects the malignant potential of lesions with multiple foci of invasion since they are all classified by the largest single focus of invasion. De Mascarel et al. have noted that microinvasive foci consisting of single cells have no impact on outcome while those comprising cohesive groups of cells are associated with a demonstrable increase in distant recurrence and death [60].

Multicentricity and Multifocality of Ductal Carcinoma In Situ

Multicentricity is generally defined as DCIS in a quadrant other than the quadrant in which the original DCIS (index quadrant) was diagnosed. There must be normal breast tissue separating the two foci. However, definitions of multicentricity vary among investigators. Hence, the reported incidence of multicentricity also varies. Rates from 0 to 78 % [7, 55, 61, 62], averaging about 30 %, have been reported. Twenty-five years ago, the 30 % average rate of multicentricity was used by surgeons as the rationale for mastectomy in patients with DCIS.

Holland et al. [63] evaluated 82 mastectomy specimens by taking a whole-organ section every 5 mm. Each section was radiographed. Paraffin blocks were made from every radiographically suspicious spot. In addition, an average of 25 blocks were taken from the quadrant containing the index cancer; random samples were taken from all other quadrants, the central subareolar area, and the nipple. The microscopic extension of each lesion was verified on the radiographs. This technique permitted a three-dimensional reconstruction of each lesion. This study demonstrated that most DCIS lesions were larger than expected (50 % were greater than 50 mm), involved more than one quadrant by continuous extension (23 %), but most importantly, were unicentric (98.8 %). Only one of 82 mastectomy specimens (1.2 %) had "true" multicentric distribution with a separate lesion in a different quadrant. This study suggests that complete excision of a DCIS lesion is possible due to unicentricity but may be extremely difficult due to larger than expected size. In a recent update, Holland reported whole-organ studies in 119 patients, 118 of whom had unicentric disease [64]. This information, when combined with the fact that most local recurrences are at or near the original DCIS, suggests that the problem of multicentricity per se is not important in the DCIS treatment decision-making process.

Multifocality is defined as separate foci of DCIS within the same ductal system. The studies of Holland et al. [63, 64] and Noguchi et al. [65] suggest that a great deal of multifocality may be artifactual, resulting from looking at a three-dimensional arborizing entity in two dimensions on a glass slide. It would be analogous to saying that the branches of a tree were not connected if the branches were cut at one plane, placed separately on a slide, and viewed in cross-section [53]. Multifocality may be due to small gaps of DCIS or skip areas within ducts as described by Faverly et al. [43]. Multifocality is more easity recognized when a serial sequential tissue processing technique as opposed to random sampling is employed.

Detection and Diagnosis

The importance of quality mammography cannot be overemphasized. Currently, most patients with DCIS (more than 90 %) present with a nonpalpable lesion detected by mammography. The most common mammographic finding is microcalcification, frequently clustered and generally without an associated soft-tissue abnormality. More than 80 % of DCIS patients exhibit microcalcifications on preoperative mammography. The patterns of these microcalcifications may be focal, diffuse, or ductal, with variable size and shape. Patients with comedo DCIS tend to have "casting calcifications." These are linear, branching, and bizarre and are almost pathognomonic for comedo DCIS [66] (Fig. 15.3). It is important to note that many DCIS with prominent comedonecrosis fail to exhibit mammographic microcalcifications, and among others, microcalcification is seen only intermittently.

Thirty-two percent of noncomedo lesions in this series did not have mammographic calcifications, making them more difficult to find and the patients more difficult to follow, if treated conservatively. When noncomedo lesions are calcified, they tend to have fine granular powdery calcifications or crushed stone-like calcifications (Fig. 15.4).

A major problem confronting surgeons relates to the fact that calcifications do not always map out the entire DCIS lesion, particularly those of the noncomedo

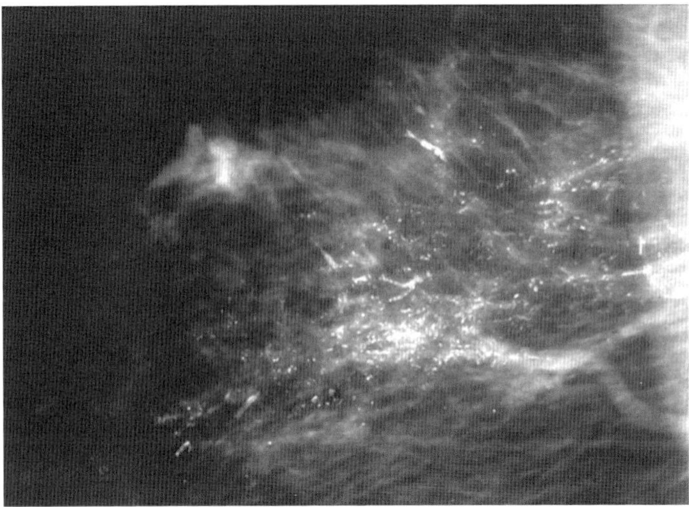

Fig. 15.3 Mediolateral mammography in a 43-year-old woman shows irregular branching calcifications. Histopathology showed high-grade comedo DCIS, Van Nuys group 3

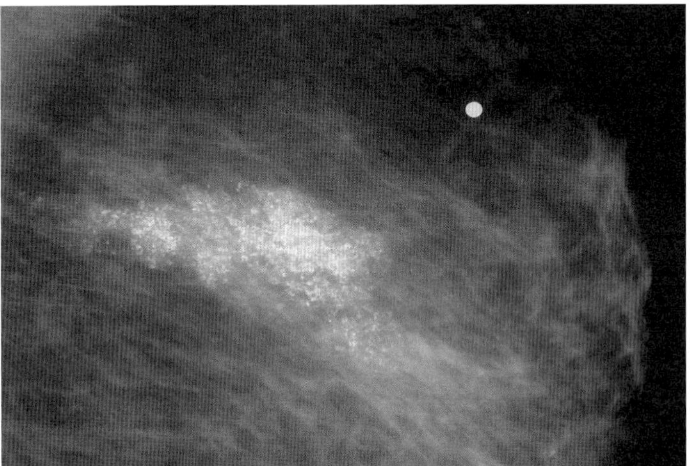

Fig. 15.4 Crushed stone type calcifications

type. Even though all the calcifications are removed, in some cases, noncalcified DCIS may be left behind. Conversely, in some patients, the majority of the calcifications are benign and map out a lesion bigger than the true DCIS lesion. In other words, the DCIS lesion may be smaller, larger, or the same size as the calcifications that lead to its identification. Calcifications more accurately approximate the size of high-grade comedo lesions than low-grade noncomedo lesions [63].

Before mammography was common or of good quality, most DCIS was usually clinically apparent, diagnosed by palpation or inspection; it was gross disease. Gump et al. divided DCIS by method of diagnosis into gross and microscopic disease [59]. Similarly, Schwartz et al. divided DCIS into two groups: clinical and subclinical [33]. Both researchers thought patients presenting with a palpable mass, a nipple discharge, or Paget's disease of the nipple required more aggressive treatment. Schwartz believed that palpable DCIS should be treated as though it were an invasive lesion. He suggested that the pathologist simply has not found the area of invasion. Although it makes perfect sense to believe that the change from nonpalpable to palpable disease is a poor prognostic sign, our group has not been able to demonstrate this for DCIS. In our series, when equivalent patients (by size and nuclear grade) with palpable and nonpalpable DCIS were compared, they did not differ in the rate of local recurrence or mortality.

If a patient's mammogram shows an abnormality, most likely, it will be microcalcifications, but it could be a nonpalpable mass or an architectural distortion. At this point, additional radiologic workup needs to be performed. This generally includes compression mammography and magnification views. Ultrasonography should be performed on all calcifications that require biopsy to rule out the presence of a mass that can be biopsied with ultrasound guidance. Magnetic resonance imaging (MRI) has become increasingly popular and if often used to map out the size and shape of biopsy proven DCIS lesions or invasive breast cancers and to rule out other foci of multifocal, multicentric or contralateral cancer.

Biopsy and Tissue Handling

If radiologic work-up shows an occult lesion that requires biopsy, there are multiple approaches: fine-needle aspiration biopsy (FNAB), core biopsy (with various types and sizes of needles), and directed surgical biopsy using guide wires or radioactive localization. FNAB is generally of little help for nonpalpable DCIS. With FNAB, it is possible to obtain cancer cells, but because there is insufficient tissue, there is no architecture. So, although the cytopathologist can say that malignant cells are present, the cytopathologist cannot say whether or not the lesion is invasive.

Stereotactic core biopsy became available in the early 1990s, and is now widely used. Dedicated digital tables make this a precise tool. Currently large gauge vacuum assisted needles are the tools of choice for diagnosing DCIS. Ultrasound guided biopsy also became popular in the 1990s but is of less value for DCIS since most DCIS lesions do not present with a mass that can be visualized by ultrasound. All suspicious microcalcifications should be evaluated by ultrasound since a mass will be found in 5–15 % [9].

Open surgical biopsy should only be used if the lesion cannot be biopsied using minimally invasive techniques. This should be a rare event with current image-guided biopsy techniques and occur in less than 5 % of cases [9, 67]. Currently, at Hoag Memorial Hospital Presbyterian, open biopsy is performed for diagnostic purposes in only 1 % of patients and we treat more than 700 new breast cancer patients per year. Needle localization segmental resection should be a critical part of the treatment regimen not the diagnosis [67].

Whenever needle localization excision is performed, whether for diagnosis or treatment, intraoperative specimen radiography and correlation with the preoperative mammogram are mandatory. Margins should be inked or dyed and specimens should be serially sectioned and a second X-ray of the slices should be obtained. The tissue sections should be arranged and processed in sequence. Pathologic reporting should include a description of all architectural subtypes, a determination of nuclear grade, an assessment of the presence or absence of necrosis, the measured extent of the lesion, and the margin status with measurement of all margins and, in particular, the closest margin [68–70].

Tumor size should be determined by direct measurement or ocular micrometry from stained slides for smaller lesions. For larger lesions, a combination of direct measurement and estimation, based on the distribution of the lesion in a sequential series of slides, should be used. The proximity of DCIS to an inked margin should be determined by direct measurement or ocular micrometry. The closest single distance between any involved duct containing DCIS and an inked margin should be reported.

If the lesion is large and the diagnosis unproven, either stereotactic or ultrasound-guided vacuum-assisted biopsy should be the first step. If the patient is motivated for breast conservation, a multiple-wire-directed oncoplastic excision can be planned. This will give the patient her best chance at two opposing goals: clear margins and good cosmesis. The best chance at completely removing a large lesion is with a large initial excision. The best chance at good cosmesis is with a small initial excision. It is the surgeon's job to optimize these opposing goals. A large quadrant resection should not be performed unless there is histologic proof of malignancy. This type of resection may lead to breast deformity, and should the diagnosis prove to be benign, the patient will have undergone needless surgery.

Removal of nonpalpable lesions is best performed by an integrated team of surgeon, radiologist, and pathologist. The radiologist who places the wires and interprets the specimen radiograph must be experienced, as must the surgeon who removes the lesion, and the pathologist who processes the tissue.

Treatment

For most patients with DCIS, there will be no single correct treatment. There will generally be a choice. The choices, although seemingly simple, are not. As the choices increase and become more complicated, frustration increases for both the patient and her physician [71, 72].

Counseling the Patient with Biopsy-Proven Ductal Carcinoma In Situ

It is never easy to tell a patient that she has breast cancer. But is DCIS really cancer? From a biologic point of view, DCIS is unequivocally cancer. But when we think of cancer, we generally think of a disease that, if untreated, runs an inexorable course toward death. That is certainly not the case with DCIS [54]. We must emphasize to the patient that she has an incomplete cancerous lesion, a preinvasive lesion, which at this time is not a threat to her life. In our series of 1,585 patients with DCIS, the breast cancer specific mortality rate is 0.5 % at 12-years. Numerous other DCIS series [73–78] confirm an extremely low mortality rate.

Patients often ask why there is any mortality rate at all if DCIS is truly a noninvasive lesion. If DCIS recurs as an invasive lesion and the patient goes on to die from metastatic breast cancer, the source of the metastases is clear, the invasive disease. But what about the patient who undergoes mastectomy, only DCIS is found, and sometime later develops metastatic disease or a patient who is treated with breast preservation who never develops a local invasive recurrence but still dies of metastatic breast cancer? The latter patients probably had an invasive focus with established metastases at the time of their original treatment but the invasive focus was missed during routine histopathologic evaluation. Routine examination of mastectomy material is inadequate for patients with DCIS. A more thorough and methodical approach utilizing specimen radiography is required. No matter how carefully and thoroughly a specimen in examined, it is still a sampling process and a small focus of invasion can be missed.

One of the most frequent concerns expressed by patients once a diagnosis of cancer has been made is the fear that the cancer has spread. We are able to assure patients with DCIS that no invasion was seen microscopically and the likelihood of systemic spread is minimal.

The patient needs to be educated that the term "breast cancer" encompasses a wide range of lesions of varying degrees of aggressiveness and lethal potential. The patient with DCIS needs to be reassured that she has a minimal lesion and that she is likely going to need some additional treatment, which may include surgery, radiation therapy, an antiestrogen, or some combination of those modalities. She needs reassurance that she will not need chemotherapy, that her hair will not fall out, and that it is highly unlikely that she will die from this lesion. She will, of course, need careful clinical follow-up.

Endpoints for Patients with DCIS

When evaluating the results of treatment for patients with breast cancer, a variety of endpoints must be considered. Important endpoints include local recurrence (both invasive and DCIS), regional recurrence (such as the axilla), distant recurrence, breast cancer-specific survival, overall survival, and quality of life. The importance of each endpoint varies depending on whether the patient has DCIS or invasive breast cancer

When treating invasive cancer, the most important endpoints are distant recurrence and breast cancer-specific survival; in other words, living or dying from breast cancer. For invasive breast cancer, a variety of different systemic treatments have been shown to significantly improve survival. These include a wide range of chemotherapeutic regimens, endocrine treatments, immunologic therapies, and others. Variations in local treatment were incorrectly thought not to affect survival. [23, 79]. They do, however, affect local recurrence and local invasive recurrence affect survival. Meta-analyses have shown that for every four local recurrences prevented, one breast cancer death is also prevented [80, 81]

DCIS is similar to invasive breast cancer in that variations in local treatment affect local recurrence, but no study to date has shown a significant difference in distant disease-free or breast cancer-specific survival, regardless of any treatment (systemic or local) and no study is likely to show a difference since there are so few breast cancer deaths in patients with pure DCIS. The most important outcome measure, breast cancer-specific survival, is essentially the same no matter what local or systemic treatment is given. Consequently, local recurrence has become the most commonly used endpoint when evaluating treatment for patients with DCIS.

A meta-analysis of four randomized DCIS trials comparing excision plus radiation therapy versus excision alone was published in 2007 [77]. It contained 3,665 patients. Radiation therapy decreased local recurrence by a statistically significant 60 % but overall survival was slightly (but statistically insignificantly) worse in the radiotherapy group with a relative risk of 1.08 These data are dissimilar to those of the Early Breast Cancer Trialists' Collaborative Group and deserve further analysis [80, 81]. Half of the recurrences in the meta-analysis were DCIS and could not possibly affect survival. Of the remaining invasive recurrences, 80–90 % are cured by early detection and treatment. This should result in a slight trend toward a lower survival for the excision alone group just as would be expected from the Early Breast Cancer Trialists' Collaborative Group. But exactly the opposite was seen, a nonsignificant trend toward a better survival in the excision only patients. The authors of the meta-analysis felt that with longer follow-up, the higher local recurrence rate for excision alone will likely result in a lower overall survival at some point in time. But for the time being, that has not happen and a small detrimental effect secondary to radiation therapy must be considered a possibility.

Local recurrences are clearly important to prevent in patients treated with DCIS. They are demoralizing. They often lead to mastectomy and if they are invasive, they upstage the patient and are a threat to life. But protecting DCIS patients from local recurrence must be balanced against the potential detrimental effects of the treatments given.

Following treatment for DCIS, 40–50 % of all local recurrences are invasive. About 10–20 % of DCIS patients who develop local invasive recurrences develop distant metastases and die from breast cancer [82, 83]. Long-term, this could translate into a mortality rate of about 0.5 % for patients treated with mastectomy, 1–2 % for conservatively treated patients who receive radiation therapy (if there is no mortality associated with radiation therapy) and 2–3 % for patients treated with excision alone. In order to save their breasts, many patients are willing to accept this theoretic, and as of now statistically unproven, small absolute risk associated with breast conservation therapy.

Treatment Options

Mastectomy

Mastectomy is, by far, the most effective treatment available for DCIS if our goal is simply to prevent local recurrence. Most mastectomy series reveal local recurrence rates of approximately 1 % with mortality rates close to 0 [84]. In our mastectomy series of 539 patients, none of whom received radiation therapy or tamoxifen, we have had 10 local recurrences (8 invasive and 2 DCIS). One of the patients with an invasive local recurrence developed metastatic disease. In addition, two other patients developed metastatic breast cancer without developing a local recurrence. The absolute rate of distant recurrence was 0.6 %.

But, mastectomy is an aggressive form of treatment for patients with DCIS. It clearly provides a local recurrence benefit but only a theoretical survival benefit. It is, therefore, often difficult to justify mastectomy, particularly for otherwise healthy women with screen-detected DCIS, during an era of increasing utilization of breast conservation for invasive breast carcinoma. Mastectomy is indicated in cases of true multicentricity (multi-quadrant disease) and when a unicentric DCIS lesion is too large to excise with clear margins and an acceptable cosmetic result.

Genetic positivity for one of the breast cancer associated genes (BRCA1, BRCA2) is not an absolute contraindication to breast preservation but many patients who are genetically positive and who develop DCIS seriously consider bilateral mastectomy and salpingo-oophorectomy.

Breast Conservation

The most recently available Surveillance Epidemiology and End Results (SEER) data reveal that 74 % of patients with DCIS are treated with breast conservation. While breast conservation is now widely accepted as the treatment of choice for DCIS, not all patients are good candidates. Certainly, there are patients with DCIS whose local recurrence rate with breast preservation is so high (based on factors that will be discussed later in this chapter) that mastectomy is clearly a more appropriate treatment. However, the majority of women with DCIS diagnosed currently are candidates for breast conservation. Clinical trials have shown that local excision and radiation therapy in patients with negative margins can provide excellent rates of local control [73, 76–78, 85–88]. However, even radiation therapy may be overly aggressive since many cases of DCIS may not recur or progress to invasive carcinoma when treated by excision alone [32, 54, 89–93].

Reasons to Consider Excision Alone

There are a number of lines of reasoning that suggest that excision alone may be an acceptable treatment for selected patients with DCIS.

1. Common Usage: Excision alone is already common in spite of the randomized data that suggest that all conservatively treated patients benefit from radiation therapy. SEER Data reflect that excision alone is being used as complete treatment for DCIS in 35 % of all DCIS patients. American doctors and patients have embraced the concept of excision alone for DCIS.
2. Anatomic: Evaluation of mastectomy specimens using the serial subgross tissue processing technique reveals that most DCIS is unicentric (involves a single

breast segment and is radial in its distribution [39, 43, 63, 64, 94, 95]. Using the same technique and evaluating patients with small extent disease (≤25 mm) more clearly established that the majority of image detected DCIS can be adequately excised [32, 38]. This means that in many cases, it is possible to excise the entire lesion with a segment or quadrant resection. Since DCIS, by definition, is not invasive and has not metastasized, it can be thought of in Halstedian terms. Complete excision should cure the patient without any additional therapy. Holland and Faverly have shown that if 10 mm margins are achieved in all directions, the likelihood of residual DCIS is less than 10 % [43].

3. Biologic: Some DCIS is simply not aggressive, for example small well-excised low-grade lesions bordering on atypical ductal hyperplasia. Lesions like this carry a low potential for development into an invasive lesion, about 1 % per year at most [53, 54, 57, 89, 96, 97]. This is only slightly more than lobular carcinoma in situ (LCIS), a lesion that is routinely treated with careful clinical follow-up.
4. Pathology Errors: The differences between atypical ductal hyperplasia and low grade DCIS may be subtle. It is not uncommon for atypical ductal hyperplasia to be called DCIS. Such patients treated with excision and radiation therapy are indeed "cured of their DCIS".
5. Prospective Randomized Data: the prospective randomized DCIS trials show no difference in breast cancer-specific survival or overall survival, regardless of treatment after excision with or without breast irradiation [73, 76–78, 88]. If this is true, why not strive for the least aggressive treatment?
6. Radiotherapy may do harm: Numerous studies have shown that radiation therapy for breast cancer may increase mortality from both lung cancer and cardiovascular disease [98–102]. Current radiotherapy techniques, which make use of CT planning, make every attempt to spare the heart and lungs from radiation exposure but long-term date are not available. If there is no proof that breast irradiation for patients with DCIS improves survival and there is proof that radiation therapy may cause harm, it makes perfect sense to spare patients from this potentially dangerous treatment whenever possible.
7. Radiation therapy is expensive, time consuming, and is accompanied by significant side effects in a small percentage of patients (cardiac, pulmonary, etc.) [103]. Radiation fibrosis continues to occur but it is less common with current techniques than it was during the 1980s. Radiation fibrosis changes the texture of the breast and skin, makes mammographic follow-up more difficult, and may result in delayed diagnosis if there is a local recurrence. This will become much less of a problem if intraoperative radiation therapy (IORT) becomes a proven modality for DCIS [104].
8. Some series show that there are more invasive recurrences in irradiated patients than in nonirradiated patients. In our own series, 39 % of excision only patients who recurred, recurred with invasive disease whereas 56 % of irradiated patients who recurred, recurred with invasive disease ($p<0.01$). This is true in the series of Schwartz et al. [92] and Wong et al. [105]. In our series, the median time to

recur after excision alone was 23 months while after excision and irradiation, it was 58 months ($p<0.01$). This delay in the diagnosis of recurrence may contribute to the increased rate of local invasive recurrence in irradiated patients.

9. If radiation therapy is given for the initial DCIS, it cannot be given again, at a later time, if there is a small invasive recurrence. In general, in favorable patients, we prefer to withhold radiation therapy initially and only give it to the few that ultimately recur with invasive disease. The use of radiation therapy with its accompanying skin and vascular changes make skin-sparing mastectomy, if needed in the future, more difficult to perform.
10. Using commonly available histopathologic parameters, we can do better than the gold standard for local recurrence established by the prospective randomized trials. The "gold standard" for irradiated patients is a 16 % local recurrence rate at 12 years. This was established by the NSABP B-17 Trial [73, 85–87, 106]. Using tools such as the USC/Van Nuys Prognostic Index, it is possible to select patients with low scores ranging from 4 to 6. These patients recur at a rate of 6 % or less at 12 years without radiation therapy.
11. Finally, within the 2008 NCCN (National Comprehensive Cancer Network) Guidelines, excision without radiation therapy (excision alone) has been added as an acceptable treatment for selected DCIS patients with low risk of recurrence [107]. Excision alone is now accepted and mainstream for favorable patients with DCIS

Distant Disease and Death

When a patient with DCIS, previously treated by any modality, develops a local invasive recurrence, followed by distant disease and death due to breast cancer, this stepwise progression makes sense. The patient has been upstaged by her local invasive recurrence. The invasive recurrence becomes the source of metastatic disease and death is now a possibility.

In contrast, when a previously treated patient with DCIS develops distant disease and there has been no invasive local recurrence, a completely different sequence of events must be postulated. This sequence implies that invasive disease was present within the original lesion but was never discovered and was already metastatic at the time of the original diagnosis. The best way to avoid missing an invasive cancer is with complete sequential tissue processing at the time the original lesion is treated. Nevertheless, even the most extensive evaluation may miss a small focus of invasion.

If, during histopathologic evaluation, even the tiniest invasive component is found, this patient can no longer be classified as having DCIS. She has invasive breast cancer and she needs to be treated as such. She will need sentinel node biopsy, radiation therapy if treated conservatively, and appropriate medical oncologic consultation and aftercare.

The Prospective Randomized Trials

All of the prospective randomized trials have shown a significant reduction in local recurrence for patients treated with radiation therapy compared with excision alone but no trial has reported a survival benefit, regardless of treatment [73, 76, 77, 85–88, 106, 108–111].

Only one trial has compared mastectomy with breast conservation for patients with DCIS and the data were only incidentally accrued. The National Surgical Adjuvant Breast Project (NSABP) performed protocol B-06, a prospective randomized trial for patients with invasive breast cancer [61, 112]. There were three treatment arms: total mastectomy, excision of the tumor plus radiation therapy, and excision alone. Axillary nodes were removed regardless of the treatment assignment.

During central slide review, a subgroup of 78 patients was confirmed to have pure DCIS without any evidence of invasion [61]. After 83 months of follow-up, the percent of patients with local recurrences were as follows: zero for mastectomy, 7 % for excision plus radiation therapy, and 43 % for excision alone [113]. In spite of these large differences in the rate of local recurrence for each different treatment, there was no difference among the three treatment groups in breast cancer-specific survival.

Contrary to the lack of trials comparing mastectomy with breast conservation, a number of prospective randomized trials comparing excision plus radiation therapy with excision alone for patients with DCIS have been performed: the NSABP (protocol B-17) [85], the European Organization for Research and Treatment of Cancer (EORTC), protocol 10,853 [88], the United Kingdom, Australia, New Zealand DCIS Trial (UK Trial) [76], and the Swedish Trial [78].

The results of NSABP B-17 were updated in 1995 [109], 1998; [87], 1999 [86], 2001 [73] and 2011 [106]. In this study, more than 800 patients with DCIS excised with clear surgical margins were randomized into two groups: excision alone versus excision plus radiation therapy. The main endpoint of the study was local recurrence, invasive or noninvasive (DCIS). The definition of a clear margin was non-transection of the DCIS.

After 15 years of follow-up, there was a statistically significant, 50 % decrease in local recurrence of both DCIS and invasive breast cancer in patients treated with radiation therapy. The overall local recurrence rate for patients treated by excision alone was 35 % at 15 years. For patients treated with excision plus breast irradiation, it was 19.8 %, a relative benefit of 43 % [106]. There was no difference in distant disease-free or overall survival in either arm. These data led the NSABP to confirm their 1993 position and to continue to recommend postoperative radiation therapy for all patients with DCIS who chose to save their breasts. This recommendation was clearly based primarily on the decreased local recurrence rate for those treated with radiation therapy and secondarily on the potential survival advantage it might confer.

The early results of B-17, in favor of radiation therapy for patients with DCIS, led the NSABP to perform protocol B-24 [86]. In this trial, more than 1,800 patients with DCIS were treated with excision and radiation therapy, and then randomized to receive either tamoxifen or placebo. After 15 years of follow-up, 16.6 % of patients treated with placebo had recurred locally, whereas, only 13.2 % of those treated with tamoxifen had recurred [106]. The difference, while small, was statistically significant for invasive local recurrence but not for noninvasive (DCIS) recurrence. A recent analysis of the subset of B24 patients known to be estrogen receptor-positive has shown no significant difference in ipsilateral in situ or invasive recurrence [114]. Again, there was no difference in distant disease-free or overall survival in either arm of the B-24 Trial.

The EORTC results were published in 2000 [88, 108]. This study was essentially identical to B-17 in design and margin definition. More than 1,000 patients were included. The data were updated in 2006 [110]. After 10 years of follow-up, 15 % of patients treated with excision plus radiation therapy had recurred locally compared with 26 % of patients treated with excision alone, results similar to those obtained by the NSABP at the same point in their trial. As in the B-17 Trial, there was no difference in distant disease-free or overall survival in either arm of the EORTC Trial. In the initial report, there was a statistically significant increase in contralateral breast cancer in patients who were randomized to receive radiation therapy. This was not maintained when the data were updated.

The United Kingdom, Australia, New Zealand DCIS Trial (UK Trial) was published in 2003 [76] and updated in 2011 [111]. This trial, which involved more than 1,694 patients, performed a two by two study in which patients could be randomized into two separate trials within a trial. The patients and their doctors chose whether to be randomized in one or both studies. After excision with clear margins (same non-transection definition as the NSABP), patients were randomized to receive radiotherapy (yes or no) and/or to tamoxifen versus placebo. This yielded four subgroups: excision alone, excision plus radiation therapy, excision plus tamoxifen, and excision plus radiation therapy plus tamoxifen. After a median follow-up of 12.7 years, those who received radiation therapy obtained a statistically significant decrease in ipsilateral breast tumor recurrence similar in magnitude to the ones shown by the NSABP and EORTC. Tamoxifen significantly reduced the incidence of ipsilateral DCIS recurrences but not invasive recurrences. It reduced the incidence of new contralateral breast cancers in a magnitude similar to NSABP B-24. As with the NSABP and the EORTC, there was no difference in survival, regardless of treatment, in any arm of the UK DCIS trial.

The Swedish DCIS Trial randomized 1,067 patients into two groups: excision alone versus excision plus radiation therapy. 1,046 have been followed for a mean of 8 years. Microscopically clear margins were not mandatory. 22 % of patients had microscopically unknown or involved margins. The cumulative incidence of local recurrence at 10-years was 21.6 % for excision only and 10.3 % for excision plus radiation therapy. There were 15 distant metastases and breast cancer related deaths in the excision only arm and 18 in the excision plus radiation therapy (p=ns) [78, 115].

All of these trials support the same conclusions. They all show that radiation therapy decreases local recurrence by a relative 50 % and they all show no survival benefit, regardless of treatment. Two trials show a decrease in local recurrence and contralateral breast cancer attributable to tamoxifen.

In 2007, Viani et al. published a meta-analysis of the four prospective randomized DCIS trials comparing excision alone with excision plus radiation therapy [77]. Three thousand six hundred and sixty-five patients were available for analysis. Pooled data revealed a 60 % reduction of both invasive and DCIS recurrences ($p<0.00001$) with the addition of radiation therapy. There was, however, no decrease in distant metastases in those who received radiation therapy nor was there any survival benefit. Patients with high-grade lesions and involved margins received the most benefit from radiation therapy.

Limitations of the Prospective Randomized Trials

The randomized trials were designed to answer a single broad question: does radiation therapy decrease local recurrence? They have accomplished that goal. All have clearly shown that, overall, radiation therapy decreases local recurrence, but they cannot identify in which subgroups the benefit is so small, that the patients can be safely treated with excision alone.

Many of the parameters considered important in predicting local recurrence (tumor size, margin width, nuclear grade, etc.) were not routinely collected prospectively during the randomized DCIS trials. In addition, the trials did not specifically require the marking of margins or the measurement of margin width. The exact measurement of margin width was present in only 5 % of the EORTC pathology reports [108]. The NSABP did not require size measurements and many of their pathologic data were determined by retrospective slide review. In the initial NSABP report, more than 40 % of patients had no size measurement [85]. Unfortunately, if margins were not inked and tissues not completely sampled and sequentially submitted, then these predictive data can never be determined accurately by retrospective review.

The relative reduction in local recurrence seems to be the same in all four trials—about 50–60 % for any given subgroup at any point in time. What does this relative reduction mean? If the absolute local recurrence rate is 30 % at 10 years for a given subgroup of patients treated with excision alone, radiation therapy will reduce this rate by approximately 50 %, leaving a group of patients with a 15 % local recurrence rate at 10 years. Radiation therapy seems indicated for a subgroup with such a high local recurrence rate. But consider a more favorable subgroup, a group of patients with a 6–8 % absolute recurrence rate at 10 years. These patients receive only a 3–4 % absolute benefit. We must irradiate 100 women to see a 3–4 % decrease in local recurrence. Here, we must ask whether the benefits are worth the risks and costs involved.

Radiation therapy is expensive, time consuming, and is accompanied by significant side effects in a small percentage of patients (cardiac, pulmonary, etc.) [103]. Radiation fibrosis continues to occur but it is less common with current techniques than it was in the past. Radiation fibrosis changes the texture of the breast and skin, makes mammographic follow-up more difficult, and may result in delayed diagnosis if there is a local recurrence. The use of radiation therapy for DCIS precludes its use if an invasive recurrence develops at a later date. The use of radiation therapy with its accompanying skin and vascular changes make skin-sparing mastectomy, if needed in the future, more difficult to perform.

Most importantly, if we give radiation therapy for DCIS, we must assume all of these risks and costs without any proven distant disease-free or breast cancer specific survival benefits. The only proven benefit will be a decrease in local recurrence. It is important, therefore, to carefully examine the need for radiation therapy in all conservatively treated patients with DCIS. The NSABP has agreed that all patients with DCIS may not need postexcisional radiation therapy [73]. The problem is how to accurately identify those patients. If we can identify subgroups of patients with DCIS in which the probability of local recurrence after excision alone is low, they may be the patients where the costs, risks, and side effects of radiotherapy outweigh the benefits.

In spite of the randomized data, which suggest that all conservatively treated patients benefit from radiation therapy, American doctors and patients have embraced the concept of excision alone. 2003 Surveillance Epidemiology and End Results (SEER) data reveal that 74 % of patients with DCIS were treated with breast conservation. Almost half of these conservatively treated patients were treated with excision alone. When all patients with DCIS are considered, 26 % received mastectomy, 39 % excision plus radiation therapy, and 35 % were treated with excision alone. It is clear that both American doctors and American patients are not blindly following the results and the recommendations of the prospective trials. Based on data and treatment trends, in 2008, the NCCN (National Comprehensive Cancer Network) added excision alone as an alternative treatment for patients with favorable DCIS and has maintained the recommendation in all yearly updates [107].

A prerequisite to calculation of the USC/VNPI is a reproducible method of determining the size or extent of DCIS in any surgical resection and evaluating margin widths. Additionally, since any focus of invasion would change the classification, great care to exclude microinvasion must be utilized in examining the resected tissue. Earlier studies [13, 32, 38] and the Van Nuys database from its inception have employed a serial subgross sequential method of tissue examination. Briefly, this requires that an oriented, selectively inked resection is sliced into uniformly thick segments and that specimen radiography is employed again to evaluate these segments. These are then processed in sequence in specifically identified cassettes to permit a three-dimensional reconstruction of the extent of disease and to thoroughly evaluate any margin involvement.

Although this approach for DCIS is now the recommended protocol of the College of American Pathologists [68, 116], this was not the case in the late 1970s through most of the 1990s. There was a great reluctance to expend pathology resources and professional time on an approach that was not seen as useful, but rather as a cost drain.

Defining a process as DCIS alone; that is, without invasion, and calculating the size and margin width is only possible for a resection that is entirely processed. The inability of the randomized trials to replicate the USC/VNPI is a reflection of the predominant pathologic technique employed by them—partial sampling. The latter approach works reasonably well for larger invasive carcinomas, but cannot determine size or margin width for a microscopic grossly invisible lesion which often exhibits an intermittent distribution within the resection and only focally demonstrates microcalcification. The randomized trials of DCIS were not empowered to define prognostic factors that are widely recognized as pertinent for DCIS. Additionally, the USC/VNPI is based on careful mammographic or other imaging correlation with the pathology, an approach which was largely missing from the prospective trial protocols [73, 76, 77, 85–88, 106, 108–111].

Many retrospective attempts to evaluate the USC/VNPI and some recent prospective studies [105] also fail because of their inability to precisely define the prognostic factors; i.e., the lack of an adequate pathologic approach. In fact, the current practice standards for mammographically detected and excised DCIS were not met by any of the randomized trials.

Predicting Local Recurrence in Conservatively Treated Patients with DCIS

There is now sufficient, readily available information that can aid clinicians in differentiating patients who significantly benefit from radiation therapy after excision from those who do not. These same data can point out patients who are better served by mastectomy because recurrence rates with breast conservation are unacceptably high even with the addition of radiation therapy.

Our research [32, 36, 38, 40, 97, 117, 118] and the research of others [35, 44, 90, 91, 109, 119] has shown that various combinations of nuclear grade, the presence of comedo-type necrosis, tumor size, margin width, and age are all important factors that can be used to predict the probability of local recurrence in conservatively treated patients with DCIS.

The Original Van Nuys Prognostic Index (VNPI) and Its Updated Version, the USC/VNPI

In 1995, the Van Nuys DCIS pathologic classification, based on nuclear grade and the presence or absence of comedonecrosis, was developed [40] (Fig. 15.1). Nuclear grade and comedo-type necrosis reflect the biology of the lesion, but neither alone or nor together are they adequate as the guidelines in the treatment decision-making process. Tumor size and margin width reflect the extent of disease, the adequacy of surgical treatment, and the likelihood of residual disease, and are of paramount importance.

The challenge was to devise a system using these variables (all independently important by multivariate analysis) that would be clinically valid, therapeutically useful, and user-friendly. The original Van Nuys Prognostic Index (VNPI) [37, 120] was devised in 1996 by combining tumor size, margin width and pathologic classification (determined by nuclear grade and the presence or absence of comedo-type necrosis). All of these factors had been collected prospectively in a large series of DCIS patients who were selectively treated (nonrandomized) [121].

A score, ranging from one for lesions with the best prognosis to three for lesions with the worst prognosis, was given for each of the three prognostic predictors. The objective with all three predictors was to create three statistically different subgroups for each, using local recurrence as the marker of treatment failure. Cut-off points (for example, what size or margin width constitutes low, intermediate or high risk of local recurrence) were determined statistically, using the log rank test with an optimum p-value approach.

Size Score

A score of 1 was given for a small tumors 15 mm or less, 2 was given for intermediate sized tumors 16–40 mm and 3 was given for large tumors 41 mm or more in diameter. The determination of size required complete and sequential tissue processing along with mammographic/pathologic correlation. Size was determined over a series of sections rather than on a single section and is the most difficult parameter to reproduce. If a 3 cm specimen is cut into ten blocks, each block is estimated to be 3 mm thick. If a lesion measuring 5 mm in maximum diameter on a single slide appears in and out of seven sequential blocks, it is estimated to be 21 mm (3 mm×7) in maximum size, not 5 mm, as measured on a single slide. The maximum diameter on a single slide was the way size was measured for most of the patients in the prospective randomized trials.

Margin Score

A score of 1 was given for widely clear tumor-free margins of 10 mm or more. This was often achieved by re-excision with the finding of no residual DCIS or only focal residual DCIS in the wall of the biopsy cavity. A score of 2 was given for intermediate margins of 1–9 mm and a score of 3 for margins less than 1 mm (involved or close margins).

Pathologic Classification Score [40, 122]

A score of 3 was given for tumors classified as group 3 (high grade lesions), 2 for tumors classified as group 2 (non-high grade lesions with comedo-type necrosis), and a score of 1 for tumors classified as group 1 (non-high grade lesion without comedo-type necrosis). The classification is diagrammed in Fig. 15.1.

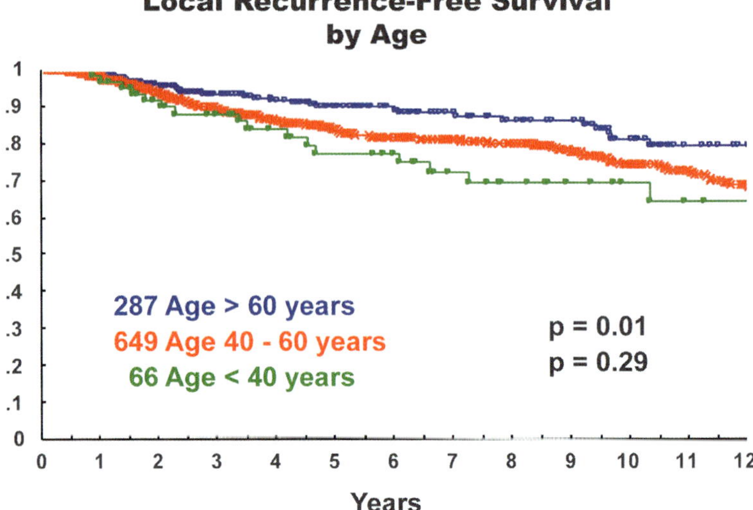

Fig. 15.5 Probability of local recurrence-free survival by age group for 1,046 breast conservation patients

The final formula for the original Van Nuys Prognostic Index (VNPI) became:

$$\text{VNPI} = \text{pathologic classification score} + \text{margin score} + \text{size score}$$

The University of Southern California/Van Nuys Prognostic Index (USC/VNPI)

By early 2001, a multivariate analysis at the University of Southern California revealed that age was also an independent prognostic factor and that it should be added to the VNPI with a weight equal to that of the other factors [117, 123, 124].

An analysis of our local recurrence data by age revealed that the most appropriate break points for our data were between ages 39 and 40 and between ages 60 and 61 (Fig. 15.5). Based on this, a score of 3 was given to all patients 39 years old or younger, a score of 2 was given to patients aged 40–60, and a score of 1 was given to patients 61 or older. The new scoring system for the USC/VNPI is shown in Table 15.1. The final formula for the USC/Van Nuys Prognostic Index became:

$$\text{USC / VNPI} = \text{pathologic classification score} + \text{margin score} + \text{size score} + \text{age score}$$

Scores range from 4 to 12. The patients least likely to recur after conservative therapy had a score of 4 or 5 (small, low grade, well-excised lesions in older

Table 15.1 The USC/Van Nuys prognostic index scoring system

Score	1	2	3
Size (mm)	≤15	16–40	≥41
Margins (mm)	≥10	1–9	<1
Pathologic classification	Non-high grade without necrosis	Non-high grade with necrosis	High grade with or without necrosis
Age (years)	≥61	40–60	≤39

One to three points are awarded for each of four different predictors of local breast recurrence (size, margins, pathologic classification, and age). Scores for each of the predictors are totaled to yield a VNPI score ranging from a low of 4 to a high of 12

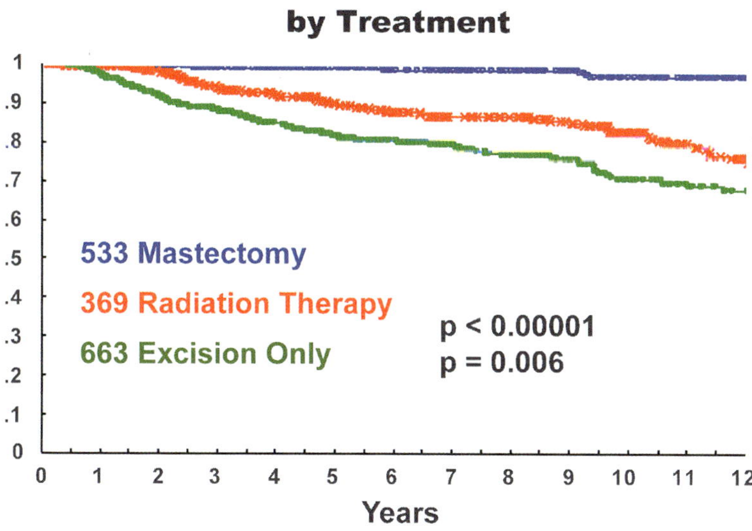

Fig. 15.6 Probability of local recurrence-free survival by treatment for 1,585 patients with DCIS

women). The patients most likely to recur had a score of 11 or 12 (large, poorly excised, high grade lesions in younger women). The probability of recurrence increased as the USC/VNPI score increased.

Updated Results Using the USC/VNPI

Through 2011, our group treated 1,585 patients with pure DCIS. 539 patients were treated with mastectomy and are generally not included in the analyses that use local recurrence as the endpoint since there were so few local recurrences in mastectomy patients. All patients are included in Fig. 15.6 with analyses local recurrence by treatment, Fig. 15.7 which analyses breast cancer specific survival by

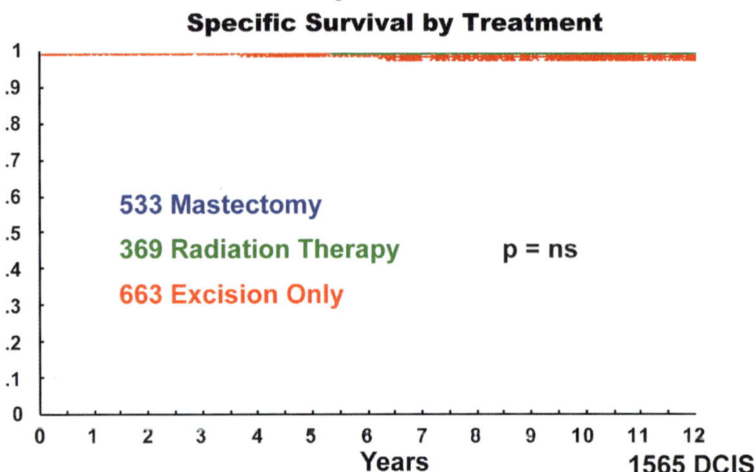

Fig. 15.7 Probability of breast cancer specific survival by treatment for 1,585 patients with DCIS

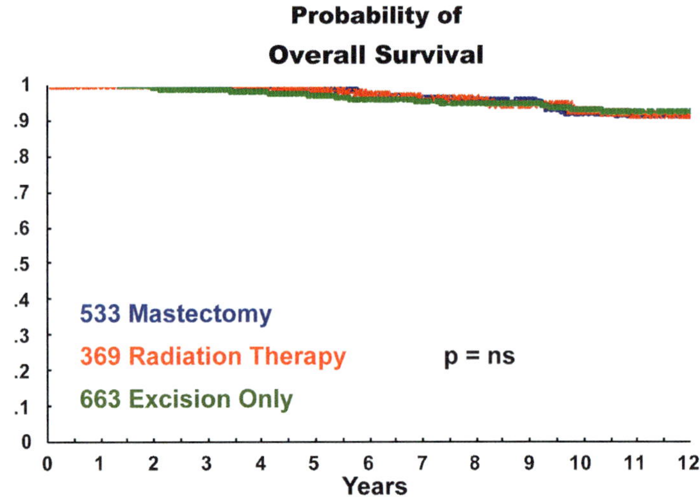

Fig. 15.8 Probability of overall survival by treatment for 1,585 patients with DCIS

treatment, and Fig. 15.8 which analyses overall survival by treatment . In addition, the mastectomy patients have their own separate recurrence analysis by USC/VNPI Score below.

1,046 patients were treated with breast conservation: 669 by excision alone and 377 by excision plus radiation therapy. The average follow-up for all patients was 85 months: 82 months for mastectomy, 109 months for excision plus radiation therapy, and 74 months for excision alone.

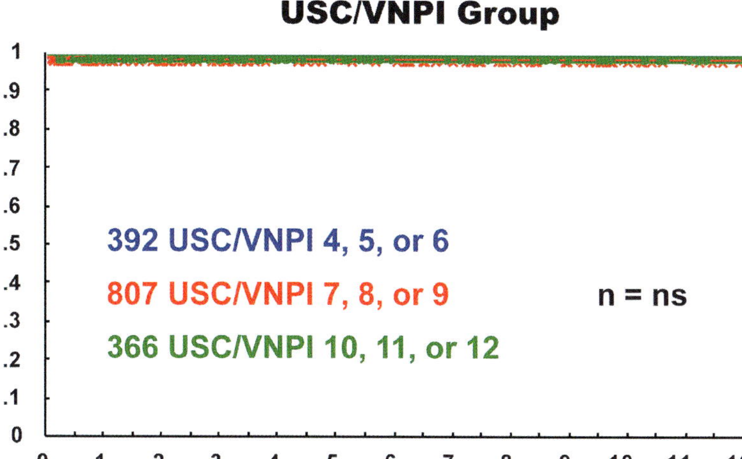

Fig. 15.9 Probability of breast cancer specific survival survival for 1,047 breast conservation patients grouped by USC/Van Nuys Prognostic Index score (4, 5, or 6 versus 7, 8, or 9 versus 10, 11, or 12)

There were 196 local failures, 92 of which (40 %) were invasive. The probability of local failure was reduced, overall, by 60 %, if radiation therapy was given, a result almost identical to the prospective randomized trials. The local recurrence-free survival is shown by treatment in Fig. 15.6. As expected, at any point in time, mastectomy had the lowest probability of local recurrence and excision alone had the highest.

Two patients developed distant metastases without ever developing a local recurrence. Both had palpable, HER2 positive, high-grade DCIS measuring 6 cm or more. Both were young, 28 and 49. Both were treated by mastectomy and immediate reconstruction. Using the USC/VNPI, one scored 11, the other 12. The mastectomy specimens were extensively serially sectioned and sequentially embedded. Neither frank invasion nor microinvasion could be found.

Seven patients treated with radiation therapy developed local recurrences (six in the same quadrant and one in a different quadrant) followed by distant metastases. Six of those patients have died from breast cancer. Three patients treated with excision alone developed local invasive recurrence followed by metastatic disease, one of whom died from breast cancer.

Seventy-eight additional patients have died from other causes without evidence of recurrent breast cancer. The 12-year actuarial overall survival, including deaths from all causes is 90 %. It is virtually identical for all three treatment groups and for all three USC/VNPI groups (Fig. 15.9).

The local recurrence-free survival for all 1,046 breast conservation patients is shown by tumor size in Fig. 15.10, by margin width in Fig. 15.11, by pathologic classification in Fig. 15.2 and by age in Fig. 15.5.

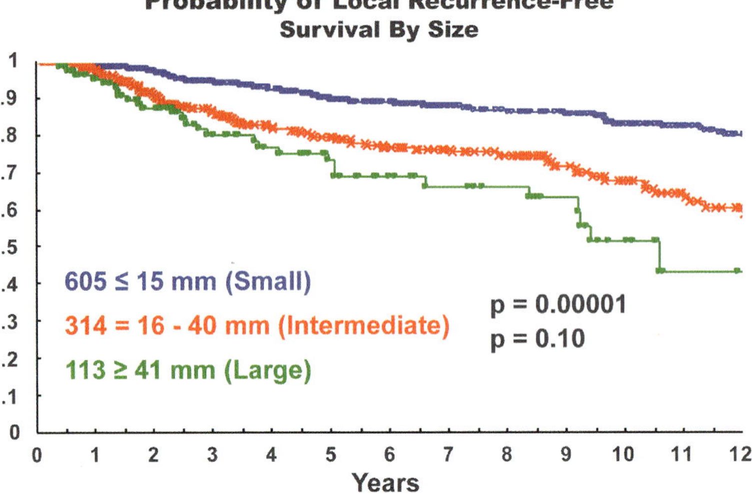

Fig. 15.10 Probability of local recurrence-free survival by tumor size for 1,047 breast conservation patients

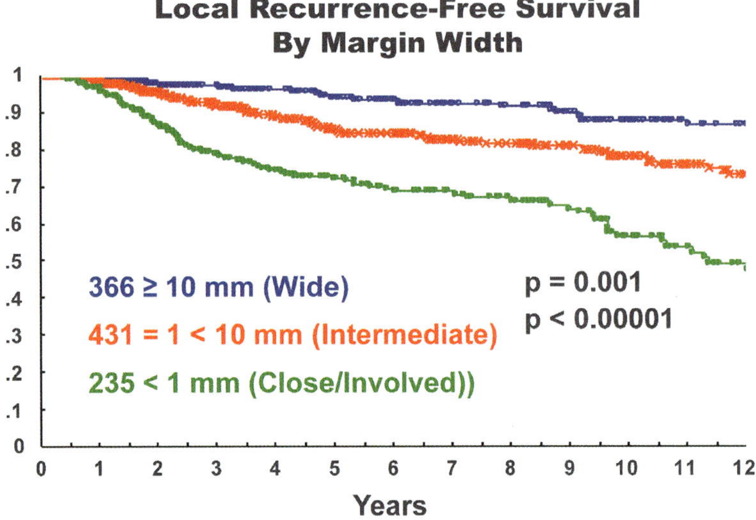

Fig. 15.11 Probability of local recurrence-free survival by margin width for 1,047 breast conservation patients

Figure 15.12 groups patients with low (USC/VNPI=4, 5, or 6), intermediate (USC/VNPI=7, 8, or 9), or high (USC/VNPI=10, 11, or 12) risks of local recurrence together. Each of these three groups is strongly statistically different from one another.

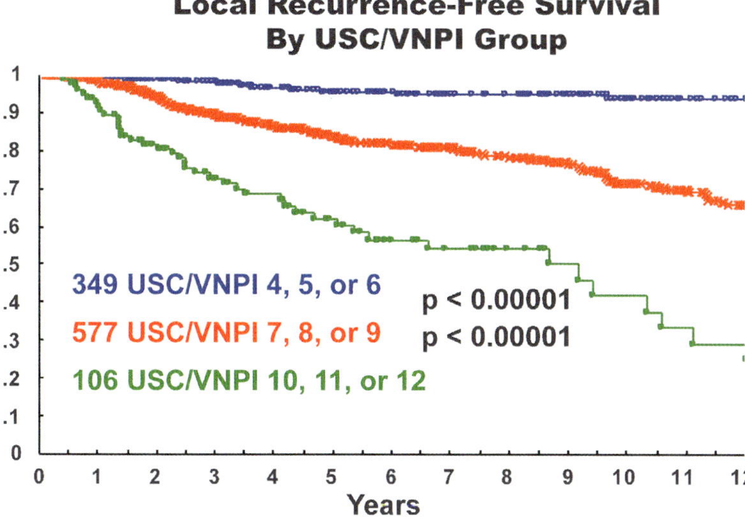

Fig. 15.12 Probability of local recurrence-free survival for 1,047 breast conservation patients grouped by USC/Van Nuys Prognostic Index score (4, 5, or 6 versus 7, 8, or 9 versus 10, 11, or 12)

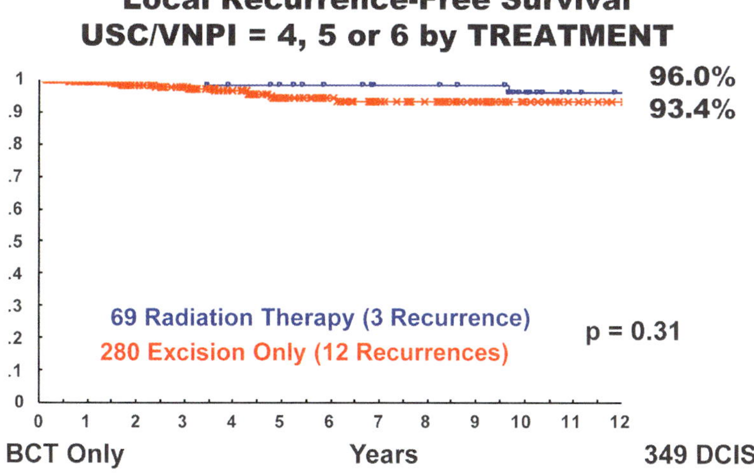

Fig. 15.13 Probability of local recurrence-free survival by treatment for 354 breast conservation patients with USC/Van Nuys Prognostic Index scores of 4, 5, or 6)

Patients with USC/VNPI scores of 4, 5 or 6 do not show a significant local recurrence-free survival benefit from breast irradiation (Fig. 15.13) (p=NS). The 12-year local recurrence rate for patients who score 4, 5, or 6 and who are treated with excision alone is 6.6 %. For those treated with excision plus radiation, it is 3.0 %, a 55 % relative reduction but only a 3.6 % absolute reduction.

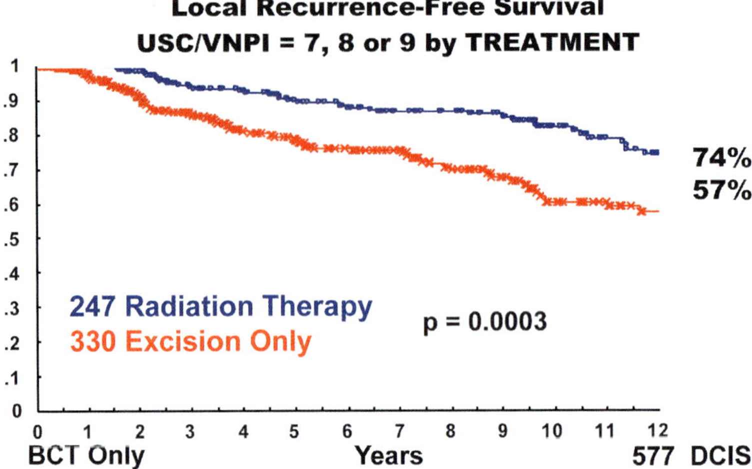

Fig. 15.14 Probability of local recurrence-free survival by treatment for 585 breast conservation patients with USC/Van Nuys Prognostic Index scores of 7, 8, or 9

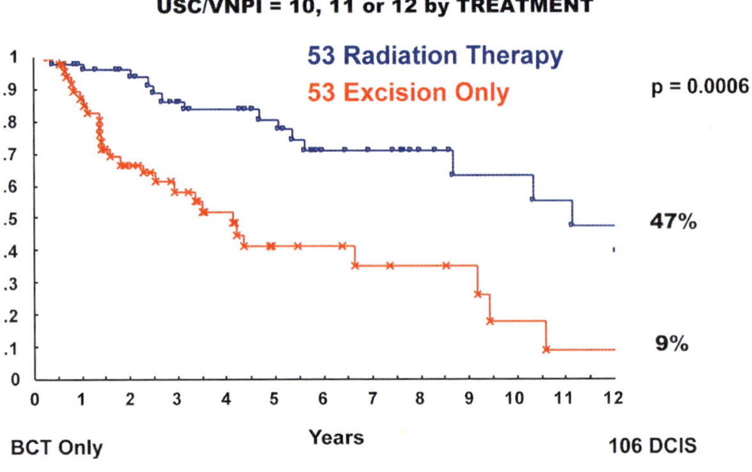

Fig. 15.15 Probability of local recurrence-free survival by treatment for 107 breast conservation patients with Modified USC/Van Nuys Prognostic Index scores of 10, 11, or 12

Patients with USC/VNPI 7, 8, or 9, are benefited by irradiation (Fig. 15.14). There is a statistically significant decrease in the probability of local recurrence, averaging 15 % throughout the curves, for irradiated patients with intermediate USC/VNPI scores compared to those treated by excision alone ($p=0.0003$). Figure 15.15 divides patients with a USC/VNPI of 10, 11, or 12 into those treated by excision plus irradiation and those treated by excision alone. Although the difference between the two groups is highly significant ($p = 0.0006$), conservatively treated DCIS patients with a USC/VNPI of 10, 11, or 12 recur at an extremely high rate even with radiation therapy.

Fine Tuning the USC/VNPI

The USC/VNPI is an algorithm, based on a rigid pathology protocol, which permits reproducible prospective quantification of measurable prognostic factors known to be important in predicting local recurrence in patients with DCIS. When originally published in 1996 [37] the Index was based on 333 patients and treatment recommendations were grouped by scores:

Excision alone for those who scored 4–6
Excision plus radiation therapy for those who scored 7–9
Mastectomy for those who scored 10–12

With more than four and a half times as many patients and nearly twice the follow-up since originally developed, sufficient numbers exist for analysis by individual score (4–12), stratified by margin width, rather than by groups of scores [125]. Since current *NCCN Treatment Guidelines* have been amended to include excision alone as an acceptable alternative but without listing any selection criteria, analysis by USC/VNPI score has become increasingly valuable [107].

The current series (1,585 patients with pure DCIS), was analyzed by:

1. Individual USC/VNPI scores (4 through 12)
2. Multiple margin widths (1, 3, 5 and 10 mm)
3. Treatment (excision plus radiation therapy versus excision alone)
4. Treatment needed to achieve a local recurrence probability of less than 10 %, 15 %, 20 %, or 25 % at 12-years

Table 15.2 illustrates the treatment and margin width necessary to achieve a probability of local recurrence of 20 % or less at 12-years and was derived using the Kaplan-Meier method. As the acceptable local recurrence probability is adjusted up or down, the treatment recommendations change.

To achieve a local recurrence probability of less than 20 % at 12-years, these data support excision alone for all patients scoring 4, 5 or 6, regardless of margin width and patients who score 7 but have margin widths ≥3 mm. Excision plus RT is appropriate for patients who score 7 and have margins <3 mm, for patients who score 8 and have margins ≥3 mm, and for patients who score 9 and have margins ≥5 mm. Mastectomy is appropriate for patients who score 8 and have margins <3 mm, who score 9 and have margins <5 mm and for all patients who score 10, 11 or 12, regardless of margin width. The value of the USC/VNPI has been confirmed by numerous studies and is the only tool currently available to aid in the treatment decision-making process [126] .

Table 15.2 USC/VNPI Score and treatment required to achieve a local recurrence rate Less than 20 % at 12-years

USC/VNPI score	No. of patients 1,585	Treatment needed	12-year recurrence (%)
All 4, 5 or 6	397	Excision alone	≤6.6
7, Margins ≥3 mm	180	Excision alone	15
7, Margins <3 mm	116	Excision + radiation	19
8, Margins ≥3 mm	116	Excision + radiation	11
8, Margins <3 mm	175	Mastectomy	0
9, Margins ≥5 mm	49	Excision + radiation	19
9, Margins <5 mm	192	Mastectomy	0
All 10, 11 or 12	369	Mastectomy	7

Table 15.3 Mastectomy patients divided into those who scored 4–9 versus 10–12

USC/VNPI score	4–9	10–12	*P* value
N	277	262	
Ave age	55	47	<0.001
Ave size	27 mm	61 mm	<0.001
Ave nuclear grade	2.05	2.73	<0.000
Local recurrence only	1	8	0.02
Local recurrence then metastatic	0	1	NS
Metastatic only	0	2	NS
# Inv recur	1	9	0.01
Prob recur at 12 years	0.2 %	7.2 %	<0.001

Using the USC/VNPI in Patients Undergoing Mastectomy

Patients with DCIS who are treated with mastectomy seldom recur locally or with metastatic disease. We questioned whether the USC/VNPI could predict these infrequent events. There are 539 patients with pure DCIS treated with mastectomy in this series. Average follow-up was 82 months. 12 patients developed recurrences: 2 metastatic without local recurrence, 1 metastatic with a preceding local recurrence, and 9 local recurrences without metastatic disease. 10 of 12 recurrences were invasive; two were DCIS. All 12 patients who recurred had multifocal disease; 9/12 had multicentric disease (in multiple quadrants). Using the USC/VNPI, patients scoring 4–9 are compared with those scored 10–12 in Table 15.3.

DCIS patients scoring 10–12 using the USC VNPI were significantly more likely to develop recurrence after mastectomy compared with patients scoring 4–9. At particularly high risk were young patients with large high-grade tumors and close or involved mastectomy margins. These data can be used when counseling a patient who is considering post-mastectomy radiation therapy.

Current Treatment Trends

In the current era of evidence-based medicine, it is reasonable to interpret the prospective randomized data as support that all conservatively treated patients with DCIS should receive post-excisional radiation therapy. However, in spite of these data, the number of patients with DCIS being treated with excision alone continues to increase. 2003 SEER data revealed that approximately one third of all patients with DCIS in the USA are now being treated with excision alone [16].

As an aid to the complex treatment decision-making process, the USC/VNPI can be used as a starting point to suggest reasonable treatment options supported by local recurrence data. The USC/VNPI divides patients with DCIS into three groups with differing probabilities of local recurrence after breast conserving surgery. Although there is an apparent treatment choice for each group, excision alone for patients who score 4–6, excision plus radiation therapy for patients who score 7–9, and mastectomy for those who score 10–12, the USC/VNPI is offered only as a guideline, a starting place for discussions with patients.

The Use of Margin Width as the Sole Predictor of Local Recurrence

Determining size has always been the most difficult part of the USC/VNPI. Our method computes size over a series of sections (the overall extent) rather than on a single slide (unless the measurement on a single slide is larger) and correlates this with the mammographic findings. For example, if a 6 by 4 mm DCIS appears in and out of 7 consecutive sections and the blocks are on average 3 mm wide, the diameter of this lesion would be recorded as a 21 mm DCIS (7 blocks × 3 mm average block width) in our database. In many other databases, it would be a 6 mm DCIS, the largest diameter on a single section.

By way of example, when the NSABP reviewed their pathologic material for the B-17 study, 75–90 % of their cases were measured at 10 mm or less in extent [73, 127]. The NSABP reported tumor size as the largest diameter on a single slide. While this is clearly the simplest and most reproducible way to measure DCIS, it is often an underestimation. Compare the NSABP sizes with our cases where only 40 % (452/1,032) of our conservatively treated patients had DCIS lesions measuring 10 mm or less. It is unlikely that the NSABP had twice as many smaller cases than a single group devoted to diagnosing and treating DCIS. Rather, the explanation probably lies in the way tissue was processed and the method used to estimate tumor size. In all likelihood, both groups treated tumors of similar size.

Due to the difficulty of estimating size, in 1997, we began evaluating the possibility of using margin width as the sole predictor of local recurrence, as a surrogate for the USC/VNPI [118]. The rationale was based on a multivariate analysis where patients with margin widths less than 1 mm had a ninefold increase in the

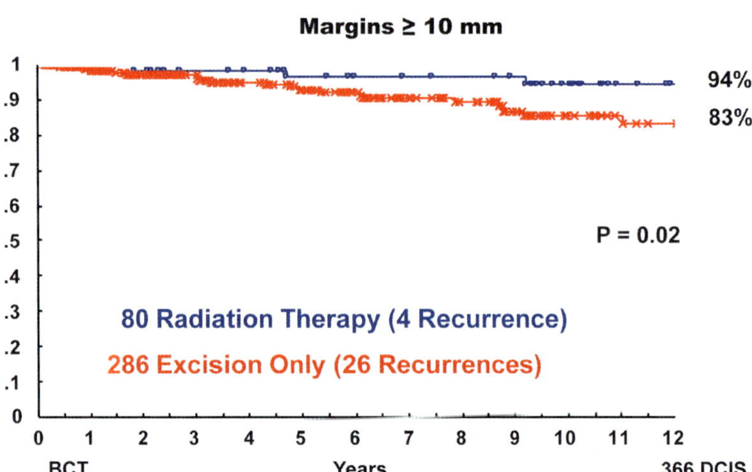

Fig. 15.16 Probability of local recurrence-free survival by treatment for 372 breast conservation patients with margins widths ≥10 mm

probability local recurrence compared with patients who had 10 mm or more margin widths. Narrow margin width was the single most powerful predictor of local failure.

In the current data set presented here, there were 372 patients with margin widths of 10 mm or more, 30 of whom (8 %) have developed a local recurrence (4 in the radiotherapy group and 26 within the excision only group) (Fig. 15.16). The local recurrence benefit for radiation therapy is significant ($p=0.02$). In spite of this, the actuarial local recurrence rate at 12-years, for those treated with excision alone was only 17 %, almost the same at that reported by the NSABP at 12 years for all patients treated with excision plus radiation therapy [73].

There were 354 patients with USC/VNPI scores of 4, 5, or 6, 15 of whom (3 %) have developed a local recurrence (3 in the radiotherapy group and 12 within the excision only group) (Fig. 15.13). The USC/VNPI is a better predictor of local recurrence than margin width alone (half as many recurrences) and it should be, since it is based on 5 predictive factors, including margin width. Nevertheless, there are so few recurrences among patients with widely clear margins that for all practical purposes, margin width can be used by itself as a surrogate for the USC/VNPI.

Treatment of the Axilla for Patients with DCIS

In 1986, our group suggested that axillary lymph node dissection be abandoned for DCIS [128]. In 1987, the NSABP made axillary node dissection for patients with DCIS optional, at the discretion of the surgeon. Since that time, we have published a series of papers that continue to show that axillary node dissection is not indicated for patients with DCIS [129, 130]. To date, our group had performed a total of 795 node evaluations, 3 of which (0.4 %) contained positive nodes by H and E staining. Two of those patients, both with macromets, were treated with adjuvant chemotherapy. Both were alive and well without local or distant recurrence at 8 and 10 years after their initial surgery (both had mastectomies and invasive cancer was likely missed during the serial sectioning of their specimens). The third patient had a cluster of 40 cells discovered by immunohistochemical staining and then retrospectively they were seen on H&E. This patient was not upstaged and was not treated with chemotherapy.

Frykberg et al., in their review of the management of DCIS, compiled the data of nine studies with a total of 754 patients. The incidence of axillary lymph node metastasis for patients with DCIS was 1.7 % [131].

Sentinel Node Biopsy for DCIS

Through 2011, we have performed 402 sentinel node biopsies for patients with DCIS. 10 (2.5 %) were positive by IHC only, two were positive by IHC and H&E (around 200 cells) and the rest ($n=390$) were negative by both IHC and H&E. In every positive case there were only a small number of positive cells (range 4–200). In no case were any patients upstaged to stage II nor were any treated with chemotherapy. All are alive and well without distant recurrence with follow-up ranging from a few months to 15.2 years (average 3.3 years).

Not all IHC positive cells are cancer cells. Some may merely by cytokeratin positive debris. Their morphology must be closely evaluated.

Our policy for sentinel node biopsy in patients with DCIS is as follows. We perform it for all patients with DCIS who are undergoing a mastectomy. We perform it if the DCIS is an upper outer quadrant high-grade lesion and the sentinel node can be easily removed through the same incision. We also remove a sentinel node if the DCIS is palpable or greater than 4 cm on mammography and/or MRI, or there is questionable microinvasion on core biopsy.

Summary

DCIS is now relatively common, and its frequency is increasing. Most of this is due to better and more frequent mammography available to a greater proportion of the female population.

Not all microscopic DCIS will progress to clinical cancer, but if a patient has DCIS and is not treated, she is more likely to develop an ipsilateral invasive breast cancer than is a woman without DCIS.

The high grade comedo subtype of DCIS is more aggressive and malignant in its histologic appearance and is more likely to be associated with subsequent invasive cancer than the lower grade noncomedo subtypes. High grade Comedo DCIS is more likely to have a high S-phase, overexpress HER2/neu, and show increased thymidine labeling as compared with noncomedo DCIS. Comedo DCIS treated conservatively is also more likely to recur locally than noncomedo DCIS. However, separation of DCIS into two groups by architecture is an oversimplification and does not reflect the biologic potential of the lesion as well as stratification by nuclear grade and comedo-type necrosis.

Most DCIS detected today will be nonpalpable. It will be detected by mammographic calcifications. It is not uncommon for DCIS to be larger than expected by mammography, to involve more than a quadrant of the breast, and to be unicentric in its distribution.

Preoperative evaluation should include mammography (preferably digital) with compression magnification and ultrasonography. MRI is becoming increasingly more popular and we obtain an MRI on every patient diagnosed with any form of breast cancer.

Reexcision often yields a poor cosmetic result and the overall plan should be to avoid them whenever possible. The initial breast biopsy should be an image-guided needle biopsy.

After establishment of the diagnosis, the patient should be counseled. If she is motivated for breast conservation, the surgeon and radiologist should plan the procedure carefully, using multiple wires to map out the extent of the lesion. The first attempt at excision is the best chance to get a complete excision with a good cosmetic result.

When considering the entire population of patients with DCIS without subset analyses, the prospective randomized trials have shown that post-excisional radiation therapy can reduce the relative risk of local recurrence by about 50 % for conservatively treated patients. But in some low-risk DCIS patients, the costs may outweigh the potential benefits. In spite of a relative 50 % reduction in the probability of local recurrence, the absolute reduction may be only a few percent. Moreover the local recurrence rate at 15 years for NSABP-B17's irradiated arm is 20 % [106]. While local recurrence is extremely important, breast cancer-specific survival is the most important endpoint for all patients with breast cancer, including patients with DCIS, and no DCIS trial has ever shown a survival benefit for radiation therapy when compared with excision alone. Moreover, radiation therapy is not without financial and physical cost. Because of this, in recent years, an increasing number of selected patients with DCIS have been treated with excision alone. Excision alone has now become an acceptable form of treatment for selected patients in the 2008 NCCN Guidelines.

The University of Southern California/Van Nuys Prognostic Index (USC/VNPI) uses five independent predictors to predict the probability of local recurrence after conservative treatment for DCIS, these include tumor size, margin width, nuclear grade, age, and the presence or absence of comedonecrosis. In combination, they can be used as an aid to identify subgroups of patients with extremely low probabilities of local recurrence after excision alone, for example, patients who score 4, 5 or 6 using the USC/VNPI. If size cannot be accurately determined, margin width by itself can be used as a surrogate for the USC/VNPI, although it is not quite as good.

Oncoplastic surgery combines sound surgical oncologic principles with plastic surgical techniques. Coordination of the two surgical disciplines may help to avoid poor cosmetic results after wide excision and may increase the number of women who can be treated with breast-conserving surgery by allowing larger breast excisions with more acceptable cosmetic results. Oncoplastic surgery requires cooperation and coordination of surgical oncology, radiology, and pathology. Oncoplastic resection is a therapeutic procedure not a breast biopsy and is performed on patients with a proven diagnosis of breast cancer. New oncoplastic techniques that allow for more extensive excisions can be used to achieve both acceptable cosmesis and widely clear margins, reducing the need for radiation therapy in many cases OF DCIS.

The decision to use excision alone as treatment for DCIS should only be made if complete and sequential tissue processing has been used and the patient has been fully informed and has participated in the treatment decision-making process.

The Future

Our knowledge of DCIS genetics and molecular biology is increasing at a remarkably rapid rate. Future studies are likely to identify molecular markers that will allow us to differentiate DCIS with an aggressive potential from DCIS that is merely a microscopic finding. Once we can identify DCIS that will soon develop the potential to invade and metastasize from DCIS that will not, the treatment selection process will become much simpler.

References

1. Siegel R, Naishadham D, Jemal A. Cancer statistics 2013. CA Cancer J Clin. 2013;63:11–30.
2. Burstein HJ, Polyak K, Wong JS, Lester SC, Kaelin CM. Ductal carcinoma in situ of the breast. N Engl J Med. 2004;350(14):1430–41.
3. Seth A, Kitching R, Landberg G, Xu J, Zubovits J, Burger A. Gene expression profiling of ductal carcinomas in situ and invasive breast tumors. Anticancer Res. 2003;23:2043–51.
4. Porter D, Lahti-Domenici J, Keshaviah A, et al. Molecular markers in ductal carcinoma in situ of the breast. Mol Cancer Res. 2003;1:362–75.
5. Ma XS, Alunga R, Tuggle J, et al. Gene expression profiles of human breast cancer progression. Proc Natl Acad Sci USA. 2003;100:5974–9.
6. Page D, Anderson T. Diagnostic histopathology of the breast. New York: Churchill Livingstone; 1987.
7. Patchefsky A, Schwartz G, Finkelstein S, et al. Heterogeneity of intraductal carcinoma of the breast. Cancer. 1989;63:731–41.
8. Nemoto T, Vana J, Bedwani R, Baker H, McGregor F, Murphy G. Management and survival of female breast cancer: results of a national survey by the American college of surgeons. Cancer. 1980;45:2917–24.
9. Silverstein M, Lagios M, Recht A, et al. Image-detected breast cancer: state of the art diagnosis and treatment. J Am Coll Surg. 2005;201:586–97.

10. Tabar L, Smith RA, Vitak B, et al. Mammographic screening: a key factor in the control of breast cancer. Cancer J. 2003;9(1):15–27.
11. Duffy SW, Tabar L, Smith RA. Screening for breast cancer with mammography. Lancet. 2001;358(9299):2166. author reply 2167–2168.
12. Silverstein MJ, Cohlan B, Gierson E, et al. Duct carcinoma in situ: 227 cases without microinvasion. Eur J Cancer. 1992;28(2/3):630–4.
13. Lagios MD. Duct carcinoma in situ: pathology and treatment. Surg Clin North Am. 1990;70:853–71.
14. Ashikari R, Hadju S, Robbins G. Intraductal carcinoma of the breast. Cancer. 1971; 28:1182–7.
15. Silverstein MJ. Ductal carcinoma in situ of the breast. Annu Rev Med. 2000;51:17–32.
16. Baxter N, Virnig B, Durham S, Tuttle T. Trends in the treatment of ductal carcinoma in situ of the breast. J Natl Cancer Inst. 2004;96:443–8.
17. Silverstein MJ. The Van Nuys breast center—the first free-standing multidisciplinary breast center. Surg Oncol Clin N Am. 2000;9(2):159–75.
18. Veronesi U, Saccozzi R, Del Vecchio M, et al. Comparing radical mastectomy with quadrantectomy, axillary dissection and radiotherapy in patients with small cancers of the breast. N Engl J Med. 1981;305:6–10.
19. Van Dongen J, Bartelink H, Fentiman I, et al. Randomized clinical trial to assess the value of breast-conserving therapy in stage I and II breast cancer, EORTC 10801 trial. J Natl Cancer Inst Monogr. 1992;11:15–8.
20. Veronesi U, Banfi A, Salvadori B, et al. Breast conservation is the treatment of choice in small breast cancer: long-term results of a randomized trial. Eur J Cancer. 1990;26:668–70.
21. Fisher B, Redmond C, Poisson R, et al. Eight-year results of a randomized clinical trial comparing total mastectomy and lumpectomy with or without radiation therapy in the treatment of breast cancer. N Eng J Med. 1989;320:822–8.
22. Veronesi U, Cascinelli N, Mariani L, et al. Twenty-year follow-up of a randomized study comparing breast-conserving surgery with radical mastectomy for early breast cancer. N Engl J Med. 2002;347:1227–32.
23. Fisher B, Anderson S, Bryant J, et al. Twenty-year follow-up of a randomized trial comparing total mastectomy, lumpectomy, and lumpectomy plus irradiation for the treatment of invasive breast cancer. N Engl J Med. 2002;347:1233–41.
24. Tavassoli F. Intraductal carcinoma. In: Tavassoli FA, editor. Pathology of the breast. Norwalk, CT: Appleton and Lange; 1992. p. 229–61.
25. Aasmundstad T, Haugen O. DNA Ploidy in intraductal breast carcinomas. Eur J Cancer. 1992;26:956–9.
26. Meyer J. Cell kinetics in selection and stratification of patients for adjuvant therapy of breast carcinoma. Natl Cancer Inst Monogr. 1986;1:25–8.
27. Allred D, Clark G, Molina R, et al. Overexpression of HER-2/neu and its relationship with other prognostic factors change during the progression of in situ to invasive breast cancer. Hum Pathol. 1992;23:974–9.
28. Barnes D, Meyer J, Gonzalez J, Gullick W, Millis R. Relationship between c-erbB-2 immunoreactivity and thymidine labelling index in breast carcinoma in situ. Breast Cancer Res Treat. 1991;18:11–7.
29. Bartkova J, Barnes D, Millis R, Gullick W. Immunhistochemical demonstration of c-erbB-2 protein in mammary ductal carcinoma in situ. Hum Pathol. 1990;21(11):1164–7.
30. Liu E, Thor A, He M, Barcos M, Ljung B, Benz C. The HER2 (c-erbB-2) oncogene is frequently amplified in in situ carcinomas of the breast. Oncogene. 1992;7:1027–32.
31. van de Vijver M, Peterse J, Mooi WJ, et al. Neu-protein overexpression in breast cancer: association with comedo-type ductal carcinoma in situ and limited prognostic value in stage II breast cancer. N Engl J Med. 1988;319:1239–45.
32. Lagios M, Margolin F, Westdahl P, Rose N. Mammographically detected duct carcinoma in situ. Frequency of local recurrence following tylectomy and prognostic effect of nuclear grade on local recurrence. Cancer. 1989;63:619–24.

33. Schwartz G, Finkel G, Carcia J, Patchefsky A. Subclinical ductal carcinoma in situ of the breast: treatment by local excision and surveillance alone. Cancer. 1992;70:2468–74.
34. Silverstein MJ, Waisman J, Gierson E, et al. Radiation therapy for intraductal carcinoma: is it an equal alternative? Arch Surg. 1991;126:424–8.
35. Solin L, Yeh I, Kurtz J, et al. Ductal carcinoma in situ (intraductal carcinoma) of the breast treated with breast-conserving surgery and definitive irradiation. Correlation of pathologic parameters with outcome of treatment. Cancer. 1993;71:2532–42.
36. Silverstein MJ, Barth A, Waisman J, et al. Predicting local recurrence in patients with intraductal breast carcinoma (DCIS). Proc Am Soc Clin Oncol. 1995;14:117.
37. Silverstein MJ, Poller D, Craig P, et al. A prognostic index for ductal carcinoma in situ of the breast. Cancer. 1996;77:2267–74.
38. Lagios M, Westdahl P, Margolin F, Rose M. Duct carcinoma in situ: relationship of extent of noninvasive disease to the frequency of occult invasion, multicentricity, lymph node metastases, and short-term treatment failures. Cancer. 1982;50:1309–14.
39. Holland R, Peterse J, Millis R, et al. Ductal carcinoma in situ: a proposal for a new classification. Semin Diagn Pathol. 1994;11(3):167–80.
40. Silverstein MJ, Poller D, Waisman J, et al. Prognostic classification of breast ductal carcinoma-in-situ. Lancet. 1995;345:1154–7.
41. Jensen J, Handel N, Silverstein M, et al. Glandular replacement therapy (GRT) for intraductal breast carcinoma (DCIS). Proc Am Soc Clin Oncol. 1995;14:138.
42. Jensen J, Handel N, Silverstein M. Glandular replacement therapy: an argument for a combined surgical approach in the treatment of noninvasive breast cancer. Breast J. 1996;2:121–3.
43. Faverly D, Burgers L, Bult P, Holland R. Three dimensional imaging of mammary ductal carcinoma is situ: clinical implications. Semin Diagn Pathol. 1994;11(3):193–8.
44. Poller D, Silverstein M, Galea M, et al. Ductal carcinoma in situ of the breast: a proposal for a new simplified histological classification association between cellular proliferation and c-erbB-2 protein expression. Mod Pathol. 1994;7:257–62.
45. Bellamy C, McDonald C, Salter D, Chetty U, Anderson T. Noninvasive ductal carcinoma of the breast: the relevance of histologic categorization. Hum Pathol. 1993;24:16–23.
46. Sloane J, Ellman R, Anderson T, Brown C, Coyne J, Dallimore N. Consistency of histopathological reporting of breast lesions detected by breast screening: findings of the UK national external quality assessment (EQA) scheme. Eur J Cancer. 1994;10:1414–9.
47. Bryan B, Schnitt S, Collins L. Ductal carcinoma in situ with basal-like phenotype: a possible precursor to invasive basal-like breast cancer. Mod Pathol. 2006;19:617–21.
48. Tamimi R, Baer H, Maroti J, et al. Comparison of molecular phenotypes of ductal carcinoma in situ and invasive breast cancer. Breast Cancer Res. 2008;10:R67.
49. Hannemann J, Velds A, Halfwerk J, et al. Classification of ductal carcinoma in situ by gene expression profiling. Breast Cancer Res. 2006;8:R61.
50. Solin L, Gray R, Baehner F, et al. A quantitative multigene RT-PCR assay for predicting recurrence risk after surgical excision alone without irradiation for ductal carcinoma in situ (DCIS): a prospective validation study of the DCIS score from ECOG E5194. Cancer Res. 2011;71(24 Suppl):Abstract No. S4–06.
51. Kerlikowske K, Molinaro AM, Gauthier ML, Berman H, et al. Biomarker expression and risk of subsequent tumors after initial ductal carcinoma in situ diagnosis. J Natl Cancer Inst. 2010;102:627–37.
52. Rudloff U, Jacks L, Goldberg J, Wynveen C, et al. Nomogram for predicting the risk of local recurrence after breast-conserving surgery for ductal carcinoma in situ. J Clin Oncol. 2010;28:3762–9.
53. Page D, Rogers L, Schuyler P, Dupont W, Jensen R. The natural history of ductal carcinoma in situ of the breast. In: Silverstein MJ, Recht A, Lagios M, editors. Ductal carcinoma in situ of the breast. 2nd ed. Philadelphia, PA: Lippincott, Williams and Wilkins; 2002. p. 17–21.
54. Sanders M, Schuyler P, Dupont W, Page D. The natural history of low-grade ductal carcinoma in situ of the breast in women treated by biopsy only revealed over 30 years of long-term follow-up. Cancer. 2005;103:2481–4.

55. Rosen P, Senie R, Schottenfeld D, Ashikari R. Noninvasive breast carcinoma: frequency of unsuspected invasion and implications for treatment. Ann Surg. 1989;1979:377–82.
56. Alpers C, Wellings S. The prevalence of carcinoma in situ in normal and cancer-associated breast. Hum Pathol. 1985;16:796–807.
57. Page D, Dupont W, Roger L, Landenberger M. Intraductal carcinoma of the breast: follow-up after biopsy only. Cancer. 1982;49:751–8.
58. Schuh M, Nemoto T, Penetrante R, Rosner D, Dao T. Intraductal carcinoma: analysis of presentation, pathologic findings, and outcome of disease. Arch Surg. 1986;121:1303–7.
59. Gump F, Jicha D, Ozzello L. Ductal carcinoma in situ (DCIS): a revised concept. Surgery. 1987;102:190–5.
60. de Mascarel I, MacGrogan G, Mathoulin-Pelissier S, Soubeyran I, et al. Breast ductal carcinoma in situ with microinvasion. A definition supported by long-term study 1248 serially sectioned ductal carcinomas. Cancer. 2002;94:2134–42.
61. Fisher E, Sass R, Fisher B, et al. Pathologic findings from the national surgical adjuvant breast project (protocol 6) i. Intraductal carcinoma (DCIS). Cancer. 1986;57:197–208.
62. Simpson T, Thirlby R, Dail D. Surgical treatment of ductal carcinoma in situ of the breast: 10 to 20 year follow-up. Arch Surg. 1992;127:468–72.
63. Holland R, Hendriks J, Verbeek A, Mravunac M, Schuurmans S. Extent, distribution, and mammographic/histological correlations of breast ductal carcinoma in situ. Lancet. 1990;335:519–22.
64. Holland R, Faverly D. Whole organ studies. In: Silverstein MJ, Recht A, Lagios M, editors. Ductal carcinoma in situ of the breast, vol 2. Philadelphia, PA: Lippincott, Williams and Wilkins; 2002;240–248.
65. Noguchi S, Aihara T, Koyama H, Motomura K, Inaji H, Imaoka S. Discrimination between multicentric and multifocal carcinomas of breast through clonal analysis. Cancer. 1994;74: 872–77.
66. Tabar L, Dean P. Basic principles of mammographic diagnosis. Diagn Imaging Clin Med. 1985;54:146–57.
67. Silverstein M. Where's the outrage. J Am Coll Surg. 2009;208:78–9.
68. Lester SC, Bose S, Chen YY, et al. Protocol for the examination of specimens from patients with ductal carcinoma in situ of the breast. Arch Pathol Lab Med. Jan 2009;133(1):15–25.
69. Lester SC, Connolly JL, Amin MB. College of American pathologists protocol for the reporting of ductal carcinoma in situ. Arch Pathol Lab Med. Jan 2009;133(1):13–4.
70. Consensus Conference Committee. Consensus Conference on the classification of ductal carcinoma in situ. Cancer. 1997;80:1798–802.
71. Silverstein MJ. Intraductal breast carcinoma: two decades of progress? Am J Clin Oncol. 1991;14(6):534–7.
72. Silverstein MJ. Noninvasive breast cancer: the dilemma of the 1990s. Obstet Gynecol Clin North Am. 1994;21(4):639–58.
73. Fisher B, Land S, Mamounas E, Dignam J, Fisher E, Wolmark N. Prevention of invasive breast cancer in women with ductal carcinoma in situ: an update of the national surgical adjuvant breast and bowel project experience. Semin Oncol. 2001;28(4):400–18.
74. Fentiman I, Fagg N, Millis R, Haywood J. In situ ductal carcinoma of the breast: implications of disease pattern and treatment. Eur J Surg Oncol. 1986;12:261–6.
75. Solin L, Kurtz J, Fourquet A, et al. Fifteen year results of breast conserving surgery and definitive breast irradiation for treatment of ductal carcinoma in situ of the breast. J Clin Oncol. 1996;14:754–63.
76. Coordinating UK. Committee on Cancer Research (UKCCCR) Ductal Carcinoma in Situ (DCIS) Working Party. Radiotherapy and tamoxifen in women with completely excised ductal carcinoma in situ of the breast in the UK, Australia, and New Zealand: randomised controlled trial. Lancet. 2003;362:95–102.
77. Viani GA, Stefano EJ, Afonso SL, et al. Breast-conserving surgery with or withour radiotherapy in women with ductal carcinoma in situ: a meta-analysis of randomized trials. Radiat Oncol. 2007;2:28–39.

78. Emdin SO, Granstrand B, Ringberg A, et al. SweDCIS: radiotherapy after sector resection for ductal carcinoma in situ of the breast. Results of a randomised trial in a population offered mammographic screening. Acta Oncol. 2006;45:536–43.
79. Fisher B, Jeong J, Anderson S, Bryant J, Fisher E, Wolmark N. Twenty-five year follow-up of a randomized trial comparing radiacal mastectomy, total mastectomy, and total mastectomy followed by irradiation. N Engl J Med. 2002;347:567–75.
80. Group EBCTC. Effects of radiotherapy and differences in the extent of surgery for early breast cancer on local recurrence and on 15-year survival. Lancet. 2005;366:2087–106.
81. Group EBTC. Effect of radiotherapy after breast-conserving surgery on 10-year recurrence and 15-year breast cancer death: meta-analysis of individual patient data for 10,801 women in 17 randomized trials. Lancet. 2011;378:771–84.
82. Silverstein MJ, Lagios M, Martino S, et al. Outcome after local recurrence in patients with ductal carcinoma in situ of the breast. J Clin Oncol. 1998;16:1367–73.
83. Romero L, Klein L, Ye W, et al. Outcome after invasive recurrence in patients with ductal carcinoma in situ of the breast. Am J Surg. 2004;188:371–6.
84. Swain S. Ductal carcinoma in situ—incidence, presentation and guidelines to treatment. Oncology. 1989;3:25–42.
85. Fisher B, Costantino J, Redmond C, et al. Lumpectomy compared with lumpectomy and radiation therapy for the treatment of intraductal breast cancer. N Engl J Med. 1993;328: 1581–6.
86. Fisher B, Dignam J, Wolmark N, et al. Tamoxifen in treatment of intraductal breast cancer: national surgical adjuvant breast and bowel project B-24 randomized controlled trial. Lancet. 1999;353:1993–2000.
87. Fisher B, Dignam J, Wolmark N, et al. Lumpectomy and radiation therapy for the treatment of intraductal breast cancer: findings from national surgical adjuvant breast and bowel project B-17. J Clin Oncol. Feb 1998;16(2):441–52.
88. Julien J, Bijker N, Fentiman I, et al. Radiotherapy in breast conserving treatment for ductal carcinoma in situ: first results of EORTC randomized phase III trial 10853. Lancet. 2000;355:528–33.
89. Page D, Dupont W, Rogers L, Jensen R, Schuyler P. Continued local recurrence of carcinoma 15–25 years after a diagnosis of low grade ductal carcinoma in situ of the breast treated only by biopsy. Cancer. 1995;76:1197–200.
90. Zafrani B, Leroyer A, Fourquet A, et al. Mammographically detected ductal in situ carcinoma of the breast analyzed with a new classification. A study of 127 cases: correlation with estrogen and progesterone receptors, p53 and c-erbB-2 proteins, and proliferative activity. Semin Diagn Pathol. 1994;11(3):208–14.
91. Schwartz G. The role of excision and surveillance alone in subclinical DCIS of the breast. Oncology. 1994;8(2):21–6.
92. Schwartz G. Treatment of subclinical ductal carcinoma in situ of the breast by local excision and surveillance: an updated personal experience. In: Silverstein MJ, Recht A, Lagios M, editors. Ductal carcinoma in situ of the breast. 2nd ed. Philadelphia, PA: Lippincott, Williams and Wilkins; 2002. p. 308–21.
93. Silverstein M. Ductal carcinoma in situ of the breast: 11 reasons to consider treatment with excision alone. Womens Health. 2008;4:565–77.
94. Holland R, Faverly D. Whole organ studies. Baltimore, MD: Williams and Wilkins; 1997.
95. Holland R, Hendriks J. Microcalcifications associated with ductal carcinoma in situ: mammographic-pathologic correlation. Semin Diagn Pathol. 1994;11(3):181–92.
96. Page D, Dupont W, Roger L, Rados M. Atypical hyperplastic lesions of the female breast. A log-term follow-up study. Cancer. 1985;55:2698–708.
97. Lagios M. Controversies in diagnosis, biology, and treatment. Breast J. 1995;1:68–78.
98. Group EBCTC. Favorable and unfavorable effects on long-term survival of radiotherapy for early breast cancer: an overview of the randomized trials. Lancet. 2000;2006:1757–70.
99. Giordano S, Kuo Y, Freeman J, et al. Risk of cardiac death after adjuvant radiotherapy for breast cancer. J Natl Cancer Inst. 2005;97:419–24.

100. Darby S, McGale P, Taylor C, Peto R. Long-term mortality from heart disease and lung cancer after radiotherapy for early breast cancer: prospective cohort study of about 300,000 women un US SEER cancer registries. Lancet Oncol. 2005;6:557–65.
101. Zablotska L, Neugut A. Lung carcinoma after radiation therapy in women treated with lumpectomy or mastectomy for primary breast carcinoma. Cancer. 2003;97:1404–11.
102. Darby S, McGale P, Peto R, et al. Mortality from cardiovascular disease more than 10 years after radiotherapy for breast cancer: nationwide cohort study of 90,000 Swedish women. BMJ. 2003;326:256–7.
103. Recht A. Randomized trial overview. In: Silverstein MJ, Recht A, Lagios M, editors. Ductal carcinoma in situ of the breast. 2nd ed. Philadelphia, PA: Lippincott, Williams and Wilkins; 2002. p. 414–9.
104. Vaidya J, Joseph D, Tobias J, et al. Targeted intraoperative radiotherapy versus whole breast radiotherapy for breast cancer (TARGIT-A trial): an international, prospective, randomised, non-inferiority phase 3 trial. Lancet. 2010;376:91–102.
105. Wong J, Kaelin C, Troyan S, et al. Prospective study of wide excision alone for ductal carcinoma in situ of the breast. J Clin Oncol. 2006;24(7):1031–6.
106. Wapnir I, Dignam J, Fisher B, et al. Long-term outcomes of invasive ipsilateral breast tumor recurrences after lumpectomy in NSABP B-17 and B-24 randomized clinical trials for DCIS. J Natl Cancer Inst. 2011;103(6):478–88.
107. Carlson RW, Allred DC, Anderson BO, et al. NCCN clincal practice guidelines in oncology: breast cancer. 2008. www.nccn.org.
108. Bijker N, Peterse J, Duchateau L, et al. Risk factors for recurrence and metastasis after breast-conserving therapy for ductal carcinoma in situ: analysis of European Organization for Research and Treatment of Cancer Trial 10853. J Clin Oncol. 2001;19:2263–71.
109. Fisher E, Constantino J, Fisher B, et al. Pathologic findings from the national surgical adjuvant breast project (NSABP) protocol B-17. Cancer. 1995;75:1310–9.
110. Bijker N, Meijnen P, Peterse J, et al. Breast conserving treatment with or without radiotherapy in ductal carcinoma in situ: ten-year results of European Organization for Research and treatment of Cancer Randomized Phase III Trial 10853—A study by the EORTC Breast Cancer Cooperative Group and EORTC Radiotherapy Group. J Clin Oncol. 2006;24:1–8.
111. Cuzick J, Sestak I, Pindler S, et al. Effect of tamoxifen and radiotherapy in women with locally excised ductal carcinoma in situ: long-term results from the UK/ANZ DCIS trial. Lancet Oncol. 2011;12(1):21–9.
112. Fisher B, Bauer M, Margolese R, et al. Five-year results of a randomized clinical trial comparing total mastectomy and lumpectomy with or without radiation therapy in the treatment of breast cancer. N Eng J Med. 1985;312:665–73.
113. Fisher E, Lemming R, Andersen S, Redmond C, Fisher B. Conservative management of intraductal carcinoma (DCIS) of the breast. J Surg Oncol. 1991;47:139–47.
114. Allred D, Anderson SJ, Paik S, et al. Adjuvant Tamoxifen reduces subsequent breast cancer in women with estrogen receptor-positive ductal carcinoma in situ: a study based on NSABP protocol B24. J Clin Oncol. 2012;30:1268–73.
115. Holmberg L, Garmo H, Granstrand B. Absolute risk reductions for local recurrence after postoperative radiotherapy after sector rsection for ductal carcinoma in situ of the breast. J Clin Oncol. 2008;26:1247–52.
116. Lester SC, Connolly JL, Amin MB. College of American pathologists protocol for the reporting of ductal carcinoma in situ. Arch Pathol Lab Med. 2009;133(1):13–4.
117. Silverstein MJ. The university of southern california/Van Nuys prognostic index for ductal carcinoma in situ of the breast. Am J Surg. 2003;186:337–43.
118. Silverstein MJ, Lagios M, Groshen S, et al. The influence of margin width on local control in patients with ductal carcinoma in situ (DCIS) of the breast. N Engl J Med. 1999;340: 1455–61.
119. Ottesen G, Graversen H, Blichert-Toft M, Zedeler K, Andersen J. Ductal carcinoma in situ of the female breast. Short-term results of a prospective nationwide study. Am J Surg Pathol. 1992;16:1183–96.

120. Silverstein MJ, Lagios M, Craig P, et al. The Van Nuys prognostic index for ductal carcinoma in situ. Breast J. 1996;2:38–40.
121. Silverstein MJ, Lagios M, Recht A, editors. Ductal carcinoma in situ of the breast. 2nd ed. Philadelphia, PA: Lippincott, Williams and Wilkins; 2002.
122. Poller D, Silverstein MJ. The Van Nuys ductal carcinoma in situ: an update. In: Silverstein MJ, Recht A, Lagios M, editors. Ductal carcinoma in situ of the breast. Secondth ed. Philadelphia, PA: Lippincott, Williams and Wilkins; 2002. p. 222–33.
123. Silverstein MJ, Buchanan C. Ductal carcinoma in situ: USC/Van Nuys prognostic index and the impact of margin status. Breast. 2003;12:457–71.
124. Silverstein MJ. The university of southern california/Van Nuys prognostic index. In: Silverstein MJ, Recht A, Lagios M, editors. Ductal carcinoma in situ of the breast. 2nd ed. Philadelphia, PA: Lippincott, Williams and Wilkins; 2002. p. 459–73.
125. Silverstein MJ, Lagios M. Choosing treatment for patients with ductal carcinoma in situ: fine tuning the University of southern California/Van Nuys Prognostic Index. J Natl Cancer Inst Monogr. 2010;41:193–6.
126. Di Saverio S, Catena F, Santini D, et al. 259 Patients with DCIS of the breast applying USC/Van Nuys prognostic index: a retrospective review with long term follow up. Breast Cancer Res Treat. 2008;109(3):405–16.
127. Fisher E, Dignam J, Tan-Chie E, et al. Pathologic findings from the National Adjuvant Breast Project (NSABP) eight-year update of Protocol B-17: intraductal carcinoma. Cancer. 1999;86:429–38.
128. Silverstein MJ, Rosser R, Gierson E, et al. Axillary Lymph node dissection for intraductal carcinoma—is it indicated? Cancer. 1987;59:1819–24.
129. Silverstein MJ. An argument against routine use of radiotherapy for ductal carcinoma in situ. Oncology. 2003;17(11):1511–46.
130. Silverstein MJ, Barth A, Poller D, et al. Ten-year results comparing mastectomy to excision and radiation therapy for ductal carcinoma in situ of the breast. Eur J Cancer. 1995;31A(9):1425–7.
131. Frykberg E, Masood S, Copeland E, Bland K. Duct carcinoma in situ of the breast. Surg Gynecol Obstet. 1993;177:425–40.

Chapter 16
The Surgical Management of Invasive Breast Cancer

Beth C. Freedman, Alyssa Gillego, and Susan K. Boolbol

The surgical treatment of breast cancer has evolved significantly over the past century. Prior to the 1890s patients diagnosed with breast cancer succumbed to their disease. William Halstead [1] is credited with development of the radical mastectomy, the first surgical treatment for breast cancer. Over the next 120 years advances in breast cancer screening and surgery led to the discovery of smaller, often nonpalpable, breast cancers. The radical or Halstead mastectomy, involves resection of breast, pectoralis major and minor muscles, and axillary lymph nodes. Halstead reported a 3 % local recurrence rate and 40 % 5 year survival. This surgery carried great morbidity and lymphedema was a frequent sequela. This remained the gold standard for breast cancer surgery from the 1890s to the mid-twentieth century. At this time, surgeons recognized the functional and cosmetic morbidity of the Halstead mastectomy and sought an alternative.

In 1948 Patey and Dyson [2] published their series of women who underwent the first version of the modified radical mastectomy. Their operation removed the breast, pectoralis minor muscle, and axillary lymph nodes, but left the pectoralis major muscle intact. They reported no difference in disease free survival or overall survival in patients who underwent a modified radical mastectomy compared with the radical mastectomy group. However, other surgeons were simultaneously advocating more radical surgical techniques including dissection of the internal mammary lymph nodes. In the late 1960s, Jerome Urban [3] and Everett Sugarbaker [4] described the extended radical mastectomy which involved resection of the breast, pectoralis major and minor muscles, axillary lymph nodes, and internal mammary lymph node chain.

B.C. Freedman, M.D.
Department of Breast Surgery, St. Luke's Roosevelt Hospital Center, New York, NY, USA

A. Gillego, M.D.
Department of Surgery, Beth Isreal Medical Center, New York, NY, USA

S.K. Boolbol, M.D., F.A.C.S. (✉)
Division of Breast Surgery, Appel-Venet Comprehensive Breast Service, Beth Israel Medical Center, 10 Union Square East, Suite 4E, New York, NY 10003, USA
e-mail: SBoolbol@chpnet.org

D.S. Francescatti and M.J. Silverstein (eds.), *Breast Cancer: A New Era in Management*,
DOI 10.1007/978-1-4614-8063-1_16,

The present day modified radical mastectomy was popularized by Hugh Auchincloss [5] in 1970. Auchincloss noted no difference in disease free survival and overall survival when both pectoralis muscles are left intact. This operation is still performed today for locally advanced invasive breast cancer. Debate over the appropriate surgical treatment led to a call for scientific evidence. Breast cancer treatment was further revolutionized in 1977 when the results of the National Surgical Adjuvant Breast Project (NSABP) B-04 clinical trial were published. Patients were compared in randomized fashion to radical mastectomy to total mastectomy with or without chest wall irradiation. The NSABP B-04 showed no significant difference in overall survival between these groups [6]. This pivotal trial established that total mastectomy with or without radiation was equivalent to a radical mastectomy with regard to overall survival.

The NSABP B-06 was a prospective randomized trial comparing the overall survival and recurrence free survival in patients who underwent total mastectomy, segmental mastectomy, or segmental mastectomy followed by breast irradiation [7] Fischer concluded segmental mastectomy followed by breast radiation was an acceptable treatment for early stage breast cancer. Twenty-year follow-up revealed 14.3 % locoregional recurrence rate in the segmental mastectomy with radiation arm versus 10.2 % in the total mastectomy arm. These results further validated segmental mastectomy with radiation as a treatment for early stage breast cancer [8]. In Milan, Veronesi and colleagues [9] conducted a randomized trial comparing the long term outcomes of patients who underwent a radical mastectomy with those who underwent breast conserving surgery followed by radiotherapy. Twenty-year follow-up was reported and they concluded no significant difference in the rate of distant metastases and overall survival between the two groups [10]. These landmark studies confirmed breast conserving surgery is equivalent to total mastectomy with regards to overall survival.

In conclusion since the development of the Halstead radical mastectomy more than 120 years ago, great strides have been made in the surgical management of breast cancer. Many breast cancers are detected at an early stage, and are often treated by breast conservation. Recent surgical advances and popularization of oncoplastic techniques have evolved, further improving the cosmetic outcome after lumpectomy. This chapter will review the role of surgery in the treatment of invasive breast cancer.

Invasive Breast Cancer

The two most common types of invasive mammary carcinoma are invasive ductal carcinoma and invasive lobular carcinoma. Other less common types of breast cancer include tubular, mucinous, medullary, and papillary carcinomas of the breast.

Infiltrating Ductal Carcinoma

Infiltrating or invasive ductal carcinoma is the most common form of invasive breast cancer, representing 80 % of all invasive breast cancers. Physical examination may reveal a spectrum of findings ranging from a benign exam to a palpable mass, skin thickening or dimpling, nipple inversion, or lymphadenopathy. Mammographically, invasive cancer may present in many ways, such as an increased density, architectural distortion, nodularity, a mass or microcalcifications. Grossly, invasive cancers have a wide range of appearances.

Microscopic features which are examined include tubule formation, nuclear pleomorphism, and mitotic activity. Each of the three features is graded from 1 to 3, and a total sum is obtained. A score of 3–5 represents a well differentiated or grade 1 carcinoma. A score of 6–7 represents a moderately differentiated or grade 2 carcinoma. A score of 8–9 represents a poorly differentiated or grade 3 carcinoma. This grading system offers prognostic significance, as patients with grade 1 tumors have significantly better survival than those with grade 2 and grade 3 tumors [11].

Infiltrating Lobular Carcinoma

Infiltrating lobular carcinoma is the second most common histology, accounting for 10 % of invasive breast cancers. At presentation, invasive lobular carcinoma may be multifocal, and the incidence of bilateral synchronous tumors is as high as 20 % in some series [12]. Physical examination frequently reveals very subtle findings such as induration or a fullness of the breast. The mammographic findings of invasive lobular carcinoma may appear as an asymmetric density, architectural distortion or microcalcifications. It is not uncommon to have subtle or vague findings either on physical exam or imaging, often leading to underestimation of the extent of disease.

Histologic analysis characteristically reveals loosely cohesive neoplastic cells invading the breast stroma in single file, a feature referred to as Indian filing. This growth pattern creates linear strands of tumor cells, which likely accounts for the vague, indeterminate findings seen on exam and imaging studies. Lobular carcinoma is characterized by the loss of a cellular adhesion protein known as epithelial cadherin or E-cadherin. This leads to the loose pattern of cells seen histologically. Staining for E-cadherin is performed to differentiate between ductal and lobular carcinomas. Invasive lobular carcinoma will be negative for E-cadherin or downregulated in 95 % of cases [13–15]. Invasive ductal carcinoma and ductal carcinoma in situ will characteristically stain positive for E-cadherin [16]. Lobular carcinomas typically express estrogen and progesterone receptors (ER/PR), and usually do not express the human epidermal growth factor receptor protein (HER2/neu) [17].

Special Breast Carcinomas

There are several less common types of breast cancer histologies, and these usually have improved prognosis when compared to ductal carcinomas. Among the most common are tubular, cribriform, mucinous, medullary, and papillary carcinomas. Tubular carcinoma usually has limited metastatic potential and excellent prognosis. Pathologic review demonstrates proliferation of glands and tubules in a single layer without a myoepithelial layer. These tumors generally have low nuclear grade, and when associated with in situ disease, the DCIS is also of low nuclear grade [10]. Invasive cribriform carcinoma also has an excellent prognosis. Histologically, a cribriform or fenestrated growth pattern is seen. It is often observed in conjunction with tumors that have tubular patterns as well. The lack of a myoepithelial layer distinguishes invasive cribriform carcinoma from cribriform DCIS [10]. Mucinous or colloid carcinoma is more commonly seen in patients after the sixth decade [18]. On gross examination these tumor specimens are soft, well-circumscribed masses with a gelatinous consistency. Histologically, tumor cells are seen in clusters within pools of extracellular mucin. These tumors have a favorable prognosis. Some studies report 100 % 10-year survival, compared to 60 % for mixed mucinous and infiltrating ductal tumors [18]. Mucinous carcinomas are traditionally ER and PR positive, and HER2/neu negative. Medullary carcinomas often have an aggressive appearance and are often classified as grade 3 tumors [19]. Most commonly it presents as a palpable mass in the upper outer quadrant of the breast, frequently with palpable axillary lymph nodes. On histologic examination, however, the lymph nodes usually reveal benign reactive changes. Medullary carcinomas are tumors which grow in a characteristic syncitial pattern and often have a surrounding moderate lymphoplasmacytic infiltrate [20]. ER and PR status are usually negative or low (0–30 %), and HER2 is generally negative. Despite these poor prognostic indicators, some studies indicate these cancers have a favorable prognosis [19, 21]. Invasive papillary carcinoma comprises less than 1–2 % of all breast cancers, and is more commonly seen in postmenopausal women. Similar to medullary carcinoma, patients can present with palpable axillary lymphadenopathy, but this is commonly due to benign reactive changes [22].

Staging

The staging of invasive breast cancer is based on the TNM classification system of the American Joint Committee on Cancer (AJCC) [23]. The tumor size (T), lymph node status (N), and the presence or absence of distant metastases (M) determines the treatment plan and prognosis of the patient. Stage 1 and 2 tumors are considered early breast cancer, and are usually treated with partial mastectomy followed by whole breast radiation. Axillary lymph node involvement is commonly seen in Stage 3 patients. These cancers are considered locally advanced, and can be considered for neoadjuvant chemotherapy followed by surgery. Patients with Stage 4 breast cancer have distant metastases beyond the breast and regional lymph nodes.

Mastectomy

The Halstead radical mastectomy was performed on women with breast cancer for almost 100 years. Removal of the breast, regional lymph nodes, and underlying muscles was the preferred surgical treatment for breast cancer for nearly a decade. This approach was based on the assumption that breast cancers spread in centrifugal fashion, invading adjacent tissue, and then near-by lymph nodes. Complications from the operation were great, and women often suffered from large wounds, lymphedema, and chronic pain. The radical mastectomy underwent numerous modifications as surgeons sought to combine oncologic integrity with less morbid procedures. Patey and Dyson [2] found no difference in overall survival when the pectoralis major muscle was preserved. Madden [24] described preservation of both the pectoralis major and minor muscles, and reported no difference in survival when compared to radical mastectomy. In 1964 Crile [25] recommended excision of the axillary lymph nodes only when they appeared to be grossly involved. In 1991 Toth and Lampert [26] were the first surgeons to describe skin-sparing mastectomy. Preservation of the skin allows for improved reconstruction techniques and better cosmetic result. Retrospective studies comparing skin-sparing mastectomy to standard mastectomy show no difference in recurrence or overall survival [27, 28]. Today, a wide variety of surgical procedures are performed to treat breast cancer. These include total mastectomy with or without reconstruction, modified radical mastectomy, partial mastectomy, sentinel node biopsy, and axillary lymph node dissection.

Total mastectomy is performed for locally advanced breast cancer or diffuse disease. Examples of diffuse disease include muticentric tumors or wide-spread DCIS. Total mastectomy is also performed for inflammatory breast cancer. Women with large tumor to breast ratio may require a mastectomy. A comprehensive review of breast imaging and preoperative image-guided biopsies are essential in all patients with breast cancer [29]. Consultation with a plastic surgeon prior to mastectomy will help determine a patient's appropriate type of reconstruction. Laboratory work-up should include complete blood count, chemistry, liver function panel, and alkaline phospatase level. Staging work-up is reserved for patients who present as clinical stage 3 or for symptomatic patients whose complaints may indicate systemic metastasis. Staging work-up includes CT scan of the chest, abdomen, and pelvis, along with bone scan.

If a patient is not an appropriate candidate for reconstruction, total mastectomy is performed by making a large skin ellipse around the nipple-areola complex. A skin-sparing approach is used for patients who are undergoing reconstruction. This incision can be extended medially or laterally to improve exposure during the procedure or allow greater access to the axilla during a dissection. The incision is deepened through the dermis and subcutaneous tissue, and an avascular plane between the overlying skin and underlying gland is identified. Mastectomy flaps can be created with sharp dissection using a scalpel or scissors, or with electrocautery. The plane is followed to the borders of the breast, while attempting to remove all breast parenchyma. The breast is dissected to the anatomic borders of the breast: the sternum medially, the clavicle superiorly, the latissimus muscle laterally, and the inframammary fold or rectus sheath insertion inferiorly. The result is a well-vascularized skin flap. Careful hemostasis is achieved and drains are placed prior to closing the wound. One should try to avoid leaving redundant skin on the chest wall, as a smooth, even surface facilitates wearing of breast prosthesis in a more comfortable fashion. The gland is excised off the chest wall, taking care to include the pectoralis major fascia with the specimen. The breast is handled gently throughout the operation and aggressive manipulation of tissue should be avoided. The specimen is oriented with sutures to help aid pathologic margin analysis. Palpation of the mastectomy flaps should be followed with excision of any additional suspicious tissue.

Recently, surgeons have embarked on nipple-sparing mastectomy and nipple and areola-sparing mastectomy. When performing these procedures, intraoperative analysis of the ductal tissue in the nipple can be performed. There are several methods to achieving this goal. One method involves gently inverting the nipple by the surgeon's forefinger and the ductal tissue is then sharply dissected from the skin. Another method is to sharply dissect the plane deep to the nipple and evaluate this tissue intraoperatively. Some surgeons will place a marker on the nipple bed for orientation purposes for the pathologist. Simmons and colleagues [30] reported on a series of nipple- and areola-sparing mastectomies. In their series, they found a nipple involvement rate of 10 %. Laronga et al. [31] reported a 3 % nipple involvement rate. If intraoperative analysis of the ductal tissue in the nipple is performed and the tissue is found to contain a malignancy, subsequent resection of the nipple-areola complex (NAC) is mandatory. In a retrospective study evaluating 353 nipple-sparing mastectomies, the NAC was preserved in 96.7 % of cases performed [32]. Few patients will retain sensation of the nipple, and both partial and complete nipple loss can be seen. Sacchini [33] published a review of 192 nipple-sparing procedures with a median of 24.6 month follow-up. No patients had involvement of the NAC on pathologic review. Nipple loss in this series was 11 %. Two patients had a local recurrence, but neither recurrence was in the NAC. Careful patient selection remains the key aspect in performing these operations.

Breast Conserving Surgery

In the 1970's increasing use of mammography led to the detection of smaller tumors in the breast, and women were therefore diagnosed at an earlier stage. Surgeons sought to perform less radical surgery and explored the possibility of offering partial mastectomy as an appropriate treatment for breast cancer. Numerous studies were designed to validate the role of breast conserving surgery (BCS). Today, breast conserving surgery is performed for early stage breast cancer. As previously mentioned, the two landmark trails which established partial mastectomy as a treatment for early stage breast cancer were published by Fisher [7] and Veronesi [9]. Fisher and colleagues conducted the NSABP B-06 trail from 1976 to 1984. This phase III trial enrolled 1,600 women with tumors 4 cm or less, and randomized them into three treatment arms. The three arms compared were modified radical mastectomy, partial mastectomy with axillary dissection, and partial mastectomy with axillary dissection and whole breast radiation. Twenty-year follow-up showed higher rate of locoregional recurrence in the group who underwent partial mastectomy with radiation compared to the group who underwent a modified radical mastectomy [8]. However, equivalent disease-free and overall survival was seen in these two groups. Veronesi [9] compared radical mastectomy to quadrantectomy with axillary dissection and radiation. In this study, 701 women with tumors 2 cm or less were randomized. Local recurrence in the radical mastectomy arm was 2.3 %, compared to 8.8 % local recurrence in the quadrantectomy arm. However, 20-year follow-up showed no difference in distant metastasis or overall survival in the two groups. These two pivotal studies helped establish breast conserving surgery as an acceptable and oncologically sound operation for the treatment for early stage breast cancer. It also provided clear evidence for the essential role of radiation in breast conserving procedures.

Breast conserving surgery plus radiation is the preferred treatment for early stage breast cancer; however, contraindications to BCS include prior radiation to the chest, pregnancy, and history of collagen vascular disease. Women with breast cancer and a history of Hodgkin's lymphoma treated with mantle radiation to the chest traditionally undergo mastectomy. Pregnancy is an absolute contraindication to radiation; therefore, pregnant women with breast cancer are treated with mastectomy. However, if a woman is diagnosed with breast cancer in the third trimester of pregnancy, she can undergo partial mastectomy and go on to receive radiation after delivery. Collagen vascular disease, such as lupus and scleroderma, is a relative contraindication to breast conservation because these patients may experience adverse effects to radiation. Another relative contraindication to breast conserving surgery is large tumor to breast ratio. Resection of a large amount of skin or removal of a significant amount of breast volume in women with small breasts may result in a large deformity with unacceptable cosmetic outcome. These patients should undergo oncoplastic reconstruction or mastectomy. Mastectomy should also be performed in patients who despite multiple re-excisions, continue to have positive margins. Inability to clear margins when attempting to perform a lumpectomy is an indication for mastectomy.

A wide variety of techniques and approaches are used when performing partial mastectomy. For nonpalpable breast lesions, an image-guided biopsy should be performed when possible. A marking clip should be placed by the radiologist or surgeon at the site of the image-guided biopsy. A localization wire should be placed at the site of a nonpalpable lesion or adjacent to a marking clip in the breast prior to performing a partial mastectomy. The wire can be placed using mammographic or sonographic guidance. The use of a localization wire for nonpalpable lesions requires careful review of a patient's imaging with the radiologist. Resection of the cancer with a margin of surrounding breast tissue requires thoughtful planning, with presence of the localization images in the operating suite for review during the procedure. Radiographic verification of the tumor or marking clip in the specimen excised is critical. Another consideration when performing a partial mastectomy is the placement and type of surgical incision. Incisions should ideally be made directly above the area of concern in order to avoid bringing the tumor through unaffected tissue. For tumors located in the superior aspect of the breast, incisions can be made in horizontal or radial fashion. Radial incisions are used for tumors located in the inferior aspect of the breast. An inframmary approach can be used for small tumors located near the breast fold. Occasionally, an incision along the inferior aspect of the areola can be created and extended medially or laterally depending on the location of the tumor.

Given the proven oncologic safety of breast conservation, the field of oncoplastic surgery has emerged to optimize cosmetic results. Oncoplastic surgery encompasses use of adjacent tissue transfer, replacement of resected breast volume with the use of autologous flaps, as well as contralateral balancing procedures. Patients who are candidates for an oncoplastic operation are women who require resection of a large volume of tissue or skin. A multidisciplinary approach is critical and must be coordinated between the breast surgeon, plastic surgeon, breast imager, and radiation oncologist [34].

Axillary Staging

Staging of the axilla is mandatory for patients with invasive carcinoma who undergo either a breast conserving operation or total mastectomy. Women who present with clinically palpable lymph nodes should undergo a needle biopsy by palpation or an image-guided biopsy. Specht et al. [35] reported on 106 patients with clinically suspicious axillary nodes, and found a false positive rate of 41 %. Women diagnosed with early stage breast cancer (T1 or T2) should undergo sentinel lymph node (SLN) biopsy [36]. Studies show that sentinel lymph node (SLN) biopsy is appropriate in patients with T3 tumors [37, 38]. Patients with T4 tumors or inflammatory breast cancer are not considered candidates for SLN biopsy and should undergo axillary node dissection [39].

The lymph nodes of the axilla are designated level 1, level 2, and level 3 according to their location relative to the pectoralis minor muscle. Level 1 nodes are lateral to the muscle, level 2 nodes are beneath the muscle, and level 3 nodes are medial to the muscle. Historically, surgical management of breast cancer involved excision of the breast and all level 1, 2, and 3 lymph nodes. In 1992 Morton [40] first introduced the use of lymphatic mapping and SLN biopsy in the management of melanoma. Giuliano and colleagues [41] then applied Morton's sentinel lymph node technique to breast cancer. The NSABP B-32 study is the largest prospective randomized trial which examined the role of sentinel lymph node biopsy in invasive breast carcinoma [36]. This phase III trial randomized 5,611 women to two arms. The women were randomized to sentinel node biopsy with axillary lymph node dissection or sentinel node biopsy with axillary dissection only if the sentinel node(s) had metastatic disease. Blue dye was used in combination with radiotracer to identify sentinel nodes. There was no statistically significant difference in 8-year overall survival between the two arms. The overall survival in the SLN biopsy with completion axillary dissection group was 91.8 %, and the overall survival was 90.3 % in the group of women who had SLN biopsy and axillary dissection only when the SLN was positive. Rates of locoregional recurrence and disease-free survival were also equivalent in the two groups.

Various techniques for performing sentinel lymph node biopsy for breast cancer have been described. One can use blue dye, radiotracer, or a combination of both blue dye and radiotracer [42]. Typically, technetium sulfur colloid (Tc99) is the radiotracer agent used. Lymphoscintigraphy is not necessary after injection of the isotope, except in the case of a patient who has had axillary surgery or staging in the past [43]. These patients should have lymphoscintigraphy to observe for mapping of the tracer into an axillary node [44]. The two most commonly used dyes when performing a sentinel node biopsy are methylene blue and isosulfan blue (Lymphazurin 1 %). The rate of allergic reaction to isosulfan blue dye was 1.6 % and the rate of hypotension was 0.5 % in a series reported by Montgomery and colleagues [45]. If blue dye is used, a volume of 1–3 mL should be injected into the subareolar lymphatic plexus behind the nipple [41]. A single intradermal dose of Tc99 should be injected into the upper outer periareolar skin [46]. The American Society of Clinical Oncology (ASCO) recommends using both blue dye and radiotracer to increase the rate of sentinel lymph node identification [42]. In a series by Kim et al. [47] the SLN identification rate was 96 % and the false negative rate was 7 %. A hand-held gamma probe is used to identify an area in the axilla with the highest counts. A small incision is made along the inferior aspect of the hair-bearing area of the axilla, the clavipectoral fascia is incised, and the axilla is exposed. An axillary node is considered a sentinel lymph node if it is blue, demonstrates increased gamma uptake, or is noted to have a count more than 10 % of the highest of node. A critical portion of the sentinel lymph node procedure is palpation of the axilla and excision of any firm or abnormal appearing lymph nodes.

The surgical complications which can result from axillary lymph node dissection are well-documented. Patients can suffer debilitating consequences such as chronic pain, lymphedema, and nerve injury. Devastating surgical morbidity which can result from axillary dissection and low rates of axillary recurrence led surgeons to attempt to identify women who may not benefit from complete axillary lymph node dissection. In 2010 Guiliano and colleagues [48] reported the results of the American College of Surgeons Oncology Group (ACOSOG) Z0011 trial. This study randomized 891 women with positive sentinel lymph nodes into two groups. One group of women with positive SLN biopsies had an axillary dissection, and the other group with positive SLN biopsies did not undergo an axillary dissection. All women in the study had T1 or T2 disease, were clinically lymph-node negative, and underwent lumpectomy with whole-breast radiation. Women with T3 or T4 disease, multicentric tumors, and 3 or more positive sentinel lymph nodes were excluded. At median follow-up of 6.3 years, 5-year overall survival was 92.5 % in women who did not have an axillary dissection and 91.8 % in women who had an axillary lymph node dissection. The rate of locoregional recurrence in the women who did not have an axillary dissection was 1.8 %, and the rate of locoregional recurrence in the women who had an axillary dissection was 3.6 %. This was not statistically significant. Adjuvant systemic therapy was administered to 97 % of women who did not have a node dissection, and to 96 % of women who had a complete axillary dissection. All women in the study received whole breast radiation with standard tangential fields.

Equivalent recurrence rates and overall survival rates in the two groups indicate that perhaps local control is not improved by axillary lymph node dissection, and dissection may be omitted for patients who fit the Z11 criteria.

If performed, a complete axillary dissection should encompass the level 1 and level 2 lymph nodes [49]. The approach to an axillary node dissection may either be through a separate axillary incision or through the same incision used for the breast operation. The clavipectoral fascia is identified and divided. The pectoralis muscles are retracted upward and medially during the dissection in order to access level 2 of the axilla. The specimen removed should include the tissue from the lateral border of the pectoralis muscles to the anterior border of the latissimus dorsi muscle. The superior border of resection is the inferior aspect of the axillary vein. Low-dosage electrocautery should be used cautiously in the axilla. The thoracodorsal and long thoracic vessels and nerves should be identified and preserved. The thoracodorsal nerve innervates the serratus anterior and injury results in weak shoulder abduction. The long thoracic nerve innervates the latissimus dorsi muscle and injury results in a winged scapula deformity. When possible the intercostobrachial nerves should also preserved in order to avoid numbness along the undersurface of the upper arm. Closed-suction drains are placed at the surgeon's discretion.

Summary

The management of breast cancer has undergone a dramatic evolution over the last century. The history of breast cancer is rich in large, elegant trials and therefore the approach to the disease should be evidence-based. The treatment of breast cancer requires a thorough examination of the patient's breast imaging and review of the preoperative workup. Image-guided biopsy should be performed prior to surgery. Selection of the type of surgery and systemic therapy entails consideration of both disease presentation and patient factors. Complete oncologic resection and achievement of negative margins is essential. Treatment of breast cancer should be coordinated by a multidisciplinary team and tailored to the individual patient.

References

1. Halstead WS. The results of operations for the cure of cancer of the breast performed at the Johns Hopkins Hospital from June, 1889, to January, 1894. Ann Surg. 1894;20(5):497–555.
2. Patey DH, Dyson WH. The prognosis of carcinoma of the breast in relation to the type of operation performed. Br J Cancer. 1948;2:7–13.
3. Urban JA. Extended radical mastectomy for breast cancer. Am J Surg. 1970;1963(106):366–404.
4. Sugarbaker ED. Extended radical mastectomy: its superiority in the treatment of breast cancer. JAMA. 1964;187(2):96–9.
5. Auchincloss H. Modified radical mastectomy: why not? Am J Surg. 1970;119(5):506–9.

6. Fisher B, Montague E, Redmond C, et al. Comparison of radical mastectomy with alternative treatments for primary breast cancer. A first report of results from a prospective randomized clinical trial. Cancer. 1977;39:2827–39.
7. Fisher B, Bauer M, Margolese R, et al. Five-year results of a randomized clinical trial comparing total mastectomy and segmental mastectomy with or without radiation in the treatment of breast cancer. N Engl J Med. 1985;312(11):665–73.
8. Fisher B, Anderson S, Bryant J, et al. Twenty-year follow-up of a randomized trial comparing total mastectomy, lumpectomy and lumpectomy plus irradiation for the treatment of invasive breast cancer. N Engl J Med. 2002;347:1233–41.
9. Veronesi U, Saccozzi R, Del Vecchio M, et al. Comparing radical mastectomy with quadrantectomy, axillary dissection, and radiotherapy in patients with small cancers of the breast. N Engl J Med. 1981;305:6–11.
10. Veronesi U, Cascinelli N, Mariani E, et al. Twenty-year follow-up of a randomized study comparing breast-conserving surgery with radical mastectomy for early breast cancer. N Engl J Med. 2002;347:1222–32.
11. Elston CW, Ellis IO. Pathologic prognostic factors in breast cancer I: the value of histologic grade in breast cancer. Experience from a large study with long-term follow-up. Histopathology. 1991;19:403–10.
12. Dixon M, Anderson TJ, Page DL, et al. Infiltrating lobular carcinoma of the breast: an evaluation of the incidence and consequence of bilateral disease. Br J Surg. 1983;70(9):513–6.
13. Holland R, Hendricks J. Microcalcifications associated with ductal carcinoma in situ: mammographic pathologic correlation. Semin Diagn Pathol. 1994;11:181.
14. Solin LJ, Fourquet A, Vicini FA, et al. Salvage treatment for local recurrence after breast conserving surgery and radiation as initial treatment for mammographically detected ductal carcinoma in situ of the breast. Cancer. 2001;91:1090–7.
15. Lagios MD. The Lagios experience. In: Silverstein MJ, editor. Ductal carcinoma in situ of the breast. Philadelphia, PA: Lippincott Williams and Wilkins; 2002. p. 303–7.
16. De Leeuw WJ, Berx G, Vos CB, et al. Simultaneous loss of E-cadherin and catenins in invasive lobular breast cancer and in lobular carcinoma in situ. J Pathol. 1997;183(4):404–11.
17. Porter PL, Garcia R, Moe R, et al. C-erb-2 oncogene protein in situ and invasive lobular breast neoplasia. Cancer. 1991;68(2):331–4.
18. Fentiman IS, Millis RR, Smith P, et al. Mucoid breast carcinomas: histology and prognosis. Br J Cancer. 1997;75(7):1061–5.
19. Pedersen L, Zedeler K, Holck S, et al. Medullary carcinoma of the breast. Prevalence and prognostic importance of clinical risk factors in breast cancer. Eur J Cancer. 1995;31(13–14):2289–95.
20. Ellis IO, Schnitt SJ, Sastre-Garau X, Bussolati G. In: Tavassoli FA, Devilee P, editors. Tumours of the breast and female genital organs. Lyon: IARC Press; 2003. p. 13–59.
21. Bloom HJ, Richardson WW, Field JR. Host resistance and survival in carcinoma of breast: a study of 104 cases of medually carcinoma in a series of 1,411 breast cancer followed for 20 years. BMJ. 1970;3(716):181–8.
22. Fisher ER, Palekar AS, Redmond C, Barton B, Fisher B. Pathologic findings from the National Surgical Adjuvant Breast Project (Protocol No.4) VI. Invasive papillary cancer. Am J Clin Pathol. 1980;73(3):313–22.
23. American Joint Committee on Cancer. AJCC cancer staging manual. 7th ed. New York, NY: Springer; 2010. p. 347–76.
24. Madden JL, Kandalaft S, Bourque RA. Modified radical mastectomy. Ann Surg. 1972;175(5):624–34.
25. Crile Jr G. Results of simplified treatment of breast cancer. Surg Gynecol Obstet. 1964;118:517–23.
26. Toth BA, Lappert P. Modified skin incision for mastectomy: the need for plastic surgical input in preoperative planning. Plast Reconstr Surg. 1991;87(6):1048–53.
27. Simmons RM, Fish SK, Gayle L, et al. Local and distant recurrence rates in skin-sparing mastectomies compared with non-skin-sparing mastectomies. Ann Surg Oncol. 1999;6(7):676–81.

28. Meretoja TJ, Rasia S, Von Smitten KAJ, et al. Late results of skin-sparing mastectomy followed by immediate breast reconstruction. Br J Surg. 2007;94(10):1220–5.
29. Clarke-Pearson E, Jacobson AF, Boolbol SK, et al. Quality assuarance initiative at one institution for minimally invasive breast biopsy as initial diagnostic technique. J Am Coll Surg. 2009;208(1):75–8.
30. Simmons RM, Brennan M, Christos P, et al. Analysis of nipple/areola involvement with mastectomy: can the areola be preserved? Ann Surg Oncol. 2002;9:165–8.
31. Laronga C, Kemp B, Johnston D, et al. The incidence of occult nipple-areola complex involvement in breast cancer patients receiving skin-sparing mastectomy. Ann Surg Oncol. 1999;66:609–13.
32. De Alcantara FP, Capko D, Barry JM, et al. Nipple-sparing mastectomy for breast cancer and risk-reducing surgery: the Memorial Sloan-Kettering cancer center experience. Ann Surg Oncol. 2011;18:3117–22.
33. Sacchini V, Pinotti JA, Barros AC, et al. Nipple-sparing mastectomy for breast cancer and risk reduction: oncologic or technical problem? J Am Coll Surg. 2006;203:704–14.
34. Holmes DR, Schooler W, Smith R. Oncoplastic approaches to breast conservation. Int J Breast Cancer. 2011;2011:303879.
35. Specht MC, Fey JV, Borgen PI, Cody HS. Is the clinically positive axilla in breast cancer really a contraindication to sentinel node biopsy? J Am Coll Surg. 2005;200(1):10–4.
36. Krag DN, Anderson SJ, Juilian TB, et al. Sentinel-lymph-node resection compared with conventional axillary-lymph-node dissection in clinically node-negative patients with breast cancer: overall survival findings from the NSABP B-32 randomised phase 3 trial. Lancet Oncol. 2010;11(10):927–33.
37. Chung MH, Ye W, Guiliano AE. Role for sentinel lymph node dissection in the management of large (≥5cm) invasive breast cancer. Ann Surg Oncol. 2001;8(9):688–92.
38. Wong SL, Chao C, Edwards MJ, et al. Accuracy of sentinel lymph node biopsy for patients with T2 and T3 breast cancers. Am Surg. 2001;67(6):522–6.
39. Hidar S, Bibi M, Gharbi O, et al. Sentinel lymph node biopsy after neoadjuvant chemotherapy in inflammatory breast cancer. Int J Surg. 2009;7(3):272–5.
40. Morton DL, Wen DR, Wong JH, et al. Technical details of intraoperative lymphatic mapping for early stage melanoma. Arch Surg. 1992;127:392–9.
41. Giuliano AE, Kirgan DM, Guenther JM, Morton DL. Lymphatic mapping and sentinel lymphadenectomy in breast cancer. Ann Surg. 1994;220:391–8.
42. Lyman GH, Giuliano AE, Somerfield MR, et al. American Society of Clinical Oncology guideline recommendations for sentinel lymph node biopsy in early-stage breast cancer. J Clin Oncol. 2005;23(30):7703–20.
43. McMasters KM, Wong SL, Tuttle TM, et al. Preoperative lymphoscintigraphy for breast cancer does not improve the ability to identify axillary sentinel lymph nodes. Ann Surg. 2000;231(5):724–31.
44. Barone JL, Feldman SM, Estabrook A, et al. Reoperative sentinel lymph node biopsy in patients with locally recurrent breast cancer. Am J Surg. 2007;194:491–3.
45. Montgomery LL, Thorne AC, Van Zee KJ, et al. Isosulfan blue reactions during sentinel lymph node mapping for breast cancer. Anesth Analg. 2002;95(2):385–8.
46. Boolbol SK, Fey JV, Borgen PI, et al. Intradermal isotope injection: a highly accurate method of lymphatic mapping in breast carcinoma. Ann Surg Oncol. 2001;8(10):20–4.
47. Kim T, Guiliano AE, Lyman GH. Lymphatic mapping and sentinel lymph node biopsy in early-stage breast carcinoma. Cancer. 2006;106:4–16.
48. Giuliano AE, Hunt KK, Ballman KV, et al. Axillary dissection vs. no axillary dissection in women with invasive breast cancer and sentinel node metastasis: a randomized clinical trial. JAMA. 2011;305(6):569–75.
49. Kodama H, Nio Y, Iguchi C, Khan N. Ten-year follow-up results of a randomized controlled study comparing level 1 versus level 3 axillary lymph node dissection for primary breast cancer. Br J Cancer. 2006;95(7):811–6.

Chapter 17
Surgical Management of the Axilla

Jennifer H. Lin, Catherine M. Dang, and Armando E. Giuliano

Past: Axillary Lymph Node Dissection

Early theories of breast cancer by W. Sampson Handley and William Halsted suggested that breast cancer was a disease which spread in an orderly progression from primary tumor to regional lymphatics then to distant metastatic sites. In 1882, Halsted performed the first radical mastectomy, which included the removal of the pectoralis major muscle, pectoralis minor, complete axillary lymph node dissection (ALND), and even supraclavicular lymph node dissection, in an attempt to achieve extensive locoregional control and thus yield the greatest cure rates [1]. This concept of sequential tumor spread was disputed by Fisher in the 1970s, who suggested that breast cancer was a systemic disease at the time of diagnosis, requiring systemic treatment rather than just locoregional surgical control. Fisher's studies on the mechanism of metastases, which demonstrated that tumor dissemination involved both the lymphatic and vascular systems of the breast, suggested that treatment aimed at the removal of nodal metastases was unlikely to improve survival [2].

The Halstedian concept was scientifically challenged by Fisher's National Surgical Adjuvant Breast and Bowel Project (NSABP) B-04 prospective randomized clinical study, which compared (a) radical mastectomy to (b) simple mastectomy with nodal and chest wall irradiation to (c) simple mastectomy alone. This study with 25 years of follow-up, which showed no difference in overall survival between the three treatment arms, demonstrated that the variations in treatment of locoregional disease did not affect survival [3]. This pivotal trial became the backbone of current surgical management of the breast and, more recently, the axilla today.

J.H. Lin, M.D.
Department of Surgical Oncology, John Wayne Cancer Institute, Santa Monica, CA, USA

C.M. Dang, M.D. • A.E. Giuliano, M.D., F.A.C.S., F.R.C.S.E.D. (✉)
Department of Surgery, Cedars-Sinai Medical Center, 310 N. San vicente Blvd., Los Angeles, CA, USA
e-mail: Armando.guiliano@cshs.org

D.S. Francescatti and M.J. Silverstein (eds.), *Breast Cancer: A New Era in Management*, DOI 10.1007/978-1-4614-8063-1_17, © Springer Science+Business Media New York 2014

Present: Sentinel Lymph Node Biopsy

Axillary nodal status is the most significant factor predictive of long-term survival in patients with breast cancer. Prior to the development of the sentinel lymph node biopsy (SLNB) technique, nodal status was traditionally determined by levels I and II axillary lymph node dissection. However, the association of axillary dissection with significant morbidity, including pain, lymphedema, cosmetic deformity, nerve injury, and increased risk of infection, prompted evaluation of a less-morbid and less-invasive technique for identification of nodal disease. In 1994, a large study established the concept of sentinel node biopsy [4]. The development and acceptance of SLNB has since revolutionized treatment. SLNB has now replaced ALND as a highly accurate and less-morbid axillary staging procedure in patients with clinically node-negative early-stage breast cancer.

Technique and Methods of Localization

This technique was first described by Morton in 1992 for clinical stage I cutaneous melanoma [5]. SLNB is based on the hypothesis that the first node draining the primary tumor reflects the tumor status of the regional lymphatic nodal basin. The sentinel node was localized by an intradermal injection at the tumor site with radiolabelled colloid or vital blue dye, or both together, and was highly predictive of the status of the remaining lymph nodes in that basin. In 1991, a feasibility study to establish the technique and efficacy of lymphatic mapping and sentinel lymph node dissection in breast cancer patients was begun in patients with breast cancer [4]. In this landmark study, 174 consecutive patients with any stage breast cancer requiring axillary dissection had 1 % isosulfan blue dye in various volumes and times injected peri-tumorally prior to lymph node dissection. This technique for sentinel node identification had not been established and evolved during the study. Even without a defined technique, the procedure was predictive of the tumor status of the axillary basin in 109/114 patients (96 %) in whom a sentinel node was identified; false negative 5/42 (11.9 %).

Subsequent studies have shown that the sentinel lymph node can be identified by injection of blue dye (isosulfan blue or methylene blue), radiolabelled colloid, or a combination of the two. When radiolabelled-colloid is used, technetium-99m labeled sulfur colloid is injected into the peritumoral, intradermal, or subareolar area about 2–24 h preoperatively. Typically, 0.5 mCi of filtered 99mTc sulfur colloid in a volume of 0.5 cm^3 is used. A lymphoscintigram can then be performed to document the drainage pattern of the breast lymphatics to the regional lymph nodes, and the area over these nodes can be marked by the nuclear medicine physician preoperatively to facilitate sentinel node identification and skin incision placement by the surgeon. Intra-operative detection with a hand-held gamma probe further aids in localizing the sentinel lymph nodes by emitting an audible signal. The number of "hot" nodes removed is dependent on several variables including timing of injection, concentration of radiolabelled colloid, and definition of a "hot" radioactive node. A radioactive node can be defined as the node with the greatest absolute counts, a 10:1 ratio of sentinel node to background, a fourfold reduction in count after sentinel node removal, or a 10-s count greater than 25. Many surgeons feel that all sentinel nodes with counts greater than 10 % of the node with the highest absolute count should be removed. This guideline has been validated at Memorial Sloan Kettering Cancer Center and has shown that it correctly identifies 98.3 % of positive nodes in patients with multiple sentinel nodes [6]. Injection of technetium-99m labeled sulfur colloid and lymphoscintigraphy has the advantage of identification of extra-axillary lymphatic drainage, including supraclavicular, infraclavicular, and internal mammary nodes. Furthermore, it can be very useful in identifying alternative lymphatic drainage and sentinel lymph nodes in patients who have had prior axillary surgery. Most surgeons find the use of both blue dye and radioisotope to be easier and more successful than either alone.

The types of vital blue dye most commonly used for lymphatic mapping are isosulfan blue dye and methylene blue. Isosulfan blue dye has a documented risk of allergic and anaphylactic reactions, and can cause rash, hives, urticaria, pruritis, and hypotension in up to 3 % of patients. Alternatively, while methylene blue is less costly and has a lower risk of allergic reactions, it has been known to cause skin and nipple necrosis when injected intradermally. For this reason, it should be used in a 1:2 dilution and intradermal injection should be avoided. Efficacy is equivalent between methylene blue and isosulfan blue [7–11].

Several studies have compared the success rate of sentinel lymph node dissection with blue dye, radiocolloid, or a combination of both. Morrow et al performed a randomized trial comparing the use of blue dye alone compared with blue dye plus radiocolloid, and identified no significant advantage to the combined technique [12]. It has also been shown, however, that the accuracy of SLNB depends heavily on the proficiency of the surgeon, and most surgeons rely on both dye and isotope to identify a sentinel node. In the past, the American Society of Breast Surgeons guidelines supported performing 20 cases of SLNB with backup ALND, with an identification rate of 85 % and a false-negative rate less than 5 %, in order to become proficient at SLNB. Currently, most surgeons are trained in the technique in residency or fellowship.

There is no consensus regarding the ideal sites for dye or radioactive colloid injection. Peritumoral [4, 13], intradermal [14, 15], subdermal [16], and subareolar [17, 18] injections have been found to be equally effective in localizing the sentinel lymph node. Peritumoral injections have been found to better identify internal mammary nodal drainage [15, 19–22], and subareolar injections are preferred for multicentric disease [23]. Several studies have reported high identification and concordance rates for subareolar injection of blue dye and/or radiocolloid. The disadvantage of a subareolar and dermal injection of vital blue dye is that it can cause prolonged blue discoloration of the skin and even permanent tattooing.

The number of nodes removed during sentinel node biopsy is most commonly 1–3 regardless of technique [24]. In the Axillary Mapping Against Nodal Axillary Clearance (ALMANAC) study, the group found that 99.6 % of the node-positive patients had metastases detected within the first 4 sentinel nodes removed. The false negative rate in patients with 1 sentinel node removed was 10 %, compared to 1 % when 3 or more sentinel nodes were removed, suggesting that removal of more than four sentinel nodes is unnecessary [25].

Several studies have identified patient characteristics associated with difficulty in sentinel node identification. Age greater than 70 years and increased BMI were associated with increased SLND failure in the American College of Surgeons Oncology Group (ACOSOG) Z0010 trial [26]. In the ALMANAC study, factors associated with decreased sentinel node identification were age >50 years, increased BMI, tumors outside of the upper outer quadrant, non-visualization of nodes on preoperative lymphoscintigraphy, or an interval of 12 h or more between radioisotope injection and sentinel node biopsy [25].

Any additional palpable or clinically suspicious nodes that are neither blue nor hot should also be removed, because cancer-filled nodes may not take up dye or colloid. If the sentinel node is not identified, a full axillary lymph node dissection should be performed.

In 2005, the American Society of Clinical Oncology (ASCO) provided guidelines for sentinel lymph node biopsy in early-stage breast cancer [27]. While these recommendations remain in effect, most surgeons do not strictly adhere to these guidelines and are doing sentinel node biopsies in select cases for T3 or T4 tumors, high grade DCIS in breast-conserving surgery (BCS), suspicious palpable axillary nodes, prior axillary surgery, prior non-oncologic breast surgery, and prior preoperative systemic therapy (see Table 17.1).

Controversial Circumstances

Pregnancy

The safety and test performance of SLNB during pregnancy has not been fully evaluated; however, radiolabelled colloids are safe based on the rapid clearance and uptake of the colloid into the reticuloendothelial system. Data has demonstrated that the dose of radiation to the fetus is minimal. Recent studies have confirmed the safety of SLNB during pregnancy using low-dose lymphoscintigraphy (10 MBq on average) with (99m)Tc, advising a 1-day protocol to reduce the time and dose of radiation [28–30]. Blue dye should not be used during pregnancy, as it currently is classified as a category C drug and there is limited data on its teratogenic effects. Furthermore, its use has a possible risk of anaphylactic maternal reaction, which can be harmful for the fetus [30]. While some centers do offer lymphoscintigraphy and SLNB for pregnant patients, some surgeons prefer routine elective ALND. Alternatively, the SLNB procedure can be delayed until postpartum if the patient is close to term.

Table 17.1 2005 ASCO guideline recommendations for sentinel lymph node biopsy in Early-Stage Breast Cancer

Clinical circumstances	Recommendations for use of sentinel node biopsy	Level of evidence
T1 or T2 tumors	Acceptable	Good
T3 or T4 tumors	Not recommended	Insufficient
Multicentric tumors	Acceptable	Limited
Inflammatory breast cancer	Not recommended	Insufficient
DCIS with mastectomy	Acceptable	Limited
DCIS without mastectomy	Not recommended except for large DCIS (>5 cm) on core biopsy or with suspected or proven microinvasion	Insufficient
Suspicious, palpable axillary nodes	Not recommended	Good
Older age	Acceptable	Limited
Obesity	Acceptable	Limited
Male breast cancer	Acceptable	Limited
Pregnancy	Not recommended	Insufficient
Evaluation of internal mammary lymph nodes	Acceptable	Limited
Prior diagnostic or excisional breast biopsy	Acceptable	Limited
Prior axillary surgery	Not recommended	Limited
Prior non-oncologic breast surgery (reduction or augmentation mammoplasty, breast reconstruction, etc.)	Not recommended	Insufficient
After preoperative systematic therapy	Not recommended	Insufficient
Before preoperative systematic therapy	Acceptable	Limited

While these recommendations remain in effect, most surgeons do not strictly adhere to these guidelines and are doing sentinel node biopsies in select cases for T3 or T4 tumors, high-grade DCIS in breast-conserving surgery (BCS), suspicious palpable axillary nodes, prior axillary surgery, prior non-oncologic breast surgery, and prior preoperative systemic therapy

Lyman GH, ASCO Guideline recommendations, J Clin Oncol. 2005 [27]

Special Situations

DCIS

SLNB is generally not recommended for patients with DCIS; however, in certain clinical circumstances, sentinel node staging may be performed in order to avoid a second operation. While 5–15 % of patients with DCIS will have involved sentinel nodes, virtually all have micrometastases or isolated tumor cells of no significance [31–33]. SLNB is recommended for patients with DCIS when a mastectomy is indicated or when immediate reconstruction is planned, as axillary staging by SLNB is no longer possible if an invasive tumor is subsequently found. To avoid a second operation on the axilla if invasive cancer is found, selective use of SLNB is recommended in patients with large (>4 cm) or high-grade DCIS diagnosed with core needle biopsy who are having BCS [27]. Invasive cancer will subsequently be found upon excision in 10–20 % of patients with DCIS diagnosed by core biopsy.

Male Breast Cancer

Although the diagnosis of breast cancer in men is often delayed, resulting in presentations with more advanced tumors, relative survival by stage of disease is similar to that for women [34]. Thus, the most common surgical procedure for male breast cancer is modified radical mastectomy followed by radiation therapy for large tumors or those with nodal metastases [35]. Numerous small institutional studies support the feasibility and accuracy of SLNB in male breast cancer patients [36–38]. As in women, sentinel node analysis has been shown to be a reliable tool in male breast cancer patients, sparing a significant number of patients unnecessary axillary lymph node dissections [39].

Prior Axillary Surgery

The success of SLNB after prior axillary surgery has been previously thought to be decreased due to the disruption of the lymphatic drainage pattern. Multiple recent studies have shown that reoperative SLNB is feasible in the setting of local recurrence after previous BCS and axillary surgery [40–42] with the success of identifying a sentinel node being inversely related to the number of nodes removed previously [43]. In patients who have had a previous complete axillary dissection, the success of reoperative SLNB has been reported to be between 29 and 38 % [43, 44]. Non-axillary drainage has been found in 11–30 % of reoperative SLNB patients after a prior complete axillary dissection [41, 43]. Lymphoscintigraphy, in addition to dye-directed lymphatic mapping, is necessary in these scenarios to aid in identifying aberrant non-axillary lymphatic drainage patterns [43, 45, 46].

Multicentric Lesions

Multicentric cancer, defined as distinct cancers occurring in different quadrants of the same breast, or at a distance of more than 2–5 cm from each other, occurs in approximately 10 % of cases. Some concerns regarding SLNB in this setting are due to the possibility that multiple foci of the cancer might drain to different lymph nodes and increase the false-negative rate of the procedure. Anatomically, the embryologic development of the lymphatic pathways support the notion that the entire breast drains through the same axillary node or nodes [47]. Studies have shown greater success in identifying the sentinel nodes in these patients with acceptable false-negative rates using subdermal [48], intradermal [21], and subareolar [17] injections over peritumoral injection. Recent data following 5-year results of a large single-institution series have demonstrated that the rate of axillary recurrence is acceptably low following SLNB in multicentric disease, thus confirming the use of SLNB as a standard procedure in this setting [49].

Suspicious Palpable Axillary Lymph Nodes

Most SLNB studies have excluded patients with clinically positive axillary nodes. While ALND is the standard of care in patients with suspicious palpable axillary lymph nodes, determination of metastatic disease in the axilla by clinical exam is often unreliable. Previous studies have shown that clinical examination of the axilla can be inaccurate and falsely positive in up to 41 % of patients [50]. In these circumstances, axillary ultrasound and ultrasound-guided needle biopsy is a reliable technique which can be used to guide axillary management [51]. Alternatively, patients with suspicious nodes can undergo SLNB, with the clinically suspicious nodes removed and evaluated as sentinel nodes regardless of whether they take up blue dye or radiolabeled colloid.

Prophylactic Mastectomy

The popularity of prophylactic mastectomy has more than doubled between 1998 and 2003 in the SEER database [52]. The risk of discovering an occult breast cancer in a prophylactic mastectomy specimen is approximately 5 % in high-risk women [53, 54]. Additionally, in patients with a history of breast cancer, the risk of developing a contralateral breast cancer is about 0.5–1 % per year [55–57]. However, the widespread use of hormonal therapy may reduce the risk to less than 0.5 % [58]. Because the ability to perform a SLNB is lost if an occult breast cancer is discovered in a prophylactic mastectomy specimen, some surgeons advocate the use of SLNB at the time of prophylactic mastectomy in high-risk patients. While routine SLNB is not warranted in all patients undergoing prophylactic mastectomy, it may be considered in higher risk patients such as older women, patients with invasive lobular carcinoma or LCIS [59], or those with ambiguous imaging abnormalities. Patients with locally advanced primary breast cancers [54] and inflammatory breast cancer [60] may be advised to undergo a SLNB at the time of contralateral prophylactic mastectomy due to a significantly increased risk of crossover metastasis. Overall, in patients undergoing prophylactic mastectomy associated with early-stage disease, SLNB is not indicated. Patients with undiagnosed imaging abnormalities on ultrasound or MRI may be candidates for SLNB where the breast with the abnormality is removed prophylactically.

Neoadjuvant Chemotherapy

The timing of when to perform SLNB with neoadjuvant chemotherapy (NAC) is still under considerable debate. Neoadjuvant chemotherapy can downstage locally advanced breast cancers, making many patients good candidates for BCS. Additionally, neoadjuvant chemotherapy can downstage the axillary lymph nodes in a considerable proportion of patients [61, 62] (30–40 %) and can lead to clearance of microscopic nodal disease. At M.D. Anderson Cancer Center, investigators reported that up to 23 % of patients with locally advanced breast cancer with axillary metastases were cleared of cytologically positive axillary nodes after four cycles of doxorubicin-based neoadjuvant chemotherapy [63]. Occult metastases were discovered with IHC stain on an additional 10 % of the negative nodes.

The feasibility and accuracy of SLNB after neoadjuvant chemotherapy remains controversial despite the increasing use of neoadjuvant chemotherapy for operable breast cancer. There are concerns that SLNB after NAC may decrease the accuracy of identification of the sentinel node and increase the chance of a false-negative finding [64, 65]. The false-negative rates of sentinel nodes after NAC have been reported to be between 0 and 33 % in several single-institution series [66–77]. Several meta-analyses have shown that SLNB after neoadjuvant chemotherapy in clinically node-negative patients has an acceptable sentinel node identification rate and false-negative rate [78] (see Table 17.2).

The largest series examining the feasibility of SLNB after NAC was completed as part of the NSABP B-27 trial [79]. 428 patients treated with NAC underwent SLNB with either radioactive colloid, lymphazurin blue dye, or both. The success rate for identification of the sentinel nodes was 84.8 %. Although further data is needed to fully evaluate the role of SLNB after neoadjuvant chemotherapy, the study suggested that the technique of SLNB can be best applicable to those patients who demonstrate a complete clinical response after NAC.

Advocates in favor of performing SLNB before NAC argue that the status of the axillary nodes can be obtained without the potential confounding effects of NAC [80]. Furthermore, the information from axillary staging before NAC is important in determining which patients will subsequently need a completion axillary dissection or axillary nodal radiation. Tumor-negative sentinel node patients can avoid ALND, while those with tumor-involved sentinel nodes prior to NAC ultimately will undergo ALND after chemotherapy [77, 81]. Currently there is no convincing evidence that patients with abnormal axillary nodes who receive NAC and then have a negative sentinel lymph node following treatment can be spared ALND. NAC is thought to affect axillary staging by causing fibrosis and obstruction of tumor-involved lymphatic channels, thus leading to inaccurate mapping. The response of lymph nodes to chemotherapy may occur nonuniformly, limiting the accuracy of the SLNB in this setting [24]. Additionally, because NAC may clear microscopic disease in axillary lymph nodes, the long-term clinical significance of negative findings on SLNB after NAC is unknown. This has implications in clinical decision-making for further axillary treatment, such as the need for completion ALND, post-mastectomy radiation, and radiation fields after lumpectomy. The real question remains the fate of patients who have positive nodes that have converted to negative with neoadjuvant chemotherapy and do not undergo ALND.

After consideration of the available data on SLNB and NAC, an algorithm for pre-NAC axillary evaluation has been suggested, avoiding the situation in which

Table 17.2 Studies of sentinel lymph node biopsy after neoadjuvant chemotherapy.

Author	Year	No. of patients	Mapping failure (%)	FNR (%)
Takei	2012	105	0	6
Canavese	2011	64	6	5
Schwartz	2010	79	1	4
Hunt	2009	575	3	6
Classe	2009	195	10	12
Tausch	2008	167	15	8
Gimbergues	2008	129	6	14
Yu	2007	127	9	8
Newman	2007	54	2	9
Lee	2007	219	6	16
Shen	2007	69	7	25
Yamamoto	2007	20	0	14
Tanaka	2006	70	10	3
Kinoshita	2006	77	6.50	11
Mamounas	2005	428	15	11
Jones	2005	36	19	11
Kang	2004	54	28	11
Shimazu	2004	47	6	12
Lang	2004	53	6	4
Patel	2004	42	5	0
Reitsamer	2003	30	13	7
Piato	2003	42	2.40	17
Vigario	2003	37	3	39
Miller	2002	35	14	0
Julian	2002	34	9	0
Stearns	2002	34	15	14
Haid	2001	33	12	0
Fernandez	2001	40	10	20
Tafra	2001	29	7	0
Breslin	2000	51	18	12
Cohen	2000	38	18	17

Adapted from: Chung A, Giuliano AE. Axillary staging in the neoadjuvant setting. Ann Surg Oncol 2010;17:2401–10 [77]

patients with positive nodes converted to negative do not get ALND [77]. Patients with clinically suspicious nodes can be advised to undergo needle biopsy, while those with clinically negative nodes can undergo sentinel node biopsy prior to neoadjuvant treatment to assess the true status of the axilla.

To date, there have been no randomized trials investigating SLNB in the setting of NAC. The ACOSOG Z1071 trial is currently accruing patients with T1-4, N1-2, M0 breast cancer who will undergo preoperative NAC followed by SLNB and ALND. The primary objective is to determine the false-negative rate for sentinel nodes in women with node-positive breast cancer at initial diagnosis who have a SLNB performed after NAC [82]. This study, however, does not answer the important question of the untreated axilla after conversion from positive to negative.

The current ASCO guidelines have concluded that there is insufficient data to recommend SLNB or suggest appropriate timing of SLNB in patients undergoing NAC. The Panel also emphasizes that a SLNB should only be performed in the setting of clinically negative axillary lymph nodes.

Other Circumstances

SLNB should not be performed in inflammatory breast cancer, because the subdermal lymphatics can be partially obstructed and contain tumor emboli. This lymphatic abnormality has led to an unacceptably high false-negative SLNB rate [75]. Thus, for patients with inflammatory breast cancer, an ALND should be performed.

In older age and obesity, the accurate identification of the sentinel node decreases with increasing age and body mass; however, advanced age and BMI are not a contraindication for SLNB.

Indications for Completion Axillary Lymph Node Dissection

Axillary node dissection, with the removal of levels I and II nodes, remains the standard for patients with grossly palpable axillary nodes or needle-biopsy proven axillary node involvement. A completion axillary node dissection should be done when clinically suspicious nodes are still present in the axilla after all sentinel nodes have been removed. ALND should also be done when the SLNB procedure fails or is technically unsatisfactory [27].

Currently, the ASCO guidelines from 2005 recommend routine ALND for micrometastases (>0.2 to ≤2 mm and/or more than 200 cells) found on SLNB, regardless of method of detection. However, recent data from the ACOSOG Z0010 and Z0011 trials suggest that a completion axillary node dissection is not necessary in all women found with tumor-involved sentinel nodes under certain circumstances. Data from Z0011 suggest that ALND is only necessary in women who undergo BCS with planned whole-breast irradiation who are found to have three or more tumor-involved sentinel lymph nodes (macrometastases) or have extranodal extension [33, 83]. Women undergoing mastectomy who are found with tumor-involved sentinel nodes still require completion axillary node dissections [83].

Indications for Sentinel Node Biopsy Only: Management of Node-Negative Patients

Current guidelines recommend that patients with tumor-free sentinel nodes be adequately treated with SLNB only without further ALND. This is supported by data from several randomized controlled trials with long-term follow-up comparing axillary failure rates for SLNB and ALND. These studies have demonstrated low axillary recurrence in patients who underwent SLNB only in node-negative patients. Veronesi recently reported a 10-year follow up comparing outcomes in 516 patients at a single-institution randomized to SLNB alone versus SLNB with routine completion ALND if the sentinel node was negative. The study showed no difference between the two groups with respect to disease-free survival (DFS) (89.9 % in the SLNB alone arm vs. 88.8 % in the SLNB + ALND arm); the overall survival (OS) was slightly greater in the SLNB alone arm (93.5 % vs. 89.7 % in the SLNB + ALND arm), but this was not statistically significant ($P=0.15$) [84].

The NSABP B-32 is the largest randomized surgical trial designed to answer the question of whether SLNB in patients with sentinel lymph node-negative breast cancer is equivalent to ALND with regard to regional control, DFS, OS [32]. Between 1999 and 2004, 5,611 women in 80 centers in Canada and the USA with clinically node negative invasive breast cancer, undergoing either lumpectomy or mastectomy, were randomized to SLNB + ALND versus SLNB alone (followed by ALND if the sentinel node was positive on H&E staining). 3,986 had pathologically negative sentinel node and follow-up information. After a mean follow-up time of 95.6 months, there were 309 deaths. The 5-year overall survival was 96.4 % (SLNB + ALND) versus 95.0 % (SLNB alone) and 8-year estimates are 91.8 % versus 90.3 % (HR 1.19, 95 % CI: 0.95–1.49, $p=0.13$). DFS (651 events) was 89.0 % (SLNB + ALND) versus 88.6 % (SLNB alone) at 5 years, 82.4 and 81.5 % at 8 years. There were 8 regional node recurrences as first events in the SLNB + ALND group, and 14 in the SLNB alone group ($p=0.22$). Both groups had less than 1 % regional recurrences as first events. The B-32 results confirmed the low rate of regional-node recurrences after SLNB as previously reported in non-randomized studies. This study demonstrated no significant difference in OS, DFS, and regional control among patients treated with SLNB followed by ALND or SLNB alone in patients with histopathologically tumor-free sentinel nodes. This large multicenter randomized study proved that SLNB alone with no further ALND is appropriate, safe, and effective therapy for patients with sentinel node-negative breast cancer.

Management of Patients with Sentinel Node Micrometastases or Isolated Tumor Cells

SLNB has dramatically changed the approach to early-stage breast cancer by allowing minimally invasive nodal staging and more intensive examination of the sentinel nodes. This has led to the detection of micrometastases (greater than 0.2 mm and/or more than 200 cells, but none greater than 2.0 mm) and isolated tumor cells (ITCs, defined as small clusters of cells not greater than 0.2 mm, or non-confluent or nearly confluent clusters of cells not exceeding 200 cells in a single histologic lymph node cross section) of uncertain significance according to the AJCC Breast Cancer Staging, seventh edition [85]. Although current guidelines from ASCO recommend completion axillary dissection when micrometastatic disease is found regardless of the method of detection [27], recent studies show this to be unnecessary.

The ACOSOG Z0010, accruing from 1999 to 2003, is one of the largest prospective trials to assess immunochemically detected metastases in the sentinel lymph nodes and bone marrow of women with early-stage breast cancer [33]. This multicenter observational study determined the prevalence and significance of occult metastases in the sentinel nodes and bone marrow of patients who underwent BCS, SLNB, and whole breast irradiation for treatment of T1 or T2, clinically node-negative breast cancer. 5,210 patients underwent BCS and SLNB. Occult metastases discovered by immunohistochemistry (IHC) were found in 349 (10.5 %) of 3,326 sentinel lymph nodes which were hematoxylin and eosin (H&E) negative. Of 3,413 bone marrow specimens examined by immunocytochemistry, 104 (3.0 %) were positive for occult metastases. Over a median of 6.3 years, among women undergoing BCS, SLNB, and whole breast irradiation, occult sentinel lymph node metastases were not significantly associated with differences in overall survival, disease-free survival, or recurrence when compared to patients with IHC-negative sentinel nodes. 5-year rates of overall survival for patients with IHC-negative sentinel nodes were 95.7 % (95 % CI, 95.0–96.5 %) versus 95.1 % (95 % CI, 92.7–97.5 %; $P=0.64$) in patients with IHC-positive sentinel nodes. Corresponding 5-year rates of disease-free survival were 92.2 % (95 % CI, 91.1–93.2 %) and 90.4 % (95 % CI, 87.2–93.8 %, $P=0.82$), respectively. Occult bone marrow metastases were found to be significantly associated with increased mortality. At 5 years, mortality rates were 5 % (95 % CI, 4.2–5.7 %) for patients with immunocytochemistry-negative bone-marrow specimens versus 9.9 % (95 % CI, 3.9–15.5 %) for those with immunocytochemistry-positive specimens on univariable analysis. This finding was not statistically significant on multivariable analysis. The authors concluded that in this study, sentinel node IHC-detected metastases appear to have no significant impact on overall survival among women receiving BCS for T1/T2 N0 M0 breast cancer, whereas occult bone marrow metastases, although rare, were associated with decreased survival. The routine examination of sentinel nodes by IHC was not supported in this study.

A secondary aim of the NSABP B-32 trial was to determine whether patients with occult micrometastases and ITCs have worse survival compared to patients with negative axillary lymph nodes, assessed by both H&E and IHC analysis [86]. The pathologically H&E negative sentinel lymph nodes in 3,887 patients were centrally evaluated for occult metastases by H&E and IHC analysis. In the 3,887 patients, occult metastases were detected in 15.9 % (11.1 % ITC, 4.4 % micrometastases, 0.4 % macrometastases). They found a statistically significant difference between patients with and without occult metastases in overall survival (94.6 % vs. 95.8 %, $p=0.03$), disease-free survival (86.4 % vs. 89.2 %, $p=0.02$), and distant disease-free survival (89.7 % vs. 92.5 %, $p=0.04$), respectively. Occult metastases were an independent prognostic variable in patients with sentinel nodes that were negative on initial examination, and were associated with a small but statistically significant 1.2 % decrease in 5-year overall survival, 2.8 % decrease in disease-free survival, and 2.8 % decrease in distant disease-free survival. While the NSABP B-32 trial showed a small but significant difference in 5-year overall survival in patients with occult sentinel node metastases, this difference was concluded to be insufficient to affect systemic treatment or justify routine immunohistochemistry. These findings are congruent with the conclusions of Z0010. Most patients in the Z0010 trial and NSABP B-32 trial received adjuvant systemic therapy, which demonstrates practice patterns independent of immunohistochemical findings.

The International Breast Cancer Study Group (IBCSG) Trial 23-01, which completed accrual in 2010, compares ALND versus SLNB only in patients with micrometastases (≤2.0 mm) in the sentinel node. Nine hundred and thirty-four patients with tumors 5 cm or less and clinically negative nodes were enrolled between 2001 and 2010. 75 % underwent BCS and 25 % underwent mastectomy. At a median follow-up of 57 months, a preliminary update demonstrated no difference in DFS (87.0 % vs. 88.4 %, $p=0.48$) or OS (97.6 % and 98.0 %, $p=0.35$) between the ALND and SLNB arms, respectively, supporting the results of Z0011 [87].

Z0010 demonstrated that IHC-detected occult metastases are not associated with survival differences in women undergoing BCS with the earliest stages of breast cancer. While long-term follow-up may eventually reveal small differences in outcome, these are likely to be of no clinical significance, as demonstrated by the NSABP B-32 trial. Findings of these two trials, which are confirmed by the preliminary results of the IBCSG trial 23-01, have important implications for current clinical practice in the management of sentinel node micrometastases and ITCs. These patients should not have additional surgery (completion axillary lymph node dissection) or systemic therapy solely based on the findings of micrometastases or ITCs in a sentinel node.

Management of Patients with Sentinel Node Macrometastases: Is Axillary Lymph Node Dissection Necessary?

Although ALND has been shown to provide excellent local control and prognostic information, the morbidity of the procedure, including paresthesias, shoulder pain, weakness, lymphedema, and axillary web syndrome, has been well-documented with no clear impact on survival [88]. Furthermore, only those patients with additional tumor-involved axillary nodes will theoretically benefit from the ALND. The sentinel node is found to be the only involved axillary node in approximately 50 % of the patients with a clinically negative axilla [4, 16, 89]. As a result, the necessity of ALND in all patients with a tumor-involved sentinel node has been questioned.

An early study, the NSABP B-04 trial, randomized clinically node-negative women to radical mastectomy, total mastectomy with axillary irradiation, or total mastectomy alone without axillary treatment. 38 % of women who had ALND were found to have nodal metastases. Because the women in the study were randomly assigned to the treatment groups, it is estimated that 38 % of the women who underwent total mastectomy alone had positive nodes that were not treated. In this group, only about half developed clinically evident axillary recurrence as a first event. These patients all had palpable tumors and did not receive adjuvant systemic therapy—therefore no treatment effect could account for the lack of clinical progression of the axillary nodal metastases in the group with no axillary treatment. This suggests that not all axillary metastases ultimately progress to become clinically evident [90]. Several retrospective studies have reported low axillary recurrence rates in women with positive sentinel nodes who did not have a completion ALND [91–93].

There are several modern randomized trials of axillary treatment in patients undergoing BCS and tangential field whole-breast irradiation demonstrating low axillary failure rates. In BCS patients who were randomized to ALND versus observation, after a median follow-up of 5 years, 0 % versus 1.8 % respectively had axillary failure [94]. In BCS patients randomized to axillary radiation therapy versus observation, after median follow-up of 5.3 years, axillary failure rates were 0.5 % versus 1.5 %, respectively [95]. In a study of BCS patients randomized to ALND versus axillary radiation therapy, axillary failure rates were 1 % versus 3 %, respectively [96]. The IBCSG trial 10-93 randomized patients to ALND versus no axillary dissection, demonstrating axillary failure rates of 1 % versus 3 %, respectively, at a median follow-up of 6.6 years. All patients were treated with tamoxifen, 33 % had BCS with radiotherapy, and 23 % had BCS without radiotherapy [97]. In these randomized trials, there were no significant differences in survival between the two treatment arms.

A non-randomized retrospective analysis of consecutive prospectively recruited elderly patients with early breast cancer, who underwent BCS with or without axillary dissection, demonstrated a low cumulative 15-year incidence of axillary failure in the no axillary dissection group: 5.8 % overall and 3.7 % for T1 patients [98].

To determine the necessity for ALND in patients with sentinel node macrometastases, the ACOSOG Z0011 trial randomized breast cancer patients with H&E-detected sentinel node metastases to SLNB alone versus ALND [83]. The women enrolled had clinical T1 or T2 invasive breast cancer, no palpable lymphadenopathy, and 1 or 2 sentinel nodes containing macrometastases (identified using H&E) who underwent BCS and received tangential field whole-breast irradiation. No axillary-specific radiation was given. 96 % of the patients received adjuvant systemic therapy (chemotherapy and/or hormonal therapy). The median number of lymph nodes removed was 17 in the ALND group and 2 in the SLND group.

In the ALND group, 27 % had additional nodal metastases removed by ALND beyond those found with SLNB alone, including 10 % of patients with sentinel node micrometastasis who had macroscopically involved non-sentinel nodes removed. Despite this, the axillary recurrence rates for both groups were similar: 0.9 % in the SLNB group alone and 0.5 % in the ALND group ($p=0.45$). Furthermore, the use of SLNB alone compared with ALND did not result in statistically inferior survival. At a median follow-up of 6.3 years, the 5-year OS was similar between the 2 groups (92.5 % in the SLNB-alone group vs. 91.8 % in the ALND group), and the DFS did not differ significantly between treatment groups as well (83.9 % in the SLND-alone group vs. 82.2 % in the ALND group). In this non-inferiority designed study, SLNB alone was not inferior to SLNB + ALND for women with H&E-detected sentinel node metastases.

The results of this trial indicate that women with 1 or 2 positive sentinel nodes and clinical T1–T2 tumors undergoing BCS with whole-breast radiation therapy followed by systemic therapy do not benefit from the addition of ALND in terms of local control, disease-free survival, or overall survival. These results are not applicable to those treated with mastectomy, partial breast irradiation, prone radiation, neoadjuvant chemotherapy, nor in those with T3 cancers, more than 2 tumor-involved sentinel nodes, or extranodal extension. These recommendations are reflected in the most recent 2012 National Comprehensive Cancer Network (NCCN) guidelines for surgical axillary staging [99].

Can Radiation Replace Surgery in Local Control of the Axilla in Breast Cancer?

The well-documented morbidities of ALND and limited impact on survival have prompted many investigators to explore alternative methods of axillary treatment in patients with clinically negative nodes, including radiation, systemic therapy, and axillary observation [94–97]. Standard breast tangential radiation treats approximately 80 % of level I and 50 % of level II axillary nodes to 95 % of the prescribed dose, while systemic therapy contributes to local control. ACOSOG Z0011 has demonstrated the efficacy of tangential breast radiation alone when compared to axillary dissection for patients with tumor-involved sentinel nodes [100].

As mentioned previously, several randomized studies have been completed demonstrating the efficacy of axillary radiation [95, 96, 101]. The largest study randomized 658 patients with clinically node-negative early breast cancer undergoing BCS and breast irradiation to ALND versus axillary radiotherapy. At 15 years, survival rates were identical (73.8 % vs. 75.5 %, respectively) and there was no statistically significant difference in axillary failure between the groups (1 % vs. 3 %, respectively; $p=.04$). There was no difference in recurrence rates in the breast or supraclavicular and distant metastases between the two groups [96]. Veronesi similarly demonstrated low axillary failure rates in patients with clinically node-negative early breast cancer who were randomized to no axillary treatment (1.5 %) versus axillary radiation (0.5 %). 5-year disease-free survival was 96.0 % without significant differences between the two groups [95].

The European Organisation for Research and Treatment of Cancer (EORTC) 10981 AMAROS (After Mapping of the Axilla: Radiotherapy or Surgery) trial is a phase III study comparing completion ALND and axillary radiation therapy (ART) in patients with tumor-involved sentinel nodes. All patients have operable invasive breast cancer (between 5 and 50 mm in size) with clinically normal regional nodes. The objective of this study is to prove equivalence of the two treatment modalities for locoregional control in the setting of a tumor-involved sentinel node.

The study completed accrual in April 2010 with 4,828 patients included. A first analysis in 2008 evaluated the first 2,000 patients enrolled with unifocal breast cancer (5–30 mm) and clinically negative lymph nodes. This showed no significant difference in the administration of adjuvant systemic therapy between the ALND and ART groups. These results support the hypothesis that the administration of adjuvant chemotherapy is mainly based on tumor characteristics, patient characteristics, and SLNB status, and that knowledge of further nodal involvement is redundant [102].

A new EORTC trial, the POWER trial (Positive Sentinel Node: Wait & See, Excision, or Radiotherapy), is planned to follow the AMAROS trial. The main objective of this trial is to analyze axillary recurrence rates in patients with sentinel node micrometastases if no further axillary therapy is offered.

Summary

The development of SLNB for invasive breast cancer in 1994 has profoundly changed the management of breast cancer. It has replaced ALND as a highly accurate and less-morbid axillary staging procedure in patients with clinically node-negative early-stage breast cancer. It is widely accepted that SLNB without further ALND is adequate in patients with tumor-negative sentinel nodes. In tumor-positive sentinel nodes, completion ALND is currently believed to offer prognostic information, prevent axillary local recurrence, and possibly render a small survival benefit. However, ACOSOG Z0011 has challenged whether ALND is necessary for tumor-positive sentinel nodes in patients undergoing BCS and whole-breast irradiation with adjuvant systemic treatment for early-stage tumors. In these patients, ALND did not improve survival compared to SLNB alone. The role of axillary staging is likely to become less important in the future as genomic analysis of primary tumors dictate the need for adjuvant systemic therapy and ALND becomes less often used.

References

1. Halsted WS. The results of operations for the cure of cancer of the breast performed at the Johns Hopkins Hospital from June 1889 to January 1894. Ann Surg. 1894;20:497–555.
2. Fisher B, Fisher ER. The interrelationship of hematogenous and lymphatic tumor cell dissecmination. Surg Gynecol Obstet. 1966;122:791–8.
3. Fisher B, Montague E, Redmond C, et al. Comparison of radical mastectomy with alternative treatments for primary breast cancer. A first report of results from a prospective randomized clinical trial. Cancer. 1977;39:2827–39.
4. Giuliano AE, Kirgan DM, Guenther JM, Morton DL. Lymphatic mapping and sentinel lymphadenectomy for breast cancer. Ann Surg. 1994;220:391–8.
5. Morton DL, Wen DR, Wong JH, et al. Technical details of intraoperative lymphatic mapping for early stage melanoma. Arch Surg. 1992;127:392–9.
6. Chung A, Yu J, Stempel M, et al. Is the "10 % rule" equally valid for all subsets of sentinel-node-positive breast cancer patients? Ann Surg Oncol. 2008;15:2728–33.
7. Lyew MA, Gamblin TC, Ayoub M. Systemic anaphylaxis associated with intramammary isosulfan blue injection used for sentinel node detection under general anesthesia. Anesthesiology. 2000;93:1145–6.
8. Kuerer HM, Wayne JD, Ross MI. Anaphylaxis during breast cancer lymphatic mapping. Surgery. 2001;129:119–20.
9. Wilke LG, McCall LM, Posther KE, et al. Surgical complications associated with sentinel lymph node biopsy: results from a prospective international cooperative group trial. Ann Surg Oncol. 2006;13:491–500.

10. Blessing WD, Stolier AJ, Teng SC, et al. A comparison of methylene blue and lymphazurin in breast cancer sentinel node mapping. Am J Surg. 2002;184:341–5.
11. Thevarajah S, Huston TL, Simmons RM. A comparison of the adverse reactions associated with isosulfan blue versus methylene blue dye in sentinel lymph node biopsy for breast cancer. Am J Surg. 2005;189:236–9.
12. Morrow M, Rademaker AW, Bethke KP, et al. Learning sentinel node biopsy: results of a prospective randomized trial of two techniques. Surgery. 1999;126:714–20.
13. Albertini JJ, Lyman OH, Cox C, et al. Lymphatic mapping and sentinel node biopsy in the patient with breast cancer. JAMA. 1996;276:1818–22.
14. Borgstein PJ, Meijer S, Pijpers R. Intradermal blue dye to identify sentinel lymph-node in breast cancer. Lancet. 1997;349:1668–9.
15. Linehan DC, Hill AD, Akhurst T, et al. Intradermal radiocolloid and intraparenchymal blue dye injection optimize sentinel node identification in breast cancer patients. Ann Surg Oncol. 1999;6:450–4.
16. Veronesi U, Paganelli G, Galimberti V, et al. Sentinel-node biopsy to avoid axillary dissection in breast cancer with clinically negative lymph-nodes. Lancet. 1997;349(9069):1864–7.
17. Klimberg VS, Rubio IT, Henry R, et al. Subareolar versus peritumoral injection for location of the sentinel lymph node. Ann Surg. 1999;229(6):860–4.
18. Kern KA. Sentinel lymph node mapping in breast cancer using subareolar injection of blue dye. J Am Coll Surg. 1999;198:539–45.
19. Povoski SP, Olson JO, Young DC, et al. Prospective randomized clinical trial comparing intradermal, intraparenchymal, and subareolar injection routes for sentinel lymph node mapping and biopsy in breast cancer. Ann Surg Oncol. 2006;13(11):1412–21.
20. Rodier JF, Velten M, Wilt M, et al. Prospective multicentric randomized study comparing periareolar and peritumoral injection of radiotracer and blue dye for the detection of sentinel lymph node in breast sparing procedure: FRANSENODE trial. J Clin Oncol. 2007;25(24):3664–9.
21. McMasters KM, Wong SL, Martin RC 2nd RC, et al. Dermal injection of radioactive colloid is superior to peritumoral injection for breast cancer sentinel lymph node biopsy: results of a multiinstitutional study. Ann Surg. 2001;233:676–87.
22. Martin R, Derossis AM, Fey J, et al. Intradermal isotope injection is superior to intramammary in sentinel node biopsy for breast cancer. Surgery. 2001;130(3):432–8.
23. Schrenk P, Wayand W. Sentinel-node biopsy in axillary lymph-node staging for patients with multicentric breast cancer. Lancet. 2001;357:122.
24. Samphao S, Eremin JM, El-Sheemy M. Management of the axilla in women with breast cancer: current clinical practice and a new selective targeted approach. Ann Surg Oncol. 2008;15:1282–96.
25. Goyal A, Newcombe RG, Mansel RE. Axillary lymphatic mapping against nodal axillary clearance (ALMANAC) Trialists Group. Clinical relevance of multiple sentinel nodes in patients with breast cancer. Br J Surg. 2005;92:438–42.
26. Posther KE, McCall LM, Blumencranz PW, et al. Sentinel node skills verification and surgeon performance: data from a multicenter clinical trial for early-stage breast cancer. Ann Surg. 2005;242:593–9.
27. Lyman GH, Giuliano AE, Somerfield MR, et al. American Society of Clinical Oncology guideline recommendations for sentinel lymph node biopsy in early-stage breast cancer. J Clin Oncol. 2005;23:7703–20.
28. Gentilini O, Cremonesi M, Trifiro G, et al. Safety of sentinel node biopsy in pregnant patients with breast cancer. Ann Oncol. 2004;15:1348–51.
29. Gentilini O, Cremonesi M, Toesca A. Sentinel lymph node biopsy in pregnant patients with breast cancer. Eur J Nucl Med Mol Imaging. 2010;37:78–83.
30. Khera SY, Kiluk JV, Hasson DM, et al. Pregnancy-associated breast cancer patients can safely undergo lymphatic mapping. Breast J. 2008;14:250–4.
31. Morrow M, Basset LW, et al. Standard for the management of ductal carcinoma in situ of the breast (DCIS). CA Cancer J Clin. 2002;52:256–76.

32. Krag DN, Anderson SJ, Julian TB, et al. Sentinel-lymph-node resection compared with conventional axillary-lymph-node dissection in clinically node-negative patients with breast cancer: overall survival findings from the NSABP B-32 randomised phase 3 trial. Lancet Oncol. 2010;11:927–33.
33. Giuliano AE, Hawes D, Ballman KV, et al. Association of occult metastases in sentinel lymph nodes and bone marrow with survival among women with early-stage invasive breast cancer. JAMA. 2011;306:385–93.
34. Giordano SH, Cohen DS, Buzdar AU, et al. Breast carcinoma in men: a population-based study. Cancer. 2004;101:51–7.
35. Cutuli B. Strategies in treating male breast cancer. Expert Opin Pharmacother. 2007;8:193–202.
36. Port ER, Fey JV, Cody 3rd HS, et al. Sentinel lymph node biopsy in patients with male breast carcinoma. Cancer. 2001;91:319–23.
37. Albo D, Ames FC, Hunt KK, et al. Evaluation of lymph node status in male breast cancer patients: a role for sentinel lymph node biopsy. Breast Cancer Res Treat. 2003;77:9–14.
38. Gentilini O, Chagas E, Zurrida S, et al. Sentinel lymph node biopsy in male patients with early breast cancer. Oncologist. 2007;12:512–5.
39. Korde LA, Zujewski JA, Kamın L, et al. Multidisciplinary meeting on male breast cancer: summary and research recommendations. J Clin Oncol. 2010;28:2114–22.
40. Taback B, Nguyen P, Hansen N, Edwards GK, Conway K, Giuliano AE. Sentinel lymph node biopsy for local recurrence of breast cancer after breast-conserving therapy. Ann Surg Oncol. 2006;13:1099–104.
41. Barone JL, Feldman SM, Estabrook A, et al. Reoperative sentinel lymph node biopsy in patients with locally recurrent breast cancer. Am J Surg. 2007;194:491–3.
42. Cox CE, Furman BT, Kiluk JV, et al. Use of reoperative sentinel lymph node biopsy in breast cancer patients. J Am Coll Surg. 2008;207:57–61.
43. Port ER, Garcia-Etienne CA, Park J, et al. Reoperative sentinel lymph node biopsy: a new frontier in the management of ipsilateral breast tumor recurrence. Ann Surg Oncol. 2007;14:2209–14.
44. Kaur P, Kiluk JV, Meade T, et al. Sentinel lymph node biopsy in patients with previous ipsilateral complete axillary lymph node dissection. Ann Surg Oncol. 2011;18:727–32.
45. Intra M, Trifiro G, Viale G. Second biopsy of axillary sentinel lymph node for reappearing breast cancer after previous sentinel lymph node biopsy. Ann Surg Oncol. 2005;12:895–9.
46. Intra M, Trifiro G, Galimberti V, et al. Second axillary sentinel node biopsy for ipsilateral breast tumour recurrence. Br J Surg. 2007;94:1216–9.
47. Mariani G, Moresco L, Viale G, et al. Radioguided sentinel lymph node biopsy in breast cancer surgery. J Nucl Med. 2001;42:1198–215.
48. Veronesi U, Paganelli G, Viale G, et al. Sentinel lymph node biopsy and axillary dissection in breast cancer: results in a large series. J Natl Cancer Inst. 1999;91:368–73.
49. Gentilini O, Veronesi P, Botteri E, et al. Sentinel lymph node biopsy in multicentric breast cancer: five-year results in a large series from a single institution. Ann Surg Oncol. 2011;18:2879–84.
50. Specht MC, Fey JV, Borgen PI, Cody 3rd HS. Is the clinically positive axilla in breast cancer really a contraindication to sentinel lymph node biopsy? J Am Coll Surg. 2005;200:10–4.
51. Krishnamurthy S, Sneige N, Bedi DG, et al. Role of ultrasound-guided fine-needle aspiration of indeterminate and suspicious axillary lymph nodes in the initial staging of breast carcinoma. Cancer. 2002;95(5):982–8.
52. Tuttle TM, Habermann EB, Grund EH, et al. Increasing use of contralateral prophylactic mastectomy for breast cancer patients: a trend toward more aggressive surgical treatment. J Clin Oncol. 2007;25:5203–9.
53. Hartmann LC, Schaid DJ, Woods JE, et al. Efficacy of bilateral prophylactic mastectomy in women with a family history of breast cancer. N Engl J Med. 1999;340:77–84.
54. Laronga C, Lee MC, McGuire KP, et al. Indications for sentinel lymph node biopsy in the setting of prophylactic mastectomy. J Am Coll Surg. 2009;209:746–52.

55. Rosen PP, Groshen S, Kinne DW, et al. Contralateral breast carcinoma: an assessment of risk and prognosis in stage I (T1N0M0) and stage II (T1N1M0) patients with 20-year follow-up. Surgery. 1989;106:904–10.
56. Peto J, Mack TH. High constant incidence in twins and other relatives of women with breast cancer. Nat Genet. 2000;26:411–4.
57. Healey EA, Cook EF, Orav EJ, et al. Contralateral breast cancer: clinical characteristics and impact on prognosis. J Clin Oncol. 1993;11:1545–52.
58. Nichols HB, Berrington de González A, Lacey JV Jr JV, et al. Declining incidence of contralateral breast cancer in the United States from 1975 to 2006. J Clin Oncol. 2011;29:1564–9.
59. Boughey JC, Khakpour N, Meric-Bernstam F, et al. Selective use of sentinel lymph node surgery during prophylactic mastectomy. Cancer. 2006;107:1440–7.
60. Nasser SM, Smith SG, Chagpar AB. The role of sentinel node biopsy in women undergoing prophylactic mastectomy. J Surg Res. 2010;164:188–92.
61. Fisher B, Brown A, Mamounas E, et al. Effect of preoperative chemotherapy on local-regional disease in women with operable breast cancer: findings from National Surgical Adjuvant Breast and Bowel Project B-18. J Clin Oncol. 1997;15(7):2483–93.
62. Bear HD, Anderson S, Brown A, et al. National Surgical Adjuvant Breast and Bowel Project Protocol B-27. The effect on tumor response of adding sequential preoperative docetaxel to preoperative doxorubicin and cyclophosphamide: preliminary results from National Surgical Adjuvant Breast and Bowel Project Protocol B-27. J Clin Oncol. 2003;21:4165–74.
63. Kucrcr HM, Sahin AA, Ilunt KK, ct al. Incidence and impact of documented eradication of breast cancer axillary lymph node metastases before surgery in patients treated with neoadjuvant chemotherapy. Ann Surg. 1999;230:72–8.
64. Newman LA, Pernick NL, Adsay V, et al. Histopathologic evidence of tumor regression in the axillary lymph nodes of patients treated with preoperative chemotherapy correlates with breast cancer outcome. Ann Surg Oncol. 2003;10:734–9.
65. Buchholz TA, Hunt KK, Whitman GJ. Neoadjuvant chemotherapy for breast carcinoma: multidisciplinary considerations of benefits and risks. Cancer. 2003;98:1150–60.
66. Nason KS, Anderson BO, Byrd DR, et al. Increased false negative sentinel node biopsy rates after preoperative chemotherapy for invasive breast carcinoma. Cancer. 2000;89:2187–94.
67. Breslin TM, Cohen L, Sahin A, et al. Sentinel lymph node biopsy is accurate after neoadjuvant chemotherapy for breast cancer. J Clin Oncol. 2000;18:3480–6.
68. Fernández A, Cortés M, Benito E, et al. Gamma probe sentinel node localization and biopsy in breast cancer patients treated with a neoadjuvant chemotherapy scheme. Nucl Med Commun. 2001;22:361–6.
69. Haid A, Tausch C, Lang A, et al. Is sentinel lymph node biopsy reliable and indicated after preoperative chemotherapy in patients with breast carcinoma? Cancer. 2001;92:1080–4.
70. Julian TB, Dusi D, Wolmark N. Sentinel node biopsy after neoadjuvant chemotherapy for breast cancer. Am J Surg. 2002;184:315–7.
71. Miller AR, Thomason VE, Yeh IT, et al. Analysis of sentinel lymph node mapping with immediate pathologic review in patients receiving preoperative chemotherapy for breast carcinoma. Ann Surg Oncol. 2002;9:243–7.
72. Piato JR, Barros AC, Pincerato KM, et al. Sentinel lymph node biopsy in breast cancer after neoadjuvant chemotherapy. A pilot study. Eur J Surg Oncol. 2003;29:118–20.
73. Jones JL, Zabicki K, Christian RL, et al. A comparison of sentinel node biopsy before and after neoadjuvant chemotherapy: timing is important. Am J Surg. 2005;190:517–20.
74. Tanaka Y, Maeda H, Ogawa Y, et al. Sentinel node biopsy in breast cancer patients treated with neoadjuvant chemotherapy. Oncol Rep. 2006;15:927–31.
75. Stearns V, Ewing CA, Slack R, et al. Sentinel lymphadenectomy after neoadjuvant chemotherapy for breast cancer may reliably represent the axilla except for inflammatory breast cancer. Ann Surg Oncol. 2002;9:235–42.
76. Newman EA, Sabel MS, Nees AV, et al. Sentinel lymph node biopsy performed after neoadjuvant chemotherapy is accurate in patients with documented node-positive breast cancer at presentation. Ann Surg Oncol. 2007;14:2946–52.

77. Chung A, Giuliano A. Axillary staging in the neoadjuvant setting. Ann Surg Oncol. 2010;17: 2401–10.
78. Xing Y, Foy M, Cox DD, Kuerer HM, Hunt KK, Cormier JN. Meta-analysis of sentinel lymph node biopsy after preoperative chemotherapy in patients with breast cancer. Br J Surg. 2006;93:539–46.
79. Mamounas EP, Brown A, Anderson S, et al. Sentinel node biopsy after neoadjuvant chemotherapy in breast cancer: results from National Surgical Adjuvant Breast and Bowel Project Protocol B-27. J Clin Oncol. 2005;23:2694–702.
80. Sabel MS, Schott AF, Kleer CG, et al. Sentinel node biopsy prior to neoadjuvant chemotherapy. Am J Surg. 2003;186:102–5.
81. Amersi F, Hansen NM. The benefits and limitations of sentinel lymph node biopsy. Curr Treat Options Oncol. 2006;7:141–51.
82. Boughey JC, Ota D, Nelson H. Reconciling the axillary staging controversy in neoadjuvant treatment of breast cancer. Bull Am Coll Surg. 2011;96:47–8.
83. Giuliano AE, McCall L, Beitsch P, et al. Locoregional recurrence after sentinel lymph node dissection with or without axillary dissection in patients with sentinel lymph node metastases: the American College of Surgeons Oncology Group Z0011 randomized trial. Ann Surg. 2010;252:426–32.
84. Veronesi U, Viale G, Paganelli G, et al. Sentinel lymph node biopsy in breast cancer: ten-year results of a randomized controlled study. Ann Surg. 2010;251:595–600.
85. Edge SB, Byrd DR, Compton CC, et al., editors. AJCC cancer staging manual. 7th ed. New York, NY: Springer, 2010, p. 347–76.
86. Weaver DL, Ashikaga T, Krag DN, et al. Effect of occult metastases on survival in node-negative breast cancer. N Engl J Med. 2011;364:412–21.
87. Galimberti V. Update of IBCSG trial 23-01 to compare axillary dissection versus no axillary dissection in patients with clinically node negative breast cancer and micrometastases in the sentinel node. San Antonio Breast Conference 2011.
88. Orr RK. The impact of prophylactic axillary node dissection on breast cancer survival – a Bayesian meta-analysis. Ann Surg Oncol. 1990;6:109–16.
89. Van Zee KJ, Manasseh DM, Bevilacqua JL, et al. A nomogram for predicting the likelihood of additional nodal metastases in breast cancer patients with a positive sentinel node biopsy. Ann Surg Oncol. 2003;10:1140–51.
90. Fisher B, Jeong JH, Anderson S, et al. Twenty-five-year follow-up of a randomized trial comparing radical mastectomy, total mastectomy, and total mastectomy followed by irradiation. N Engl J Med. 2002;347:567–75.
91. Fant JS, Grant MD, Knox SM, et al. Preliminary outcome analysis in patients with breast cancer and a positive sentinel lymph node who declined axillary dissection. Ann Surg Oncol. 2003;10:126–30.
92. Guenther JM, Hansen NM, DiFronzo LA, Giuliano AE, Collins JC, Grube BL, et al. Axillary dissection is not required for all patients with breast cancer and positive sentinel nodes. Arch Surg. 2003;138:52–6.
93. Bilimoria KY, Bentrem DJ, Hansen NM, et al. Comparison of sentinel lymph node biopsy alone and completion axillary lymph node dissection for node-positive breast cancer. J Clin Oncol. 2009;27:2946–53.
94. Martelli G, Boracchi P, De Palo M, et al. A randomized trial comparing axillary dissection to no axillary dissection in older patients with T1N0 breast cancer: results after 5 years of follow-up. Ann Surg. 2005;242:1–6.
95. Veronesi U, Orecchia R, Zurrida S, et al. Avoiding axillary dissection in breast cancer surgery: a randomized trial to assess the role of axillary radiotherapy. Ann Oncol. 2005;16:383–8.
96. Louis-Sylvestre C, Clough K, Asselain B, et al. Axillary treatment in conservative management of operable breast cancer: dissection or radiotherapy? Results of a randomized study with 15 years of follow-up. J Clin Oncol. 2004;22:97–101.

97. Rudenstam CM, Zahrieh D, Forbes JF, et al. International Breast Cancer Study Group. Randomized trial comparing axillary clearance versus no axillary clearance in older patients with breast cancer: first results of International Breast Cancer Study Group Trial 10-93. J Clin Oncol. 2006;24:337–44.
98. Martelli G, Miceli R, Daidone MG, et al. Axillary dissection versus no axillary dissection in elderly patients with breast cancer and no palpable axillary nodes: results after 15 years of follow-up. Ann Surg Oncol. 2011;18:125–33.
99. NCCN Clinical Practice Guidelines in Oncology, Breast Cancer (version 2.2012). www.nccn.org.
100. Giuliano AE, Hunt KK, Ballman KV, et al. Axillary dissection vs. no axillary dissection in women with invasive breast cancer and sentinel node metastasis: a randomized clinical trial. JAMA. 2011;305:569–75.
101. Spruit PH, Siesling S, Elferink MA, et al. Regional radiotherapy versus an axillary lymph node dissection after lumpectomy: a safe alternative for an axillary lymph node dissection in a clinically uninvolved axilla in breast cancer. A case control study with 10 years follow up. Radiat Oncol. 2007;30:2.
102. Straver ME, Meijnen P, van Tienhoven G, et al. Role of axillary clearance after a tumor-positive sentinel node in the administration of adjuvant therapy in early breast cancer (AMAROS). J Clin Oncol. 2010;28:731–7.

Chapter 18
Radiotherapy of the Breast

Frederick M. Dirbas, Darius S. Francescatti, and Amanda B. Francescatti

Overview

Lumpectomy, or breast conservation surgery (BCS), followed by approximately 6 weeks of daily whole-breast radiation therapy (WB-XRT) has been available for several decades as an alternative to mastectomy for the local therapy of women with early stage breast cancer. The long-term safety and effectiveness of BCT compared with mastectomy has been confirmed through prospective, randomized trials conducted in the USA and Europe (Table 18.1) [1–6]. Local recurrence after BCS + WB-XRT (the combination of BCS and WB-XRT is known as breast conservation therapy, BCT) is slightly more common than after mastectomy but there is no difference in overall survival. This makes breast conservation an appealing option for many women. A recent study demonstrated that 63 % of women treated for breast cancer in the USA select breast BCT [7]. Overall, the availability of breast conservation therapy has expanded treatment options and enhanced the lives of many women diagnosed with breast cancer who otherwise would have been forced to choose mastectomy.

Retrospective analyses have demonstrated that the vast majority of local recurrences after BCT are near the site of the original tumor (Table 18.2) [8–11]. Such recurrences are commonly known as "true recurrences" or "marginal misses." True recurrences are distinguished from recurrences elsewhere in the breast which are referred to as "new primaries" or "elsewhere failures" [12]. True recurrences are

F.M. Dirbas (✉)
Stanford Cancer Institute, 900 Blake Wilbur Dr, Stanford, CA 94304, USA
e-mail: dirbas@stanford.edu

D.S. Francescatti • A.B. Francescatti, M.S.
Department of Surgery, Rush University Medical Center,
1653 West Congress Parkway, Chicago, IL 60612, USA

D.S. Francescatti and M.J. Silverstein (eds.), *Breast Cancer: A New Era in Management*,
DOI 10.1007/978-1-4614-8063-1_18,

Table 18.1 Survival for patients undergoing mastectomy or breast conservation therapy (BCT) in randomized studies (from Dirbas et al., Cancer Biotherapy 2004)

	Survival*		Local recurrence		
Trial [ref.]	Mastectomy	BCT	Mastectomy	BCT	Median f/u
Milan I [1]	58.8 %	58.3 %	2.3 %	8.8 %	20 year
NSABP BO6 [2]	47 %	46 %	10.1 %	14.3 %	20.8/20.7 year, resp.
Danish [3]	79 %	82 %	3.7 %	2.6 %[a]	40 month
EORTC[b] [4]	60.0 %	54.9 %	12.2 %	19.7 %[a]	13.4 year
Gustave-Roussy [5]	49 %	60 %	9.9 %	15.9 %[a]	22.7/22.1 year, resp.
NCI/NIH [6]	58 %	53 %	0.0 %	27 %[a]	18.4 year

*p = NS for all

[a]Involved surgical margins accepted after breast conservation

[b]Survival rates at 13 years; locoregional recurrence rates, rather than local recurrence rates

Table 18.2 Incidence of true recurrences after breast conservation surgery (BCS) in prospective studies (from Dirbas et al., Cancer Biotherapy 2004)

		BCS		
Trial [ref.]	*n*	True recurrences	%	Median f/u (months)
Ontario [8]	421	93/108	86.1	43
Swedish (Uppsala-Orebro) [9]	194	8/11	72.7	27.5
Milan III [10]	273	48/56	85.7	109
NSABP BO6 [11] (first events only)	636	40/57	70.2	125

Table 18.3 Incidence of elsewhere failures after breast conservation surgery (BCS) in prospective studies (from Dirbas et al., Cancer Biotherapy 2004)

	BCS		BCT		
Trial [ref.]	*n*	%	*n*	%	Median f/u (months)
NSABP-B06 [11]	17/636	2.7	24/629	3.8	125
Milan [10]	8/273	2.9	2/294	0.7	109
Swedish (Uppsala-Orebro) [9]	3/194	1.5	1/187	0.5	31
Ontario [8]	15/421	3.6	4/416	1	43

BCS breast conservation surgery, *BCT* breast conservation therapy

much more common than elsewhere failures. Studies have demonstrated that delivery of WB-XRT markedly reduces the risk of true recurrences, but does not appear to impact the low rate of elsewhere failures (Table 18.3) [8–11]. This observation has raised questions regarding the merits of targeting the entire breast with radiation and has suggested a possible role for more limited radiation targeting the breast tissue immediately around the surgical resection cavity.

This more focused approach to post-surgical breast irradiation has become referred to as accelerated, partial breast irradiation (APBI). With APBI, radiation is targeted to the margin of breast tissue surrounding the lumpectomy cavity rather than the whole breast (hence "partial"). With a smaller target volume, the radiation dose can be escalated and delivered over a shorter time period (hence "accelerated").

There are currently two general approaches to APBI. The first approach is a BID treatment over 5 days accomplished with either interstitial brachytherapy or intracavitary brachytherapy or limited-field external beam radiotherapy (typically 3 dimensional conformal radiotherapy, or 3D-CRT). The second approach involves a single, very large radiation dose delivered intraoperatively to the lumpectomy cavity margins while the patient is asleep in the operating room (intraoperative radiotherapy, or IORT).

If successful, APBI would be more convenient to patients, would provide less radiation exposure to normal tissues, and could potentially lower treatment costs. General principles of APBI, as well as recent trends in patient selection, surgical technique, and radiation delivery are the focus of this chapter.

Rationale for APBI

Initial randomized studies comparing BCT to mastectomy were designed to compare rates of local recurrence and survival [13, 14]. Retrospective evaluation of these trials demonstrated that approximately 70–90 % of in breast recurrences take place near the original tumor site. Such "true recurrences" usually manifest within 5–7 years of the original resection [15]. WB-XRT markedly reduces true recurrences. New primaries in the breast, or "elsewhere failures," are less common and do not appear markedly altered by WB-XRT. These elsewhere failures occur at a slow, fairly consistent rate over the patient's lifetime: they extended beyond the typical 5 to 7-year time frame within which most true recurrences take place. In fact, elsewhere failures appear to be distinct events that temporally mirror the development of new primaries in the contralateral breast. It is important to note that there is some ambiguity in defining a true recurrence vs. an elsewhere failure as there are no strict physical, imaging, or molecular markers that can absolutely distinguish the two. Nonetheless, these general observations regarding true recurrences and elsewhere failures are widely accepted.

The timing, location, probability, and effective reduction with led investigators to initiate trials that directed post-surgical radiation to the breast tissue surrounding the surgical cavity. Due to the smaller target, radiation doses could be escalated. The mathematical tool that enables radiation physicists to adjust dose and schedule this way while achieving the same radiobiologic effect on potential residual cancer cells and normal tissue is the linear quadratic equation [16]. This formula includes tissue-specific variables, the α/β ratio, which represents tumor sensitivity to radiation and normal tissue tolerance by the target organ, such as the breast. In this way, radiation physicists have been able to develop treatment plans that reduced the whole breast radiation treatment time from 6 weeks to a partial breast approach given over 1–5 days with the same anticipated effects on residual microscopic tumor and normal breast tissue.

Early Efforts with APBI

Early attempts at partial breast irradiation were attempted in four trials that used multiple approaches: interstitial brachytherapy catheters; "limited field" external beam radiotherapy; and single fraction IORT. Local recurrence rates in these studies were unacceptably high: two of the studies demonstrated ipsilateral breast tumor recurrence (IBTR) rates of 15–37 % with by 6 years of follow-up [17–20]. In these early APBI trials, recurrence rates were even higher in some patient subsets, particularly those with invasive lobular cancer or extensive ductal carcinoma in situ. This stood in contrast to randomized studies with BCT using WB-XRT which demonstrated IBTR rates at 0.5–1 % per year. Interest in APBI waned with the publication of these recurrence rates.

Importantly, tissue side effects/toxicity was not a factor in any of early APBI trials with short- or long-term follow-up.

Subsequent review of these original APBI studies exposed major gaps in study design. There were: wide variations in patient selection; inconsistent surgical technique; and potential inaccuracies in radiation targeting. More specifically, many patients did not have preoperative mammography to assist in defining extent of disease or presence of satellite lesions. Often patients received gross "tumorectomies" of palpable disease rather than excision to tumor-free margins. Surgical pathology was incomplete or unavailable for some patients. For patients receiving either brachytherapy or external beam approaches, radiation treatments were targeted visually to the skin incision, rather than visualization of the cavity using ultrasound (US) or computed tomography (CT) guidance. In the single fraction IORT pilot study, patients with large tumors and multiple involved nodes were included. These are all scenarios that can contribute to high IBTR rates whether one follows lumpectomy with APBI or WB-XRT. To some extent these approaches represented a perspective that focused, high-dose radiation could, or would, effectively eliminate residual tumor foci more effectively compared with WB-XRT. This was not the case. Rather than a test of APBI, these early studies were a proving ground for the importance of patient selection, surgical technique, and radiation treatment planning with APBI.

Later APBI trials addressed these concerns [21, 22]. Phase I/II studies with modified APBI approaches have since demonstrated local recurrence rates comparable to those seen historically with WB-XRT [23]. Several professional societies, in particular the consensus guidelines from the American Society for radiation Oncology have since published guidelines for APBI that have refined patient selection, surgical technique, and radiation treatment planning: it is believed these criteria can enable patients to achieve IBTR rates with APBI comparable to those seen with conventional 6-week WB-XRT [24].

Patient Selection in APBI

There are multiple patient selection criteria to be considered (Table 18.4).

Age: Local recurrence rates following BCS decrease with age [25]. The biological reasons have not been fully elucidated. Among current APBI trials, some

Table 18.4 Patients "suitable" for APBI if all criteria are present (from Smith et al. [24])

Factor	Criterion
Patient factors	
Age	>60 year
BRCA1/2 mutation	Not present
Pathologic factors	
Tumor size	≤2 cm[a]
T stage	T1
Margins	Negative by at least 2 mm
Grade	Any
LVSI	No[b]
ER status	Positive
Multicentricity	Unicentric only
Multifocality	Clinically unifocal with total size ≤2.0 cm[c]
	Histology
	Invasive ductal or other favorable subtypes[d]
Pure DCIS	Not allowed
EIC	Not allowed
Associated LCIS	Allowed
Nodal factors	
N stage	pN0 (i−, i+)
Nodal surgery	SN Bx or ALND[e]
Treatment factors	
Neoadjuvant therapy	Not allowed

Criteria are derived from data (when available) and conservative panel judgment

APBI accelerated partial-breast irradiation, *LVSI* lymph–vascular space invasion, *ER* estrogen receptor, *DCIS* ductal carcinoma in situ, *EIC* extensive intraductal component, *LCIS* lobular carcinoma in situ, *SN Bx* sentinel lymph node biopsy, *ALND* axillary lymph node dissection

[a]The size of the invasive tumor component as defined by the American Joint Committee on Cancer

[b]The finding of possible or equivocal LVSI should be disregarded

[c]Icroscopic multifocality allowed, provided the lesion is clinically unifocal (a single discrete lesion by physical examination and ultrasonography/mammography) and the total lesion size (including foci of multifocality and intervening normal breast parenchyma) does not exceed 2 cm

[d]Favorable subtypes include mucinous, tubular, and colloid

[e]Pathologic staging is not required for DCIS

investigators have duly set the lower age cut-off at 40. Others suggest that only post-menopausal candidates are appropriate. Only the ongoing, randomized NSABP B-39 trial permits enrollment of women under age 40: in this NSABP study, women 19 or older may be considered candidates [26]. Some have suggested there is a point at which radiation may not be necessary at all: clinical data suggests that women >age 70 with T1, endocrine sensitive tumors may experience such a small increase in local recurrence without radiation that BCS and tamoxifen alone are adequate [27]. In this

Table 18.5 "Cautionary" group: any of these criteria should invoke caution and concern when considering APBI (from Smith et al. [24])

Factor	Criterion
Patient factors	
Age	50–59 year
Pathologic factors	
Tumor size	2.1–3.0 cm[a]
T stage	T0 or T2
Margins	Close (<2 mm)
LVSI	Limited/focal
ER status	Negative[b]
Multifocality	Clinically unifocal with total size 2.1–3.0 cm[c]
Histology	Invasive lobular
Pure DCIS	≤3 cm
EIC	≤3 cm

Abbreviations as in Table 18.4

[a]The size of the invasive tumor component as defined by the American Joint Committee on Cancer [72]

[b]Patients with ER-negative tumors are strongly encouraged to enroll in the National Surgical Adjuvant Breast and Bowel Project B-39/Radiation Therapy and Oncology Group 04-13 clinical trial

[c]Microscopic multifocality allowed, provided the lesion is clinically unifocal (a single discrete lesion by physical examination and ultrasonography/mammography) and the total lesion size (including foci of multifocality and intervening normal breast parenchyma) falls between 2.1 and 3.0 cm

CALBG study, at 10 years follow-up, 4 % of patients had succumbed to breast cancer related causes while 28 % died of other causes: 1 % of patients who had lumpectomy and WB-XRT then tamoxifen experienced an IBTR, while 10 % of patients with lumpectomy and tamoxifen alone experienced an IBTR. While this trial's results are used as a guide in discussing treatment options with patients, most physicians take into account the overall health and potential longevity of the patient before making a no radiation/radiation recommendation: most specialists are still recommending post-lumpectomy radiation for patients over age 70 who are in excellent health. ASTRO consensus guidelines consider women ≥age 50 as "cautionary" candidates (Table 18.5), while women above age 60 are considered "suitable" for APBI.

Preoperative workup: All APBI candidates should undergo conventional workup with physical exam, diagnostic mammography, and ultrasound as indicated. Breast magnetic resonance imaging (MRI) is considered by some to be a valuable adjunct in identifying prospective APBI candidates [28–30]. The goal of MRI in APBI candidates is to better define extent of disease, identify occult multifocal or multicentric lesions, and optimize chances for single-stage surgical resection. Fewer excisions will produce a smaller surgical cavity and a smaller radiation target volume regardless of which APBI approach is used. The benefits of single-stage excision are most critical for patients receiving APBI with single fraction IORT as one of the key benefits of this approach is the concept of 1 operation/1 radiation dose treatment: if a patient were to have close or positive margins, additional surgery and/or WB-XRT might be needed (with the IORT used as the boost dose). Suspicious lesions identified elsewhere in the breast by physical exam or imaging should be biopsied preoperatively with percutaneous techniques or excised at the time of lumpectomy for patients considering any of the 5-day forms of APBI. For patients considering single fraction IORT, suspicious satellite lesions should be sampled before surgery. APBI is generally contraindicated for almost all patients with multifocal disease and all patients with multicentric disease due to the potential for further satellite lesions and out of concern for such patients having a tendency to be at higher risk for local recurrence. The only APBI trial openly permitting limited multifocal disease is the ongoing NSABP B-39 trial.

Tumor size: Most clinical trials have utilized upper limits of tumor size of 2–3 cm. Multiple studies have demonstrated that large tumor size is associated with increased trends towards local recurrence. Furthermore, increasing tumor size leads to larger lumpectomy cavities which are problematic for all forms of APBI as larger tumor size requires larger volume excisions, which in turn leads to larger target volumes: as target volume increases, so does tissue toxicity due to the higher doses used with APBI. Such toxicity may manifest as adverse cosmetic results, fat necrosis, pain, etc. At this time, patients with locally advanced tumors are not considered optimal candidates for APBI even with a pCR. Efforts have been made to identify tumors that are so small that no radiation is necessary: to date, these studies have failed to identify a group of patients that does not receive significant benefit from post-lumpectomy radiation [31].

Surgical margins: All breast specimens and nodes in patients considering APBI should be evaluated by pathologists with considerable experience with breast disease. Tumor-free margins are critical: "tumorectomies" are unacceptable. An "optimal" tumor free margin has not been determined [32]. Most studies require or at least advise a tumor-free margin of 2 mm, while the NSABP B-39 study follows the traditional NSABP "no tumor on ink" paradigm.

Nodal status: Lymph node involvement has historically been associated with trends towards increased IBTR rates. Nodal involvement is considered by many a contraindication for APBI and has been deemed "unsuitable" by ASTRO criteria (Table 18.6). Institutional and registry data are conflicting [33, 34]. The NSABP B-39 trial permits enrollment of women with up to three involved nodes.

Tumor histology: Most APBI studies have focused on patients with pure invasive ductal cancer (IDC) or IDC mixed with limited ductal carcinoma in situ (DCIS). Extensive intraductal components (EIC) and invasive lobular cancer are considered a high risk feature for local recurrence and suboptimal for APBI [18]. Few studies have enrolled substantial numbers of patients with pure DCIS or invasive lobular cancer. Nonetheless, there is also conflicting institutional and registry data on the relative importance of these tumor factors as well [35, 36].

Table 18.6 Patients "unsuitable" for APBI outside of a clinical trial if any of these criteria are present (from Smith et al. [24])

Factor	Criterion
Patient factors	
Age	<50 year
BRCA1/2 mutation	Present
Pathologic factors	
Tumor size[a]	>3 cm
T stage	T3-4
Margins	Positive
LVSI	Extensive
Multicentricity	Present
Multifocality	If microscopically multifocal >3 cm in total size or if clinically multifocal
Pure DCIS	If >3 cm in size
EIC	If >3 cm in size
Nodal factors	
N stage	pN1, pN2, pN3
Nodal surgery	None performed
Treatment factors	
Neoadjuvant therapy	If used

Abbreviations as in Table 18.4
If any of these factors are present, the Task Force recommends against the use of APBI outside of a prospective clinical trial
[a]The size of the invasive tumor component as defined by the American Joint Committee on Cancer [72]

Tumor biology: Molecular profiling using intrinsic subset criteria (luminal A/B, basal, and so forth.) has emerged as a potentially meaningful factor in local recurrence, and hence has become a topic of interest with respect to patient selection for APBI. Further work needs to be done to understand whether profiling could lead to omission of post-surgical radiation or help identify optimal candidates [37]. Patients with luminal A tumors appear to have very low local recurrence rates and represent an optimal cohort for APBI [38]. Of note, most "profiling" studies to date have used immunohistochemistry surrogates rather than true gene expression profiling analyses to categorize tumor phenotype: there is a 10–15 % discordance between tumor profiling with IHC vs. tumor profiling through gene expression analysis [39].

Results from ongoing Phase II and especially Phase III studies should shed further light on the importance of each of these variables in patient selection.

Surgical Technique in APBI

Role of the surgeon: Surgeons play a critical role in APBI [40]. Often the surgeon is the first specialist to introduce the concept to potential candidates, educating patients regarding treatment options, and helping match each patient with an optimal treatment plan, whether it be BCS with conventional WB-XRT, BCS with APBI, BCS alone, neoadjuvant chemotherapy, or mastectomy. Patients considering APBI are ideally identified prior to resection of the tumor. This will ensure a thorough preoperative evaluation, enhance collaborative planning with colleagues in radiology and radiation oncology, and optimize chances of single-stage resection with tumor-free margins. For potential APBI candidates pre-surgical consultation with the treating radiation oncologist is ideal.

Tumor localization: Should a patient decide to pursue APBI, any and all localization tools should be used to maximize chances for single stage resection to tumor free margins and to minimize resection volume. This is accomplished, as possible, with the potential use of guidewires (X-ray, ultrasound, or MRI guided localization), radioactive seeds (ROLL technique), skin markers, and/or intraoperative ultrasound. Surgical specimens should always be oriented. This may not only facilitate efforts at re-excision, but may also guide the radiation oncologist to "high-risk" cavity margins. This author prefers resection of the specimen as a single piece of tissue rather than routine use of shaved margins. Should inspection, palpation, or imaging of the surgical specimen suggest a close margin, however, additional shave margins are taken as needed to help avoid a return to the OR for re-excision. Rarely, frozen section is performed intraoperatively to assess specimen edges. Ideally the index lesion is located centrally within the resection specimen such that the subsequent irradiation of cavity margins leads to symmetric coverage of tissue "at risk."

Location of skin incision: Placement of the skin incision over the lesion may help guide post-surgical radiation with most forms of APBI by more clearly identifying the lumpectomy cavity vs. surrounding edema. Location of the incision over tumor is more critical for APBI to facilitate single-stage excision and accurate targeting of radiation.

Clip placement: With most forms of APBI intraoperative clip placement at lumpectomy cavity margins prior to skin closure can be of great benefit for identifying the cavity on subsequent CT scans [41, 42]. However, clips should be avoided when balloon devices are to be used as the clips can lead to balloon rupture. Clips are not necessary for single fraction IORT as the cavity margins are identified by direct visualization by the surgeon in the operating room.

Use of sentinel node biopsy: Sentinel node biopsy (SNB) should be performed in all women with invasive breast cancer considering APBI in order to stage the axilla (see patient selection, above). Nodal involvement is associated with slightly higher IBTR rates and falls in ASTRO's "unsuitable" category.

APBI and ACOSOG Z0011: The ACOSOG Z-0011 study demonstrated that women who underwent lumpectomy and SNB for T1 or T2 invasive breast cancer and had 2 or fewer involved sentinel nodes did not benefit from a completion axillary node dissection (cALND) providing they subsequently received appropriate systemic therapy and WB-XRT [43]. The ACOSOG Z-0011 study did not enroll women who received lumpectomy and APBI. This study's findings therefore are not directly applicable to patients considering APBI. As noted above, ASTRO guidelines consider any nodal involvement "unsuitable" for APBI.

The successful implementation of APBI relies on close cooperation between breast imaging, the surgical team, pathologists, and radiation oncologists. Poorly selected patients, poorly executed excisions, unnecessarily large or irregular surgical cavities, improper device placement, or poor radiation treatment planning can all undermine long-term treatment success.

The following section reviews the specific methods for delivering APBI. Each approach has slightly different technical requirements from the surgical and radiation oncology teams.

APBI Techniques

Overview

In general, there is no APBI technique that is optimal for any given patient. Part of the art of APBI is identifying patients appropriately and following that which approach is best for the patient at hand.

Brachytherapy

The first successful APBI implementation relied on interstitial brachytherapy [44]. Accurate in delivery of radiation, but technically challenging, interstitial brachytherapy techniques rely on the placement of a series of catheters placed in parallel through-and-through the breast around the surgical cavity. Low-dose-rate (LDR) sources were used initially, while interstitial brachytherapy teams now utilizes high-dose-rate (HDR) seeds delivered and distributed between and among the catheters with an HDR afterloading machine.

Successful interstitial brachytherapy paved the way for the development of intracavitary brachytherapy devices: rather than 10–20 catheters placed around the surgical cavity as with interstitial brachytherapy, intracavitary devices are usually a single catheter designed to lay within the surgical cavity. Device placement is faster, more comfortable, and can be accomplished any breast surgeon, rather than depending on access to the far more limited number of radiation oncologists who have training and experience with interstitial breast brachytherapy. The MammoSite was the first intracavitary device: it received FDA approval in 2005. This balloon device has a single channel through which the radioactive source can be delivered: single channel systems permit several dwell positions, but is quite limited in specifying dose distribution compared with the hundreds of dwell positions possible with interstitial brachytherapy. As the number of dwell positions increases, the radiation oncologist is better able to target cavity margins and avoid toxicity to skin and deep structures, such as muscle and rib. To address this concern, multichannel intracavity devices were developed. Some multichannel devices are balloon based, others not. Multichannel, intracavitary devices allow for greater control over radiation delivery with the convenience of a single skin entry point.

Most brachytherapy approaches utilize a treatment schedule of 34 Gy given in divided doses of 3.4 Gy BID over 5 days with a minimum of 6 h between treatments.

3D Conformal Radiotherapy

3D-CRT utilizes multiple external beams typically delivered via a linear accelerator that converge on the limited target volume around the lumpectomy cavity. 3D-CRT can be combined with other techniques, such as breathing synchronization, to further minimize target volume and dose to normal tissue. Variations on APBI with 3D-CRT include APBI with intensity modulated radiotherapy (IMRT) and APBI using protons.

Most 3D-CRT approaches utilize a treatment schedule of 38.5 Gy given in divided doses of 3.85 Gy BID over 5 days with a minimum of 6 h between treatments.

IORT

IORT delivers the entire therapeutic radiation treatment in a single dose through the open surgical incision while the patient is under anesthesia in the operating room. There are two major approaches to delivering single-fraction breast IORT. The ELIOT approach uses a collimator placed at the opening of the skin incision to direct high energy electrons to the target volume of cavity margins. The TARGIT approach relies on placement of a low energy brachytherapy sphere within the surgical cavity.

The single radiation dose for IORT is typically 20–21 Gy.

Detailed Review of APBI Techniques

APBI with Interstitial Brachytherapy

APBI with interstitial brachytherapy is accomplished via a series of catheters placed in parallel which pass through the surgical cavity and surrounding breast tissue (Fig. 18.1). The catheters may be placed at the time of surgery, or as a separate

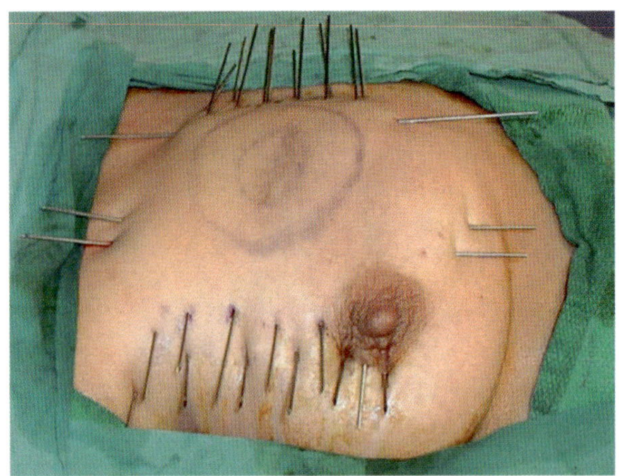

Fig. 18.1 An ultrasound-guided implant illustrating: (1) triangulation between the superficial and deep planes, where the superficial needles are in between pairs of deep needles, and (2) the use of crossing needles at right angles and between the two planes, at the periphery of the target volume, benefiting dosimetry in the "*z*-plane" of the implant and avoiding medial sources too close to the skin (From Dirbas/Scott Conner, Chapter 68) [73]

invasive procedure postoperatively. Approximately 1 dozen catheters or more are placed into the breast tissue in two to three parallel rows using a free-hand approach or with a template "guide." A CT scan is then performed to determine the relative position of the catheters in relation to the surgical cavity. Simulation software is used to determine dwell positions and durations for the Iridiium-192 seed in order to deliver the appropriate radiation dose to cavity margins while minimizing toxicity to surrounding tissue. In combination with special software, the dwell time and sequential positioning of the radioactive seed is controlled by a device known as an HDR afterloader (Fig. 18.2). Although the area around each dwell position is a "hot spot" at risk for developing toxicity, one of the great benefits of interstitial brachytherapy is that several hundred dwell positions are utilized as the seed can be placed at a series of locations in each of many catheters. The target volume for radiation delivery is 1.5 cm around the lumpectomy cavity, with restrictions placed on radiation delivery to skin and chest wall. The most commonly used treatment plan delivers a total of 34 Gy in 3.4 Gy fractions delivered twice daily over 5 days. After treatment is complete, catheters are removed. Despite the somewhat disturbing appearance of the catheters while they are in place, there is remarkably little evidence of the catheters in long-term follow-up. Phase I/II studies have validated this approach as being safe and yielding comparable results to historical controls for WB-XRT [45, 46].

The disadvantages of this approach are: the potential for dose inhomogeneity due to hot spots that can lead to skin and rib toxicity, including telangiectasia, poor cosmetic outcome, and rib fracture; the need for a very invasive procedure after completion of breast surgery; and the limited availability of radiation oncologists with the training to place the brachytherapy catheters and deliver the treatment appropriately.

While interstitial brachytherapy remains popular among some radiation oncologists, overall use is shifting in favor of other APBI approaches.

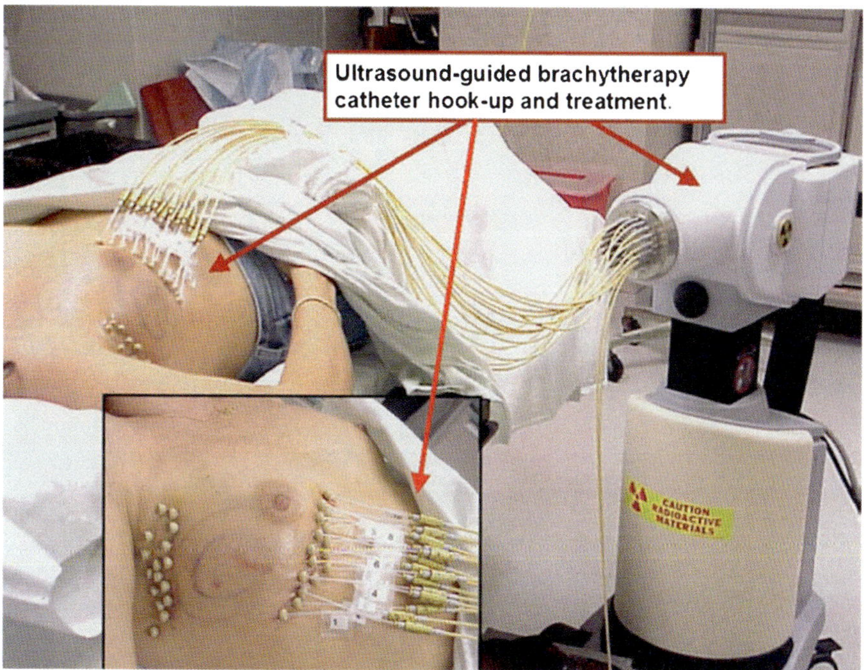

Fig. 18.2 After CT-based 3D brachytherapy treatment planning, the patient is connected to high dose rate remote afterloader for treatment (From Dirbas/Scott Conner, Chapter 68) [73]

APBI with Intracavitary Brachytherapy

Single-Channel Intracavitary Brachytherapy

The MammoSite® (Hologic, Inc. Bedford, MA), the first intracavitary brachytherapy device, was broadly accepted as a considerably easier way to deliver APBI compared with interstitial brachytherapy (Fig. 18.3). In initial studies, the device was placed at the time of lumpectomy either: (a) directly via the lumpectomy incision; (b) percutaneously through a separate entry site at the time of lumpectomy; or (c) percutaneously away from the lumpectomy site as an office procedure weeks after the operation when final pathology was available. The device is now most commonly placed postoperatively in the office or procedure room setting. Once placed and inflated a planning CT is performed (Fig. 18.4). Initially a single dwell position at the center of the balloon catheter was utilized. Subsequently, multiple dwell positions were utilized along the single channel and a variety of balloon shapes were then introduced to improve options for cavity and balloon conformance (Fig. 18.5). Phase I/II studies have supported the balloon brachytherapy concept as a reasonable alternative to interstitial brachytherapy [47].

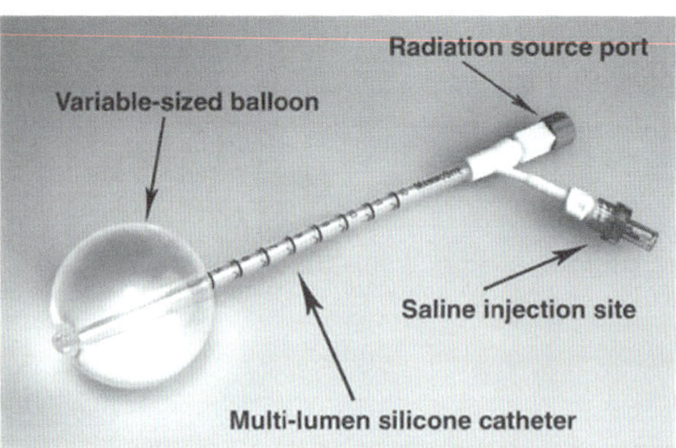

Fig. 18.3 The MammoSite™ brachytherapy device (Courtesy of Hologic, Inc.)

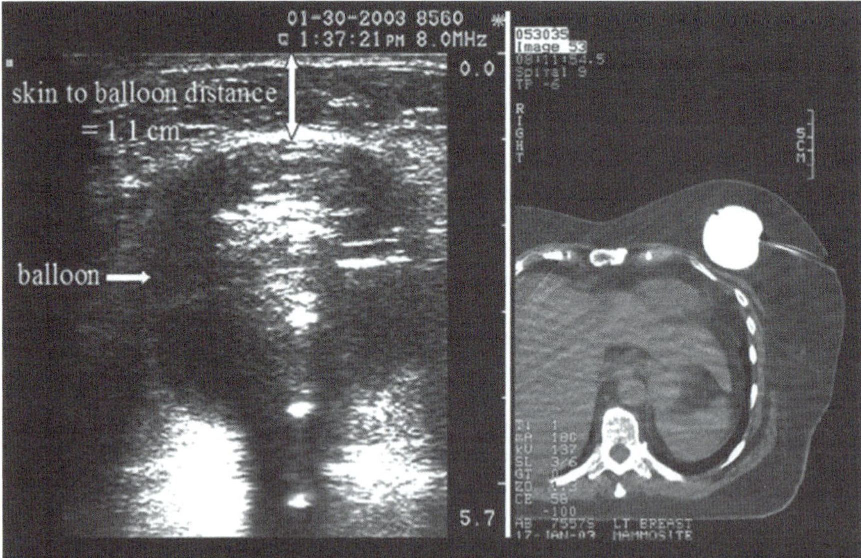

Fig. 18.4 Sonographic and CT imaging of the indwelling inflated catheter confirming balloon symmetry and skin spacing (Courtesy of Springer) [73]

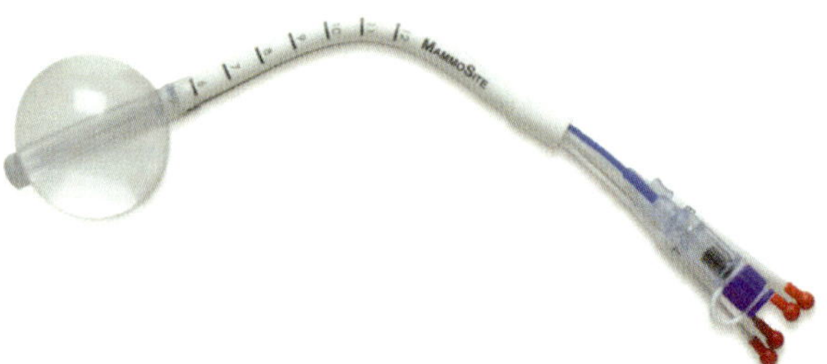

Fig. 18.5 The MammoSite™ Multilumen System (Courtesy of Hologic, Inc.)

The device has limitations aside from the limited number of dwell positions. It does not deliver radiation symmetrically if there air or fluid pockets separating the balloon surface from the cavity margins. Early experience demonstrated that patients could be prone to skin injury if precautions were not taken to ensure a minimum 7 mm distance between the balloon surface and skin. There are isolated case reports of angiosarcoma developing after use of this device [48].

Balloon brachytherapy with the MammoSite, more than any other device, enabled the rapid adoption of APBI among breast specialists.

The target volume is a 1.5 cm rim of breast tissue around the surgical cavity, excepting skin and rib, treating to a total dose of 34 Gy over a 5-day period using BID dosing at 3.4 Gy per fraction. Some effort has been made to compress this treatment from 5 to 2 days [49].

The apparent initial success of APBI, predominantly with the MammoSite balloon catheter, was recently challenged by a retrospective SEER database review which suggested that use of APBI after lumpectomy subsequently led to an increase in mastectomies compared with lumpectomy followed by conventional WB-XRT [50]. Some have considered the study design flawed. Investigators compared outcomes from a period when a novel device was in its first few years of widespread use, in the absence of more refined guidelines such as those now available from ASTRO. There was also no mechanism to evaluate the experience or skill of the surgical or radiation oncology teams using brachytherapy, while patients receiving lumpectomy and WB-XRT almost certainly were treated using algorithms and techniques employed for decades. More clarity regarding outcomes from APBI and WB-XRT will be available from ongoing phase III clinical trials.

Use of the MammoSite has decreased over time as multichannel devices have come to market (see below).

Multichannel Intracavitary Brachytherapy

While the single channel, balloon based MammoSite brachytherapy systems introduced a simplified method for offering APBI, the single channel could not tailor dose delivery with the precision of interstitial brachytherapy.

This observation encouraged the development of newer intracavitary brachytherapy designs that incorporated multiple channels. One of these incorporates multiple channels as part of a balloon type device (CONTURA® Multi-Lumen Balloon (MLB) Catheter, SenoRx, Inc., Bard Biopsy Systems, Tempe, AZ) with a separate channel to aspirate air or seroma surrounding the balloon (something the MammoSite was not capable of accomplishing) (Fig. 18.6). Another multichannel device omits the balloon component while retaining multiple channels (Savi®, Cianna Medical, Aliso Viejo, CA) (Fig. 18.7). A third device, ClearPath® (Huiheng Medical, Inc., Shenzen China), offered multiple channels while omitting the balloon component: at the time of this writing this device is not clear if this device is commercially available in the USA (Fig. 18.8).

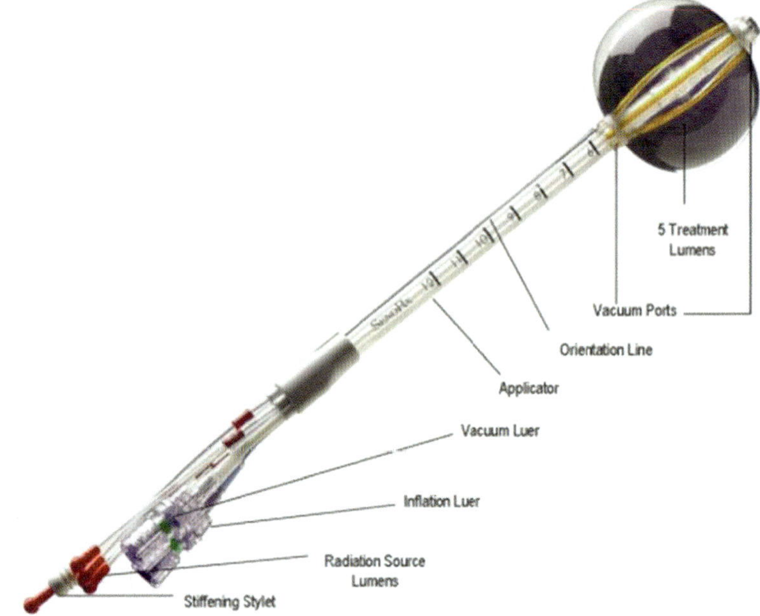

Fig. 18.6 The Contura balloon applicator (Courtesy of SenoRx, Inc.)

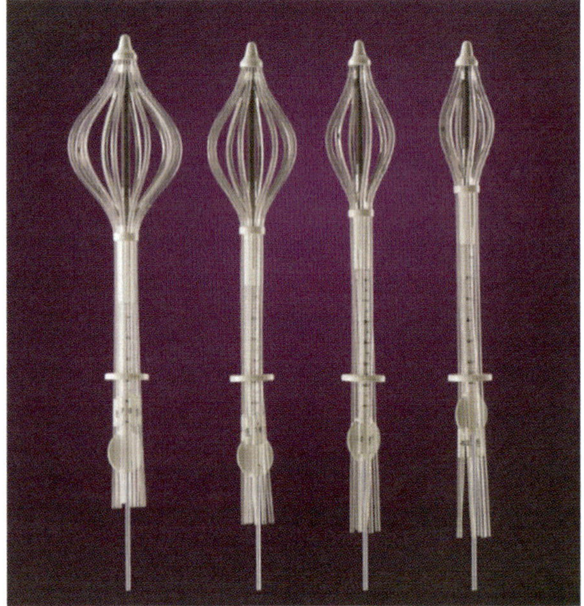

Fig. 18.7 SAVI device (Courtesy of Cianna Medical, Inc.)

a

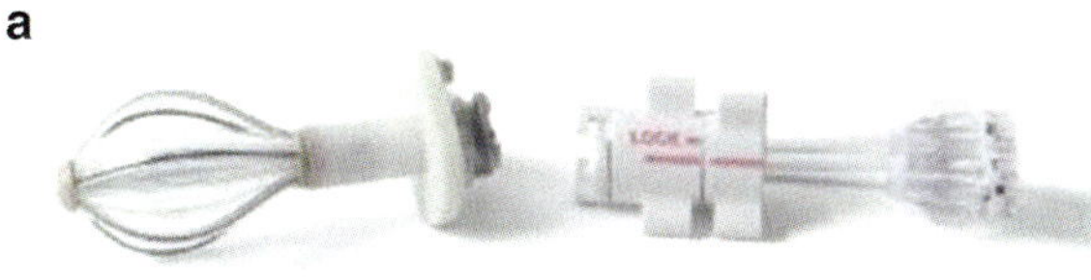

b

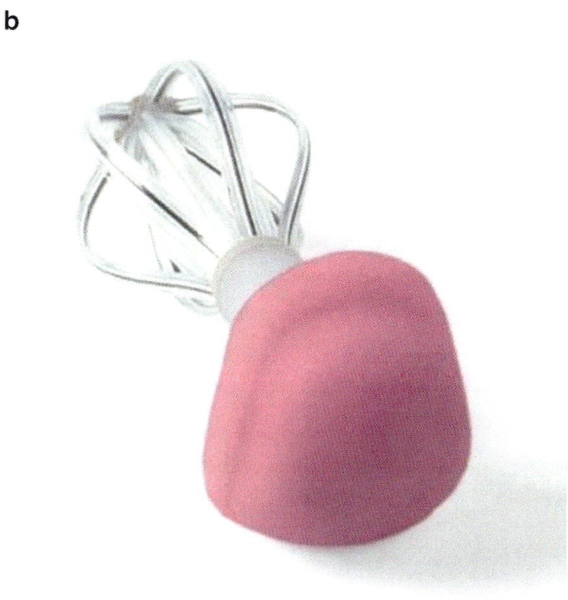

Fig. 18.8 ClearPath® device (**a**) the base detached (**b**) a cap placed over the HDR channels (Huiheng Medical, Inc.)

Multichannel, intracavitary devices may be placed at the time of surgery or postoperatively as a separate procedure when final pathology is known in much the same way as the MammoSite is deployed, i.e., by the surgeon in an office or procedure room setting. As with interstitial brachytherapy and single-channel intracavitary brachytherapy, Iridium-192 is used as the radiation source and an HDR afterloader is used to control seed deployment. The target volume is a 1.5 cm rim of breast tissue around the surgical cavity, excepting skin and rib, treating to a total dose of 34 Gy over a 5-day period using BID dosing at 3.4 Gy per fraction. Results from Phase I/II studies with multichannel brachytherapy devices compare favorably with those of the single channel MammoSite and historical controls using WB-XRT [51–53]. Efforts are underway to compress this treatment schedule from 5 days to 2 [54].

APBI with 3D Conformal RT

Most radiation oncologists do not employ brachytherapy as part of their practice. This initially hampered adoption of APBI among radiation oncologists. To make APBI more accessible to the radiation oncology community, radiation oncologists

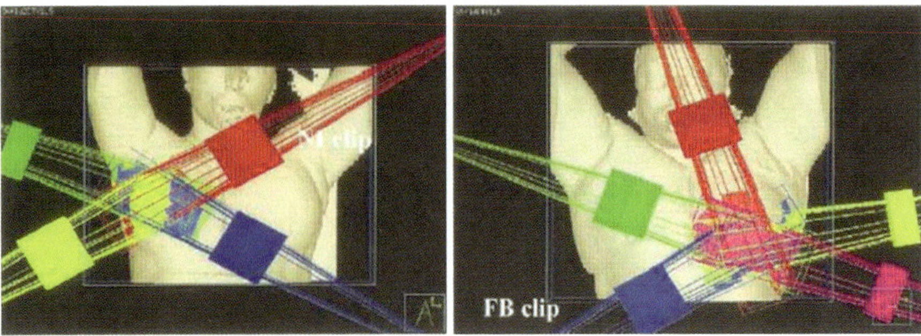

Fig. 18.9 Typical 4-field arrangement for right-sided lesions and 5-field arrangement for left-sided lesions [53]

at William Beaumont Hospital (WBH) developed an approach which modified external beam WB-XRT technique. Instead of using the traditional two-tangent approach normally used to cover the entire breast with conventional WB-XRT, 3D-CRT as developed by WBH relied on multiple beams converging on the planning target volume from at different angles to minimize exposure of surrounding structures to radiation [55] (Fig. 18.9).

There are a number of 3D-CRT techniques that have been promoted. The 3D-CRT approach most commonly targets a 1.5 cm margin around the surgical cavity, adds 5 mm for daily set-up variation, and then another 5 mm for respiratory motion, for a total treatment margin around the cavity of 2.5 cm. Variations include active or passive breathing synchronization, different beam angles, etc. [56]. IMRT, a more complex external beam approach, has been used by some [57]. Others have investigated APBI with protons and even the CyberKnife® (CyberKnife Robotic Radiosurgery System, Sunnyvale, CA) has been explored [58, 59]. Most external beam treatments use 3D-CRT are typically given to a total dose of 38.5 Gy over a 5 day period, with BID doses therefore of 3.85 Gy per fraction. 3D-CRT potentially enables any radiation oncologist with a linear accelerator to deliver APBI.

Most treat patients in the typical supine position while others treat in the prone position [60]. While differing from the traditional supine position, the prone position may help avoid radiation to heart and lung, and may be particularly helpful in patients with very large breasts.

The primary benefit of 3D-CRT is the avoidance of a brachytherapy device which requires special training and has been associated with worse cosmesis, increases in chronic seroma and infection, the inconvenience of another invasive procedure after the lumpectomy, and an indwelling foreign body for a minimum of 5 days.

The primary toxicity concern with APBI using 3D-CRT or related approaches is the larger volume of breast tissue exposed to radiation compared with interstitial and intracavitary brachytherapy. As volume increases, so does toxicity. Most 3D-CRT approaches utilize a cut-off in terms of volume of breast treated/entire breast volume.

Several phase II institutional studies suggested that APBI with 3D-CRT could also be associated with poor cosmetic outcome and other side effects. with 3D-CRT [61]. The NSABP performed an interim analysis of NSABP B-39 data: toxicity was not increased. Early results from the Phase III Canadian RAPID trial were favorable for APBI using 3D-CRT [62]. However, updated results presented at ASTRO 2012 (publication pending) indicated a poorer cosmetic result with 32 % of patients in the APBI arm having a fair or poor cosmetic result as compared with 19 % of patients in the WB-XRT arm at 2.3 years of follow-up, while these assessments were 33 and 13 % for the more limited number of patients who had reached 5 years of follow-up.

APBI with 3D-CRT would certainly make PBI accessible to many women who receive post lumpectomy RT.

APBI with Intraoperative Radiotherapy (IORT)

IORT most completely fulfills the potential benefits of accelerated, partial breast irradiation. With single fraction breast IORT the entire dose of APBI is delivered to cavity margins in one dose at the time of surgery through the open surgical incision by direct visualization of cavity margins directly visualized in the OR by the surgeon and radiation oncologist working together. The most common dose to the cavity margins of 21 Gy is felt to be radiobiologically similar to other forms of post-lumpectomy radiation: interstitial brachytherapy (BID × 5 days, 34 Gy total), 3D-CRT (BID × 5 days, 38.5 Gy total), or WB-XRT (1.8–2 Gy/day over approximately 5 ½ weeks plus a boost dose of 10 Gy for 60 Gy total).

There are currently two methods that have undergone extensive evaluation for single fraction IORT. These are the ELIOT (ELectron IntraOperative radioTherapy) technique and the TARGIT (TARGeted Intraoperative radioTherapy) approach. There are key differences between these two approaches. The ELIOT technique uses a megavoltage radiation source using high energy electrons with deep tissue penetration. This is delivered via with a collimator to the target volume. The TARGIT approach uses a low energy (50 kV) orthovoltage radiation source with rapid dose fall-off. This is delivered by a spherical applicator placed within the lumpectomy cavity. Used to a lesser degree are: collimator based, single-fraction IORT with high energy (200 kV) orthovoltage radiation; the H.A.M applicator which uses an HDR source; and intraoperative electronic brachytherapy catheter system which uses a low energy 50 kV source.

IORT: ELIOT and Other Collimator Based Approaches

In 1999, the European Institute of Oncology (EIO) began using high energy electrons to deliver breast IORT. Modeling initial studies on earlier trials in the USA and France, in which 10 Gy had been delivered intraoperatively to lumpectomy cavity margins as a planned "boost" dose, the EIO ultimately escalated using IORT solely as the 10 Gy boost dose to single fraction doses of 15, 17, 19, then finally 21 Gy in a pilot study of 102 patients in which the larger doses were used as the entire course of post-BCS radiation (The EIO uses a quadrantectomy, rather than lumpectomy, ostensibly removing more breast tissue around the tumor). The 21 Gy dose was delivered using a mobile linear accelerator using high energy electrons, typically 6–11 MeV [63].

Following the pilot study, in 2001 the EIO launched a prospective randomized study comparing single fraction IORT with conventional WB-XRT. Patients were selected based on tumor size, absence of evidence of multifocality, negative nodes via intraoperative analysis, and other criteria. Patients who desired single fraction IORT but did not meet study criteria were enrolled in a registry trial [64].

The EIO technique for IORT included a quadrantectomy including resection of skin and pectoralis fascia. In order to allow mobility to the surrounding breast tissue so it could be approximated as a target, the quadrantectomy was followed by mobilization of the surrounding breast tissue from the pectoralis muscle and the skin. A lead-aluminum plate combination was then placed at the base of the surgical cavity as a "beam stopper," followed by temporary approximation of the lumpectomy cavity margins with sutures over the lead-aluminum plate. This beam stopper prevented exit dose to muscle or rib, as well as deeper structures such as the heart and lungs. A cylindrical collimator was then inserted through the open surgical incision and placed upon the approximated cavity margins under direct visualization: there was no "guessing" what margins represented the edges of the surgical cavity. The collimator was aligned with a high energy electron source and 21 Gy delivered to the cavity margins over a matter of minutes. The high energy electrons were able to deliver a significant dose of radiation deeply into the breast tissue around the surgical cavity. After radiation delivery is complete, the radiation device is removed, approximating breast sutures are cut and removed, as are the lead-aluminum plates. Depending on the size of the cavity, a drain may be placed to help minimize seroma formation.

Preliminary results from this trial were presented at the Milan Breast Cancer meeting in June 2012 but have not been published. When all 1,822 patients treated with single fraction IORT (both on and off-protocol) were analyzed by ASTRO guideline criteria, the cohort which met the "suitable" ASTRO criteria had a 1.5 % IBTR rate at 5 years of follow-up [65]. The group is now offering single fraction IORT to patients meeting ASTRO consensus guidelines.

Using a similar technique to the EIO, a team from Verona recently reported single fraction breast IORT with high energy electrons in a cohort of 226 patients with only a single local recurrence reported at a mean follow-up of 46 months [66]. Other institutions have reported similar initial results with carefully selected patients undergoing single fraction IORT with this approach [67].

At Stanford, we have used single fraction breast IORT since 2002 with the same collimator based approach. Our radiation source was initially a 200 kV Philips orthovoltage system, more recently converting to the Mobetron system using 7–11 MeV electrons: we have seen two recurrences in 55 patients since beginning our trial. The open incision, after lumpectomy, with cavity margins approximated is seen in Fig. 18.10, and with the collimator in place in Fig. 18.11.

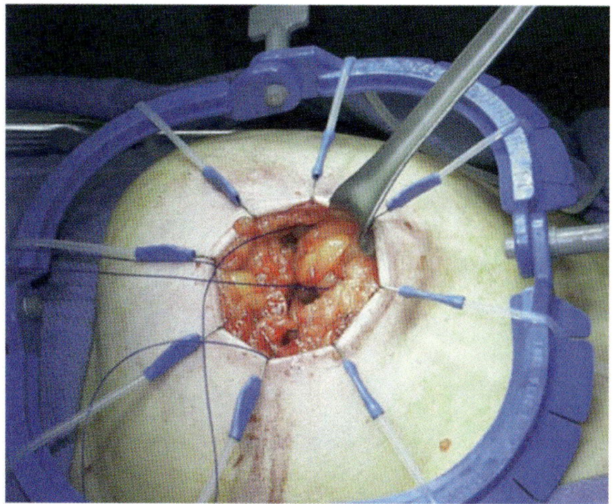

Fig. 18.10 IORT showing lumpectomy cavity and target volume

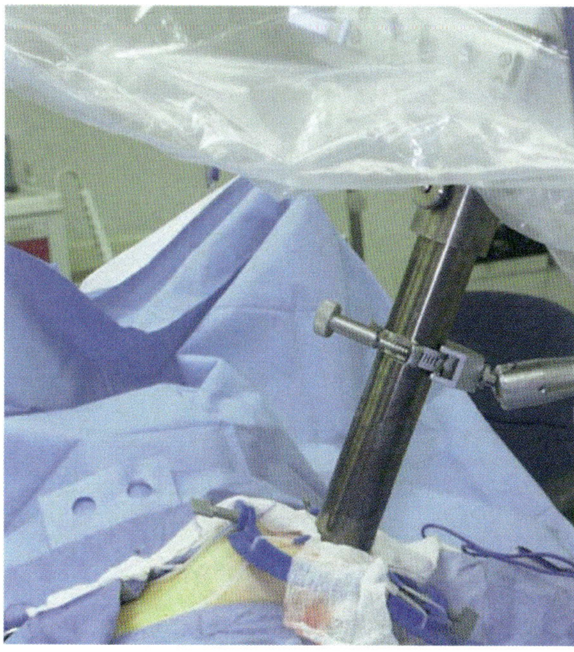

Fig. 18.11 IORT with collimator in place

The strength of single fraction breast IORT is the obvious convenience of no additional radiation treatments; direct vision of cavity margins; lack of implanted hardware, and potential radiobiologic advantages of the high dose delivered. Potential downsides of this approach are the relatively limited number of machines available worldwide for performing the technique, delivery of radiation in the absence of final pathology; and the lack of a visual record of the target volume actually receiving radiation.

Since the EIO first reported results, several institutions have begun using the EIO technique. The three most common cited concerns over this and other single fraction approaches are: the delivery of radiotherapy in the absence of final pathology status; long term effectiveness; and toxicity. Regarding the absence of final pathology, most groups have adopted the approach of returning the patient to the OR as needed to achieve clear margins, then following the IORT "boost" dose, delivering WB-XRT. Regarding long term effectiveness, data from the ELIOT, TARGIT (see below), and other phase III trials will be critical. Regarding toxicity, there are few reports of long term toxicity using single fraction breast IORT despite the large dose utilized. The most current version of the system as used in the ELIOT trial is Novac 11 (New Radiant Technology, Rome, IT). The megavoltage IORT system most commonly used in the USA is the Mobetron (IntraOp Medical, Sunnyvale, CA).

IORT: TARGIT and Other Brachytherapy Approaches

Rather than using radiation that is directed through the open skin incision, IORT may be accomplished by placing a device inside the lumpectomy cavity, hence IORT with brachytherapy.

The most commonly used system for IORT with a brachytherapy device is the Intrabeam. In contrast to the high energy electrons used at the EIO and other facilities, the Intrabeam uses a 50 kV source, often referred to as "soft" X-rays.

IORT with the Intrabeam® (Carl Zeiss Meditec, Germany) was introduced in 1995 [68]. After a lumpectomy or similar BCS procedure is performed, the Intrabeam device is brought to the OR table. The X-ray source is coupled with an appropriately sized applicator, then the applicator is lowered into the surgical cavity (Fig. 18.12). Tungsten shields may be placed to protect adjacent structures that might be harmed by radiation, such as muscle/rib and skin. After the shields are placed, and the applicator is inserted into the breast, a purse-string suture is placed which draws the breast tissue in close approximation with the applicator surface. While the dose delivered to breast tissue adjacent to the applicator is 20 Gy, dose fall off is quite considerable such that at 1 cm from the applicator surface the dose is approximately 5 Gy. This rapid fall-off in dose is a major concern with the Intrabeam source. The 50 kV energy delivered via the most commonly used applicator, 3.5 cm, is approximately 20–30 min.

Since the Intrabeam device was introduced, a multi-institutional, prospective randomized trial, the TARGIT study, was developed to compare this single fraction APBI technique with conventional WB-XRT. In the TARGIT study each participating institution has been allowed to determine inclusion/exclusion criteria. Patients who are deemed "high risk" due to involved margins, re-excision, and/or involved nodes, among other variables, may subsequently receive WB-XRT, yet remain in the single fraction IORT arm as part of an "intent to treat" analysis. 15–20 % of the patients in "IORT" arm of this study actually received WB-XRT after receiving IORT. The TARGIT study, based on data presented at the San Antonio Breast Cancer Symposium in December 2013, had accrued 3,451 patients, with 1,679 patients eligible for evaluation treated in the single fraction ("intent to

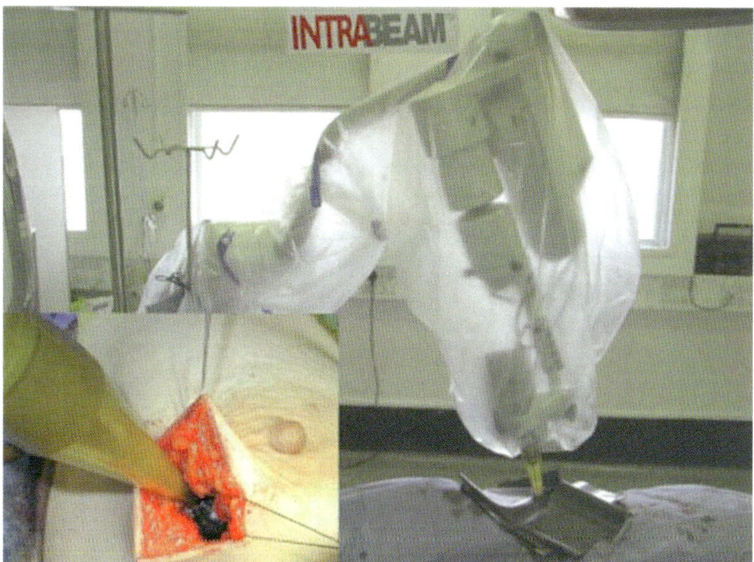

Fig. 18.12 Intrabeam system in place

treat") arm, and 1696 patients randomized to WB-XRT. Results showed approximately a 3 % higher absolute recurrence rate for those patients reaching 5 years of follow-up. The investigators noted a much smaller difference for those patients with PR positive tumors.

Another 50 kV device is the Axxent® electronic brachytherapy system (Axxent® eBx System) from iCad (Figs. 18.13 and 18.14). The Axxent system is much like the MammoSite balloon catheter in concept. However, the energy source is a 2.2 cm miniature x-ray tube that is powered from a standard electrical outlet. This eliminates the need for a radioactive source, or extensive lead shielding of the room in which treatment is delivered. The Axxent system can be placed at the time of surgery, or postoperatively once pathology is known. While the configuration of the device is similar to the MammoSite, dosimetry from the Axxent system is similar to the Intrabeam, as both share a 50 kV source, with 20 Gy delivered at the applicator surface and rapid fall-off at 1 cm to approximately 5 Gy. The key benefit of the Axxent system is the ability to deliver IORT without the need for a radiation seed such as Iridium-192. The Axxent device is a relatively new device. Single institution series have reported results that compare favorably with other brachytherapy devices [69].

Both the Intrabeam and Axxent IORT devices are quite mobile and are easy to deploy. As with other forms of IORT, the target is seen under direct vision, ensuring that radiation is delivered exactly to surgical cavity margins. Concern exists over the rapid dose fall off from the surface of the respective applicators: neither the Intrabeam nor the Axxent system provide the same target volume coverage as interstitial, intracavitary, or 3D-CRT approaches, or high-energy electron IORT as with the ELIOT approach. Whether this is ultimately a factor in local recurrence will be proven in

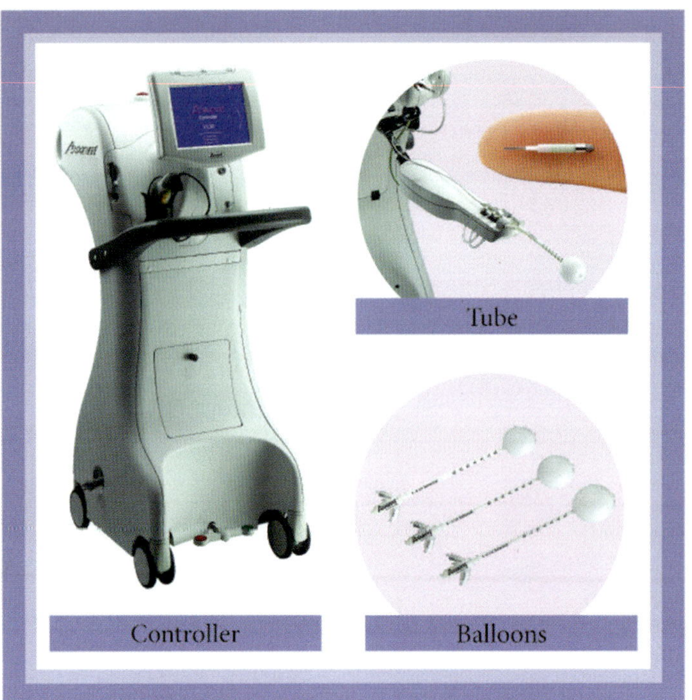

Fig. 18.13 Axxent system

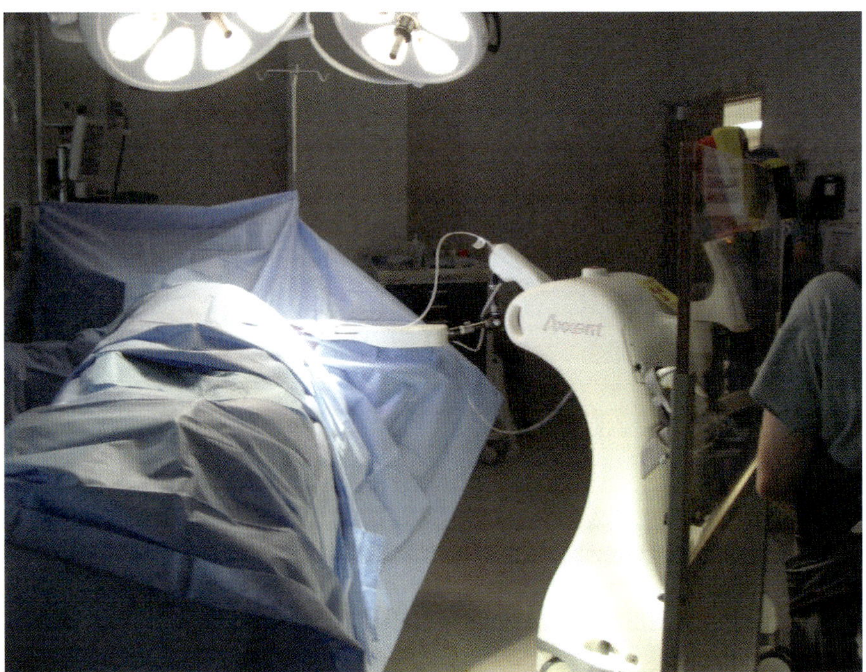

Fig. 18.14 Operating room setup

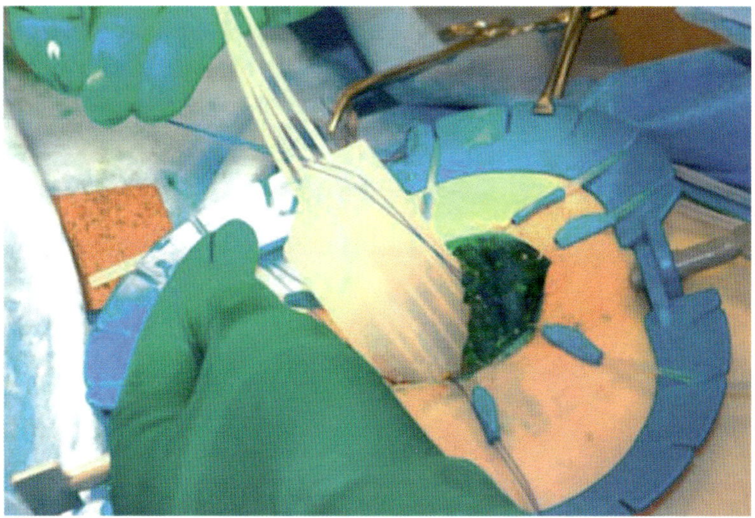

Fig. 18.15 H.A.M. applicator in place

clinical trials. Because of the low energy sources, treatment times for the Intrabeam system is approximately 20–30 min, and treatment time for the Axxent system, on average, is 10 min. Varying slightly for both systems based on applicator size.

IORT: HDR, Brachytherapy Approach

Investigators at Memorial Sloan Kettering Cancer Center conducted a clinical trial using a multichannel silastic applicator, the H.A.M. device, connected to an HDR afterloader (Fig. 18.15). The MSKCC group used this approach in a limited fashion on a trial basis. Skin toxicity led to a decrease in dose and alteration of technique to protect skin. Due to the limited availability of the device and alternative methods for performing single—fraction IORT this technique has not been widely adopted. Nonetheless, IBTR rates were low as was overall toxicity [70].

Interest in APBI with IORT is increasing. The US Centers for Medicaid and Medicare services introduced new CPT codes and increased reimbursement for IORT in December 2012.

Clinical Trials with APBI

At present, there are multiple clinical trials with APBI. Phase III trials have the greatest impact. Only one has published long term results. Other studies have been completed with publication of long-term results pending. Numerous ongoing phase I/II studies are in progress which will continue to suggest modifications to patient selection, surgical technique, and radiation delivery [71] (Table 18.7).

Table 18.7 Major phase III APBI trials

	NCI Hungary	TARGIT	ELIOT	NSABP B39/RTOG 3804/ SWOG	CIHR RAPID	GEC-ESTRO
Targ/Act acrual	258	3,451	1,306	Target 4,300	2,123	Target 1,170
Study arms	WB vs. HDR brachy or 3D-CRT	WB vs. IORT (some with boost)	WB vs. IORT	WB 50–50.5 Gy with optional boost to 60–66.6 Gy brachytherapy 34 Gy, or MammoSite 34 Gy, or 3D conformal RT 38.5 Gy	WB 42.5 Gy in 16 fractions (50 Gy large breasts/25 fractions). Boost permitted if high risk, 10 Gy in four or five fractions	WB 50.4 plus 10 Gy boost, vs. HDR/PDR brachytherapy. HDR in 32 Gy or 30 Gy, PDR 50 Gy
Age	>40	≥35	≥48	≥18	>40	≥40
Stage	I, II	I, II	I, II	0, I, II	0, I, II	0, I, II
Tumor size	≤2 cm	T1–T3	≤2.5 cm	≤3 cm	≤3 cm	≤3 cm
Unifocal/ multifoc al	Unifocal	Unifocal	Unifocal	Multifocal within one quadrant, and no more than 4 cm apart	Unifocal	Unifocal
Histology	IDC	IDC	IDC, ILC	All	DCIS or IDC	Stage 0 low risk or, 1 or 2 invasive
Nodes	cN0, pN0, or pN1mi	cN0	N0, N1	1–3 pos nodes	Negative or ITC	N0
Exclusion	ILC, pure DCIS	ILC, EIC	Multifocal	life exp <10 year	BRCA 1/2 , ILC	LVI, EIC
Excision margin	Negative	Negative	Negative	Microscopically clear	Microscopically clear	5 mm DCIS, 2 mm invasive
RT margin	2 cm	1 cm	1–3 cm	2.5 cm	Similar to B39, 2.5 cm	2–3 cm margin

3D-CRT Three-dimensional conformal radiotherapy, *CIHR RAPID* Canadian Institutes of Health Research Radiation Therapy for Accelerated Partial Breast Irradiation Trial, *DCIS* ductal carcinoma in situ, *EIC* extensive intraductal carcinoma (DCIS), *ELIOT* electron intraoperative radiotherapy technique, *GEC-ESTRO* Groupe Européen de Curiethérapie and European Society for Therapeutic Radiology and Oncology, *HDR* high dose rate, *IDC* invasive ductal carcinoma, *ILC* invasive lobular carcinoma, *IORT* intraoperative radiotherapy, *ITC* isolated tumor cells, *LVI* lymphovascular invasion, *mi* micrometastasis, *NCI* National Cancer Institute, *PDR* pulsed dose rate, *TARGIT* targeted intraoperative radiotherapy, *WB* whole breast radiotherapy

Summary

Should APBI be demonstrated safe and effective with long-term follow-up, women with early stage breast cancer will have a third option for local management of disease. In addition to mastectomy, BCS followed by whole breast radiation, a third option of BCS followed by APBI will make treatment shorter and even more appealing.

Intraoperative Breast Radiotherapy Utilizing Electronic Brachytherapy: Surgical Technique

A.B. Francescatti and D.S. Francescatti

The operative technique described is that used for the Xoft Axxent© system in the delivery of single fraction radiotherapy to the surgical bed after breast conserving surgery for early stage breast cancer. The technique is similar to that used with other systems such as Intrabeam©.

The utilization of electronic brachytherapy in the operating room as a means for the delivery of radiotherapy following partial mastectomy (lumpectomy) in breast conserving surgery provides both patient and surgeon a number of advantages.

The patient will benefit either by the administration of a complete radiotherapeutic dose (single fraction) to the tumor bed thus avoiding any postoperative radiotherapy or will receive a "boost" dose to the surgical cavity that will decrease both the time expended and number of postoperative radiation treatments needed to complete therapy.

For the surgeon, the use of electronic brachytherapy (eBx) in the operating room offers additional practical advantages not realized by other delivery systems used in intra-operative radiotherapy. Because of the low energy employed in standard 50 kV systems, no infrastructure changes are required to the standard operating room for its performance. Because of this, regulatory requirements for the use of eBx in the operating room are markedly reduced. Although the intraoperative treatment time using an electron system is reduced (approximately 2 min), eBx systems can deliver a complete radiotherapeutic single fraction treatment in as little as 8 min with logistical advantages not shared by Linac Systems©; these include ease of portability of the eBx system from department to department, room to room, or facility to facility. Because the surgical cavity is exposed, both the skin as well as deeper structures that include the pectoralis muscle, ribs and thoracic cavity and its contents can be easily shielded utilizing surgical techniques prior to the delivery of radiotherapy.

Additionally, because of the mobility of both the controller and docking arm, flexibility is provided to the operating team in the approach angle to the operative site utilized for docking the system to the balloon applicator for the delivery of radiotherapy. The angle and direction of the balloon applicator inserted at operation can take any direction or angle exiting the surgical cavity. This will provide for practically an unlimited approach angle that can be taken by the oncology team in docking the controller to the balloon applicator. In addition, during the delivery of radiotherapy anesthesiology can remain at the head of the operating table during treatment by simply remaining behind a rolling shield placed between the patient and ventilator controls.

The technique for placement of the balloon applicator post lumpectomy is straight forward but does require attention to detail critical to preparing the surgical field for single fraction radiotherapy.

Operative Technique

This description of the procedure for delivery of breast IORT utilized for the Axxent© system closely parallels other eBx systems in use.

After completion of the partial mastectomy (lumpectomy) for early stage cancer of the breast, the surgical team must prepare the surgical bed for placement of the balloon applicator. This process is divided into the following important steps:

1. Negative margin status is first established prior to radiotherapy employing any of a number of methodologies that the treating team feels appropriate.
2. One hundred percent applicator balloon surface apposition to the circumferential surface of the surgical cavity.

Once the lumpectomy specimen has been removed, an inflatable "sizer" (foley catheter) is utilized to determine the optimal fill volume of the treatment balloon applicator that will be placed prior to treatment. The sizer is used to assure breast tissue to balloon wall apposition. Appositional conformance can be checked both visually by the operating team in real time and/or by utilizing intraoperative ultrasound. More sophisticated imaging techniques can be employed if desired. Importantly, the final fill volume of the sizer is carefully measured and is used to determine the ideal dosimetric calculations to deliver 20 Gy to the tissue/balloon surface. As an example, an applicator sized to a diameter of 4 cm delivers 20 Gy at the surface of the balloon and approximately 7 Gy at 1 cm distal to the balloon surface. A larger diameter balloon will require additional treatment time while delivering the same dose at the surface of the balloon and at 1 cm. The duration of treatment is a function of balloon applicator diameter and source output and can be calculated preoperatively by the physicist for any balloon diameter determined appropriate by the surgical team. When the exact diameter of the surgical cavity has been determined by the "sizer" as measured by the fill volume, this information is easily and quickly uploaded into the controller by the radiation oncologist/physicist team prior to the start of radiation treatment. Treatment dosimetry predicated on various balloon sizer volumes can be predetermined prior to the surgical procedure and captured on flash drives and utilized at the time of operation.

3. Shielding of the underlying Pectoralis musculature, ribs, lung, and heart from non-targeted radiation exposure.

The depth of surgical excision for a cancerous lesion may extend to the retro mammary fatty layer separating the posterior surface of the breast from the fascia of the pectoralis musculature. If this is the case, this potential space can be dissected in a circumferential fashion around the circumference of the cavity to a lateral depth of approximately two centimeters in order to create a "lip" of breast tissue at the base of the surgical cavity. Flexible or rigid shielding material can be used at the base of the lumpectomy cavity to protect deeper structures. As an example, a malleable sheet of lead, previously sterilized, approximately 5 mm in thickness, can be cut at the operating table to conform to the "sized" diameter of the surgical cavity with the addition of a 1 cm rim of shielding beyond the sized diameter. This "shield" is now placed by inserting it at the base of the surgical cavity, i.e., positioned on the Pectoralis fascia. The shield is inserted under the "lip" of mobilized breast tissue in a circumferential fashion so that breast tissue will, with inflation of the balloon applicator, be in total apposition to the surface of the applicator with the shield laying beneath both breast and balloon applicator. If breast tissue should remain on the "floor" of the lumpectomy cavity after excision of the cancer, this remaining breast tissue must be treated and a shield is not used. An added benefit to the mobilization of breast tissue at this stage is realized if an oncoplastic closure is chosen.

4. Protecting the skin from non-targeted radiation exposure.

Because the skin is sensitive to radiation damage, it must be protected. The Axxent system© offers the surgeon flexibility of choice in choosing how to best protect the skin from unwanted radiation. Because of the flexibility of the controller arm utilized for docking to the balloon applicator that is placed in the surgical cavity, virtually any angle above the plane of the incision including the vertical can be accessed for treatment. Additionally, the balloon applicator shaft can exit the cavity in any circumferential direction relative to the incisional site. Flexibility in approach to the patient and delivery of radiation therapy is thus assured. In the incisional approach any number of surgical spacing methods can be employed to either shield the at-risk skin or distance the skin from the source of radiation. Alternatively a percutaneous approach permits the exit of the balloon applicator shaft in a 360° arc around the circumference of the lumpectomy cavity and at any angle from the perpendicular. This approach can be utilized readily in procedures where tunneling is used to remove the cancerous area to obtain a more beneficial cosmetic result. Either approach facilitates the unencumbered and rapid docking of controller to applicator shaft without unneeded vertical overhang. By temporarily closing the incision over the balloon applicator, the distance between the applicator balloon surface and epidermis can now be determined prior to the start of radiation therapy. This determination is done either by physical measurement and/or via intraoperative ultrasound examination in real time. The distance between the balloon applicator surface and epidermis must be at least 1 cm.

5. Delivery of radiotherapy and completion of the surgical procedure.

Sterile overdraping is now placed over the operative field and an exit site through the drape created for the applicator shaft. This in turn is secured to the over drape with a sterile adhesive sheet. The distal portion of the balloon applicator can be handled in a non-sterile fashion by the radiation oncologist/physicist for delivery of treatment while the operative field remains sterile. The Axxent© dose delivery time will add, depending on the applicator balloon diameter, an average of 10 min of operating time. Preparations during the procedure, i.e., determining the appropriate size applicator to be used, placing shielding if necessary and checking balloon integrity will add an additional 10–15 min to operating room time. Once radiotherapy has been delivered the applicator balloon is deflated and is removed in concert with the overdrape, thus exposing the protected sterile operative field.

With the withdrawal of the balloon applicator and removal of the overdrape, the surgical team returns and completes the procedure in their usual fashion.

References

1. Veronesi U, Cascinelli N, Mariani L, et al. Twenty-year follow-up of a randomized study comparing breast-conserving surgery with radical mastectomy for early breast cancer. N Engl J Med. 2002;347:1227–32.
2. Fisher B, Anderson S, Bryant J, et al. Twenty-year follow-up of a randomized trial comparing total mastectomy, lumpectomy, and lumpectomy plus irradiation for the treatment of invasive breast cancer. N Engl J Med. 2002;347:1233–41.
3. Blichert-Toft M, Rose C, Andersen J, et al. Danish randomized trial comparing breast conservation therapy with mastectomy: six years of life-table analysis. Danish Breast Cancer Cooperative Group. J Natl Cancer Inst Monogr. 1992;11:19–25.
4. van Dongen J, Voogd A, Fentiman I, et al. Long-term results of a randomized trial comparing breast-conserving therapy with mastectomy: European Organization for Research and Treatment of Cancer 10801 trial. J Natl Cancer Inst. 2000;92:1143–50.
5. Arriagada R, Le M, Guinebretiere J, Dunant A, Rochard F, Tursz T. Late local recurrences in a randomised trial comparing conservative treatment with total mastectomy in early breast cancer patients. Ann Oncol. 2003;14:1617–22.
6. Poggi M, Danforth D, Sciuto L, et al. Eighteen-year results in the treatment of early breast carcinoma with mastectomy versus breast conservation therapy: the National Cancer Institute Randomized Trial. Cancer. 2003;98:697–702.
7. Chagpar A, Kaufman C, J C, C B, T G, Winchester D. What's influencing breast conservation rates in the United States. San Antonio Breast Cancer Symposium; 2012 Dec 15: Cancer Research; 2012. p. 122s.
8. Clark R, McCulloch P, Levine M, et al. Randomized clinical trial to assess the effectiveness of breast irradiation following lumpectomy and axillary dissection for node-negative breast cancer. J Natl Cancer Inst. 1992;84:683–9.
9. Uppsala-Orebro Breast Cancer Study Group. Sector resection with or without postoperative radiotherapy for stage I breast cancer: a randomized trial. J Natl Cancer Inst. 1990;82:277–82.
10. Veronesi U, Marubini E, Mariani L, et al. Radiotherapy after breast-conserving surgery in small breast carcinoma: long-term results of a randomized trial. Ann Oncol. 2001;12:997–1003.
11. Fisher B, Anderson S. Conservative surgery for the management of invasive and noninvasive carcinoma of the breast: NSABP trials. National Surgical Adjuvant Breast and Bowel Project. World J Surg. 1994;18:63–9.

12. Recht A, Silver B, Schnitt S, Connolly J, Hellman S, Harris J. Breast relapse following primary radiation therapy for early breast cancer. I. Classification, frequency and salvage. Int J Radiat Oncol Biol Phys. 1985;11:1271–6.
13. Fisher B, Redmond C, Poisson R, et al. Eight-year results of a randomized clinical trial comparing total mastectomy and lumpectomy with or without irradiation in the treatment of breast cancer. N Engl J Med. 1989;320:822–8.
14. Veronesi U, Del Vecchio M, Greco M, et al. Conservative treatment for breast cancer of limited extent. Results of a randomized trial. Isr J Med Sci. 1981;17:928–31.
15. Recht A, Silen W, Schnitt S, et al. Time-course of local recurrence following conservative surgery and radiotherapy for early stage breast cancer. Int J Radiat Oncol Biol Phys. 1988;15:255–61.
16. Jones B, Dale R, Deehan C, Hopkins K, Morgan D. The role of biologically effective dose (BED) in clinical oncology. Clin Oncol (R Coll Radiol). 2001;13:71–81.
17. Fentiman I, Poole C, Tong D, et al. Inadequacy of iridium implant as sole radiation treatment for operable breast cancer. Eur J Cancer. 1996;32A:608–11.
18. Ribeiro G, Magee B, Swindell R, Harris M, Banerjee S. The Christie Hospital breast conservation trial: an update at 8 years from inception. Clin Oncol (R Coll Radiol). 1993;5:278–83.
19. Proulx G, Hurd T, Lee R, Stomper P, Podgorsak M, Edge S. Intraoperative radiation therapy (IORT) to the tumor bed only for breast cancer: technique and outcome. Radiol Oncol. 2001;35:35–41.
20. Dodwell DJ, Dyker K, Brown J, et al. A randomised study of whole-breast vs. tumour-bed irradiation after local excision and axillary dissection for early breast cancer. Clin Oncol (R Coll Radiol). 2005;17:618–22.
21. Vicini FACP, Fraile M, Gustafson GS, Edmundson GK, Jaffray DA, Benitez P, et al. Low-dose-rate brachytherapy as the sole radiation modality in the management of patients with early-stage breast cancer treated with breast-conserving therapy: preliminary results of a pilot trial. Int J Radiat Oncol Biol Phys. 1997;38:301–10.
22. King TAJJ, Kuske RR. Long term results of wide field brachytherapy as the sole method of radiation after segmental mastectomy for tis, T1, T2 breast cancer. Am J Surg. 2000;180: 299–304.
23. Vicini F, Kestin L, Chen P, Benitez P, Goldstein N, Martinez A. Limited-field radiation therapy in the management of early-stage breast cancer. J Natl Cancer Inst. 2003;95:1205–10.
24. Smith BD, Arthur DW, Buchholz TA, et al. Accelerated partial breast irradiation consensus statement from the American Society for Radiation Oncology (ASTRO). Int J Radiat Oncol Biol Phys. 2009;74:987–1001.
25. Veronesi U, Luini A, Galimberti V, Zurrida S. Conservation approaches for the management of stage I/II carcinoma of the breast: Milan Cancer Institute trials. World J Surg. 1994;18: 70–5.
26. Sanghani M, Wazer DE. Patient selection for NSABP B-39/RTOG 0413: have we posed the right questions in the right way? Brachytherapy. 2007;6:119–22.
27. Hughes KS, Schnaper LA, Berry D, et al. Lumpectomy plus tamoxifen with or without irradiation in women 70 years of age or older with early breast cancer. N Engl J Med. 2004;351: 971–7.
28. Horst KC, Ikeda D, Birdwell RL, et al. Breast magnetic resonance imaging alters patient selection for accelerated, partial breast irradiation. Int J Radiat Oncol Biol Phys. 2005;63:S4–5.
29. Kimple RJ, Klauber-DeMore N, Kuzmiak CM, et al. Local control following single-dose intraoperative radiotherapy prior to surgical excision of early-stage breast cancer. Ann Surg Oncol. 2011;18:939–45.
30. Horst KC, Ikeda DM, Fero KE, Daniel BL, Goffinet DR, Dirbas FM. Breast magnetic resonance imaging alters patient selection for accelerated partial breast irradiation. Am J Clin Oncol. 2012 Dec 27. [Epub ahead of print].
31. Fisher ER, Costantino JP, Leon ME, et al. Pathobiology of small invasive breast cancers without metastases (T1a/b, N0, M0): National Surgical Adjuvant Breast and Bowel Project (NSABP) protocol B-21. Cancer. 2007;110:1929–36.

32. Singletary SE. Surgical margins in patients with early-stage breast cancer treated with breast conservation therapy. Am J Surg. 2002;184:383–93.
33. Shah C, Wilkinson JB, Shaitelman S, et al. Impact of lymph node status on clinical outcomes after accelerated partial breast irradiation. Int J Radiat Oncol Biol Phys. 2012;82:e409–14.
34. Dekhne N, Shah C, Wilkinson JB, et al. Axillary lymph node failure in patients treated with accelerated partial breast irradiation. Cancer. 2012;118:38–43.
35. Jeruss JS, Kuerer HM, Beitsch PD, Vicini FA, Keisch M. Update on DCIS outcomes from the American Society of Breast Surgeons accelerated partial breast irradiation registry trial. Ann Surg Oncol. 2011;18:65–71.
36. Goyal S, Vicini F, Beitsch PD, et al. Ductal carcinoma in situ treated with breast-conserving surgery and accelerated partial breast irradiation: comparison of the Mammosite registry trial with intergroup study E5194. Cancer. 2011;117:1149–55.
37. Demirci S, Broadwater G, Marks LB, Clough R, Prosnitz LR. Breast conservation therapy: the influence of molecular subtype and margins. Int J Radiat Oncol Biol Phys. 2012;83:814–20.
38. Miyamoto DT, Harris JR. Molecular predictors of local tumor control in early-stage breast cancer. Semin Radiat Oncol. 2011;21:35–42.
39. Nguyen B, Cusumano PG, Deck K, et al. Comparison of molecular subtyping with BluePrint, MammaPrint, and TargetPrint to local clinical subtyping in breast cancer patients. Ann Surg Oncol. 2012;19:3257–63.
40. Beitsch PD, Hodge CW, Dowlat K, et al. The surgeon's role in breast brachytherapy. Breast J. 2009;15:93–100.
41. Coles CE, Wilson CB, Cumming J, et al. Titanium clip placement to allow accurate tumour bed localisation following breast conserving surgery: audit on behalf of the IMPORT Trial Management Group. Eur J Surg Oncol. 2009;35:578–82.
42. Landis DM, Luo W, Song J, et al. Variability among breast radiation oncologists in delineation of the postsurgical lumpectomy cavity. Int J Radiat Oncol Biol Phys. 2007;67:1299–308.
43. Giuliano AE, Hunt KK, Ballman KV, et al. Axillary dissection vs. no axillary dissection in women with invasive breast cancer and sentinel node metastasis: a randomized clinical trial. JAMA. 2011;305:569–75.
44. King T HD, Cederbom G, Champaign J, Smetherman D, Kuske R, Farr G, Bolton J, Fuhrman G. Image-guided core-needle breast biopsy has no impact on local tumor control in patients treated with breast conservation therapy. 1999 SSO Plenary Session 1999.
45. Shah C, Antonucci JV, Wilkinson JB, et al. Twelve-year clinical outcomes and patterns of failure with accelerated partial breast irradiation versus whole-breast irradiation: results of a matched-pair analysis. Radiother Oncol. 2011;100:210–4.
46. Kuske R, Winter K, Arthur D, et al. A phase II trial of brachytherapy alone following lumpectomy for stage I or II breast cancer: initial outcomes of RTOG 9517. JCO. 2004;23:18.
47. Keisch M, Arthur DW. Current perspective on the mammosite radiation therapy system—a balloon breast brachytherapy applicator. Brachytherapy. 2005;4:177–80.
48. Andrews S, Wilcoxon R, Benda J, Jacobson G. Angiosarcoma following MammoSite partial breast irradiation. Breast Cancer Res Treat. 2010;124:279–82.
49. Wallace M, Martinez A, Mitchell C, et al. Phase I/II study evaluating early tolerance in breast cancer patients undergoing accelerated partial breast irradiation treated with the mammosite balloon breast brachytherapy catheter using a 2-day dose schedule. Int J Radiat Oncol Biol Phys. 2010;77:531–6.
50. Smith GL, Xu Y, Buchholz TA, et al. Association between treatment with brachytherapy vs. whole-breast irradiation and subsequent mastectomy, complications, and survival among older women with invasive breast cancer. JAMA. 2012;307:1827–37.
51. Brown S, McLaughlin M, Pope DK, et al. A dosimetric comparison of the Contura multilumen balloon breast brachytherapy catheter vs. the single-lumen MammoSite balloon device in patients treated with accelerated partial breast irradiation at a single institution. Brachytherapy. 2011;10:68–73.
52. Lu SM, Scanderbeg DJ, Barna P, Yashar W, Yashar C. Evaluation of two intracavitary high-dose-rate brachytherapy devices for irradiating additional and irregularly shaped volumes of breast tissue. Med Dosim. 2012;37:9–14.

53. Njeh CF, Saunders MW, Langton CM. Accelerated partial breast irradiation (APBI): a review of available techniques. Radiat Oncol. 2010;5:90.
54. Khan AJ, Dale RG, Arthur DW, Haffty BG, Todor DA, Vicini FA. Ultrashort courses of adjuvant breast radiotherapy: wave of the future or a fool's errand? Cancer. 2012;118:1962–70.
55. Baglan K, Sharpe M, Jaffray D, et al. Accelerated partial breast irradiation using 3D conformal radiation therapy (3D-CRT). Int J Radiat Oncol Biol Phys. 2003;55:302–11.
56. Bourgier C, Marsiglia H, Taghian A. A mixed-modality 3d-conformal accelerated partial breast irradiation technique using opposed mini-tangent photon fields and en face electrons to minimize the lung exposure to radiation: in regard to Jain et al. (Int J Radiat Oncol Biol Phys 2009;75:82-88). Int J Radiat Oncol Biol Phys. 2010;76:956–7. author reply 7.
57. Lewin AA, Derhagopian R, Saigal K, et al. Accelerated partial breast irradiation is safe and effective using intensity-modulated radiation therapy in selected early-stage breast cancer. Int J Radiat Oncol Biol Phys. 2012;82:2104–10.
58. Bush DA, Slater JD, Garberoglio C, Do S, Lum S, Slater JM. Partial breast irradiation delivered with proton beam: results of a phase II trial. Clin Breast Cancer. 2011;11:241–5.
59. Vermeulen S, Cotrutz C, Morris A, et al. Accelerated Partial Breast Irradiation: using the CyberKnife as the Radiation Delivery Platform in the Treatment of Early Breast Cancer. Front oncol. 2011;1:43.
60. Formenti SC, Hsu H, Fenton-Kerimian M, et al. Prone accelerated partial breast irradiation after breast-conserving surgery: five-year results of 100 patients. Int J Radiat Oncol Biol Phys. 2012;84(3):606–11.
61. Jagsi R, Ben-David MA, Moran JM, et al. Unacceptable cosmesis in a protocol investigating intensity-modulated radiotherapy with active breathing control for accelerated partial-breast irradiation. Int J Radiat Oncol Biol Phys. 2010;76:71–8.
62. Berrang TS, Olivotto I, Kim DH, et al. Three-year outcomes of a Canadian multicenter study of accelerated partial breast irradiation using conformal radiation therapy. Int J Radiat Oncol Biol Phys. 2011;81:1220–7.
63. Intra M, Gatti G, Luini A, et al. Surgical technique of intraoperative radiotherapy in conservative treatment of limited-stage breast cancer. Arch Surg. 2002;137:737–40.
64. Intra M, Luini A, Gatti G, et al. Surgical technique of intraoperative radiation therapy with electrons (ELIOT) in breast cancer: a lesson learned by over 1000 procedures. Surgery. 2006;140:467–71.
65. Leonardi MC, Maisonneuve P, Mastropasqua MG, et al. How do the ASTRO consensus statement guidelines for the application of accelerated partial breast irradiation fit intraoperative radiotherapy? A retrospective analysis of patients treated at the European Institute of Oncology. Int J Radiat Oncol Biol Phys. 2012;83:806–13.
66. Maluta S, Dall'Oglio S, Marciai N, et al. Accelerated partial breast irradiation using only intraoperative electron radiation therapy in early stage breast cancer. Int J Radiat Oncol Biol Phys. 2012;84:e145–52.
67. Arcangeli G, Arcangeli S, C G, et al. Intraoperative (IORT) vs. standard radiotherapy (EBRT) in breast cancer: an update of an ongoing Italian multicenter, randomized study. ISIORT Meeting Abtracts; 2008; Madrid. p. 13.
68. Vaidya J, Baum M, Tobias J, et al. Targeted intra-operative radiotherapy (Targit): an innovative method of treatment for early breast cancer. Ann Oncol. 2001;12:1075–80.
69. Ivanov O, Dickler A, Lum BY, Pellicane JV, Francescatti DS. Twelve-month follow-up results of a trial utilizing Axxent electronic brachytherapy to deliver intraoperative radiation therapy for early-stage breast cancer. Ann Surg Oncol. 2011;18:453–8.
70. Sacchini V, Beal K, Goldberg J, Montgomery L, Port E, McCormick B. Study of quadrant high-dose intraoperative radiation therapy for early-stage breast cancer. Br J Surg. 2008;95:1105–10.
71. Polgar C, Major T, Fodor J, et al. Accelerated partial-breast irradiation using high-dose-rate interstitial brachytherapy: 12-year update of a prospective clinical study. Radiother Oncol. 2010;94:274–9.
72. Greene FL, Page DL, Fleming ID. AJCC cancer staging handbook. 6th ed. New York: Springer; 2002.
73. Dirbas FM, Scott-Conner CEH. Breast surgical techniques and interdisciplinary management. New York: Springer; 2011.

Chapter 19
Systemic Therapy

Ruta Rao

Introduction

There have been many significant advances in both the understanding of breast cancer biology and the treatment of breast cancer. The systemic treatment of breast cancer at all stages can include hormonal treatment, chemotherapy and targeted therapies. It is the deeper understanding of the biology which allows us to determine which tumors will benefit from a particular treatment. We are now learning that there are different subtypes of breast cancer with different gene expression profiles and this information can be used to guide therapeutic decisions. This chapter discusses some of the recent advances in the understanding of breast cancer biology, the use of breast cancer genomics in determining breast cancer prognosis and recommending treatment, and the systemic treatment of breast cancer.

Gene Profiling in Breast Cancer

Breast cancer has been found to be a heterogeneous disease at the genetic level, and differences in gene expression affect the clinical behavior of the disease and the response to therapy. We are now learning that there are different subtypes of breast cancer with distinct gene expression profiles. This was first demonstrated by Perou and colleagues who analyzed the gene expression patterns of 65 breast cancer specimens from 42 individuals [1]. The tumors showed a wide variation in the patterns of gene expression. The patterns from two tumor samples from the same individual

R. Rao, M.D. (✉)
Department of Medicine, Rush University Medical Center, 1725 W. Harrison Street, Suite 809, Chicago, IL, USA
e-mail: ruta_d_rao@rush.edu

D.S. Francescatti and M.J. Silverstein (eds.), *Breast Cancer: A New Era in Management*,
DOI 10.1007/978-1-4614-8063-1_19,

were more similar to each other than to any other sample. They identified four intrinsic subtypes of breast cancer: estrogen receptor positive (ER+)/luminal-like, basal-like, Erb-B2+, and normal. The subtypes have been expanded to divide ER+/luminal-like into luminal A and B, and to include another subtype, claudin-low. These subtypes of breast cancer have different clinical histories and survival patterns, as well as different responses to therapy. Gene expression profiling is not yet routinely performed in the analysis of a breast tumor, so identification of these subtypes is not utilized clinically. Instead, in the clinical setting, tumors are classified based on the status of their receptors including estrogen receptor (ER), progesterone receptor (PR), and human epidermal growth factor receptor-2 (HER2). For practical purposes, the subtypes can be approximated using clinical data, but there is not a perfect correlation with the gene expression array results.

At the 12th Annual St. Gallen International Breast Cancer Conference in 2011, an Expert Panel recognized the importance of intrinsic biological subtypes and encouraged the approximation of the subtypes with clinical and pathological criteria, including ER and PR status, HER2 status and Ki-67 labeling index [2]. According to these guidelines, systemic treatment recommendations should be made based on the intrinsic subtypes. Luminal A tumors generally require only endocrine therapy. Chemotherapy is indicated for most luminal B tumors (along with endocrine therapy), for HER2-positive tumors (along with trastuzumab) and for triple negative tumors. However, there is not any phase III trial data available yet evaluating the role of intrinsic subtype classification as a predictive tool for chemotherapy benefit.

Genomic Tests in Breast Cancer

Two FDA-approved genomic tests are now available for use in the clinical setting. Oncotype Dx is a 21 gene RT-PCR assay and Mammaprint uses a 70 gene signature.

The 21 gene RT-PCR assay (Oncoytpe Dx) is performed on formalin-fixed paraffin-embedded tissue and provides prognostic and predictive information for women with lymph node negative, ER and/or PR positive breast cancer. Of the 21 genes, 16 are tumor-related and five are reference genes. An algorithm is used to determine a Recurrence Score (RS), which is divided into low risk (RS<18), intermediate-risk (RS 18–30), and high-risk (RS≥31) categories. The assay was evaluated in patients who had been treated in the prospective National Surgical Adjuvant Breast and Bowel Project (NSABP) B-14 trial [3]. RT-PCR profiles were obtained in 668 node negative, ER positive patients treated with tamoxifen. The rates of recurrence were as follows: 6.8 % (95 % CI 4.0–9.6) for low-risk, 14.3 % (95 % CI 8.3–20.3) for intermediate-risk, and 30.5 % (95 % CI 23.6–37.4) for high-risk patients. The rate in the low-risk group was significantly lower than that in the high-risk group, $p<0.001$. In addition, the study was able to show that the RT-PCR profile had a predictive power independent of age and tumor size

($p<0.001$). In an analysis of 651 tumor samples from the NSABP B-20 trial, a prospective randomized trial evaluating the benefit of the addition of chemotherapy, either cyclosphosphamide, methotrexate, and 5-flourouacil (CMF), or MF, to tamoxifen, the 21 gene RT-PCR assay was able to predict chemotherapy benefit [4]. Those with high-risk scores had a large benefit (RR 0.26, 95 % CI 0.13–0.53), whereas those with low-risk scores had minimal if any benefit (RR 1.31, 95 % CI 0.46–3.78). For the intermediate-risk scores, chemotherapy did not seem to have a large benefit, but a clinically important benefit could not be excluded. The use of this test is endorsed by the American Society of Clinical Oncology [5], the NCCN guidelines [6], and the St. Gallen International Expert Consensus [7]. According to the NCCN guidelines, the 21 gene RT-PCR assay should be considered to determine the need for adjuvant chemotherapy in patients with hormone receptor positive, HER2 negative tumors pT1b–pT3 and N0 or N1mi ($\leq$2 mm axillary nodal metastases). If the Recurrence Score (RS) is low risk (<18), adjuvant endocrine therapy alone is recommended. If the RS is intermediate Risk (18–31), chemotherapy should be considered and if it is high Risk ($\geq$31), chemotherapy is recommended [6].

Mammaprint, the 70-gene signature, is a prognostic assay for women less than 61 years of age with ER positive or negative, lymph node negative breast cancer. This test requires fresh frozen tumor tissue. The assay focuses on genes involved in proliferation, with an additional emphasis on genes involved in invasion, metastases, stromal integrity, and angiogenesis. The test gives dichotomous results, with either a high or low risk of disease recurrence. The test was developed at the Netherlands Cancer Institute. Investigators performed a supervised analysis of gene expression arrays on frozen tissue from 98 sporadic primary breast tumor samples, all from women less than 55 years old with tumors less than 5 cm and negative lymph nodes [8]. Of the 78 sporadic tumors, 34 (44 %) had distant metastases within 5 years, whereas 44 patients (66 %) did not. A set of 231 genes was identified and found to be statistically significantly associated with disease outcome, defined as the presence of distant metastases within 5 years. This group of genes was then reduced to a core group of 70 genes, with an 83 % accuracy at differentiating patients with distant disease relapse from those without relapse. The classifier correctly predicted the outcome of disease for 65 of the 78 patients (83 %), with five poor prognosis signature patients and eight good prognosis signature patients assigned incorrectly. The 70-gene signature was then validated by retrospective analysis in a number of trials. In one study of 295 patients, there was a strong correlation between the good prognosis 70-gene signatures and the absence of early distant recurrence or death [9]. The odds ratio (OR) for the development of distant metastases within 5 years in node negative patients (excluding the patients that overlapped with the prior study) was 15.3, similar to the results seen in the previous study. The prognosis profile was significantly associated with histologic grade ($p<0.001$), ER status ($p<0.001$), and age ($p<0.001$), but not the size, extent of vascular invasion, number of lymph nodes involved, or the treatment given. This study also showed that the prognosis signature was more accurate at classifying patients into a low or high risk of distant recurrence compared to standard clinical and pathological criteria. A second study was an independent validation of the 70-gene signature in 302 women who had not been treated with adjuvant systemic therapy [10]. It showed that the 70-gene signature provides independent prognostic information to the clinical and pathological risk assessment for patients with early stage breast cancer untreated with systemic therapy. A third validation study was an independent series of 123 patients, in which a multivariate analysis demonstrated that the prognosis signature was an independent prognostic factor and outperformed the clinical and pathological criteria [11]. Although it has not been sufficiently validated for clinical use, there is data to suggest that the 70-gene signature can predict responsiveness to current chemotherapy regimens. In one study, 167 patients with stage I–III breast cancer were analyzed prior to neoadjuvant chemotherapy, and the rate of pathological complete response (pCR) was used to measure chemosensitivity [12]. Pathologic complete responses were seen in 29 of the 144 patients with poor prognosis signatures and in none of the 23 patients with good prognosis signatures, $p = 0.015$. This led to the conclusion that patients with a poor prognosis signature were more sensitive to chemotherapy. Another study showed a significant survival benefit with the addition of chemotherapy in patients with the poor prognosis signature but not for those with a good prognosis signature [13].

The 70-gene signature test is FDA approved, but the American Society of Clinical Oncology stated that definitive recommendations for the use of this assay will require data from more clearly directed retrospective studies [5] or from the ongoing Microarray In Node negative Disease may Avoid ChemoTherapy trial (MINDACT), see below. The Mammaprint assay is approved for both ER-positive and ER-negative disease, but its utility in ER-negative disease is limited, because less than 10 % of those tumors have a good prognosis signature.

Prospective clinical trials to evaluate the 21-gene RT-PCR assay and the 70-gene prognosis signature in the node positive, early breast cancer population are ongoing. For the 21-gene RT-PCR assay, the TAILORx (Trial Assigning Individualized Options for Treatment (Rx)) trial has completed accrual but results have not yet been reported. This is the largest randomized adjuvant trial ever conducted, enrolling over 10,000 patients. All of the patients had the 21-gene RT-PCR assay performed, and those with RS between 11 and 25, were randomized to either hormonal therapy alone or hormonal therapy with chemotherapy. Patients with RS ≤ 10 were treated with hormonal therapy only and those with RS > 25 were given chemotherapy with hormonal therapy. Another trial, the Rx for Positive Node, Endocrine Responsive Breast Cancer (RxPONDER) trial, also known as SWOG S1007, is ongoing and opened in January 2011. Planned accrual is for 4,000 patients with early stage, hormone receptor positive, HER2 negative early stage breast cancer with 1–3 positive lymph nodes who have Recurrence Scores ≤ 25. Patients will be randomized to either chemotherapy plus endocrine therapy or endocrine therapy alone. They will be stratified into groups by RS 0–13 vs. 14–25, by menopausal status, and by axillary lymph node dissection vs. sentinel lymph node biopsy. For the 70-gene signature assay, the Microarray In Node negative Disease may Avoid ChemoTherapy (MINDACT) study is open in Europe. This is a prospective randomized study comparing the 70-gene signature to the common clinical-pathological criteria in the selection of patients for adjuvant chemotherapy. This trial opened in February 2007 and planned enrollment is 6,000 early stage breast cancer patients (T1, T2, and operable T3M0). The original focus was on lymph node negative patients, but more recently, the study was expanded to include tumors with 1–3 positive lymph nodes. Patients are assessed by the standard clinicopathologic prognostic factors included in Adjuvant! Online and by the 70-gene signature assay. If both traditional and molecular assays predict a high-risk status, the patient receives adjuvant cytotoxic chemotherapy and hormonal therapy, if the tumor is ER positive. If both assays indicate a low risk, no chemotherapy is given and ER-positive patients are given adjuvant hormonal therapy only. When there is discordance between the traditional clinicopathologic prognostic factors and the 70-gene signature prediction of risk, the patients are randomized to receive treatment based on either the genomic or the clinical prediction results. The results of these trials should provide more information to improve the use of genomic assays in early stage breast cancer.

Adjuvant Therapy

Although early stage breast cancer can be cured by surgical resection alone, some patients will still develop recurrent metastatic disease. Adjuvant therapy reduces the risk of distant recurrence and improves the overall survival rate. Adjuvant therapy has been shown to improve disease-free and overall survival in both premenopausal and postmenopausal patients up to age 70 with node-negative or node-positive disease. There are three adjuvant treatment modalities available: chemotherapy, hormonal therapy, and targeted biologic therapy such as trastuzumab. The decision about which adjuvant therapy to give has traditionally been based on clinical and pathological factors, such as tumor size, grade, presence of lymphatic vascular invasion, nodal involvement, and estrogen receptor (ER), progesterone receptor (PR), and human epidermal grown factor receptor (HER2) status.

Chemotherapy

Adjuvant chemotherapy is an important component in the treatment of early stage breast cancer, but it should be selectively given to those patients who will derive the greatest benefit. Patients are selected to receive chemotherapy based on their age, performance status, receptor status (ER, PR, HER2/neu), tumor size, tumor grade, tumor histology, and nodal involvement as well as genomic information as detailed above. Computer models, such as Adjuvant! Online (http://www.AdjuvantOnline.com) can provide accurate estimates of the benefit of chemotherapy, using patient and tumor related factors [14].

According to the guidelines from the National Cancer Comprehensive Network (NCCN), for hormone receptor-positive tumors, the decision regarding adjuvant chemotherapy should be based on the results of the 21-gene RT-PCR assay if the tumor is node negative or has micrometastatic disease in the node. Chemotherapy should be considered if the Recurrence Score (RS) is intermediate risk, and it is recommended if the RS is high risk. Chemotherapy should also be recommended if the tumor is node positive [6]. For HER2-positive tumors, chemotherapy with trastuzumab should be considered if the tumors are <0.5 cm with nodal micrometastasis or 0.6–1.0 cm with node negative or micrometastatic disease in the node. It should be recommended for all tumors that are greater than 1 cm, whether they are node negative, have micrometastatic nodal disease, or are positive nodes. For triple negative (ER, PR, and HER2 negative) tumors, chemotherapy should be considered for any tumors that have micrometastatic nodal disease or are ≥0.6 cm, regardless of nodal status.

Adjuvant Chemotherapy

The Early Breast Cancer Trialists' Collaborative Group (EBCTCG) has met every 5 years since the mid-1980s to perform a systematic review of all randomized clinical trials in early breast cancer. The 2000 meta-analysis summarized the results of randomized adjuvant trials started by 1995, and included 28,764 women in 60 trials looking at chemotherapy versus no chemotherapy and 14,470 women in 17 trials of anthracycline-containing chemotherapy versus CMF-type chemotherapy [15]. The review showed that the addition of any chemotherapy (single-agent or multiagent) reduced the risk of breast cancer recurrence by 22 % and mortality by 15 %, compared with no chemotherapy.

Prior to the widespread use of taxanes, the most commonly used adjuvant chemotherapy regimens were CMF (cyclophosphamide, methotrexate, and 5-fluorouracil) and anthracycline-based regimens. For CMF regimens, oral cyclophosphamide appears to be superior to using intravenous [16, 17]. The EBCTCG analysis demonstrated a significant 11 % reduction in the annual risk of disease recurrence and a 16 % reduction in the rate of death for anthracycline-based regimens compared to CMF [15] The regimen AC×4 (doxorubicin 60 mg/m^2, cyclophosphamide 600 mg/m^2, every 21 days) became a standard adjuvant regimen based on trials showing equivalency to CMF, with a shorter duration of treatment and less toxicity. The NSABP B-15 trial compared AC×4 to CMF×6 (cyclophosphamide 100 mg/m^2 oral daily days 1–14, methotrexate 40 mg/m^2 IV day 1 and 8, and 5-fluorouracil 600 mg/m^2 day 1 and 8, every 28 days) to AC followed in 6 months by 3 cycles of intravenous CMF in 2,194 women with node-positive breast cancer. The trial showed no differences in disease-free survival or overall survival between the groups [18]. Similarly, the NSABP B-23 trial showed no differences in disease-free survival or overall survival for AC×4 or CMF×6 (with tamoxifen given to ER-positive patients) for 2,008 women with node-negative breast cancer [19].

Adjuvant Taxane Chemotherapy

The two taxanes routinely used for the adjuvant treatment of breast cancer are paclitaxel and docetaxel. When added to anthracycline-based adjuvant regimens, taxanes have shown a survival benefit in some trials. They are included routinely in the adjuvant treatment of node-positive and high-risk, node-negative breast cancer. Reviewed here are some of the pivotal adjuvant taxane-containing trials.

The Cancer and Leukemia Group B (CALGB) 9344 trial was a phase III trial in which 3,121 women with node-positive, early stage breast cancer were randomized to AC using three different doxorubicin doses (60, 75 or 90 mg/m^2) plus cyclophosphamide 600 mg/m^2 for 4 cycles followed by randomization to paclitaxel 175 mg/m^2 every 3 weeks for 4 cycles versus no paclitaxel [20]. There was no additional benefit seen from higher doses of doxorubicin. The addition of paclitaxel improved the 5-year disease-free survival (70 % compared with 65 %) and overall survival (80 % compared with 77 %). In an unplanned subset analysis, the improvement in DFS from the addition of paclitaxel was significantly greater for patients with ER negative disease (HR 0.72, 95 % CI 0.59–0.86) compared to those with ER-positive disease (HR 0.91, 95 % CI 0.78–1.07), 94 % of whom had received tamoxifen. A second large trial, NSABP B-28, confirmed the benefit of paclitaxel in 3.060 women with node-positive, operable breast cancer. Patients were randomized to 4 cycles of AC or 4 cycles of AC followed by 4 cycles of paclitaxel (225 mg/m^2 IV every 3 weeks) [21]. The disease free survival was improved (RR 0.83, 95 % CI 0.72–0.95, $p=0.006$) with 5 year DFS 72 % vs. 76 % respectively. The improvement in OS was small and not statistically significant. The 5 year OS for both groups was 85 %. A subset analysis did not reveal any interaction between the effect of paclitaxel and the hormone receptor status or tamoxifen use. GEICAM 9906, a multicenter European trial, showed an advantage in 5 year DFS rates for 1,246 women with node-positive early stage breast cancer who received FEC (fluorouracil, epirubicin, cyclophosphamide) followed by weekly paclitaxel over those who received FEC alone: 78.5 % compared with 72.1 %, 95 % CI 1.6–11.2, $p=0.006$ [22]. There was a nonsignificant trend favoring overall survival for the paclitaxel group as well.

The CALGB 9741 trial tested the concept of dose-density, intensifying the therapy by shortening the interval between treatment cycles with the use of hematopoietic growth factors [23]. This trial had a 2×2 factorial design and compared sequential to concurrent administration of the chemotherapy as well as every 3 week to every 2 week dosing schedules. Patients ($N=2{,}005$) with node-positive breast cancer were randomized to one of four arms: sequential doxorubicin (60 mg/m^2×4) followed by paclitaxel (175 mg/m^2×4) followed by cyclophosphamide (600 mg/m^2×4) or concurrent AC (doxorubicin 60 mg/m^2, cyclophosphamide 600 mg/m^2×4) followed by paclitaxel (175 mg/m^2×4) administered every 21 days or every 14 days with filgrastim (dose-dense schedule). At a median follow-up of 36 months, there was no difference between sequential and concurrent therapy but there was an advantage to dose-dense administration, with an improvement in DFS (RR 0.74, $p=0.010$) and OS (RR 0.69, $p=0.013$). At a longer follow-up of 69 months, the benefits were less impressive (DFS HR 0.80, $p=0.01$ and OS HR 0.85, $p=0.04$) [24]. At this updated analysis, an unplanned subset analysis showed that the benefit was seen only in the ER-negative patients (DFS HR 0.76, $p=0.01$, OS HR 0.79, $p=0.04$) and not in the ER-positive patients (DFS HR 0.92, $p=$ns, OS HR 0.92, $p=$ns). It is unclear whether there is additional long-term toxicity with the dose-dense regimen. TheAML/MDS cases were similar in the two groups (five cases in the dose-dense arm, six cases in the standard arm, with an incidence approximately 0.5 % in both arms).

Also, trials have shown a benefit from the addition of docetaxel to anthracycline-based chemotherapy regimens. The Breast Cancer International Research Group (BCIRG) study 001 randomized 1,491 women with node-positive, early stage breast cancer to FAC (5-FU 500 mg/m^2, doxorubicin 50 mg/m^2, cyclosphosphamide 500 mg/m^2) or TAC (docetaxel 75 mg/m^2, doxorubicin 50 mg/m^2, cyclophosphamide 500 mg/m^2), with both regimens given every 3 weeks for 6 cycles [25]. At a median follow-up of 120 months, the TAC regimen showed an improvement in both DFS (HR 0.79, $p=0.004$) and OS (HR 0.74, $p=0.002$) [26]. Similar results were noted in the PACS 01 trial, which randomized 1,999 patients with node-positive breast cancer to IV FEC (fluorouracil 500 mg/m^2, epirubicin 100 mg/m^2, and cyclophosphamide 500 mg/m^2 on day 1 every 21 days)×6 vs. FEC×3 followed by docetaxel×3(100 mg/m^2 every 3 weeks) [27]. The addition of docetaxel improved both DFS (HR 0.82, 95 % CI 0.69–0.99, $p=0.034$) and OS (HR 0.73, 95 % CI 0.56–0.99).

The Eastern Cooperative Oncology Group (ECOG) E1199 trial compared paclitaxel and docetaxel at different schedules in the adjuvant setting. 4,950 women with node-positive or high-risk node-negative breast cancer received 4 cycles of AC (doxorubicin 60 mg/m^2, cyclosphosphamide 600 mg/m^2) every 3 weeks and were subsequently randomized to paclitaxel every 3 weeks×4 (175 mg/m^2), weekly paclitaxel×12 (80 mg/m^2), docetaxel every 3 weeks×4 (100 mg/m^2), or weekly docetaxel×12 (35 mg/m^2) [28]. When compared to the paclitaxel regimen of 175 mg/m^2 every 3 weeks, weekly paclitaxel showed an improved DFS (OR 1.27, $p=0.006$) and OS (OR 1.32, $p=0.01$), and was therefore considered to be the preferred regimen. Of note, this regimen of AC followed by weekly paclitaxel has not been compared to the dose-dense AC followed by paclitaxel regimen.

The NSABP B-30 trial randomized 5,351 women with node-positive breast cancer to one of three treatment groups: AC×4 followed by docetaxel×4, AT (doxorubicin, docetaxel)×4, or TAC (docetaxel, doxorubicin, cyclophosphamide)×4 [29]. At a median follow-up of 73 months, both DFS and OS were improved for the group treated with sequential AC followed by docetaxel. The 8 year OS was 83 % for the sequential arm compared with 79 % for AT (HR for death 0.83, $p=0.03$) and 79 % for TAC (HR for death 0.86, $p=0.09$). Eight year DFS was 74 % for AC followed by docetaxel, 69 % for AT (HR 0.80, $p=0.001$), and 69 % for TAC (HR 0.83, $p=0.01$). In contrast, the BCIRG 005 trial compared AC×4 followed by docetaxel×4 to TAC×6 and showed no significant differences in DFS or OS with a median follow-up of 65 months [30].

A meta-analysis was performed in 2008 to evaluate the benefit of the addition of taxanes to anthracycline-based regimens in early breast cancer [31]. The study included 22,903 patients from 13 randomized trials, and showed that the addition of a taxane improved both DFS (pooled HR 0.83, 95 % CI 0.79 to 0.87, $p<0.00001$) and OS (pooled HR 0.85, 95 % CI 0.79 to 0.91, $p<0.00001$). This translated into a 5-year absolute risk reduction of 5 % for DFS and 3 % for OS. To put this into perspective, anthracyclines became the gold standard for adjuvant regimens when the EBCTCG analysis showed an absolute 5 year risk reduction of approximately 3 % for both DFS and OS [15]. In the taxane meta-analysis, the risk reduction was not influenced by the type of taxane, ER expression, number of axillary metastases (1–3 nodes vs. 4 or more nodes), age/menopausal status, or administration schedule of the taxane.

One non-anthracycline based, taxane containing regimen has become a standard adjuvant chemotherapy option. It was tested in the US Oncology 9375 trial, which compared adjuvant AC (doxorubicin 60 mg/m^2, cyclophosphamide 600 mg/m^2) to TC (docetaxel 75 mg/m^2, cyclophosphamide 600 mg/m^2), each given every 3 weeks for 4 cycles [32]. This study included 1,016 women with stage I–III breast cancer; 52 % node-positive. With a median follow-up of 7 years, TC showed an improvement in DFS (81 % vs. 75 %, $p=0.033$, HR 0.74, 95 % CI 0.56–0.98) and OS (87 % vs. 82 %, $p=0.032$, HR 0.69, 95 % CI 0.50–0.97) [33]. The US Oncology group has partnered with the NSABP to conduct the three-arm NSABP B49 trial, currently open to accrual, in which node-positive and high-risk node-negative patients are randomized between 6 cycles of TAC, and 6 cycles of TC. The results of this study will help to better define the role of both TC and anthracyclines in adjuvant breast cancer treatment.

The results of the previous randomized trials have validated several active adjuvant chemotherapy regimens: dose dense AC × 4 followed by paclitaxel × 4 every 14 days with growth factor support [23], AC × 4 followed by 12 weekly doses of paclitaxel [28], FEC × 3 followed by docetaxel (100 mg/m^2 every 3 weeks) × 3 [27], TAC × 6 [25, 30, 34], and TC (docetaxel plus cyclophosphamide) [32, 33]. The NCCN has selected the following as preferred regimens: TAC, dose dense AC followed by paclitaxel given every 2 weeks, AC followed by weekly paclitaxel, TC or AC [6].

The two most common adjuvant regimens used in the United States are AC × 4 followed by a taxane (either paclitaxel or docetaxel for 4 cycles every 3 weeks or paclitaxel weekly for 12 treatments) or TAC × 6 [35]. The NSABP B-38 trial, has compared these regimens add reference: J Clin Oncol. 2012;30:abstr LBA1000. In this 3 arm trial, 4894 women with node-positive breast cancer were randomized to either TAC × 6 (given every 21 days), dose-dense AC × 4 followed by paclitaxel × 4 (given every 14 days), or dose-dense AC × 4 followed by paclitaxel and gemcitabine × 4 (given every 14 days). With a median follow up of 64 months, there was no significant difference in efficacy between the TAC and dose dense AC-paclitaxel arms, although the toxicity profiles differed. The addition of gemcitabine did not improve outcomes.

The Impact of Dose

Trials have looked at increasing the doses of chemotherapy drugs but no significant benefit has been seen. Both NSABP B-22 and B-25 compared AC and used increasing doses of cyclophosphamide, but both studies showed no differences in DFS or OS [34, 36]. Also, there was no difference in DFS or OS for increased doses of doxorubicin (60 mg/m^2, 75 mg/m^2 or 90 mg/m^2) in the CALGB 9344 trial [20]. High dose chemotherapy with hematopoietic reconstitution was extensively tested in the setting of adjuvant breast cancer. A meta-analysis of 15 trials showed a significant 13 % reduction in the risk of recurrence (HR 0.87, 95 % CI 0.81–0.93) but no significant reduction in the risk of death (HR 0.94, 95 % CI 0.87–1.02). Patients who received high dose chemotherapy had a lower survival rate after relapse [37]. Autologous stem cell transplantation following high dose chemotherapy is not considered a standard approach for the treatment of early stage breast cancer, even for those with high-risk disease, because of the toxicity and lack of survival benefit.

Dosing with Obesity

Overweight and obese women often receive chemotherapy doses based on their ideal body weight, rather than their actual body weight. These patients receive a relatively lower dose, which may result in the compromised outcomes reported in obese women [38–42]. Obese patient should receive chemotherapy doses based on their actual body weight [42].

Timing of Chemotherapy

Ideally, adjuvant chemotherapy should be started between 4 and 6 weeks after surgery, but it can be started until 12 weeks after. A retrospective analysis of 2,594 women receiving adjuvant chemotherapy for stage I and II breast cancer at the British Columbia Cancer Agency confirmed that chemotherapy was equally effective if given up to 12 weeks after definitive surgery [43]. However, the overall survival was compromised if the initiation of chemotherapy was delayed beyond 12 weeks.

HER2 Directed Therapy

Trastuzumab is a humanized monoclonal antibody that targets the human epidermal growth factor receptor 2 (HER2). HER2 is amplified and/or overexpressed in about 15–20 % of invasive breast cancers [44–46]. HER2-positive breast tumors are more aggressive and have a higher rate of recurrence than tumors that are not

HER2-positive [46, 47]. Trastuzumab provides significant clinical benefit as monotherapy and in combination with chemotherapy as either first- or second-line therapy, in patients with metastatic breast cancer [48–53].

These findings prompted trials evaluating trastuzumab in the adjuvant setting. Four large trials and several smaller trials evaluated adjuvant trastuzumab and demonstrated significant improvements in disease-free survival (36–52 % reduction in DFS events) and overall survival (33–37 % reduction in deaths), irrespective of tumor size, nodal status, hormone receptor status, or age. On the basis of these results, adjuvant trastuzumab-based chemotherapy regimens have become the standard of care for patients with HER2-positive early breast cancer. The current FDA approval for trastuzumab is as adjuvant treatment of HER2-overexpressing node positive or node negative (ER/PR negative or if ER and/or PR positive with one high risk feature, including tumor size >2 cm, age <35 or tumor grade 2 or 3) breast cancer. Trastuzumab is combined with one of three chemotherapy regimens: doxorubicin, cyclophosphamide and either paclitaxel or docetaxel, with docetaxel and carboplatin or as a single agent following multimodality anthracycline-based therapy.

The first trial to report results was a combined analysis of the data from the North Central Cancer Treatment Group (NCCTG) N9831 Intergroup trial and National Surgical Adjuvant Breast and Bowel Project (NSABP) B-31 trial in 2005 [54]. The NCCTG N9831 was a three arm trial, randomizing patients to 4 cycles of AC followed by 12 doses of weekly paclitaxel (arm A), the same chemotherapy followed by weekly trastuzumab for 52 weeks (arm B), or the same chemotherapy with weekly trastuzumab starting with the first dose of paclitaxel (arm C) followed by weekly trastuzumab to finish 52 weeks. The NSABP B-31 trial was a two arm trial randomizing patients to 4 cycles of AC followed by 4 cycles of paclitaxel every 3 weeks (arm 1) or the same chemotherapy with weekly trastuzumab starting with the first dose of paclitaxel and continuing for 52 weeks. In both trials, the trastuzumab was given as a loading dose of 4 mg/kg followed by 2 mg/kg weekly. In both trials, patients were treated with radiation therapy and endocrine therapy as appropriate. For the pooled analysis, arm A and arm 1 were combined as the control arm, and arm C and arm 2 were the treatment arm. Eligible patients had HER2- positive disease as defined as HER2 3+ on immunohistochemistry (IHC) or amplified by FISH by a central or reference laboratory. Initially both trials were for node positive women, but N9831 later allowed high risk node negative patients (tumor >2 cm and ER/PR positive or tumor >1 cm and ER/PR negative). This accounted for 14.5 % of the patients on N9831. The primary endpoint of both trials was disease-free survival (DFS). The combined analysis included 2,101 patients from B-31 and 1,944 from N9831. The initial results were reported after a median 2 year follow-up and showed a HR of 0.48 for DFS ($p<0.0001$) and HR 0.65 for overall survival (OS) ($p=0.015$). Initial results presented at the American Society of Clinical Oncology (ASCO) meeting in 2007 with a median 2.9 years of follow-up were consistent, with a HR of 0.49 for DFS ($p<0.0001$) and 0.63 for OS ($p=0.0004$) [55]. After the initial results, patients who were on the control arm were offered trastuzumab if they were still on chemotherapy or had completed it within the last 6 months. The most recent report of this data, after a median follow-up of 3.9 years, demonstrated a long-term continued benefit for the addition of trastuzumab to chemotherapy, with a HR of 0.52 for DFS ($p > 0.001$) and 0.61 for OS ($p < 0.001$) [56]. In all analyses, all subgroups appeared to benefit.

The Herceptin Adjuvant (HERA) Trial (Breast International Group [BIG] 01-01) initially reported results in 2005 [57]. This was an international open label phase 3 randomized trial. Patients were eligible if they had tumors that were HER2 overexpressed or amplified, which was confirmed centrally, node positive disease or node negative disease if the tumor size was greater than 1 cm. Patients had completed all surgical therapy, radiation therapy if appropriate and at least 4 cycles of adjuvant or neoadjuvant chemotherapy. The chemotherapy consisted of anthracycline-containing regimens in 94 %, and taxane-containing regimens in 26 %. Thirty-two percent of patients had negative nodes, and 11 % had unknown nodal status. They were randomized after the completion of their last treatment to one of three groups: observation alone, observation followed by trastuzumab for 2 years or trastuzumab for 1 year. Patients were only eligible for randomization if they had a left ventricular ejection fraction (LVEF) of ≥55 % on echocardiography or multiple gated acquisition scanning (MUGA) after the completion of chemotherapy. Trastuzumab was given with a loading dose of 8 mg/kg followed by 6 mg/kg every 3 weeks for the duration specified. The primary endpoint was disease-free survival (DFS). The first interim analysis was presented with a median follow-up of 1 year, and compared only the observation ($N = 1{,}693$) and 1 year arms ($N = 1{,}694$). This showed an unadjusted HR for an event of 0.54 ($p < 0.0001$) and an absolute benefit in DFS at 2 years of 8.4 %. There was no statistical difference in overall survival (29 deaths in the trastuzumab arm and 37 in the observation arm). In a subsequent report, with a median 2 year follow-up, the benefit in DFS persisted, with an unadjusted HR for the risk of an event of 0.64 ($p < 0.0001$) which translated into an absolute DFS benefit of 6.3 % at 3 years [58] There was also a benefit seen in OS, with an unadjusted HR for the risk of an event of 0.66 ($p = 0.0115$), resulting in an absolute OS benefit of 2.7 % at 3 years. More recently, results were published with a 4 year median follow-up [59]. In the intent-to-treat analysis of DFS, there continued to be a significant benefit favoring 1 year of trastuzumab, HR 0.76 ($p < 0.0001$). There was no significant difference in the intent-to-treat analysis of the risk of death, HR 0.85 ($p = 0.11$). This report also included analysis of the patients in the observation arm who were allowed to crossover after the first interim analysis. In the observation arm, 1,354 women were disease-free at 1 year and eligible, and of those, 52 % (885 patients) elected to do so at a median of 22.8 (range 4.5–52.7 months) after randomization. In this non-randomized comparison, the patients in the crossover arm had fewer DFS events than patients remaining in the observation arm, HR 0.68 ($p = 0.0077$). Of note, the intent-to-treat analysis is biased in favor of the observation group because patients in this arm included the crossover patients who received trastuzumab therapy.

A smaller trial, the Finland Herceptin (Fin-Her) trial, compared trastuzumab therapy for a shorter duration, albeit in a much smaller population of patients [60]. The original trial consisted of 1,010 women with node-positive or high-risk node-negative patients and randomized them to 3 cycles of docetaxel or vinorelbine. All women then received 3 cycles of fluorouracil, epirubicin, and cyclophosphamide (FEC). A subgroup of 232 women was found to have HER2-positive tumors, which was confirmed by FISH analysis at a reference laboratory. These women were randomized to receive or not to receive 9 weekly trastuzumab injections. The primary endpoint was recurrence-free survival. In the HER2-positive patients, the 3 year recurrence-free survival was improved for the patients receiving trastuzumab (HR 0.42, $p=0.01$). Final results of this trial were reported later, showing that the HR for distant recurrence or death was 0.65, $p=0.12$ [61]. There was a greater number of node-positive women among the patients assigned to the trastuzumab containing arm, when adjusted for the presence of nodal metastases, the HR for distant recurrence or death was 0.57, $p=0.047$.

The BCIRG 006 trial was the most recent of the large adjuvant trials to report results [62]. This was a unique trial as it was the only one to have a non-anthracycline containing regimen with trastuzumab. In this trial, 3,222 patients with HER2-positive, node-positive, or high-risk node-negative (29 % of patients) breast cancer were randomized to one of three regimens: adriamycin and cyclophosphamide followed by docetaxel (AC-T), the same regimen with trastuzumab started concurrently with the first dose of docetaxel (AC-T plus trastuzumab), or TCH (docetaxel, carboplatin, trastuzumab) in which the trastuzumab was started with the first dose of chemotherapy. Trastuzumab was given with a loading dose of 4 mg/kg followed by weekly doses of 2 mg/kg while concurrent with chemotherapy, then 6 mg/kg every 3 weeks to finish 1 year total of trastuzumab therapy. The primary endpoint was DFS. The median follow-up was 65 months. Both trastuzumab-containing regimens were superior to the control arm: HR for AC-T compared to AC-T plus trastuzumab was 0.64 for DFS ($p<0.001$) and 0.63 for OS ($p<0.001$), HR for AC-T compared to TCH was 0.75 for DFS ($p=0.04$) and 0.77 for OS ($p=0.04$). There were no significant differences seen in the rates of DFS or OS for the two trastuzumab-containing regimens, but the study had not been powered to detect this. Numerically, there were 29 more primary events in the TCH group compared with the AC-T plus trastuzumab (214 vs. 185). This difference in efficacy came at the cost of a highly significant increase in congestive heart failure (21 vs. 4) as well as a significantly increased risk of sustained, subclinical loss of left ventricular ejection fraction for those who received adriamycin. This study added further evidence supporting the role of adjuvant trastuzumab, and established a non-anthracycline containing regimen, TCH, as a standard of care.

One trial notably failed to demonstrate a significant improvement in DFS [63]. This was a large trial which randomized 3,010 operable, node-positive patients to an anthracycline-based chemotherapy regimen with or without docetaxel. In this trial, 528 patients had HER2-positive disease and were also randomized to 1 year of trastuzumab given every 3 weeks or observation. Trastuzumab was started after chemotherapy and radiation therapy were completed. The primary endpoint was DFS. At a median follow-up of 47 months, there was a 14 % nonsignificant reduction in the risk of relapse for women randomized to trastuzumab (HR 0.86, $p=0.41$). Possible reasons for a negative result included a small sample size or the fact that

10 % of randomized patients never received trastuzumab and 38 patients (of the 234 who received at least one dose of trastuzumab) received less than 6 months of trastuzumab. It is also possible that the concurrent administration of chemotherapy may be superior to sequential.

Sequential Versus Concurrent Trastuzumab

In the N9831 study, there was an improvement in DFS for concurrent trastuzumab compared to sequential trastuzumab, with a HR 0.77, $p = 0.02$. However, due to the low number of events, this did not cross the prespecified boundaries [56]. Although there is some controversy, with contradictory results from the PACS-04 study [63], the N9831 data support the DFS benefit seen in the HERA BIG 01-01 trial [59], but suggest that the outcome may be improved with a concurrent approach. The Adjuvant Lapatinib and/or Trastuzumab Treatment Optimisation (ALTTO) trial, which is currently accruing patients, will provide more information regarding this question.

Tumor Size

There is no established size criteria for treatment of HER2-positive tumors with chemotherapy and trastuzumab. The previously conducted adjuvant trials had very few patients with node negative tumors less than 1 cm in size. In this subgroup, there is limited data on the benefit of treatment with trastuzumab. Current NCCN guidelines do not recommend chemotherapy and trastuzumab for HER-2 positive, node negative tumors that are ≤0.5 cm [6]. Although there is limited data to confirm the benefit of treatment, recent reports have shown that HER2 amplification and overexpression is a powerful negative prognostic factor for small, node negative tumors [64, 65]. Both the NCCTG N9831 and BCIRG 006 trials showed the benefit of adding trastuzumab to chemotherapy in node-negative patients [54, 62]. Patients with small (<1 cm) node-negative disease should be informed about the risk of recurrence, as well as the availability, benefit and risks associated with treatment.

Based on these trials, the benefit of adjuvant trastuzumab has become routine clinical use. The significant improvements in both DFS (24–58 %) and OS (23–35 %) shown in these individual trials were confirmed in a meta-analysis, which demonstrated that patients with HER2-positive breast cancer derived benefit in disease-free survival, overall survival, locoregional recurrence, and distant recurrence (all $p < 0.001$) from the addition of trastuzumab to adjuvant chemotherapy [66]. Even small HER2-positive tumors seem to have a higher risk of recurrence than their HER2-negative counterparts.

Duration of Trastuzumab

The optimal duration of trastuzumab appears to be one year. A longer duration has been tested. The HERA trial reported that the 1 year and 2 year duration of trastuzumab arms were comparable in both DFS and OS, with a median follow up of 8 years [67]. A shorter duration appears not to be as beneficial. The French National Cancer Institute conducted the PHARE trial, in which 3382 patients with early stage, HER2-positive breast cancer were randomized to 6 months versus 12 months of trastuzumab. The results of this trial failed to show that 6 months of trastuzumab was not inferior to 12 months [68].

Side Effects of Chemotherapy

The most common side effects of the chemotherapy regimens used for breast cancer include alopecia, nausea and vomiting, fatigue, neutropenia and neutropenic fevers, anemia, thrombocytopenia, allergic/infusion reactions, and peripheral neuropathy. The most significant potential long-term toxicities include cardiotoxicity in patients treated with anthracyclines and the risk of secondary hematologic malignancies in patients treated with alkylating agents and anthracyclines. These risks need to be discussed with patients, but they should also be put into perspective in relation to the risk of breast cancer recurrence.

Cardiotoxicity is a well-recognized side effect of the anthracyclines. It is generally dose dependent, and is characterized by a symptomatic or asymptomatic decline in the left ventricular ejection fraction, which can result in congestive heart failure. The overall incidence of anthracycline-induced cardiotoxicity is between 1 and 5 %. Risk factors for anthracycline-induced cardiotoxicity include cumulative dose (increasing at doses >550 mg/m^2), hypertension, preexisting cardiac disease, age, prior mediastinal radiation, and female gender [69]. A retrospective cohort study of 21,106 patients diagnosed with breast cancer was performed using a commercial managed care claims database [70]. Within that group, 3,428 received anthracycline-containing chemotherapy, 7,125 received nonanthracycline-containing chemotherapy, and 10.553 did not receive chemotherapy. After adjusting for all baseline differences, the odds ratio of cardiac events compared to controls was 3.98 (95 % CI 3.27–4.85), and 1.31 (95 % CI 1.11–1.54) for anthracycline-containing chemotherapy versus nonanthracycline-containing chemotherapy cohorts. Anthracycline-induced cardiotoxicity can be potentiated by other drugs, particularly trastuzumab and possibly the taxanes.

Cytotoxic drugs, particularly alkylating agents, such as cyclophosphamide, and topoisomerase II inhibitors, such as doxorubicin, increase the risk of developing acute myeloid leukemia (AML) or myelodysplastic syndrome (MDS). In one analysis, six NSABP trials (B-15, B-16, B-18, B-22, B-23, and B-25) in which patients received doxorubicin and cyclosphosphamide were reviewed [71]. The incidence of treatment-related AML/MDS was found to be 0.5 % in all patients, but the relative risks were higher for patients undergoing more intense regimens compared with standard doses of AC. The risk also appears to be higher for older patients. A review of the Surveillance, Epidemiology and End Results (SEER)-Medicare database was conducted for women diagnosed with nonmetastatic breast cancer between 1992 and 2002 [72]. The primary endpoint was a claim with an inpatient or outpatient diagnosis of AML. Of the 64, 715 patients, 10,130 received chemotherapy and 54,585 did not. The median age was 75.6 years and the mean follow-up was 54.8 months. The absolute risk of AML at 10 years after adjuvant chemotherapy was 1.8 % vs. 1.2 % for those patients who did not receive chemotherapy. It is thought that the use of hematopoietic growth factors may increase the risk of AML/MDS as well, due to either the growth factor stimulation and/or the fact that patients are more likely to receive their chemotherapy at full dose, on time, and often with a shorter interval between cycles (dose dense). A retrospective cohort study of 5,510 women older than 65 years who received chemotherapy for stage I–III breast cancer from the SEER-Medicare database from January 1, 1991 through December 31, 1999 showed that 16 % of patients had received at least 1 cycle that included a growth factor [73]. The rate of AML/MDS was 1.16 % at least 18 months after diagnosis, 1.77 % for those treated with a growth factor versus 1.04 % for those without.

Chemotherapy-induced peripheral neuropathy is a common and serious problem, which is seen most commonly after the administration of taxane chemotherapy. Currently, there are no effective approaches for prevention or treatment. In the Eastern Cooperative Oncology Group E1199 trial, 4,950 women were treated with 4 cycles of AC and then randomized to paclitaxel every 3 weeks for 4 cycles, paclitaxel weekly for 12 cycles, docetaxel every 3 weeks for 4 cycles or docetaxel weekly for 12 cycles [74]. In a secondary analysis with a median follow-up of 95.5 months, 16–20 % of the patients developed grade 2–4 peripheral neuropathy, depending on which of the four taxane regimens they received. Peripheral neuropathy (grade 2–4, either sensory or motor) occurred in 27 % of women treated with weekly paclitaxel, in 20 % of women treated with paclitaxel every 3 weeks, and in 16 % of women treated with either docetaxel schedule.

Trastuzumab is associated with an increased incidence of asymptomatic decline in left ventricular ejection fraction (LVEF) and symptomatic congestive heart failure (CHF). The adjuvant trials had used different definitions of cardiac toxicity, and therefore, their rates of cardiac events differed slightly. The reported cardiac event rates are highest in the anthracycline-containing trastuzumab arms (1.9–3.8 %) and lowest in the TCH arm (0.4 %) [54, 57, 62]. Of note, 5.0–6.6 % of patients who completed their anthracycline-containing therapy in the NSABP B-31 and NCCTG N9831 trials were unable to receive any trastuzumab due to a drop in LVEF [54]. In a systematic and independent assessment of cardiac safety data from the NSABP B-31 and NCCTG N9831 trials, patients who received trastuzumab had a 2.0 % incidence of symptomatic heart failure events (requiring evidence of cardiac dysfunction with subjective symptoms, objective signs, and a decline in LVEF of >10 % or to an absolute LVEF <50 %) compared with 0.45 % for patients treated with chemotherapy alone at a median follow-up of 2 and 1.9 years respectively [75]. Complete or partial recovery was observed in 86.1 % of trastuzumab-treated patients. Independent predictors for cardiac events included age greater than 50 years and low ejection fraction at the start of paclitaxel chemotherapy and trastuzumab treatment. A review of data from the HERA trial, with a median 3.6 year follow-up, also reported a higher incidence of severe CHF for trastuzumab treated patients versus the observation group, 0.8 % vs. 0.0 % and confirmed significant LVEF decline in 3.6 % vs. 0.6 %, respectively [76]. Again, trastuzumab-associated cardiac dysfunction appeared to have a higher rate of reversibility than cardiac dysfunction due to an anthracycline. In the BCIRG 006 trial, the rates of CHF and cardiac dysfunction were significantly higher in the anthracycline-trastuzumab arm than in the TCH group ($p<0.001$) [62]. The rates of CHF were 2.0 % for AC-T plus trastuzumab, 0.7 % for AC-T and 0.4 % for TCH. There were also higher rates of sustained, subclinical loss of LVEF between the AC-T plus trastuzumab and TCH arms.

Cardiac monitoring is recommended for all patients receiving adjuvant trastuzumab. Recommendations in the prescribing information include a thorough cardiac assessment, including a history, physical examination and measurement of LVEF by echocardiogram or MUGA scan [77]. LVEF measurements are recommended at baseline, every 3 months during trastuzumab treatment, at the completion of treatment and every 6 months for at least 2 years after treatment. Treatment should be withheld if there is an ≥16 % absolute decrease in LVEF from pretreatment levels or an LVEF that is below the institutional limits of normal and ≥10 % from pretreatment values. Repeat measurements should be taken at 4 week intervals if trastuzumab is withheld. Treatment may be resumed within 4–8 weeks if the LVEF returns to normal and the absolute decrease from baseline is ≤15 %. Treatment should be permanently discontinued if there is a persistent decrease in LVEF (defined as lasting 8 weeks or longer).

Neoadjuvant Chemotherapy

Neoadjuvant chemotherapy, also called primary or preoperative chemotherapy, is chemotherapy given prior to definitive surgery. Chemotherapy regimens that are effective in the adjuvant setting are used in the neoadjuvant setting. The primary clinical goals are to downstage large tumors and improve surgical resectability. Neoadjuvant chemotherapy is often used in women with locally advanced disease which is initially inoperable or in women for whom a mastectomy is indicated in an attempt to make them candidates for breast conservation. It had originally been thought that the earlier initiation of systemic therapy in patients at risk for distant recurrence might improve survival, but this was not borne out in randomized clinical trials.

Several trials have compared neoadjuvant chemotherapy to standard adjuvant chemotherapy. A meta-analysis of 9 randomized trials including 3,946 patients demonstrated no statistically or clinically significant differences in death (relative risk [RR] 1.00, 95 % CI 0.90–1.12), disease progression (RR 0.99, 95 % CI 0.91–1.07) or distant disease recurrence (RR 0.94, 95 % CI 0.83–1.06) [78]. Neoadjuvant therapy was statistically significantly associated with an increased risk of locoregional disease recurrences (RR = 1.22, 95 % CI = 1.04–1.43), compared with adjuvant therapy, especially in trials where more patients in the neoadjuvant, than the adjuvant, arm received radiation therapy without surgery (RR = 1.53, 95 % CI = 1.11–2.10).

The significant neoadjuvant trials include the NSABP B-18 trial, in which 1,523 patients with clinical T1–3, N0–1 breast cancer were randomized to receive AC (doxorubicin 60 m/m^2, cyclophosphamide 600 mg/m^2) × 4 every 3 weeks as either adjuvant or neoadjuvant chemotherapy [79]. With a 9 year follow-up, there was no significant difference in overall survival (OS) (70 % in the postoperative group, 69 % in the preoperative group, $p = 0.80$) or disease-free survival (DFS) (53 % in the postoperative group, 55 % in the preoperative group, $p = 0.50$). With 16 years of follow-up, there continued to be no differences in OS or DFS [80]. However, the rate of breast conservation surgery was higher in the neoadjuvant group (68 % vs. 60 %).

The European Organization for Research and Treatment of Cancer (EORTC) 10902 trial randomized 698 patients with T1c-T4b, N0-N1 breast cancer to preoperative or postoperative FEC (fluorouracil 600 mg/m^2, epirubicin 60 mg/m^2, cyclophosphamide 600 mg/m^2) × 4 cycles [81]. At a median follow-up of 56 months, there was no difference between the groups in overall survival (hazard ratio HR = 1.16, $p = 0.38$), progression-free survival (HR 1.15, $p = 0.27$), or time to locoregional recurrence (HR 1.13, $p = 0.61$).

The NSABP B-27 trial randomized 2,411 patients with T1c-3N0 or T1-3N1 breast cancer to one of three treatments: neoadjuvant AC × 4, neoadjuvant AC × 4 followed by docetaxel × 4, or neoadjuvant AC × 4 followed by surgery followed by docetaxel × 4 after surgery [80, 82]. Neoadjuvant docetaxel improved the pathologic complete response rate (pCR) (26 % vs. 13 %, $p < 0.0001$) compared with neoadjuvant AC alone, but with a median 8 year follow-up, there was no difference in OS or DFS between any of the three groups. The achievement of pCR was associated with a significantly improved DFS (HR = 0.49) and OS (HR = 0.36).

In a patient who has pathologic residual disease after neoadjuvant chemotherapy, additional adjuvant chemotherapy is not recommended [6]. Patients should be treated with endocrine therapy and anti-HER2-neu directed therapy as appropriate based on their tumor characteristics.

Determining the response to neoadjuvant therapy can be done both clinically and pathologically. The clinical response is assessed by measuring the tumor during treatment. A clinical complete response (cCR) is defined as no palpable disease in the breast and regional lymph nodes. Imaging, including mammography, ultrasound, and MRI, may be useful as well. Pathologic response is assessed by evaluation of the surgical specimen. A pathologic complete response rate (pCR) is achieved when no residual invasive tumor is detected in the pathological specimen. In studies, however, the definitions of pCR vary, and some definitions allow noninvasive tumor in the breast and/or invasive or noninvasive tumor in the lymph nodes.

For example, the NSABP guidelines define pCR as either no invasive cancer in the breast or only noninvasive in situ cancer in the breast; the status of the lymph nodes are not included in this definition [79, 80, 82].

There is a correlation between the clinical and pathological response to neoadjuvant chemotherapy and clinical outcomes. A pathologic complete response in the breast and axilla appears to be the best predictor of long-term survival. In the NSABP B-18 trial, 9-year follow-up confirmed that patients who achieved a pCR had significantly superior disease-free and overall survival compared to those who had a cCR with residual invasive cancer on pathologic examination or to those patients who did not achieve a cCR [79, 80]. Clinical and pathological tumor response are highly prognostic even after controlling for LN status, tumor size, and patient age. Residual disease in the lymph nodes seems to indicate a worse prognosis than residual disease in breast [83]. Other factors shown to predict outcome are LN status, size of residual tumor, multifocal residual disease, LVI, and tumor cell proliferation as measured by Ki67 [84, 85].

Neoadjuvant HER2 Therapy

For patients with HER2-positive tumors, the addition of trastuzumab in the neoadjuvant setting has improved both pCR rates and event-free survival. In the Neoadjuvant Herceptin (NOAH) Trial, 228 patients with HER2-positive, locally advanced or inflammatory breast cancer were treated with neoadjuvant anthracycline-based chemotherapy and were randomized to receive trastuzumab concurrently with the neoadjuvant chemotherapy followed by adjuvant trastuzumab for a total of a year or no trastuzumab [86]. The addition of trastuzumab improved the pCR rate (43 % with trastuzumab versus 22 % without trastuzumab, $p=0.0007$) and 3 year EFS (71 % vs. 56 %, HR 0.59, $p=0.013$) but there was no difference in overall survival (87 % vs. 79 % $p=0.114$). No trials have compared neoadjuvant to adjuvant trastuzumab administration. However, based on the survival benefit seen with trastuzumab in the adjuvant setting and the increased pCR rates seen in the neoadjuvant setting, combining trastuzumab with neoadjuvant chemotherapy is recommended.

The data from three phase III trials with a total of 1,765 patients were combined for an analysis of cardiac toxicity [86–89]. The results showed that the frequency of cardiotoxicity increased when anthracycline-based chemotherapy and trastuzumab were administered concurrently (odds ratio 1.95, 95 % CI 1.16–3.29).

Dual anti-HER2 therapy with two agents may be more effective than single-agent trastuzumab. Lapatinib is an oral small molecule dual tyrosine kinase inhibitor of epidermal growth factor receptor (EGFR) and HER2. Preliminary results of the Neo-adjuvant Lapatinib and/or Trastuzumab Treatment Optimization Trial (Neo-ALLTO, BIG 01–06, EGF 106903) showed higher pCR rates with the combination of lapatinib, trastuzumab, and paclitaxel compared to either trastuzumab or lapatinib alone with paclitaxel [90]. Another study combined trastuzumab with pertuzumab, a monoclonal antibody that targets HER2 dimerization. The results of the Neoadjuvant Study of Pertuzumab and Herceptin in an Early Regimen Evaluation (NeoSphere) phase II trial showed that the combination of trastuzumab, pertuzumab, and docetaxel resulted in significantly higher pCR rates than either agent alone with docetaxel or the combination of trastuzumab and pertuzumab without docetaxel Interestingly, there was a pCR rate of 17 % for patients who received only the two antibodies, with no chemotherapy [91].

Inflammatory Breast Cancer

Inflammatory breast cancer is a rare and aggressive form of breast cancer. The classical clinical findings are diffuse erythema of the skin and edema (peau d'orange) involving at least one-third of the breast. The skin changes are due to tumor emboli within the dermal lymphatics; however, the finding of dermal lymphatic invasion is not necessary or sufficient on its own for the diagnosis, in the absence of the classical clinical findings. Inflammatory breast cancer requires a multimodality treatment approach that includes neoadjuvant chemotherapy followed by a mastectomy, and post-mastectomy radiation therapy, with anti-HER2 and/or endocrine therapy as indicated. There is no single recommended chemotherapy regimen for inflammatory breast cancer; the most commonly used chemotherapy regimens include an anthracycline and taxane combination.

Endocrine Therapy

Some of the earliest observations on the endocrine-responsiveness of breast cancer came from Dr. George Beatson who described the regression of advanced breast cancer following oophorectomy in 1896 [92]. Hormonal manipulation remains the most effective treatment for tumors that express hormone receptors (ER-estrogen receptor and PR-progesterone receptor). Since the development of tamoxifen in the 1970s, ovarian ablation has been largely replaced by pharmacologic manipulation. The hormonal therapy of breast cancer was the first form of targeted therapy ever used in the treatment of a malignancy [93].

The American Society of Clinical Oncology and the College of American Pathologists have recently published guidelines for the evaluation of hormone receptors and the use of hormonal therapy [94]. They recommend that ER and PR assays be considered positive if at least 1 % of the nuclei in the tumor cells test positive in the presence of expected reactivity of internal and external controls. Women with early stage breast cancer should be offered adjuvant hormonal therapy if they have hormone receptor-positive tumors. The absence of benefit from adjuvant endocrine therapy for women with ER-negative invasive breast cancers has been confirmed in large overviews of randomized clinical trials. In the adjuvant setting, endocrine therapy is initiated after the completion of chemotherapy and radiation therapy, if indicated.

Tamoxifen

Tamoxifen is a selective estrogen receptor modulator (SERM), and it has both partial antagonist and partial agonist activities. The antagonistic activity inhibits the growth of breast cancer cells by competitive antagonism of estrogen at the estrogen receptor (ER). The partial agonist activity can be beneficial (prevent bone demineralization in postmenopausal women) as well as harmful (increased risk of venous thromboembolic disease and uterine cancer).

Tamoxifen has been the gold standard for breast cancer therapy for over 30 years. The most recent meta-analysis from the Early Breast Cancer Trialists Collaborative Group (EBCTCG) included updated data from each trial of tamoxifen versus no adjuvant tamoxifen of approximately 5 year duration [95]. For patients with ER positive disease, tamoxifen reduced the recurrence rate by 39 % and reduced breast cancer mortality by 35 %. The reductions in the risk of recurrence were independent of patient age, nodal status, tumor grade, tumor diameter, chemotherapy use and chemotherapy timing. Tamoxifen also reduced the risks of local recurrence, contralateral breast cancer and distant recurrence (all $p<0.00001$).

The recommended dose of tamoxifen is 20 mg daily, starting after the completion of chemotherapy and radiation therapy, for a total of 5 years in women who have hormone receptor positive tumors. Common side effects of tamoxifen include hot flashes, headaches and changes in menstrual cycles in premenopausal women. More serious side effects include an increased risk of thromboembolic events and endometrial cancer. In a breast cancer prevention trial in which 13,388 women were randomized to placebo or tamoxifen for 5 years, the average annual rates of these events were 1.34 per 1,000 women for deep venous thrombosis, 0.69 per 1,000 women for pulmonary embolism, 1.03 per 1,000 women for stroke and 13.0 per 1,000 women for endometrial cancer [96]. Tamoxifen may cause a decrease in bone mineral density in premenopausal women, but is beneficial in increasing bone mineral density in postmenopausal women.

Duration of Tamoxifen

Data from the Oxford meta-analysis suggests that more than half of all breast cancer recurrences and deaths occur after 5 years of adjuvant tamoxifen; however, older studies evaluating a longer duration of tamoxifen have not shown a benefit to the continuation of tamoxifen beyond 5 years [97]. In the NSABP B-14 trial, 1,172 women with ER-positive, lymph node negative disease who remained disease-free after 5 years of tamoxifen were then randomized to either placebo or an additional 5 years of tamoxifen [97]. With a follow-up of 7 years after randomization, there was a slight advantage noted for disease-free survival (82 % vs. 78 %, $p=0.03$), recurrence-free survival (94 % vs. 92 %, $p=0.13$) and overall survival (94 % vs. 91 %, $p=0.07$) for the women who discontinued tamoxifen. The Scottish trial also showed no advantage to tamoxifen continuation beyond 5 years with a nonsignificant trend towards a worse outcome [98]. Different results were seen in two more recent trials. In the Adjuvant Tamoxifen: Longer Against Shorter (ATLAS) trial, 6846 ER positive women who had completed 5 years of tamoxifen were randomized to continue to year 10 or to stop. 10 years of tamoxifen produced further reductions in breast cancer recurrence (617 versus 711 recurrences, $p=0.002$) and breast cancer mortality (331 versus 397 deaths, $p=0.01$) as well as overall mortality (639 versus 722 deaths, $p=0.01$) [99]. A second trial, adjuvant tamoxifen treatment offers more? (aTTom), also randomized nearly 7000 women with ER-positive or unknown breast cancer, who had completed 5 years of tamoxifen, to continue to 10 years or stop. They found that the longer treatment duration group had fewer breast cancer recurrences (28 versus 32 %, $p=.003$) and reduced breast cancer mortality (392 versus 443 deaths, $p=0.06$) [100].

Aromatase Inhibitors

Although adjuvant tamoxifen is an option in postmenopausal women, aromatase inhibitors (AIs) are preferred as they have been shown to result in a greater reduction in the risk of recurrence than tamoxifen in several landmark trials. The American Society of Clinical Oncology (ASCO) recommends that postmenopausal women with hormone-receptor positive breast cancer receive an AI at some point during their adjuvant treatment. AIs can be given upfront, after 2–3 years or after 5 years of tamoxifen [101]. The optimal timing and duration of treatment with AIs has not yet been definitively established.

Aromatase is the enzyme responsible for synthesizing estrogen from androgenic substrates [102]. Aromatase inhibitors act by inhibiting this enzyme. AIs lack any partial agonist activity, and therefore are not associated with increased risks of uterine cancer or thromboembolic events. Currently, there are three aromatase inhibitors, anastrozole and letrozole, which are nonsteroidal, and exemestane, which is steroidal.

AIs as Initial Therapy

The Arimidex, Tamoxifen, Alone or in Combination (ATAC) trial was the first to show a benefit for an aromatase inhibitor, anastrozole, over tamoxifen [103–106]. This was a double-blind, randomized trial in which 9,366 postmenopausal women were randomized to anastrozole alone (1 mg), tamoxifen alone (20 mg) or the combination of both as adjuvant therapy for 5 years. After an initial analysis, the combination arm was closed due to low efficacy. The most recent published results, with a median follow-up of 120 months, showed a significantly longer disease-free survival (DFS) with anastrozole than with tamoxifen (HR 0.91, 95 % CI 0.83–0.99,

$p=0.04$). Anastrozole was also associated with a prolonged time to recurrence (HR 0.84, 95 % CI 0.75–0.93, $p=0.001$), time to distant recurrence (HR 0.87, 95 % CI 0.77–0.99, $p=0.03$) and decreased contralateral breast cancers (HR 0.68, 95 % CI 0.50–0.91, $p=0.01$). However, there was no significant difference in overall survival (HR 0.95, 95 % CI 0.84–1.06, $p=0.4$).

The Breast International Group (BIG) 1–98 trial also showed a benefit for an aromatase inhibitor, letrozole compared to tamoxifen [107]. This was a randomized, phase III, double-blind 4 arm trial in which postmenopausal women with ER and/or PR positive breast cancer were randomized to 5 years of hormonal therapy: tamoxifen, letrozole, tamoxifen for 2 years followed by letrozole for 3 years or letrozole for 2 years followed by tamoxifen for 3 years. The primary endpoint was disease-free survival (DFS). Of the 8,028 women on the trial, 4,922 were randomized to either monotherapy arm. With a median of 51 month follow-up, there was an advantage in DFS for letrozole over tamoxifen (HR 0.82, 95 % CI 0.71–0.95, $p=0.007$) [108]. When the initial results were announced, women randomized to tamoxifen monotherapy were allowed to crossover to letrozole. In an analysis with a median of 76 months follow-up in the monotherapy arm, the DFS benefit was confirmed, but there was no significant difference in overall survival between the two monotherapy arms [109]. This lack of survival benefit may have been due to treatment crossover, which occurred in 25 % of women. When this bias was adjusted for, letrozole reduced the risk of death (HR 0.82, 95 % CI 0.70–0.95) [110]. There was no significant difference in DFS with either sequential treatment arm as compared with letrozole monotherapy [109].

Sequential Adjuvant Hormonal Therapy

MA.17 was a phase III, randomized, double-blind, placebo-controlled trial in which 5,187 postmenopausal women who had completed 5 years of adjuvant tamoxifen were randomized to 5 years of therapy with letrozole versus placebo [111]. Of these women, 46 % were node-positive and 98 % were ER-positive. The primary endpoint of the trial was disease-free survival (DFS). In the updated final analysis, at a median of 2.5 years, there was a significant improvement in DFS for the women who were randomized to letrozole (HR 0.58, 95 % CI 0.45–0.76, $p>0.001$) [112]. Distant DFS was also improved (HR 0.60, 95 % CI 0.43–0.84, $p=0.002$). For the entire group, there was no difference in overall survival (OS) (HR 0.92, 95 % CI 0.57–1.19, $p=0.3$), but there was an improvement in OS for patients with positive lymph nodes (HR 0.61, 95 % CI 0.38–0.98, $p=0.04$). Because the initial interim analysis showed an improvement in DFS for the letrozole arm, the study was terminated early. At the time of unblinding, patients in the placebo arm were offered letrozole, at a median of 2.8 years from the completion of tamoxifen [113]. Of the 2,594 patients in the placebo arm, 66 % (1,579 patients) chose to start letrozole; as a group, these women were younger, had a better performance status, and were more likely to have positive nodes, axillary dissection, and adjuvant chemotherapy.

When compared to the women in the placebo arm who chose no further therapy, these women had an improvement in DFS (HR 0.37, 95 % CI 0.23–0.61, $p<0.0001$), and distant DFS (HR 0.39, 95 % CI 0.20–0.74, $p=0.004$).

Switching Adjuvant Hormonal Therapy

Some trials have employed a strategy of switching to an AI after 2–3 years of tamoxifen compared to tamoxifen alone, for a total of 5 years of therapy. The International Exemestane Study (IES) randomized 4,724 postmenopausal women with ER-positive or ER-unknown tumors, who were disease-free after 2–3 years on tamoxifen, to exemestane (25 mg daily) or tamoxifen (20 mg) daily to finish 5 years of therapy [114]. With a median follow-up of 55.7 months, there was an improvement in the primary endpoint of disease-free survival (DFS) for the women who switched to exemestane (HR 0.76, 95 % CI 0.66–0.88, $p=0.001$). The overall survival (OS) was not significantly improved for the entire group (HR 0.85, 95 % CI 0.71–1.02, $p=0.08$), but there was a significant improvement when the 122 patients who were subsequently found to have ER-negative tumors were excluded (HR 0.83, 95 % CI 0.69–1.00, $p=0.05$).

A meta-analysis was performed of 3 trials that used the strategy of switching to anastrozole, the Austrian Breast and Colorectal Cancer Study Group 8 (ABCSG 8), Arimidex-Nolvadex (ARNO 95) and Italian Tamoxifen Anastrozole (ITA) [115]. All three studies showed similar results, with a benefit in switching to an AI. These trials enrolled a total of 2009 postmenopausal women with hormone-sensitive, early-stage breast cancer. Patients who were relapse-free after 2–3 years of tamoxifen were randomized to either anastrozole (1 mg daily) or tamoxifen (20 mg daily) to complete 5 years of therapy. An advantage was seen in DFS (HR 0.59, 95 % CI 0.48–0.74, $p<0.0001$) and overall survival (HR 0.71, 95 % CI 0.52–0.98, $p=0.04$).

Trials have also compared treatment with an AI for 5 years to tamoxifen for 2–3 years followed by an AI to complete 5 years. The Tamoxifen Exemestane Adjuvant Multinational (TEAM) phase 3 trial randomized 9,229 postmenopausal women to exemestane or tamoxifen followed by exemestane, with the primary end point of DFS [116]. At 5 years, there was no difference in DFS (HR 0.97, 95 % CI 0.88–1.08; $p=0.60$). The main differences were in toxicity.

Tamoxifen versus Aromatase Inhibitors

The Early Breast Cancer Trialists' Collaborative Group conducted a meta-analyses of randomized trials of aromatase inhibitors (AIs) compared with tamoxifen either as initial monotherapy or after 2–3 years of tamoxifen [117]. There were 9,856 patients in whom AIs were compared to tamoxifen monotherapy. With a mean of 5.8 years of follow-up, the rate of disease recurrence was 9.6 % for AI versus 12.6 % for tamoxifen ($2p<0.00001$) with an absolute 2.9 % improvement. For mortality, there was a nonsignificant decrease, 4.8 % for AI versus 5.9 % for tamoxifen ($2p<0.01$) with a nonsignificant absolute 1.1 % improvement. There were 9,015 patients analyzed in switching trials. With a mean of 3.9 years of follow-up, AIs resulted in a lower rate of disease recurrence, 5.0 % for AI versus 8.1 % for tamoxifen ($p<0.00001$) with an absolute improvement of 3.1 %. There was also an improvement in mortality, 1.7 % for AI versus 2.4 % for tamoxifen ($2p<0.02$) with an absolute decrease of 0.7 %. There was no difference in benefit for patients based on age, nodal status, tumor grade or PR status.

Another independent meta-analysis of studies comparing AIs to tamoxifen examined nine randomized controlled trials, including 28,632 women, and looked at three treatment strategies: monotherapy, sequential therapy (switching) and extended therapy (after tamoxifen) [118]. Disease free survival was significantly improved for monotherapy (HR 0.89, 95 % CI 0.83–0.96, $p=0.002$) and sequential therapy (HR 0.72, 95 % CI 0.63–0.83, $p<0.00001$). There was no difference in overall survival for monotherapy (HR 0.94,95 % CI 0.82–1.08, $p=0.39$) or extended therapy (HR 0.86, 0.79–1.16, $p=0.67$) but overall survival was prolonged for patients who switched from tamoxifen to AI therapy (HR 0.78, 95 % CI 0.68–0.91, $p=0.001$).

Comparison of Different AIs

The different AIs appear to have equivalent efficacy. The MA27 trial compared anastrozole (1 mg daily) versus exemestane (25 mg daily) as initial adjuvant therapy for 5 years in 7,576 postmenopausal women with hormone receptor-positive primary breast cancer, and showed no differences in event-free survival (EFS), distant disease-free survival, disease-specific survival or overall survival [119]. The hazard ratio for EFS was 1.02, $p=0.85$, and was similar regardless of nodal status. The adjuvant Femara versus Anastrozole Clinical Evaluation (FACE) trial is ongoing. This is an open-label randomized phase III trial which will accrue 4,000 patients and compare upfront letrozole (femara) with anastrozole for up to 5 years in postmenopausal women with hormone receptor-positive, node-positive breast cancer. The primary endpoint will be DFS.

Side Effects of Aromatase Inhibitors

The most common side effects seen with the AIs are myalgias and arthralgias. In the ATAC trial, 27.8 % of women taking anastrozole reported musculoskeletal disorders compared with 21.3 % taking tamoxifen [105]. In the BIG 1–98 trial, 20.3 % of patients on letrozole versus 12.3 % on tamoxifen reported arthralgias of any grade [107]. In these large adjuvant trials, nearly 5 % of patients in the AI group discontinued therapy because of side effects. A recent study analyzing medical and pharmacy claims data from three national longitudinal databases found that adherence to adjuvant anastrozole therapy decreased from between 69 % and 78 % in year 1 to 50 % to 68 % in year 3 [120, 121]. The incidence of musculoskeletal problems may actually be higher than the rates reported in the large trials. In a survey of 200 postmenopausal women receiving AIs for early stage breast cancer, 47 % reported joint pain and 44 % reported joint stiffness [122]. The success of AI treatment depends on adherence to the regimen. Switching to another AI may be an alternative for women who are unable to tolerate the musculoskeletal side effects since patients may tolerate one AI better than another. Compared to tamoxifen, AIs have a lower incidence of venous thromboembolism and endometrial cancer, but an increased risk of bone fractures and cardiovascular disease. This was demonstrated in a meta-analysis of 7 trials that included 30,023 patients [123]. There was a decreased incidence of venous thromboembolism compared with tamoxifen (OR = 0.55, 95 % CI 0.46–0.64, $p < 0.001$); in absolute numbers, the incidence was 1.6 % for AIs and 2.8 % for tamoxifen, with an absolute difference of 1.3 %. Similarly, the risk of endometrial cancer was reduced for patients taking AIs (OR 0.34, 95 % CI 0.22–0.53, $p < 0.001$) with a frequency of 0.1 % for AIs and 0.5 % for tamoxifen. The risk of cardiovascular disease was increased in patients taking AIs (OR = 1.30, 95 % CI 1.06–1.61, $p = 0.01$) with an absolute risk of 4.2 % on AIs versus 3.4 % on tamoxifen. It is known that AIs accelerate bone loss in postmenopausal women. The risk of bone fractures were increased with AIs (OR = 1.47, 95 % CI 1.34–1.61, $p < 0.001$) with an absolute risk of 7.5 % for AIs and 5.2 % for tamoxifen. There was no difference in the incidence of cerebrovascular disease in patients receiving AIs or tamoxifen.

Premenopausal Women

Tamoxifen is the most commonly used endocrine therapy in premenopausal women with early stage breast cancer. The NCCN guidelines recommend tamoxifen with or without ovarian suppression/ablation in these patients [6]. Tamoxifen can be given for 5 years, followed by an AI, if the woman is postmenopausal at the end of 5 years. It can also be given for 2–3 years, followed by an AI to complete treatment for a total duration of 5 years or longer, if the woman is postmenopausal after 2–3 years of tamoxifen therapy.

As monotherapy, it is recommended that tamoxifen be given at a dose of 20 mg daily for 5 years.

Ovarian Suppression and Ablation

Ovarian suppression/ablation (OS/OA) can be used in the adjuvant treatment of premenopausal breast cancer. OA can be accomplished via surgery (oophorectomy) or radiation and OS can be achieved via medications (luteinizing hormone-releasing hormone (LHRH) agonists). The EBCTCG meta-analysis included nearly 8,000 women younger than 50 years of age with ER-positive or ER-unknown disease. For women who received ovarian suppression/ablation, there was a significant decrease in both the 15-year probability of breast cancer recurrence and mortality compared to those who received no ovarian treatment [15]. Another meta-analysis used LHRH-agonists alone and found that they reduced the risk of breast cancer recurrence by 28 %, but this result was not statistically significant [124]. Both of these meta-analyses suggest that ovarian suppression/ablation has a similar efficacy to chemotherapy, but the chemotherapy regimens used in these studies were often CMF, and not the current anthracycline and taxane based regimens [15, 124].

Chemotherapy combined with ovarian suppression/ablation has not been shown to be superior to chemotherapy alone [103]. In INT 0101 (E5188), 1,503 premenopausal women with lymph node-positive, hormone receptor-positive breast cancer were randomized to 6 cycles of CAF (cyclophosphamide, doxorubicin, fluorouracil) alone, CAF followed by monthly goserelin for 5 years or CAF followed by monthly goserelin plus daily tamoxifen for 5 years. With a median follow-up of 9.6 years, there was no advantage for the addition of goserelin to CAF chemotherapy. An unplanned, retrospective subset analysis suggested that the addition of tamoxifen resulted in a possible benefit in time to recurrence and disease-free survival, but not overall survival. Other trials have also confirmed that the addition of OS/OA to chemotherapy provided no additional benefit compared to chemotherapy alone [125–127].

One way that adjuvant chemotherapy may benefit premenopausal women is through the induction of early menopause. An unplanned, retrospective subset analysis of INT 0101 [128] suggested a possible benefit from ovarian suppression in patients under age 40, while patients over the age of 40 were likely to undergo menopause due to the chemotherapy alone. This benefit was also seen in two other trials [126, 127]. This potential benefit of OS/OA is currently being tested in the Suppression of Ovarian Function (SOFT) trial which compares tamoxifen to ovarian suppression plus tamoxifen to ovarian suppression plus exemestane in premenopausal women.

The data from studies combining OS/OA with tamoxifen are still emerging, and the results are unclear. Individual trials have failed to show any benefit for the addition of OS/OA to tamoxifen when compared to each agent individually [129–131]. A meta-analysis of 11,906 premenopausal, hormone receptor-positive women showed that the addition of LHRH-agonists to tamoxifen, chemotherapy or both reduced recurrence by 12.7 % ($p=0.02$) and death after recurrence by 15.1 % ($p=0.08$) but no trials has addressed an LHRH agonist versus chemotherapy with tamoxifen in both arms [124].

At least 2 large trials comparing OS/OA plus tamoxifen to chemotherapy have suggested that they are equivalent in efficacy in premenopausal women. One trial randomized 333 premenopausal women to either LHRH agonist (triptorelin 3.75 mg IM monthly) plus tamoxifen 30 mg daily for 3 years or FEC chemotherapy (fluorouracil 500 mg/m^2, epirubicin 50 mg/m^2, cyclophosphamide 500 mg/m^2 IV) every 21 days for 6 treatments and showed no difference in disease-free survival or overall survival at 7 years [132]. Another study compared 6 cycles of CMF (cyclophosphamide 100 mg/m^2 orally daily on days 1–14 with IV methotrexate 40 mg/m^2 and fluorouracil 600 mg/m^2 IV on days 1 and 8, repeated every 28 days) with 5 years of tamoxifen 30 mg daily plus ovarian suppression (via surgical oophorectomy, radiation therapy or monthly goserelin injections) in 244 pre/perimenopausal women [133]. At a median follow-up of 76 months, there was no difference in disease-free or overall survival. A third trial randomized 1,034 premenopausal women with hormone-receptor positive, stage I and II breast cancer to either 3 years of goserelin plus 5 years of daily tamoxifen 20 mg daily or 6 cycles of IV CMF chemotherapy (cyclophosphamide 600 mg/m^2, methotrexate 40 mg/m^2 and fluorouracil 600 mg/m^2 on D1 and 8 of 28 day cycles) [134]. With a median of 60 months of follow-up, the recurrence-free survival (RFS) and local RFS favored the endocrine treatment, $p=0.037$ and $p=0.015$ respectively. There was a trend for overall survival favoring endocrine therapy, but this was not significant, $p=0.195$. These trials seem to suggest that OS/OA plus tamoxifen may be sufficient for premenopausal women.

The Cancer Care Ontario (CCO) published guidelines on Adjuvant Ovarian Ablation (OA) in the Treatment of Premenopausal Women With Early-Stage Invasive Breast Cancer. These guidelines were reviewed and endorsed by ASCO [135]. They recommended that ovarian ablation should not be routinely added to systemic therapy with chemotherapy, tamoxifen, or the combination of tamoxifen and chemotherapy. They also stated that ovarian ablation alone is not recommended as an alternative to any other form of systemic therapy.

Aromatase inhibitors (AIs) are not indicated for the adjuvant treatment of premenopausal women. The use of AIs with LHRH-agonists is being studied in premenopausal women, but the data available so far does not suggest an advantage over tamoxifen+OS/OA. In the ABCSG-12 trial, there was no difference in disease-free survival for 1,803 premenopausal women randomized to goserelin and tamoxifen versus goserelin and anastrozole, HR 1.10, 95 % CI 0.78–1.53, $p=0.59$ [136]. A subsequent subset analysis of this trial based on BMI calculations showed that for overweight patients treated with anastrozole, there were significant increases in the risk of disease recurrence, HR, 1.49; 95 % CI, 0.93–2.38; $p=0.08$, and death, HR, 3.03; 95 % CI, 1.35–6.82; $p=0.004$, compared with patients treated with tamoxifen [137].

Premenopausal women can be considered for AI therapy after 2–3 years or 5 years of tamoxifen if they become menopausal during that time. Reasonable criteria for the definition of menopause include bilateral oophorectomy, age ≥60 years, age <60 years and amenorrhea for 12 months in the absence of chemotherapy, tamoxifen or ovarian suppression and FSH and estradiol in the postmenopausal range, or age <60 on tamoxifen with FSH and estradiol in the postmenopausal range. For women who are premenopausal at the start of chemotherapy, amenorrhea cannot be a reliable measure of ovarian function, so serial measurements of FSH and/or estradiol should be performed to ensure postmenopausal status prior to starting therapy with an AI [6].

Zoledronic Acid

In patients with early stage breast cancer, several studies have suggested that adjuvant bisphosphonate therapy may have antitumor and anti-metastatic properties and decrease the rates of recurrence and death [136, 138, 139]. However, two other trials suggested no benefit [140, 141]. Recently published data also shows conflicting results.

The Austrian Breast and Colorectal Cancer Study Group-12 (ABCSG-12) trial enrolled 1,803 premenopausal women with stage I–II breast cancer who received standard treatment with goserelin [136]. Preoperative chemotherapy was allowed but only approximately 5 % of patients had received it. No patients received postoperative adjuvant chemotherapy. This trial had a two-by-two factorial design in which women were randomized to tamoxifen or anastrozole with or without zoledronic acid. The initial dose of zoledronic acid was 8 mg; this was subsequently reduced to 4 mg and given every 6 months for 5 years. The primary endpoint was disease-free survival (DFS). There was no difference in DFS between patients receiving tamoxifen or anastrozole, but the addition of zoledronic acid resulted in a significant improvement in DFS compared with endocrine therapy alone: 94.0 % vs. 90.8 %, HR 0.74, 95 % confidence interval 0.46–0.91, $p=0.01$. Zoledronic acid was well-tolerated. There were three possible cases of osteonecrosis of the jaw, but the diagnosis was ruled out in all cases after a detailed review of the dental records.

The Adjuvant Zoledronic Acid to Reduce Recurrence (AZURE) trial was a randomized, open-label, phase III trial in which 3,360 patients with stage II–III (either N1 or T3–4) early stage breast cancer were randomized to standard adjuvant systemic therapy (including chemotherapy, endocrine therapy and radiation to breast, chest wall and/or regional lymph nodes as indicated) with or without zoledronic acid [77]. The zoledronic acid was given immediately after chemotherapy every 3–4 weeks at a dose of 4 mg for six treatments. It was then continued every 3 months for eight doses, then every 6 months for five additional doses, to complete a total of 5 years of therapy. The majority of patients (95.5 %) received chemotherapy and the median follow-up was 59.3 months. There was no difference in the primary endpoint of disease-free survival (DFS), with a rate of 77 % for both groups (adjusted hazard ratio (HR) in the zoledronic acid group, 0.98; 95 % CI 0.85–1.13, $p=0.79$). In a prespecified analysis, there was an improvement in postmenopausal women in DFS, 78.2 % for the zoledronic acid treatment arm versus 71.0 % for the control arm (adjusted HR 0.75, 95 % CI 0.59–0.96, $p=0.02$), and for OS, 84.6 % vs. 78.7 % (adjusted HR 0.74, 95 % confidence interval 0.55–0.98, $p=0.04$). The confirmed rate of osteonecrosis of the jaw was 1.1 % (17 cases) with another 9 suspected cases.

There were a few major differences between these two trials of adjuvant zoledronic acid. The patient populations differed. The ABCSG-12 trial had premenopausal women who were estrogen-receptor positive and treated with goserelin and either tamoxifen or anastrozole and less than 5 % of those patients received chemotherapy. In the AZURE trial, 95.5 % received chemotherapy [77, 136]. The data is still insufficient to recommend adjuvant zoledronic acid therapy as a standard of care.

Metastatic Breast Cancer

Despite advances in the treatment of early stage breast cancer, approximately 20–30 % of patients will relapse and die from metastatic disease. In addition, up to 5 % of patients have distant metastatic spread at the time of diagnosis. Metastatic disease is incurable in the vast majority of cases, but is treatable. The mean survival for patients with metastatic disease is 18–24 months [142] but survival can range from a few months to many years. This wide variation is largely due to the biological diversity of the disease, with different sensitivities and responses to treatment as well as differences in the patterns of spread. The goal of treatment of patients with metastatic disease is to prolong their duration of time free from disease-related symptoms, while minimizing toxicities from treatment. Although no randomized trials have compared systemic therapy versus best supportive care, it is assumed that treatment prolongs survival.

Systemic therapy options are determined by many factors, including patient-related factors such as age, menopausal status, performance status, severity of symptoms, previous treatments, and organ function, and disease-related factors, such as tumor biology (ER, PR and HER2 status), duration of time between primary treatment and relapse (determining sensitive versus resistant disease), presence or absence of visceral disease and burden of disease. In general, patients remain on one treat ment regimen until they experience unacceptable toxicity or disease progression.

The most commonly used agents for postmenopausal patients with hormone-receptor positive disease include tamoxifen, aromatase inhibitors (anastrozole, letrozole, exemestane), and ER-antagonists (fulvestrant). For premenopausal patients, available endocrine options include tamoxifen, ovarian ablation (via surgery, radiation therapy, or LHRH agonists) alone or with aromatase inhibitors or fulvestrant.

Chemotherapy is the treatment of choice for patients with metastatic disease who have triple-negative (ER, PR and HER2 negative) tumors as well as in those with hormone receptor-positive tumors who have progressed on one to three prior hormonal regimens, or if a rapid response to treatment is required. There is considerable debate as to whether combination chemotherapy or sequential single agent chemotherapy should be given. In general, response rates tend to be higher when a combination regimen is used, but chemotherapy combinations also cause more toxicity. Palliation of symptoms is the goal, and this increased toxicity may impair the patient's quality of life. Combination chemotherapy has not been adequately compared to using the same agents sequentially as single agents. In general, combination chemotherapy is reserved for patients with good performance status, rapidly progressive disease and evidence of visceral crisis (organ dysfunction). It is used more often in the first-line setting, as opposed to further lines of treatment, where toxicity considerations are even more important. Sequential single agent chemotherapy is often given in a lower-dose, weekly fashion, to reduce toxicity and increase tolerability.

For HER2-positive metastatic disease, regimens that include targeted agents against HER2 are the standard of care. A pivotal trial evaluated the use of trastuzumab in 469 women with HER2-overexpressing metastatic breast cancer who had been previously untreated [53]. These women were randomized to chemotherapy alone or chemotherapy combined with trastuzumab. At a median follow-up of 30 months, the survival was significantly improved for the patients who received chemotherapy plus trastuzumab compared to those who received chemotherapy alone (25.1 months vs. 20.3 months, $p=0.01$). These results were seen in the intent-to-treat analysis, which means that patients were analyzed according to the treatment group they had originally been randomized to. Therefore, despite that two-thirds of the chemotherapy alone group had crossed over to receive trastuzumab, there was still a significant survival advantage noted. This led to the FDA-approved indication for trastuzumab combined with paclitaxel for first-line treatment. Trastuzumab is also approved as a single agent in patients who have received one or more chemotherapy regimens [48]. Trastuzumab is commonly used in combination with other chemotherapy drugs as well as with aromatase inhibitors. Another anti-HER2 targeted agent is lapatinib, an oral tyrosine kinase inhibitor that targets EGFR (HER1) and HER2. Lapatinib is approved in combination with capecitabine for patients with HER2-positive breast cancer who have been previously treated with anthracyclines, taxanes, and trastuzumab [143]. Lapatinib has also shown activity in combination with other cytotoxic agents, such as paclitaxel [144] and in combination with trastuzumab without chemotherapy in women with heavily pretreated disease [145]. Two new anti-HER2 drugs were recently approved for HER2-positive metastatic breast cancer. Pertuzumab is a monoclonal antibody directed against HER2 which binds at a different site than trastuzumab. It is indicated in combination with trastuzumab and docetaxel, for patients with HER2-positive, metastatic breast cancer who have not received prior anti-HER2 therapy or chemotherapy for their metastatic disease [146]. Trastuzumab emtansine (TDM-1) is an antibody-drug conjugate which incorporates trastuzumab with DM-1, a cytotoxic. This is approved for use in metastatic, HER2-positive breast cancer patients who previously received trastuzumab and a taxane, based on the results of the EMILIA trial [147]. Promising results have been seen in trials with other anti-HER2 agents, including additional tyrosine kinase inhibitors (neratinib).

Bone metastasis is a common problem in metastatic breast cancer, seen in up to 80 % of patients. Bone metastases can result in pain, hypercalcemia, and skeletal-related events (SREs) which consist of requiring radiation therapy for pain control or to prevent a fracture, surgery to treat or prevent a fracture, a pathological fracture or spinal cord compression. The use of bone-modifying agents has been shown to reduce the incidence of SREs, and are recommended by the American Society of Clinical Oncology as pamidronate 90 mg given over at least 90 min intravenously every 3–4 weeks, zoledronic acid 4 mg given over at least 15 min intravenously every 3–4 weeks, or denosumab 120 mg given subcutaneously every 4 weeks [148].

The first drug used in this setting was pamidronate, a bisphosphonate. In two prospective, randomized, double-blind, placebo-controlled trials, 754 patients with stage IV breast cancer with bone metastases were randomized to either pamidronate or placebo infusions every 3–4 weeks [149]. For the primary endpoint of skeletal morbidity rate (events/year), there was an improvement for patients who received pamidronate (2.4 vs. 3.7, ≤ 0.001). In the pamidronate group, 51 % had skeletal complications compared with 64 % in the placebo group ($P<0.001$). The median time to first skeletal complication and pain scores were also reduced with pamidronate. Subsequently, pamidronate was compared to another bisphosphonate, zoledronic acid [150]. In breast cancer patients, zoledronic acid was significantly more effective than pamidronate, reducing the risk of SREs by an additional 20 %

($P=0.025$) compared with pamidronate. The third bone-modifying agent, denosumab, is a fully human monoclonal antibody receptor activator of nuclear factor κ-β (RANK) ligand. In a comparison to zoledronic acid, denosumab was superior in delaying time to first on-study SRE (HR 0.82; 95 % CI, 0.71–0.95; $p=0.01$ superiority) [151]. One side effect common to all of these is osteonecrosis of the jaw, and all patients should have a thorough dental examination and be counseled to maintain good oral hygiene prior to initiating therapy with a bone-modifying agent.

Summary

Major progress has been made in the field of breast cancer. The classification of breast tumors based on their gene expression profiles has allowed us to better understand their clinical behavior. We are now starting to use this knowledge to individualize therapy to tumors based on their perceived risk of recurrence. There also been significant advances in the treatment of breast cancer. Chemotherapy regimens are being refined to involve more active agents and we are learning how to give chemotherapy to those who will derive the greatest benefit. Targeted therapies are the future of breast cancer. The greatest examples are anti-estrogen and anti-HER2 therapies, which have had impressive results in improving both disease-free and overall survival when given to the appropriate early stage breast cancer patients. The contribution of clinical trials to the evolution of the field breast cancer cannot be overemphasized. For future advancements in this field, it is vital to continue enrollment to clinical trials.

References

1. Perou CM, Sorlie T, Eisen MB, et al. Molecular portraits of human breast tumours. Nature. 2000;406:747–52.
2. Goldhirsch A, Wood WC, Coates AS, et al. Strategies for subtypes—dealing with the diversity of breast cancer: highlights of the St Gallen International Expert Consensus on the Primary Therapy of Early Breast Cancer 2011. Ann Oncol. 2011;22:1736–47.
3. Paik S, Shak S, Tang G, et al. A multigene assay to predict recurrence of tamoxfien-treated, node-negative breast cancer. N Engl J Med. 2004;351:2817–26.
4. Paik S, Tang G, Shak S, et al. Gene expression and benefit of chemotherapy in women with node-negative, estrogen receptor-positive breast cancer. J Clin Oncol. 2006;24:3726–34.
5. Harris L, Fritsche H, Mennel R, et al. American Society of Clinical Oncology 2007 Update of recommendations for the use of tumor markers in breast cancer. J Clin Oncol. 2007;25:5287–312.
6. NCCN Clinical Practice Guidelines in Oncology: Breast Cancer Version 2.2011. http://www.nccn.org/professionals/physician_gls/pdf/breast.pdf. Accessed Dec 2011.
7. Goldhirsch A, Ingle JN, Gelber RD, et al. Thresholds for therapies: highlights of the St Gallen International Expert Consensus on the primary therapy of early breast cancer 2009. Ann Oncol. 2009;20:1319–29.
8. van't Veer LJ, Dai H, van de Vijver MJ, et al. Gene expression profiling predicts clinical outcome of breast cancer. Nature. 2002;415:530–6.

9. van de Vijver MJ, He YD, van't Veer LJ, et al. A gene expression signature as a predictor of survival in breast cancer. N Engl J Med. 2002;347:1999–2009.
10. Buyse M, Loi S, van't Veer L, et al. Validation and clinical utility of a 70-gene prognostic signature for women with node-negative breast cancer. J Natl Cancer Inst. 2006;98:1183–92.
11. Bueno-de-Mesquita JM, Linn SC, Keijzer R, et al. Validation of 70-gene prognosis signature in node-negative breast cancer. Breast Cancer Res Treat. 2009;117:483–95.
12. Straver ME, Glas AM, Hannemann J, et al. The 70-gene signature as a response predictor for neoadjuvant chemotherapy in breast cancer. Breast Cancer Res Treat. 2010;119:551–8.
13. Knauer M, Mook S, Rutgers EJ, et al. The predictive value of the 70-gene signature for adjuvant chemotherapy in early breast cancer. Breast Cancer Res Treat. 2010;120:655–61.
14. Adjuvant! Online. http://www.adjuvantonline.com. Accessed Dec 2011.
15. Early Breast Cancer Trialists' Collaborative Group (EBCTCG). Effects of chemotherapy and hormonal therapy for early breast cancer on recurrence and 15-year survival: an overview of the randomised trials. Lancet. 2005;365:1687–717.
16. Goldhirsch A, Coates AS, Colleoni M, et al. Adjuvant chemoendocrine therapy in postmenopausal breast cancer: cyclophosphamide, methotrexate and fluorouracil dose and schedule may make a difference. International Breast Cancer Study Group. J Clin Oncol. 1998;16:1358–62.
17. Engelsman E, Klijn JC, Rubens RD, et al. "Classical" CMF versus a 3-weekly intravenous CMF schedule in postmenopausal patients with advanced breast cancer. An EORTC Breast Cancer Co-operative Group Phase III Trial (10808). Eur J Cancer. 1991;27:966–70.
18. Fisher B, Brown AM, Dimitrov NV, et al. Two months of doxorubicin-cyclophosphamide with and without interval reinduction therapy compared with 6 months of cyclophosphamide, methotrexate, and fluorouracil in positive-node breast cancer patients with tamoxifen-nonresponsive tumors: results from the National Surgical Adjuvant Breast and Bowel Project B-15. J Clin Oncol. 1990;8:1483–96.
19. Fisher B, Anderson S, Tan-Chiu E, et al. Tamoxifen and chemotherapy for axillary node-negative, estrogen receptor-negative breast cancer: findings from National Surgical Adjuvant Breast and Bowel Project B-23. J Clin Oncol. 2001;19:931–42.
20. Henderson IC, Berry DA, Demetri GD, et al. Improved outcomes from adding sequential paclitaxel but not from escalating doxorubicin dose in an adjuvant chemotherapy regimen for patients with node-positive primary breast cancer. J Clin Oncol. 2003;21:976–83.
21. Mamounas EP, Bryant J, Lembersky B, et al. Paclitaxel after doxorubicin plus cyclophosphamide as adjuvant chemotherapy for node-positive breast cancer: results from NSABP B28. J Clin Oncol. 2005;23:3686–96.
22. Martin M, Rodriguez-Lescure A, Ruiz A, et al. Randomized phase 3 trial of fluorouracil, epirubicin, and cyclophosphamide alone or followed by paclitaxel for early breast cancer. J Natl Cancer Inst. 2008;100:805–14.
23. Citron ML, Berry DA, Cirrincione C, et al. Randomized trial of dose-dense versus conventionally scheduled and sequential versus concurrent combination chemotherapy as postoperative adjuvant treatment of node-positive primary breast cancer: first report of Intergroup Trial C9741/Cancer and Leukemia Group B Trial 9741. J Clin Oncol. 2003;21:1431–9.
24. Hudis C, Citron M, Berry D, et al. Five year follow-up of INT C9741: dose-dense chemotherapy is safe and effective. Breast Cancer Res Treat. 2005;94:20s (Suppl 1;abstr. 49).
25. Martin M, Pienkowski T, Mackey J, et al. Adjuvant docetaxel for node-positive breast cancer. N Engl J Med. 2005;352:2302–13.
26. Martin M, Mackey J, Pienkowski T, et al. Ten-year follow-up analysis of the BCIRG 001 trial confirms superior DFS and OS benefit of adjuvant TAC (docetaxel, doxorubicin, cyclophosphamide) over FAC (fluorouracil, doxorubicin, cyclophosphamide) in women with operable node-positive breast cancer. Presented at the 33rd Annual San Antonio Breast Cancer Symposium, San Antonio, TX, December 8–12, 2010(abstract S4-3).
27. Roché H, Fumoleau P, Spielmann M, et al. Sequential adjuvant epirubicin-based and docetaxel chemotherapy for node-positive breast cancer patients: the FNCLCC PACS 01 Trial. J Clin Oncol. 2006;24:5664–71.

28. Sparano JA, Wang M, Martino S, et al. Weekly paclitaxel in the adjuvant treatment of breast cancer. N Engl J Med. 2008;358:1663–71.
29. Swain SM, Jeong JH, Geyer Jr CE, et al. Longer therapy, iatrogenic amenorrhea, and survival in early breast cancer. N Engl J Med. 2010;362:2053–65.
30. Eiermann W, Pienkowski T, Crown J, et al. Phase III study of doxorubicin/cyclophosphamide with concomitant versus sequential docetaxel as adjuvant treatment in patients with human epidermal growth factor receptor 2-normal, node-positive breast cancer: BCIRG-005 trial. J Clin Oncol. 2011;29:3877–84.
31. De Laurentiis M, Cancello G, D'Agostino D, et al. Taxane-based combinations as adjuvant chemotherapy of early breast cancer: a meta-analysis of randomized trials. J Clin Oncol. 2008;26:44–53.
32. Jones SE, Savin MA, Holmes FA, et al. Phase III trial comparing doxorubicin plus cyclophosphamide with docetaxel plus cyclophosphamide as adjuvant therapy for operable breast cancer. J Clin Oncol. 2006;24:5381–7.
33. Jones S, Holmes A, O'Shaughnessy J, et al. Docetaxel with cyclophosphamide is associated with an overall survival benefit compared with doxorubicin and cyclophosphamide: 7-year follow-Up of US oncology research trial 9375. J Clin Oncol. 2009;27.1177–783.
34. Fisher B, Anderson S, Wickerham DL, et al. Increased intensification and total dose of cyclophosphamide in a doxorubicin-cyclophosphamide regimen for the treatment of primary breast cancer: findings from National Surgical Adjuvant Breast and Bowel Project B-22. J Clin Oncol. 1997;15:1858–69.
35. Perez EA. TAC—a new standard in adjuvant therapy for breast cancer? N Engl J Med. 2005;352:2346–8.
36. Fisher B, Anderson S, DeCillis A, et al. Further evaluation of intensified and increased total dose of cyclophosphamide for the treatment of primary breast cancer: findings from the National Surgical Adjuvant Breast and Bowel Project B-25. J Clin Oncol. 1999;17:3374–88.
37. Berry DA, Ueno NT, Johnson MM, et al. High-dose chemotherapy with autologous tem-cell support as adjuvant therapy breast cancer: overview of 15 randomized trials. J Clin Oncol. 2011;29:3214–23.
38. Bastarrachea J, Hortobagyi GN, Smith TL, et al. Obesity as an adverse prognostic factor for patients receiving adjuvant chemotherapy for breast cancer. Ann Intern Med. 1994;120:18–25.
39. Colleoni M, Li S, Gelber RD, et al. Relation between chemotherapy dose, oestrogen receptor expression and body-mass index. Lancet. 2005;366:1108–10.
40. Litton JK, Gonzalez-Angulo AM, Warneke CL, et al. Relationship between obesity and pathologic response to neoadjuvant chemotherapy among women with operable breast cancer. J Clin Oncol. 2008;26:4072–7.
41. Kroenke CH, Chen WY, Rosner B, Holmes MD. Weight, weight gain and survival after breast cancer diagnosis. J Clin Oncol. 2005;23:1370–8.
42. Sparreboom A, Wolff AC, Mathijssen RH, et al. Evaluation of alternate size descriptors for dose calculation of anticancer drugs in the obese. J Clin Oncol. 2007;25:4707–13.
43. Lohrisch C, Paltiel C, Gelmon K, et al. Impact on survival of time from definitive surgery to initiation of adjuvant chemotherapy for early-stage breast cancer. J Clin Oncol. 2006;24:4888–94.
44. Owens MA, Horten BC, Da Silva MM. HER2 amplification ratios by fluorescence in situ hybridization and correlation with immunohistochemistry in a cohort of 6556 breast cancer tissues. Clin Breast Cancer. 2004;5:63–9.
45. Sjogren S, Inganas M, Lindgren A, et al. Prognostic and predictive value of c-erbB-2 overexpression in primary breast cancer, alone and in combination with other prognostic markers. J Clin Oncol. 1998;16:462–9.
46. Slamon DJ, Clark GM, Wong SG, et al. Human breast cancer: correlation of relapse and survival with amplification of the HER-2/neu oncogene. Science. 1987;235:177–82.
47. Slamon DJ, Godolphin W, Jones LA, et al. Studies of the HER-2/neu proto-oncogene in human breast and ovarian cancer. Science. 1989;244:707–12.

48. Cobleigh MA, Vogel CL, Tripathy D, et al. Multinational study of the efficacy and safety of humanized anti-HER2 monoclonal antibody in women who have HER2-overexpressing metastatic breast cancer that has progressed after chemotherapy for metastatic disease. J Clin Oncol. 1999;17:2639–48.
49. Marty M, Cognate F, Maraninchi D, et al. Randomized phase II trial of the efficacy and safety of trastuzumab combined with docetaxel in patients with human epidermal growth factor receptor 2-positive metastatic breast cancer administered as first-line treatment: the M77001 study group. J Clin Oncol. 2005;23:4265–74.
50. Perez EA. Impact, mechanisms, and novel chemotherapy strategies for overcoming resistance to anthracyclines and taxanes in metastatic breast cancer. Breast Cancer Res Treat. 2009;114:195–201.
51. Vogel CL, Cobleigh MA, Tripathy D, et al. Efficacy and safety of trastuzumab as a single agent in first-line treatment of HER2-overexpressing metastatic breast cancer. J Clin Oncol. 2002;20:719–26.
52. von Minckwitz G, du Bois A, Schmidt M, et al. Trastuzumab beyond progression in human epidermal growth factor receptor 2-positive advanced breast cancer: a German Breast Group 26/Breast International Group 03-05 study. J Clin Oncol. 2009;27:1999–2006.
53. Slamon DJ, Leyland-Jones B, Shak S, et al. Use of chemotherapy plus a monoclonal antibody against HER2 for metastatic breast cancer that overexpresses HER2. N Engl J Med. 2001;344:783–92.
54. Romond EH, Perez EA, Bryant J, et al. Trastuzumab plus adjuvant chemotherapy for operable HER2positive breast cancer. N Engl J Med. 2005;353:1673–84.
55. Perez EA, Romond EH, Suman VJ, et al. Updated results of the combined analysis of NCCTG 9831 and NSABP B-31 adjuvant chemotherapy with/without trastuzumab in patients with HER2-positive breast cancer. J Clin Oncol. 2007;25:18s. abstract 512.
56. Perez EA, Romond EH, Suman VJ, et al. Four-year follow-up of trastuzumab plus adjuvant chemotherapy for operable human epidermal growth factor receptor 2-positive breast cancer: joint analysis of data from NCCTG N9831 and NSABP B-31. J Clin Oncol. 2011;29:3366–73.
57. Piccart-Gebhart MJ, Procter M, Leyland-Jones B, et al. Trastuzumab after adjuvant chemotherapy in HER2-positive breast cancer. N Engl J Med. 2005;353:1659–72.
58. Smith I, Procter M, Gelber RD, et al. 2 year follow-up of trastuzumab after adjuvant chemotherapy in HER2-positive breast cancer: a randomised controlled trial. Lancet. 2007;369:29–36.
59. Gianni L, Dafni U, Gelber RD, et al. Treatment with trastuzumab for 1 year after adjuvant chemotherapy in patients with HER2-positive early breast cancer: a 4-year follow-up of a randomised controlled trial. Lancet Oncol. 2011;12:236–44.
60. Joensuu H, Kellokumpu-Lehtinen P-L, Bono P, et al. Adjuvant docetaxel or vinorelbine with or without trastuzumab for breast cancer. N Engl J Med. 2006;354:809–20.
61. Joensuu H, Bono P, Kataja V, et al. Fluorouracil, epirubicin and cyclophosphamide with either docetaxel or vinorelbine, with our without trastuzumab, as adjuvant treatments of breast cancer: final results of the Fin Her trial. J Clin Oncol. 2009;27:5685–92.
62. Slamon D, Eiermann W, Robert N, et al. Adjuvant trastuzumab in HER2-positive breast cancer. N Engl J Med. 2011;365:1273–83.
63. Spielmann M, Roche H, Delozier T, et al. Trastuzumab for patients with axillary-node-positive breast cancer: results of the FNCLCC-PACS 04 trial. J Clin Oncol. 2009;27:6129–34.
64. Gonzalez-Angulo AM, Litton JK, Broglio KR, et al. High risk of recurrence for patients with breast cancer who have human epidermal growth factor receptor 2-positive, node negative tumors 1 cm or smaller. J Clin Oncol. 2009;27:5700–6.
65. Curigliano G, Viale G, Bagnardi V, et al. Clinical relevance of HER2 overexpression/amplification in patients with small tumor size and node-negative breast cancer. J Clin Oncol. 2009;27:5693–9.
66. Yin W, Jiang Y, Shen Z, et al. Trastuzumab in the adjuvant treatment of HER2-positive early breast cancer patients: a meta-analysis of published randomized controlled trials. PLoS One. 2011;6:e21030.

67. Goldhirsch A, Piccart-Gebhardt MJ, Procter M, et al. HERA Trial: 2 years versus 1 year of trastuzumab after adjuvant chemotherapy in women with HER2-positive early breast cancer at 8 years of median follow up. Cancer Res. 2012;72:S5–2.
68. Pivot X, Romieu G, Bonnefoi H, et al. PHARE trial results of subset analysis comparing 6 to 12 months of trastuzumab in adjuvant early breast cancer. Cancer Res. 2012;72:S5–3.
69. Theodoulou M, Seidman AD. Cardiac effects of adjuvant therapy for early breast cancer. Semin Oncol. 2003;30:730–9.
70. Choi JC, Chang JD, Seal B, et al. Risk and cost of anthracycline-induced cardiotoxicity among breast cancer patients in the United States. J Clin Oncol. 2009;27:15s. suppl; abstr 1037.
71. Smith RE. Risk for the development of treatment-related acute myelocytic leukemia and myelodysplastic syndrome among patients with breast cancer: review of the literature and the National Surgical Adjuvant Breast and Bowel Project experience. Clin Breast Cancer. 2003;4:273–9.
72. Patt DA, Duan Z, Fang S, et al. Acute myeloid leukemia after adjuvant breast cancer treatment in older women: understanding risk. J Clin Oncol. 2007;25:3871–6.
73. Hershman D, Neugut AI, Jacobson JS, et al. Acute myeloid leukemia or myelodysplastic syndrome following use of granulocyte colony-stimulating factors during breast cancer adjuvant chemotherapy. J Natl Cancer Inst. 2007;99:196–205.
74. Schneider BP, Wang M, Stearns V, et al. Relationship between taxane-induced neuropathy and clinical outcomes after adjuvant chemotherapy. J Clin Oncol 2011;29:(suppl 27; abstr 270).
75. Russell SD, Blackwell KL, Lawrence J, et al. Independent adjudication of symptomatic heart failure with the use of doxorubicin and cyclophosphamide followed by trastuzumab adjuvant therapy: a combined review of cardiac data from the National Surgical Adjuvant Breast and Bowel Project B-31 and the North Central Cancer Treatment Group N9831 clinical trials. J Clin Oncol. 2010;28:3416–21.
76. Procter M, Suter TM, de Azambuja E, et al. Longer-term assessment of trastuzumab related cardiac adverse events in the Herceptin Adjuvant (HERA) trial. J Clin Oncol. 2010;28:3422–8.
77. Coleman RE, Marshall H, Cameron D, et al. Breast-cancer adjuvant therapy with zoledronic acid. N Engl J Med. 2011;365:1396–405.
78. Mauri D, Pavlidis N, Ioannidis JP. Neoadjuvant versus adjuvant systemic treatment in breast cancer: a meta-analysis. J Natl Cancer Inst. 2005;97:188–94.
79. Wolmark N, Wang J, Mamounas E, et al. Preoperative chemotherapy in patients with operable breast cancer: nine-year results from National Surgical Adjuvant Breast and Bowel Project B-18. J Natl Cancer Inst Monogr. 2001;30:96–102.
80. Rastogi P, Anderson SJ, Bear HD, et al. Preoperative chemotherapy: updates of National Surgical Adjuvant Breast and Bowel Project Protocols B-18 and B-27. J Clin Oncol. 2008;26:778–85.
81. van der Hage JA, van de Velde CJ, Julien JP, et al. Preoperative chemotherapy in primary operable breast cancer; results from the European Organization for Research and Treatment of Cancer trial 10902. J Clin Oncol. 2001;19:4224–37.
82. Bear HD, Anderson S, Smith RE, et al. Sequential preoperative or postoperative docetaxel added to preoperative doxorubicin plus cyclophosphamide for operable breast cancer: National Surgical Adjuvant Breast and Bowel Project Protocol B-27. J Clin Oncol. 2006;24:2019–27.
83. Hennessy BT, Hortobagyi GN, Rouzier R, et al. Outcome after pathologic complete eradication of cytologically proven breast cancer axillary node metastases following primary chemotherapy. J Clin Oncol. 2005;23:9304–11.
84. Chen AM, Meric-Bernstam F, Hunt KK, et al. Breast conservation after neoadjuvant chemotherapy: the MD Anderson cancer center experience. J Clin Oncol. 2004;22:2303–12.
85. Jones RL, Salter J, A'Hern R, et al. The prognostic significance of Ki67 before and after neoadjuvant chemotherapy in breast cancer. Breast Cancer Res Treat. 2009;116:53–68.

86. Gianni L, Eiermann W, Semiglazov V, et al. Neoadjuvant chemotherapy with trastuzumab followed by adjuvant trastuzumab versus neoadjuvant chemotherapy alone, in patients with HER2-positive locally advanced breast cancer (the NOAH trial): a randomized controlled superiority trial with a parallel HER2-negative cohort. Lancet. 2010;375:377.
87. Buzdar AU, Ibrahim NK, Francis D, et al. Significantly higher pathologic complete remission rate after neoadjuvant therapy with trastuzumab, paclitaxel and epirubicin chemotherapy: results of a randomized trial in human epidermal growth factor receptor 2-positive operable breast cancer. J Clin Oncol. 2005;23:3676–85.
88. Untch M, Muscholl M, Tjulandin S, et al. First-line trastuzumab plus epirubicin and cyclophosphamide therapy in patients with human epidermal growth factor receptor 2-positive metastatic breast cancer: cardiac safety and efficacy data from the Herceptin, Cyclophosphamide and Epirubicin (HERCULES) trial. J Clin Oncol. 2010;28:1473–80.
89. Bozovic-Spasojevic I, Azim Jr HA, Paesmans M, et al. Neoadjuvant anthracycline and trastuzumab for breast cancer: is concurrent treatment safe? Lancet Oncol. 2011;12:209–11.
90. Baselga J, Bradbury I, Eidtmann H, et al. First results of the NeoALLTO trial (BIG 01-06/EGF 106093): a phase III, randomized, open-label, neoadjuvant study of lapatinib, trastuzuman, and their combination plus paclitaxel in women with HER2-positive primary breast cancer. Presented at the 33rd Annual San Antonio Breast Cancer Symposium, December 8–12, 2010;abstract S3–3.
91. Gianni L, Pienkowski T, Im Y-H, et al. Efficacy and safety of neoadjuvant pertuzumab and trastuzumab in women with locally advanced, inflammatory, or early HER2-positive breast cancer (NeoSphere): a randomised multicentre, open-label, phase 2 trial. Lancet Oncol. 2012;13:25–32.
92. Beatson GT. On the treatment of inoperable cases of carcinoma of the mamma: suggestions for a new method of treatment with illustrative cases. Lancet. 1896;148:162–5.
93. Osborne CK, Yochmowitz MG, Knight 3rd WA. The value of estrogen and progesterone receptors in the treatment of breast cancer. Cancer. 1980;46(12 Suppl):2884–8.
94. Hammond MEH, Hayes DF, Allred DC, et al. American Society of Clinical Oncology/College of American Pathologists Guideline Recommendations for Immunohistochemical Testing of Estrogen and Progesterone Receptors in Breast Cancer. J Clin Oncol. 2010;28:2784–95.
95. Early Breast Cancer Trialists' Collaborative Group (EBCTCG), Davies C, Godwin J, et al. Relevance of breast cancer hormone receptors and other factors to the efficacy of adjuvant tamoxifen: patient-level meta-analysis of randomised trials. Lancet. 2011;378:771–84.
96. Fisher B, Costantino JP, Wickerham DL, et al. Tamoxifen for prevention of breast cancer: a report of the National Surgical Adjuvant Breast and Bowel Project P-1 Study. J Natl Cancer Inst. 1998;90:1371–88.
97. Fisher B, Dignam J, Bryant J, et al. Five versus more than five years of tamoxifen for lymph node-negative breast cancer: updated findings from the National Surgical Adjuvant Breast and Bowel Project B-14 randomized trial. J Natl Cancer. 2001;93:684–90.
98. Stewart HJ, Forrest AP, Everington D, et al. Randomised comparison of 5 years of adjuvant tamoxifen with continuous therapy for operable breast cancer. The Scottish Cancer Trials Breast Group. Br J Cancer. 1996;74:297–9.
99. Davies C, Pan H, Godwin J, et al. Long-term effects of continuing adjuvant tamoxifen to 10 years versus stopping at 5 years after diagnosis of oestrogen receptor-positive breast cancer: ATLAS, a randomised trial. Lancet. 2013;381:805–16.
100. Gray RG, Rea D, Handley K, et al. aTTom: Long term effects of continuing adjuvant tamoxifen to 10 years versus stopping at 5 years in 6,953 women with early breast cancer. J Clin Oncol. 2013;31:abstr 5.
101. Burstein HJ, Prestrud AA, Seidenfeld J, et al. American Society of Clinical Oncology Clinical Practice Guideline: update on adjuvant endocrine therapy for women with hormone receptor-positive breast cancer. J Clin Oncol. 2010;28:3784–96.
102. Smith IE, Dowsett M. Aromatase inhibitors in breast cancer. N Engl J Med. 2003;348:2431–42.

103. Arimidex, Tamoxifen, Alone or in Combination (ATAC) Trialists' Group, Forbes JF, Cuzick J, et al. Effect of anastrozole and tamoxifen as adjuvant treatment for early-stage breast cancer: 100-month analysis of the ATAC trial. Lancet Oncol. 2008;9:45–53.
104. Howell A, Cuzick J, Baum M, et al. Results of the ATAC (Arimidex, Tamoxifen, Alone or in Combination) trial after completion of 5 years; adjuvant treatment for breast cancer. Lancet. 2005;365:60–2.
105. Baum M, Budzar AU, Cuzick J, et al. Anastrozole alone or in combination with tamoxifen versus tamoxifen alone for adjuvant treatment of postmenopausal women with early breast cancer: first results of the ATAC randomised trial. Lancet. 2002;359:2131–9.
106. Cuzick J, Sestak I, Baum M, et al. Effect of anastrozole and tamoxifen as adjuvant treatment for early-stage breast cancer: 10-year analysis of the ATAC trial. Lancet Oncol. 2010;11:1135–41.
107. Breast International Group (BIG) 1-98 Collaborative Group, Thürlimann B, Keshaviah A, et al. A comparison of letrozole and tamoxifen in postmenopausal women with early breast cancer. N Engl J Med. 2005;353:2747–57.
108. Coates AS, Keshaviah A, Thürlimann B, et al. Five years of letrozole compared with tamoxifen as initial adjuvant therapy for postmenopausal women with endocrine-responsive early breast cancer: update of study BIG 1-98. J Clin Oncol. 2007;25:486–92.
109. BIG 1-98 Collaborative Group, Mouridsen H, Giobbie-Hurder A, et al. Letrozole therapy alone or in sequent with tamoxifen in women with breast cancer. N Engl J Med. 2009;361:766–76.
110. Colleoni M, Giobbie-Hurder A, Regan MM, et al. Analyses adjusting for selective crossover show improved survival with adjuvant letrozole compared with tamoxifen in the BIG 1-98 study. J Clin Oncol. 2011;29:1117–24.
111. Goss PE, Ingle JN, Martino S, et al. A randomized trial of letrozole in postmenopausal women after five years of tamoxifen therapy for early-stage breast cancer. N Engl J Med. 2003;349:1793–802.
112. Goss PE, Ingle JN, Martino S, et al. Randomized trial of letrozole following tamoxifen as extended adjuvant therapy in receptor-positive breast cancer: updated findings from NCIC CTG MA.17. J Natl Cancer Inst. 2005;97:1262–71.
113. Goss PE, Ingle JN, Pater JL, et al. Late extended adjuvant treatment with letrozole improves outcome in women with early-stage breast cancer who complete 5 years of tamoxifen. J Clin Oncol. 2008;26:1948–55.
114. Coombes RC, Kilburn LS, Snowdon CF, et al. Survival and safety of exemestane versus tamoxifen after 2–3 years' tamoxifen treatment (Intergroup Exemestane Study): a randomised controlled trial. Lancet. 2007;369:559–70.
115. Jonat W, Gnant M, Boccardo F, et al. Effectiveness of switching from adjuvant tamoxifen to anastrozole in postmenopausal women with hormone-sensitive early-stage breast cancer: a meta-analysis. Lancet Oncol. 2006;7:991–6.
116. van de Velde CJ, Rea D, Seynaeve C, et al. Adjuvant tamoxifen and exemestane in early breast cancer (TEAM): a randomised phase 3 trial. Lancet. 2011;377:321–31.
117. Dowsett M, Cuzick J, Ingle J, et al. Meta-analysis of breast cancer outcomes in adjuvant trials of aromatase inhibitors versus tamoxifen. J Clin Oncol. 2010;28:509–18.
118. Josefsson ML, Leinster SJ. Aromatase inhibitors versus tamoxifen as adjuvant hormonal therapy for oestrogen sensitive early breast cancer in post-menopausal women: meta-analyses of monotherapy, sequenced therapy and extended therapy. Breast. 2010;19:76–83.
119. Goss PE, Ingle JN, Chapman J-AW, et al. Final analysis of NCIC CTG MA.27: a randomized phase III trial of exemestane versus anastrozole in postmenopausal women with hormone receptor positive primary breast cancer. Presented at the 33rd Annual San Antonio Breast Cancer Symposium, December 8-12, 2010;abstract S1-1.
120. Partridge AH, LaFountain A, Mayer E, et al. Adherence to initial adjuvant anastrozole therapy among women with early-stage breast cancer. J Clin Oncol. 2008;26:556–62.
121. Salgado B, Zivian MT: aromatase inhibitors: side effects reported by 612 women. Presented at San Antonio Breast Cancer Symposium, December 14–17, 2006, San Antonio, TX.

122. Crew KD, Greenlee H, Capodice J, et al. Prevalence of joint symptoms in postmenopausal women taking aromatase inhibitors for early-stage breast cancer. J Clin Oncol. 2007;25:3877–83.
123. Amir E, Seruga B, Niraula S, et al. Toxicity of adjuvant endocrine therapy in postmenopausal breast cancer patients: a systematic review and meta-analysis. J Natl Cancer Inst. 2011;103:1299–309.
124. LHRH-agonists in Early Breast Cancer Overview group, Cuzick J, Ambroisine L, et al. Use of luteinizing-hormone-releasing hormone agonists as adjuvant treatment in premenopausal patients with hormone-receptor-positive breast cancer: a meta-analysis of individual patient data from randomised adjuvant trials. Lancet. 2007;369:1711–23.
125. International Breast Cancer Study Group (IBCSG), Castiglione-Gertsch M, O'Neill A, et al. Adjuvant chemotherapy followed by goserelin versus either modality alone for premenopausal lymph node-negative breast cancer: a randomized trial. J Natl Cancer Inst. 2003;95:1833–46.
126. Arriagada R, Lê MG, Spielmann M, et al. Randomized trial of adjuvant ovarian suppression in 926 premenopausal patients with early breast cancer treated with adjuvant chemotherapy. Ann Oncol. 2005;16:389–96.
127. Vanhuyse M, Fournier C, Bonneterre J. Chemotherapy-induced amenorrhea: influence on disease-free survival and overall survival in receptor-positive premenopausal early breast cancer patients. Ann Oncol. 2005;16:1283–8.
128. Davidson NE, O'Neill AM, Vukov AM, et al. Chemoendocrine therapy for premenopausal women with axillary lymph node-positive, steroid hormone receptor-positive breast cancer: results from INT 0101 (E5188). J Clin Oncol. 2005;23:5973–82.
129. Robert JN, Wang M, Cella D, et al. Phase III comparison of tamoxifen versus tamoxifen with ovarian ablation in premenopausal women with axillary node-negative receptor-positive breast cancer 3 cm. Proc Am Soc Clin Oncol. 2003;22:5a.
130. Baum M, Hackshaw A, Houghton J, et al. Adjuvant goserelin in pre-menopausal patients with early breast cancer: results from the ZIPP study. Eur J Cancer. 2006;42:895–904.
131. Hackshaw A, Baum M, Fornander T, et al. Long-term effectiveness of adjuvant goserelin in premenopausal women with early breast cancer. J Natl Cancer Inst. 2009;101:341–9.
132. Roché H, Kerbrat P, Bonneterre J, et al. Complete hormonal blockage versus epirubicin-based chemotherapy in premenopausal, one to three node-positive and hormone-receptor positive, early breast cancer patients: 7-year follow-up results of the French Adjuvant Study Group 06 randomised trial. Ann Oncol. 2006;17:1221–7.
133. Boccardo F, Rubagotti A, Amoroso D, et al. Cyclophosphamide, methotrexate, and fluorouracil versus tamoxifen plus ovarian suppression as adjuvant treatment of estrogen receptor-positive pre-/perimenopausal breast cancer patients: results of the Italian Breast Cancer Adjuvant Study Group 02 randomized trial. J Clin Oncol. 2000;18:2718–27.
134. Jakesz R, Hausmaninger H, Kubista E, et al. Randomized adjuvant trial of tamoxifen and goserelin versus cyclophosphamide, methotrexate, and fluorouracil: evidence for the superiority of treatment with endocrine blockade in premenopausal patients with hormone- responsive breast cancer –Austrian Breast and Colorectal Cancer Study Group Trial 5. J Clin Oncol. 2002;20:4621–7.
135. Griggs JJ, Somerfield MR, Anderson H, et al. American Society of Clinical Oncology Endorsement of the Cancer Care Ontario Practice Guideline on Adjuvant Ovarian Ablation in the Treatment of Premenopausal Women With Early-Stage Invasive Breast Cancer. J Clin Oncol. 2011;29:3939–42.
136. Gnant M, Mlineritsch B, Schippinger W, et al. Endocrine therapy plus zoledronic acid in premenopausal breast cancer. N Engl J Med. 2009;360:679–91.
137. Pfeiler G, Königsberg R, Fesl C, et al. Impact of body mass index on the efficacy of endocrine therapy in premenopausal patients with breast cancer: an analysis of the prospective ABCSG-12 trial. J Clin Oncol. 2011;29:2653–9.

138. Diel IJ, Jaschke A, Solomayer EF, et al. Adjuvant oral clodronate improves the overall survival of primary breast cancer patients with micrometastases to the bone marrow: a long-term follow-up. Ann Oncol. 2008;19:2007–11.
139. Powles T, Paterson A, McCloskey E, et al. Reduction in bone relapse and improved survival with oral clodronate for adjuvant treatment of operable breast cancer. Breast Cancer Res. 2006;8:R13.
140. Saarto T, Vehmanen L, Virkkunen P, et al. Ten-year follow-up of a randomized controlled trial of adjuvant clodronate treatment in node-positive breast cancer patients. Acta Oncol. 2004;43:650–6.
141. Kristensen B, Ejlertsen B, Mouridsen HT, et al. Bisphosphonate treatment in primary breast cancer: results from a randomised comparison of oral pamidronate versus no pamidronate in patients with primary breast cancer. Acta Oncol. 2008;47:740–6.
142. Ellis MJ, Hayes DF, Lippman ME. Treatment of Metastatic Breast Cancer. In: Harris JR, Lippman ME, Morrow M, Osborne KC, editors. Diseases of the Breast. 3rd ed. Philadelphia, Pa: Lippincott Williams & Wilkins; 2004. p. 1102.
143. Geyer CE, Forster J, Lindquist D, et al. Lapatinib plus capecitabine for HER2-positive advanced breast cancer. N Engl J Med. 2006;355:2733–43.
144. Di Leo A, Gomez HL, Aziz Z, et al. Phase III, double-blind, randomized study comparing Lapatinib plus paclitaxel with placebo plus paclitaxel as first-line treatment for metastatic breast cancer. j clin oncol. 2008;26:5544–52.
145. O'Shaughnessy J, Blackwell KL, Burstein A, et al. A randomized study of lapatinib alone or in combination with trastuzumab in heavily pretreated HER2+ metastatic breast cancer progressing on trastuzumab therapy. J Clin Oncol 2008;26:abstr 1015.
146. Baselga J, Cortes J, Kim S, et al. Pertuzumab plus trastuzumab plus docetaxel for metastatic breast cancer. N Engl J Med. 2012;366:109–19.
147. Verma S, Miles D, Gianni L, et al. Trastuzumab emtansine for HER2 positive, advanced breast cancer. N Engl J Med. 2012;367:1783–91.
148. Van Poznak CH, Temin S, Yee GC, et al. American Society of Clinical Oncology executive summary of the clinical practice guideline update on the role of bone-modifying agents in metastatic breast cancer. J Clin Oncol. 2011;29:1221–7.
149. Lipton A, Theriault RL, Hortobagyi GN, et al. Pamidronate prevents skeletal complications and is effective palliative treatment in women with breast carcinoma and osteolytic bone metastases: long term follow-up of two randomized, placebo-controlled trials. Cancer. 2000;88:1082–90.
150. Rosen LS, Gordon D, Kaminski M, et al. Long-term efficacy and safety of zoledronic acid compared with pamidronate disodium in the treatment of skeletal complications in patients with advanced multiple myeloma or breast carcinoma: a randomized, double-blind, multicenter, comparative trial. Cancer. 2003;98:1735–44.
151. Stopeck AT, Lipton A, Body JJ, et al. Denosumab compared with zoledronic acid for the treatment of bone metastases in patients with advanced breast cancer: a randomized study. J Clin Oncol. 2010;28:5132–9.
152. Trastuzumab PI. http://www.herceptin.com/pdf/herceptin-prescribing.pdf.

Index

D.S. Francescatti and M.J. Silverstein (eds.), *Breast Cancer: A New Era in Management*, DOI 10.1007/978-1-4614-8063-1, © Springer Science+Business Media New York 2014

B

E

F

L

T

Printed by Printforce, the Netherlands